HUMAN CARCINOGENESIS

Academic Press Rapid Manuscript Reproduction

HUMAN CARCINOGENESIS

EDITED BY

Curtis C. Harris
Herman N. Autrup

Laboratory of Human Carcinogenesis
National Cancer Institute
National Institutes of Health
Bethesda, Maryland

1983

ACADEMIC PRESS
A Subsidiary of Harcourt Brace Jovanovich, Publishers
New York   London
Paris   San Diego   San Francisco   São Paulo   Sydney   Tokyo   Toronto

ACADEMIC PRESS, INC.
111 Fifth Avenue, New York, New York 10003

United Kingdom Edition published by
ACADEMIC PRESS, INC. (LONDON) LTD.
24/28 Oval Road, London NW1 7DX

Library of Congress Cataloging in Publication Data

Main entry under title:

Human carcinogenesis.

  Includes indexes.
  1. Carcinogenesis--Congresses. 2. Cancer cells--
Congresses. 3. Human cell culture--Congresses.
I. Harris, Curtis C., Date   . II. Autrup, Herman.
RC268.5.H84 1983   616.99'4071   83-3827
ISBN 0-12-327660-8

PRINTED IN THE UNITED STATES OF AMERICA

83 84 85 86   9 8 7 6 5 4 3 2 1

Contents

I. Growth and Differentiation of Human Cells

II.   Metabolism of Chemical Carcinogens, DNA Damage, and DNA Repair

III.   Tumor Promotion

IV.   Cellular Lesions Caused by Chemical Carcinogens

V.   Cellular Lesions Caused by Physical Carcinogens

VI.   Special Address

VII.   Viral Oncogenesis

VIII. Laboratory Epidemiology Studies

Contributors

Numbers in parentheses indicate the pages on which the authors' contributions begin.

Stuart A. Aaronson (609), Laboratory of Cellular and Molecular Biology, National Cancer Institute, National Institutes of Health, Bethesda, Maryland 20205

John D. Adams (809), American Health Foundation, Naylor Dana Institute for Disease Prevention, Valhalla, New York 10595

Richard H. Adamson (xix), Director, Division of Cancer Cause and Prevention, National Cancer Institute, National Institutes of Health, Bethesda, Maryland 20205

Paul A. Amstad (217), Department of Carcinogenesis, Swiss Institute of Experimental Cancer Research, CH-1066, Epalinges, Lausanne, Switzerland

Alan D. Andrews (519), Department of Dermatology, Columbia University, College of Physicians and Surgeons, New York, New York 10032

Herman Autrup (169), Carcinogen Macromolecular Interaction Section, Laboratory of Human Carcinogenesis, National Cancer Institute, National Institutes of Health, Bethesda, Maryland 20205

P. E. Barker (589), Department of Biology, Yale University, New Haven, Connecticut 06511

H. Bartsch (833), Division of Environmental Carcinogenesis, International Agency for Research on Cancer, F-69372 Lyon Cedex 08, France

Thomas Bechtold (709), Department of Pathology and Laboratory Medicine, University of Nebraska Medical Center, Omaha, Nebraska 68105

Michael A. Beckett[1] (85), Division of Cell Growth and Regulation, Dana-Farber Cancer Institute, Department of Physiology and Biophysics, Harvard Medical School, Boston, Massachusetts 02115

[1]Present address: Cambridge Research Laboratory, Ortho Diagnostic Systems, Inc., Cambridge, Massachusetts 02135.

William F. Benedict (509), Clayton Ocular Oncology Center and the Division of Hematology/Oncology, Childrens Hospital of Los Angeles, and Department of Pediatrics, University of Southern California, School of Medicine, Los Angeles, California 90027

Irene K. Berezesky (35), Department of Pathology, University of Maryland School of Medicine, Baltimore, Maryland 21201

R. Bernards (631), Department of Medical Biochemistry, Sylvius Laboratories, University of Leiden, 2333 AL Leiden, The Netherlands

William A. Blattner (913), Family Studies Section, Environmental Epidemiology Branch, National Cancer Institute, National Institutes of Health, Bethesda, Maryland 20205

Emil Bogenmann (123), Division of Hematology/Oncology, Childrens Hospital of Los Angeles, Los Angeles, California 90027

Carmia Borek (519), Departments of Radiobiology, Pathology, and Dermatology, Columbia University, College of Physicians and Surgeons, New York, New York 10032

J. L. Bos (631), Department of Medical Biochemistry, Sylvius Laboratories, University of Leiden, 2333 AL Leiden, The Netherlands

Douglas E. Brash (281), Laboratory of Biochemical Pharmacology, Dana-Farber Cancer Institute, Boston, Massachusetts 02115

Thomas C. Brown (217), Department of Carcinogenesis, Swiss Institute of Experimental Cancer Research, CH-1066 Epalinges, Lausanne, Switzerland

Klaus D. Brunnemann (809), American Health Foundation, Naylor Dana Institute for Disease Prevention, Valhalla, New York 10595

Peter A. Cerutti (217), Department of Carcinogenesis, Swiss Institute of Experimental Cancer Research, CH-1066 Epalinges, Lausanne, Switzerland

M. Crespi (833), The Regina Elena Institute for the Study and Therapy of Tumours, 00161 Rome, Italy

Janet D. Crow (371), Cell Genetics Section, Laboratory of Molecular Carcinogenesis, National Cancer Institute, National Institutes of Health, Bethesda, Maryland 20205

Channing J. Der[2] (97), Department of Microbiology, College of Medicine, University of California, Irvine, California 92717

Sushilkumar G. Devare (609), Laboratory of Cellular and Molecular Biology, National Cancer Institute, National Institutes of Health, Bethesda, Maryland 20205

B. Hugh Dorman[3] (469), Department of Pathology, University of North Carolina School of Medicine, Chapel Hill, North Carolina 27514

Magdalena Eisinger (195), Memorial Sloan-Kettering Cancer Center, New York, New York 10021

Barbara Fagg[4] (97), Department of Microbiology, College of Medicine, University of California, Irvine, California 92717

Werner W. Franke (3), Institute of Cell and Tumor Biology, German Cancer Research Center, Heidelberg, Federal Republic of Germany

[2]Present address: Dana-Farber Cancer Institute and Department of Pathology, Harvard Medical School, Boston, Massachusetts 02115.

[3]Present address: Chemical Industry Institute of Toxicology, Research Triangle Park, North Carolina 27709.

[4]Present address: Basel Institute for Immunology, CH-4005 Basel, Switzerland.

William A. Franklin (281), Laboratory of Biochemical Pharmacology, Dana-Farber Cancer Institute, Boston, Massachusetts 02115

Eileen A. Friedman (325), Memorial Sloan-Kettering Cancer Center, New York, New York 10021

Hirota Fujiki (303), National Cancer Center Research Institute, Tokyo 104, Japan

R. C. Gallo (679), Laboratory of Tumor Cell Biology, National Cancer Institute, National Institutes of Health, Bethesda, Maryland 20205

Emily Germain[5] (85), Division of Cell Growth and Regulation, Dana-Farber Cancer Institute, Department of Physiology and Biophysics, Harvard Medical School, Boston, Massachusetts 02115

James J. Goedert (913), Family Studies Section, Environmental Epidemiology Branch, National Cancer Institute, National Institutes of Health, Bethesda, Maryland 20205

Niels Græm (145), Pathological–Anatomical Institute, Kommunehospitalet, Copenhagen, Denmark

Mark H. Greene (913), Family Studies Section, Environmental Epidemiology Branch, National Cancer Institute, National Institutes of Health, Bethesda, Maryland 20205

Dezider Grunberger (195), Department of Biochemistry and Public Health, Institute of Cancer Research, Columbia University, New York, New York 10032

Pawan K. Gupta[6] (255), Fels Research Institute and the Department of Pharmacology, Temple University School of Medicine, Philadelphia, Pennsylvania 19140

Nancy J. Haley (809), American Health Foundation, Naylor Dana Institute for Disease Prevention, Valhalla, New York 10595

Hiroshi Hamada (371), Cell Genetics Section, Laboratory of Molecular Carcinogenesis, National Cancer Institute, National Institutes of Health, Bethesda, Maryland 20205

Shinji Harada (709), Department of Pathology and Laboratory Medicine, University of Nebraska Medical Center, Omaha, Nebraska 68105

Curtis C. Harris (169, 561, 941), Laboratory of Human Carcinogenesis, National Cancer Institute, National Institutes of Health, Bethesda, Maryland 20205

William A. Haseltine (281), Laboratory of Biochemical Pharmacology, Dana-Farber Cancer Institute, Boston, Massachusetts 02115

Seisuke Hattori (657), Department of Viral Oncology, Cancer Institute, Tokyo 170, Japan

Aage Haugen (561), Department of Toxicology, National Institute of Public Health, Oslo, Norway

Stephen S. Hecht (809), American Health Foundation, Naylor Dana Institute for Disease Prevention, Valhalla, New York 10595

Tadashi Hirakawa (371), Cell Genetics Section, Laboratory of Molecular Carcinogenesis, National Cancer Institute, National Institutes of Health, Bethesda, Maryland 20205

Dietrich Hoffmann (809), American Health Foundation, Naylor Dana Institute for Disease Prevention, Valhalla, New York 10595

Clara L. Horn (783), American Health Foundation, Naylor Dana Institute for Disease Prevention, Valhalla, New York 10595

[5]Present address: Albert Einstein College of Medicine, Bronx, New York 10461.

[6]Present address: Department of Chemical Carcinogenesis, Michigan Cancer Foundation, Detroit, Michigan 48201.

Chu-chieh Hsia (883), Department of Pathology, Cancer Institute, Chinese Academy of Medical Sciences, Beijing, People's Republic of China

Jeffrey R. Idle (857), Department of Pharmacology, St. Mary's Hospital Medical School, London W2 1PG, England

Peter A. Jones (123), Division of Hematology/Oncology, Childrens Hospital of Los Angeles, Los Angeles, California 90027

Takeo Kakunaga (371), Cell Genetics Section, Laboratory of Molecular Carcinogenesis, National Cancer Institute, National Institutes of Health, Bethesda, Maryland 20205

V. S. Kalyanaraman (679), Department of Cell Biology, Litton Bionetics, Inc., Kensington, Maryland 20895

David G. Kaufman (469), Department of Pathology, University of North Carolina School of Medicine, Chapel Hill, North Carolina 27514

Ruth M. Kay[7] (783), American Health Foundation, New York, New York 10017

Peter K. LeMotte[8] (545), Laboratory of Radiobiology, Harvard School of Public Health, Boston, Massachusetts 02115

John Leavitt (371), Linus Pauling Institute of Sciences and Medicine, Palo Alto, California 94306

John F. Lechner (561), *In Vitro* Carcinogenesis Section, Laboratory of Human Carcinogenesis, National Cancer Institute, National Institutes of Health, Bethesda, Maryland 20205

Howard L. Liber[9] (545), Laboratory of Radiobiology, Harvard School of Public Health, Boston, Massachusetts 02115

Judith A. Lippke (281), Laboratory of Biochemical Pharmacology, Dana-Farber Cancer Institute, Boston, Massachusetts 02115

John B. Little (545), Laboratory of Radiobiology, Harvard School of Public Health, Boston, Massachusetts 02115

Kwok Ming Lo (281), Laboratory of Biochemical Pharmacology, Dana-Farber Cancer Institute, Boston, Massachusetts 02115

S. H. Lu[10] (833), Division of Environmental Carcinogenesis, International Agency for Research on Cancer, F-69372 Lyon Cedex 08, France

Veronica M. Maher (401), Carcinogenesis Laboratory, Departments of Microbiology and Biochemistry, Michigan State University, East Lansing, Michigan 48824

Dean L. Mann (913), Office of the Director, Division of Biology and Diagnosis, National Cancer Institute, National Institutes of Health, Bethesda, Maryland 20205

Patricia L. Marion (743), Stanford University School of Medicine, Stanford, California 94305

Helen S. Maurer (709), Children's Memorial Hospital, Chicago, Illinois 60614

J. Justin McCormick (401), Carcinogenesis Laboratory, Departments of Microbiology and Biochemistry, Michigan State University, East Lansing, Michigan 48824

[7]Present address: Department of Surgery, University of Toronto, Toronto Western Hospital, Toronto, Ontario M5T 258, Canada.

[8]Present address: Department of Biology, Massachusetts Institute of Technology, Cambridge, Massachusetts 02139.

[9]Present address: Department of Nutrition and Food Science, Massachusetts Institute of Technology, Cambridge, Massachusetts 02139.

[10]Present address: Department of Chemial Etiology, Cancer Institute, Chinese Academy of Medical Sciences, Beijing, People's Republic of China.

Roger H. Miller (743), Stanford University School of Medicine, Stanford, California 94305

George E. Milo (431), Department of Physiological Chemistry and Comprehensive Cancer Center, The Ohio State University, Columbus, Ohio 43210

Roland Moll (3), Institute of Cell and Tumor Biology, German Cancer Research Center, Heidelberg, Federal Republic of Germany

Richard E. Moore (303), Department of Chemistry, University of Hawaii, Honolulu, Hawaii 96822

N. Muñoz (833), Division of Epidemiology and Biostatistics, International Agency for Research on Cancer, F-69372 Lyon Cedex 08, France

A. Linn Murphree (509), Clayton Ocular Oncology Center, and the Division of Ophthalmology, Childrens Hospital of Los Angeles, Los Angeles, California 90027, and Departments of Ophthalmology and Pediatrics, University of Southern California School of Medicine, Los Angeles, California

Karen G. Nelson (469), Department of Pathology, University of North Carolina School of Medicine, Chapel Hill, North Carolina 27514

Hugo J. Niggli (217), Department of Carcinogenesis, Swiss Institute of Experimental Cancer Research, CH-1066 Epalinges, Lausanne, Switzerland

H. Ohshima (833), Division of Environmental Carcinogenesis, International Agency for Research on Cancer, F-69372 Lyon Cedex 08, France

Ismail Parsa (451), Department of Pathology, State University of New York Downstate Medical Center, Brooklyn, New York 11203

Patricia C. Phelps (35), Department of Pathology, University of Maryland School of Medicine, Baltimore, Maryland 21201

Jacalyn H. Pierce (609), Laboratory of Cellular and Molecular Biology, National Cancer Institute, National Institutes of Health, Bethesda, Maryland 20205

M. Popovic (679), Laboratory of Tumor Cell Biology, National Cancer Institute, National Institutes of Health, Bethesda, Maryland 20205

Carl O. Povlsen[11] (145), Pathological–Anatomical Institute, Kommunehospitalet, Copenhagen, Denmark

D. Pravtcheva (589), Department of Biology, Yale University, New Haven, Connecticut 06511

David T. Purtilo (709), Department of Pathology and Laboratory Medicine, University of Nebraska Medical Center, Omaha, Nebraska 68105

E. Premkumar Reddy (609), Laboratory of Cellular and Molecular Biology, National Cancer Institute, National Institutes of Health, Bethesda, Maryland 20205

Bandaru S. Reddy (783), American Health Foundation, Naylor Dana Institute for Disease Prevention, Valhalla, New York 10595

M. S. Reitz (679), Laboratory of Tumor Cell Biology, National Cancer Institute, National Institutes of Health, Bethesda, Maryland 20205

James G. Rheinwald (85), Division of Cell Growth and Regulation, Dana-Farber Cancer Institute, Department of Physiology and Biophysics, Harvard Medical School, Boston, Massachusetts 02115

[11]Present address: Pathological–Anatomical Institute, Frederiksborg County Central Hospital, Hillerød 3400, Denmark.

James C. Ritchie (857), Department of Pharmacology, St. Mary's Hospital Medical School, London W2 1PG, England

Keith Robbins (609), Laboratory of Cellular and Molecular Biology, National Cancer Institute, National Institutes of Health, Bethesda, Maryland 20205

M. Robert-Guroff (679), Laboratory of Tumor Cell Biology, National Cancer Institute, National Institutes of Health, Bethesda, Maryland 20205

William S. Robinson (743), Stanford University School of Medicine, Stanford, California 94305

F. H. Ruddle (589), Departments of Biology and Human Genetics, Yale University, New Haven, Connecticut 06511

J. Ryan (589), Department of Human Genetics, Yale University, New Haven, Connecticut 06511

Kiyoshi Sakamoto (709), IInd Department of Surgery, Kumamoto University Medical School, Kumamota 860, Japan

Andrew J. Saladino (35), Department of Pathology, University of Maryland School of Medicine, Baltimore, Maryland 21201

M. G. Sarngadharan (679), Department of Cell Biology, Litton Bionetics, Inc., Kensington, Maryland 20895

Erika Schmid (3), Institute of Cell and Tumor Biology, German Cancer Research Center, Heidelberg, Federal Republic of Germany

P. I. Schrier (631), Department of Medical Biochemistry, Sylvius Laboratories, University of Leiden, 2333 AL Leiden, The Netherlands

J. Schuepbach (679), Laboratory of Tumor Cell Biology, National Cancer Institute, National Institutes of Health, Bethesda, Maryland 20205

Motoharu Seiki (657), Department of Viral Oncology, Cancer Institute, Tokyo 170, Japan

Richard B. Setlow (231), Biology Department, Brookhaven National Laboratory, Upton, New York 11973

Jill M. Siegfried (469), The Cancer Research Center, University of North Carolina School of Medicine, Chapel Hill, North Carolina 27514

Michael A. Sirover (255), Fels Research Institute and the Department of Pharmacology, Temple University School of Medicine, Philadelphia, Pennsylvania 19140

Eric J. Stanbridge (97), Department of Microbiology, College of Medicine, University of California, Irvine, California 92717

Masami Suganuma (303), National Cancer Center Research Institute, Tokyo 104, Japan

Takashi Sugimura (303), National Cancer Center Research Institute, Tokyo 104, Japan

Tsung-tang Sun (757), Department of Immunology, Cancer Institute, Chinese Academy of Medical Sciences, Beijing, People's Republic of China

Albert L. Sutton (469), Department of Pathology, State University of New York, Downstate Medical Center, Brooklyn, New York 11203

David C. Swan (609), Laboratory of Cellular and Molecular Biology, National Cancer Institute, National Institutes of Health, Bethesda, Maryland 20205

Gail Theall[12] (195), Department of Biochemistry and Public Health, Institute of Cancer Research, Columbia University, New York, New York 10032

[12]Present address: Haskell Laboratory, DuPont, Newark, Delaware 19711.

Takayoshi Tokiwa (561), *In Vitro* Carcinogenesis Section, Laboratory of Human Carcinogenesis, National Cancer Institute, National Institutes of Health, Bethesda, Maryland 20205

Steven R. Tronick (609), Laboratory of Cellular and Molecular Biology, National Cancer Institute, National Institutes of Health, Bethesda, Maryland 20205

Benjamin F. Trump (35, 561), Department of Pathology, University of Maryland School of Medicine, Baltimore, Maryland 21201

Leslie A. Walton (469), Department of Obstetrics and Gynecology, University of North Carolina School of Medicine, Chapel Hill, North Carolina 27514

Neng-jin Wang (757), Pathology Section, Qidong Liver Cancer Institute, Jiangsu, People's Republic of China

John H. Weisburger (783), American Health Foundation, Naylor Dana Institute for Disease Prevention, Valhalla, New York 10595

F. Wong-Staal (679), Laboratory of Tumor Cell Biology, National Cancer Institute, National Institutes of Health, Bethesda, Maryland 20205

Ernst L. Wynder (783, 809), American Health Foundation, New York, New York 10017

Mitsuaki Yoshida (657), Department of Viral Oncology, Cancer Institute, Tokyo 170, Japan

P. J. Van den Elsen[13] (631), Department of Medical Biochemistry, Sylvius Laboratories, University of Leiden, 2333 AL Leiden, The Netherlands

A. J. Van der Eb (631), Department of Medical Biochemistry, Sylvius Laboratories, University of Leiden, 2333 AL Leiden, The Netherlands

[13]Present address: Dana-Farber Cancer Institute, Harvard Medical School, Boston, Massachusetts 02115.

Foreword

In 1979 NCI and NHLBI cosponsored a conference entitled "Culture of Human Tissues and Cells"; the proceedings were published in *Methods in Cell Biology*, Volumes 21A and 21B. The focus of that meeting was more on methodology than on application. The conference, however, set the stage for the application of *in vitro* techniques to the study of human tissues and cells and, in particular, for the study of many important aspects of the process of carcinogenesis. In addition, it provided impetus for the further development of model systems for such studies.

Since that conference, remarkable progress has been made, and to review this progress is the objective of the present meeting. Among the accomplishments reviewed are the successful maintenance in culture of normal human tissues for weeks and, in some cases, for months; the development of chemically defined media; and the ability to clone and passage repeatedly isolated epithelial cells from human tissues. Because many of the technical methodological problems associated with maintaining human tissues and cells in culture have been resolved, we are now able to turn our attention to using these systems for studies of the process of carcinogenesis at the cellular and even the molecular level. For example, precise and detailed studies of differentiation in human cells and tissues are now being performed under carefully defined culture conditions, and the results of the studies will undoubtedly provide some clues as to how this process is disrupted in carcinogenesis.

The capability to maintain human cells and tissues in culture also provides the opportunity to study in relative isolation the metabolism of chemical carcinogens—both their activation and their detoxification—along with their interaction with biologically important macromolecules. Equally important in carcinogenesis is the repair of DNA damage inflicted by chemicals and other agents.

The action of tumor promoters and biological effects of transforming growth factors in human tissue and cells can now be dissected and scrutinized in a way that was previously impossible. Growth factors used by the cells for their own proliferation have been characterized, new and potent tumor promoters have been discovered in naturally occurring materials, and the differential effect of classical tumor promoters, phorbol esters, on premalignant epithelial cells is reported.

The maintenance of human cells and tissues in culture also provides the opportunity to study the process of malignant transformation by chemical and physical carcinogens as well as by oncogenic viruses. The new methodology has developed to the point where studies of the mechanisms of transformation can be performed at the cellular level and carcinogen-induced alterations in DNA and gene expression can be assessed.

We are all aware of recent progress in viral oncogenesis and of studies of this phenomenon using cultured human cells. This session will consider the role of retroviruses and adenoviruses in human oncogenesis, including a discussion of the human T-cell leukemia–lymphoma virus. Subsequent speakers will address the subject of oncogenesis by DNA viruses, in particular, EBV-induced lymphoma in immunosuppressed individuals and the relationship between hepatitis B virus and human hepatocellular carcinoma.

In the final session of this meeting, laboratory correlates of epidemiologic studies will be considered, with particular consideration given to individual, genetically determined differences in carcinogen metabolism and in susceptibility to chemical and biological carcinogens. Again, such correlations are made more cogent by the use of human tissues and cells. Clearly, they provide an important link between cancer epidemiology and the enlarging data base from carcinogenesis studies using experimental animals.

In a sense, the topics considered at the many session of this meeting summarize, in my view, what the objectives of this meeting should be. In addition to reviewing recent progress in the use of cultured human tissues and cells in carcinogenesis studies, I think it is important at this point to begin making comparisons not only *between* animal species but also between different cell types within the *same* species. I also anticipate that the participants in this meeting will highlight the role that host factors play in carcinogenesis. For example, by comparing the results of *in vitro* studies of cells from humans who are exceptionally sensitive to carcinogenic influences—such as individuals with xeroderma pigmentosum, ataxia telangiectasia, and familial malignant melanoma—with those individuals who seem to be relatively resistant to such influences, it may well be possible to develop some strategies for prevention.

In addition, I feel that carcinogenesis studies using cultured human tissues and cells may obviate some of the problems associated with extrapolating carcinogenesis data from the experimental to the human situation. The problem of risk assessment has recently received considerable attention, both scientifically and in the lay press. Clues to carcinogenic hazards provided by epidemiologic studies alone are invaluable and usually unambiguous, but almost by definition they are derived from unfortunate human experience. On the other hand, the difficulties of extrapolating data from animal studies (primarily in rodents) to humans are well known and not worth reciting here. In a sense, carcinogenesis studies using cultured human cells and tissues represent a bridge between epidemiologic studies and studies involving experimental animals. That is, they assess the carcinogenic risk of chemical, physical, and biological agents in human components without putting the composite human at risk. In addition, the *in vitro* systems provide an ideal opportunity to study in isolation specific aspects of growth differentiation, metabolism, promotion, transformation, and other phenomena related to the process of human carcinogenesis. For these reasons, I believe that the topic of this meeting is a timely one and that the results will substantially contribute to our understanding of carcinogenesis in humans.

Richard H. Adamson

Preface

Scientific opportunities generally arise when two or more areas of research converge or advances in methodology occur. Such opportunities are arising for the study of human carcinogenesis. Recently, laboratory research has provided us with critical information on the mechanism of carcinogenesis. This has been made possible in part by new technological advancements, including those in molecular and cellular biology and those allowing new methods for culturing tissues and cells. Concomitantly, epidemiology has clearly demonstrated the etiological importance of environmental exposure to carcinogens and cocarcinogens and has identified populations at high cancer risk. Cancer researchers are taking advantage of these new scientific opportunities and designing increasingly sophisticated studies in the area of biochemical and molecular epidemiology.

Human Carcinogenesis is intended to provide the reader with a collection of reviews and up-to-date reports of the ongoing investigations in this important area of research. Although it is not possible to cover this multifaceted topic completely in one volume, the spectrum of these contributions is quite broad and ranges from basic molecular to applied clinical studies. We hope that this book will encourage investigators in associated fields and younger scientists to join in these efforts to find innovative ways to prevent human cancer.

I. Growth and Differentiation of Human Cells

1

THE INTERMEDIATE FILAMENT CYTOSKELETON IN TISSUES AND IN CULTURED CELLS: DIFFERENTIATION SPECIFITY OF EXPRESSION OF CELL ARCHITECTURAL ELEMENTS

Werner W. Franke, Erika Schmid, and Roland Moll

Institute of Cell and Tumor Biology
German Cancer Research Center
Heidelberg, Federal Republic of Germany

I.   THE CYTOSKELETON AND ITS COMPONENTS

The characteristic shape and functional organization of
the eukaryotic cell is based, largely, on the defined arrangement of nonmembranous, cytoplasmic structures that resist cell
lysis and also extraction in buffers of nearly physiological
ionic strength and pH, as well as treatments with nondenaturing

detergents. Such structures are commonly subsumed under the primarily preparative term, cytoskeleton (for review see Brinkley, 1982). The importance of the contribution of cyto- skeletal components to the specific architecture of a cell is perhaps best demonstrated by the fact that, in many cells, the typical cellular morphology can still be recognized after extraction of the soluble components and membranes. The major elements of this cytoskeleton have been identified over the past two decades, the most prominent and almost ubiquitous being the 4-6-nm microfilaments containing actin polymers and 20-26-nm microtubules containing polymers of α- and β-tubulins.

Even more remarkable, however, has been the observation that, in a broad variety of vertebrate cells, the specific cell architecture is still recognizable when microfilaments and microtubules have been removed as, for example, by extrac- tion in high-salt buffers. Such cytoskeletal residues ob- tained after treatment of cells with high-salt buffers and de- tergents have been examined in greater detail, and the struc- tures observed in such preparations can be classified into two major groups, that is, membrane-associated plaques (e.g., Aaronson and Blobel, 1975; Cohen *et al.*, 1977; Drochmans *et al.*, 1978; Franke *et al.*, 1979a, 1981d; Colaco and Evans, 1981) and intermediate-sized filaments.

Intermediate-sized filaments (intermediate filaments; Ishikawa *et al.*, 1968) are filaments of 7 to 11 nm diameter that are usually unbranched, frequently several micrometers long, and characterized by a hollow core and a wall composed of a still unknown number of protofilamentous subunits (for reviews see Lazarides, 1980, 1982; Anderton, 1981; Franke *et al.*, 1982c). Filaments of this category are exceptional not only in their resistance to extraction buffers of a broad range of salt concentrations and pH values, but also by the remarkable tendency of their constituent proteins to renature rapidly and to reassemble the same type of filaments after removal of the denaturing agent (Cooke, 1976; Steinert *et al.*, 1976, 1981; Small and Sobieszek, 1977; Rueger *et al.*, 1979; Huiatt *et al.*, 1980; Cabrall *et al.*, 1981; Geisler and Weber, 1981; Renner *et al.*, 1981).

Filamentous structures of this type, albeit morphologically similar, can be formed by different subclasses of proteins that can be immunologically and biochemically distinguished, and are expressed in a manner related to cell differentiation (Bennett *et al.*, 1978; Franke *et al.*, 1978b; Hynes and Destree, 1978; for reviews see Lazarides, 1980, 1982; Franke *et al.*, 1982c; Holtzer *et al.*, 1982; Osborn *et al.*, 1982). According to their subunit proteins, seven types of intermediate filaments have so far been demonstrated (Table I). The distribution of the various subclasses of intermediate-sized filaments in various tissues has shown that their occurrence is mostly mutually exclusive and therefore of particular value for cell type diagnosis (Franke *et al.*, 1978a,b, 1979b, 1982c; Schmid *et al.*, 1979; Sun *et al.*, 1979; Osborn *et al.*, 1982). For example, filaments containing proteins related to the α-keratins of epidermis and its appendages are specific for epithelial cells (cytokeratins; Franke *et al.*, 1978a,b, 1979b; Sun and Green, 1978a; Sun *et al.*, 1979), and here their expression is usually correlated with the synthesis of desmoplakins, that is, the major proteins of the desmosomal plaque to which these filaments are often attached (Franke *et al.*, 1981d, 1983).

Only in specific cells has coexistence of two types of different constituent proteins of intermediate filaments been observed. One example is a certain subclass of vascular smooth muscle cells and the cultured hamster cell line BHK, which produce both vimentin and desmin (Starger *et al.*, 1978; Gard *et al.*, 1979; Tuszynski *et al.*, 1979; Osborn *et al.*, 1981a; Gabbiani *et al.*, 1981a; Frank *et al.*, 1982; Schmid *et al.*,

1982), and here the existence of both types of proteins in
the same filament has been shown by dissociation kinetics and
chemical cross-linking (e.g., Steinert *et al.*, 1981; Quinlan
and Franke, 1982). Similarly, astrocytes and cultured human
glioma cells contain both glial filament protein and vimentin
(Paetau *et al.*, 1979; Osborn *et al.*, 1981b; Schnitzer *et al.*,
1981; Yen and Fields, 1981), and here it has also been
shown, by chemical cross-linking (Quinlan and Franke, 1983)
and immunoelectron microscopy (Sharp *et al.*, 1982), that
both protein subunits can occur in the same filament.
Moreover, the cell type-specific expression of one class of
intermediate filaments may be lost and the cytoskeleton
altered when tissue cells are dissociated and grown in culture,
a phenomenon frequently observed with epithelial and carcinoma
cells (see later), which reminds one of the limitations of cor-
relating findings in cells grown *in vitro* to tissue cells grown
in situ.

II. THE INTERMEDIATE FILAMENT CYTOSKELETON OF TUMOR CELLS

    In general, tumor cells generally present the same type of
intermediate filament proteins as characteristic of the cell
from which they are derived. This has been shown for epithelia-
derived tumors, including carcinomas, as well as for myogenic
and nonmyogenic sarcomas, neuroblastomas, and gliomas (Bannasch
et al., 1980; Battifora *et al.*, 1980; Schlegel *et al.*, 1980;
for references see Gabbiani *et al.*, 1981b; Osborn *et al.*, 1982;
Ramaekers *et al.*, 1982). This is true for primary tumors as
well as for metastases. Immunocytochemistry using antibodies
to these filament proteins and to desmoplakins has already found
widespread application in clinical diagnosis (see references
just quoted, and Franke *et al.*, 1983).

An even finer subdivision of intermediate filament proteins has been possible with epithelial cells and carcinomas.
The cytokeratins represent a family of a number of related
polypeptides of various sizes and isoelectric variants and are
again expressed in cell type-specific patterns in the different
epithelia (Jackson *et al.*, 1980; Doran *et al.*, 1980; Winter *et
al.*, 1980; Franke *et al.*, 1981a,b,c,e, 1982c; Fuchs and Green,
1981; Milstone, 1981; Milstone and McGuire, 1981; Wu and
Rheinwald, 1981). In human tissues at least 19 different polypeptides associated with cytokeratin filaments have been distinguished and their relatedness examined by antibody binding
and peptide map analysis (for designations see Fig. 11; see also
Moll *et al.*, 1982b; Schiller *et al.*, 1982).

Even within the same epithelium, such as epidermis, different cytokeratins can be expressed in different strata
(Fuchs and Green, 1978, 1979, 1980; Bowden and Cunliffe, 1981)
or in functionally different lateral domains of skin (Drochmans
et al., 1978; Lee *et al.*, 1979; Moll *et al.*, 1982a; see these
for further references). Comparison of the specific cytokeratin polypeptide patterns of dissected benign (papillomas, basal
cell epitheliomas, adamantinomas, adenomas) and malignant (carcinomas) tumors has revealed a high degree of conservativity
of cytokeratin expression (e.g., Moll *et al.*, 1982a,b; Denk *et
al.*, 1982). For example, hepatocellular carcinomas express
the same two specific major cytokeratins as hepatocytes, and
colonic adenocarcinoma cells usually continue to produce cytokeratins Nos. 8, 18, and 19 characteristic of normal mucosal
cells of the intestinal tract. Of course, tumors derived from
stratified epithelia often do not express the whole complement
found in the multilayered normal tissue (Moll *et al.*, 1982a,b;
see Kubilus *et al.*, 1980), but this might be the result of cell
type selection during tumor development. Tumor-specific cytokeratin polypeptides, which do not occur anywhere in normal

epithelia, have not been found (Moll *et al.*, 1982a,b). This epithelial type-specific pattern of expression of cytokeratin polypeptides in carcinomas opens the possibility of identifying the cell type of origin of a given tumor by polypeptide analysis of tumor regions microdissected from biopsies (see Moll *et al.*, 1982a,b) or by immunocytochemistry using antibodies selective for one type of cytokeratins only (see Lane, 1982).

Expression of cell type-specific polypeptides is apparently not dependent on the degree of differentiation of the tumor. For example, highly differentiated adenocarcinomas may express the same cytokeratin polypeptides as undifferentiated carcinomas derived from the same organ (Moll *et al.*, 1982b).

III. CYTOSKELETAL ELEMENTS OF CULTURED CELLS AS IDENTIFIED BY
      IMMUNOFLUORESCENCE MICROSCOPY

The various cytoskeletal structures can be identified and visualized by immunofluorescence microscopy using antibodies specific for the major constitutive proteins of these structures. In tissue cells the distribution of these elements and their constituent proteins is characteristic of the special functional architecture (for examples see Franke *et al.*, 1979a,b, 1981a,e, 1982c). Such specialized organization is often lost in cultured cells. The diverse arrays of such components present in the same cultured cell are illustrated in the example of the polarized epithelial cells of the MDBK line, which contains both types of intermediate filament proteins, cytokeratin and vimentin (Fig. 1). Cytokeratin fibrils extend through most of the cytoplasm and, in cell colonies, are often oriented toward the cell-to-cell boundaries. Here they seem to be attached to certain sites at the plasma membrane (Fig. 1a),

which can be identified as desmosomes by staining with antibodies to desmoplakins (Fig. 1c). The display of cytokeratin
fibrils is different from that of the vimentin filaments
(Fig. 1b), which do not regularly attach to desmosomes (Fig.
1c).

This difference of arrays of the two types of intermediate
filaments is especially clear after treatment of the cells with
certain drugs such as colchicine and colcemid, resulting in the
selective aggregation of the vimentin filaments (Bennett *et
al.*, 1978; Franke *et al.*, 1978a, 1979c,f,g; Hynes and Destree,
1978). In various cell lines such as MDBK the arrays of both
types of intermediate filaments change dramatically during mitosis, when a large proportion of the cytokeratin and vimentin
filaments are transiently rearranged and included in spheroidal
aggregates of insoluble structures of protofilament-like dimen-
sions (Franke *et al.*, 1982b). The arrays of both types of
intermediate filaments are also different from those of the
bundles of actin-containing microfilaments decorated by actin
antibodies (also called cables or stress fibers; Fig. 1d) and
the microtubules visualized by antibodies to tubulins (Geiger
et al., 1983). Detailed three-dimensional analysis using
various combinations of antibodies in double-label immunofluorescence microscopy (e.g., Schmid *et al.*, 1983; Geiger
et al., 1983) has also shown limited regions of spatial relationships between certain cytoskeletal components such as
actin and vinculin or vimentin and tubulin (for examples see
Geiger, 1982; Singer *et al.*, 1982), but the functional implications of these relationships are not clear.

When different cultured cell lines of human origin have
been compared with respect to their intermediate filament components, four categories of cells have been distinguished.

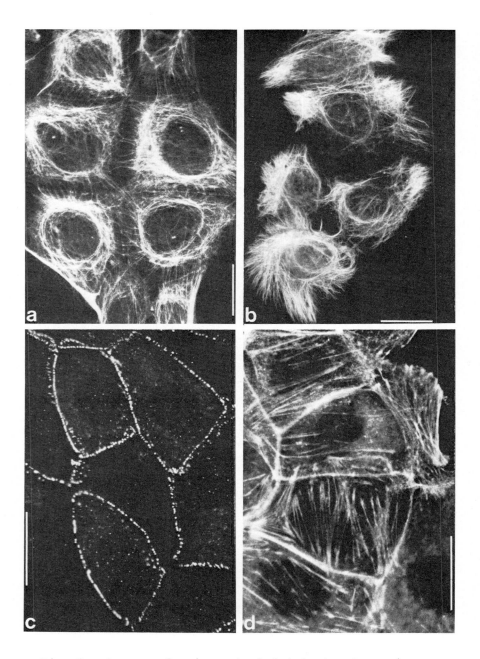

Fig. 1.   Arrays of major cytoskeletal structures in
cultured cells of a bovine kidney epithelial line (MDBK; ATCC-
CCL22) visualized by immunofluorescence microscopy using anti-

1. Mesenchymally derived cells such as embryonic fibroblasts of the WI-38 strain (Fig. 2) or endothelial cells
(Franke *et al.*, 1979b,e) contain only vimentin filaments.

2. Certain glioma cells contain both vimentin filaments
and glial filaments (Osborn *et al.*, 1981b; Sharp *et al.*,
1982; Quinlan and Franke, 1983).

3. One type of epithelia-derived cell, including carcinoma cells, corresponds to epithelial cells *in situ* in that it
only contains filaments of the cytokeratin type but not vimentin filaments (Figs. 3 and 4). Examples include cell lines
characterized by very simple cytokeratin polypeptide patterns,
such as mammary carcinoma-derived MCF-7 cells and HT-29 cells
derived from colonic adenocarcinoma, as well as cells characterized by a large complexity of cytokeratins, such as A-431
cells derived from an epidermoid carcinoma of the vulva, which
contain as many as 10 different cytokeratins (Fig. 4; see also
Fig. 9d; Moll *et al.*, 1982b). These examples also show that
epithelial cells from various types of epithelia, including
stratified squamous epithelia, can proliferate *in vitro*
without producing vimentin (see also Sun and Green, 1978b;
Fuchs and Green, 1981; Wu and Rheinwald, 1981).

4. Certain human epithelial cells contain large proportions of both cytokeratin and vimentin filaments (Franke *et
al.*, 1979f,g; Virtanen *et al.*, 1981; Osborn *et al.*, 1982),

(Fig. 1 continued) bodies to cytokeratins (a), vimentin (b),
desmoplakin (c) and actin (d). Characterization of antibodies
and preparation of cells have been presented elsewhere (see
Franke *et al.*, 1979g, 1980a, 1982b, 1983; Schmid *et al.*, 1983).
Microtubular arrays stained with tubulin antibodies and
adhaerens junctions stained with vinculin antibodies have been
shown elsewhere (Geiger *et al.*, 1983). Note the different
arrays of the various cytoskeletal elements. Many of the cytokeratin fibrils (a) are oriented toward the desmosomes of the
lateral membranes (c), whereas vimentin and actin filaments are
not. Bars are 20 μm long.

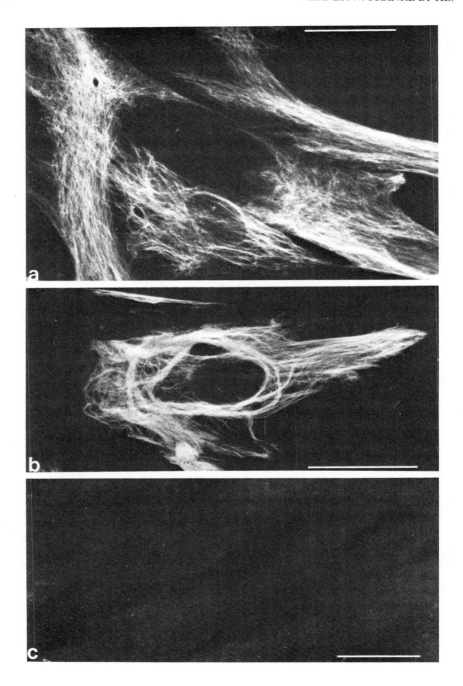

Fig. 2. Immunofluorescence microscopy of human WI-38

including authentic HeLa cells (Fig. 5) as well as many other human cell lines, some of which may actually be derived from HeLa cells such as the line "intestine 407" (ATCC-CCL6) (Fig. 6; see also following discussion). This new appearance of vimentin filaments in epithelial cells growing in culture has also been reported for various animal cell types, including murine hepatocytes and transformed keratinocytes (Franke *et al.*, 1979c,d, 1981b; Summerhayes *et al.*, 1981; Schmid *et al.*, 1983). The reason for this advent of a new type of cytoskeletal filament during culturing is not understood. It may be that the environmental change results in a relaxation from restrictions of cell differentiation, thus allowing the expression of proteins not normally produced in the tissue. Environmental influence is also indicated by observation of hormonal effects on the expression of vimentin and specific cytokeratins in cultures of bovine mammary gland-derived epithelial cells (Schmid *et al.*, 1983).

All human epithelia-derived cell cultures examined also synthesize desmoplakins (e.g., Figs. 3, 4, and 6), which are usually, at least in densely packed cell colonies, arranged in desmosomal plaques that seem to provide the attachment sites for the cytokeratin fibrils (tonofibrils). Therefore, the combined use of antibodies to both marker proteins, cytokeratins and desmoplakins, contributes to the positive identification and definition of epithelial and carcinoma cells.

(Fig. 2 continued) fibroblast cell culture after reaction with antibodies to vimentin (a and b) and cytokeratins (c). Extended fleeces of vimentin fibrils are seen (a), which can be aggregated into perinuclear bundles after treatment of the cells with colcemid (b) (see Franke *et al.*, 1979g). These cells are negative with antibodies to the other four classes of intermediate filament proteins including cytokeratins (c). Bars are 30 μm long.

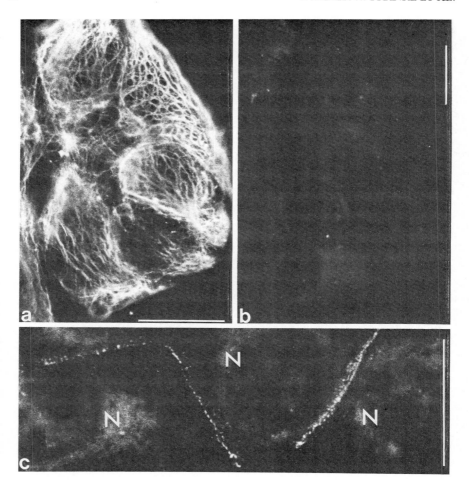

Fig. 3.   Immunofluorescence microscopy of cultured human
epithelial cells of the MCF-7 line (derived from mammary carcinoma; see Soule *et al.*, 1973) after reaction with antibodies
to cytokeratins (a), vimentin (b), and desmoplakin (c).   Epithelial cells are identified by presence of cytokeratin filaments (a) and desmosomes (dotted lines at cell boundaries in
c; N, nuclei).   This cell line does not reveal vimentin filaments (b).   Bars are 20 µm long.

Fig. 4.   Cultured human epithelial cells derived from a
stratified squamous epithelium (line A-431; from epidermoid carcinoma of vulva; cf. Fabricant *et al.*, 1977) show extended cytoplasmic arrays of cytokeratin fibrins (a) and desmosomal plaque
units (b), which are located in intercellular bridges (b),

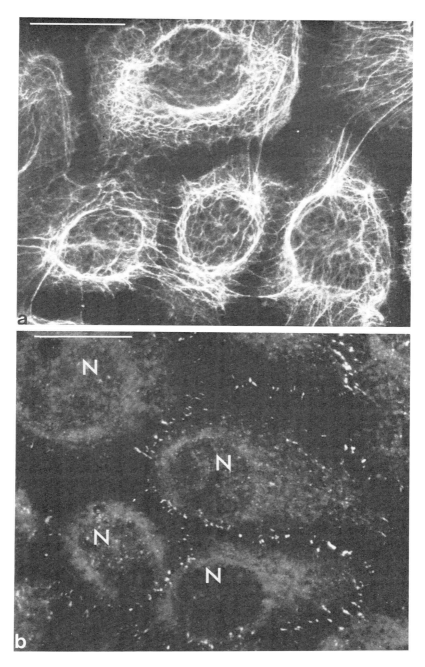

(Fig. 4 continued) visualized by immunofluorescence microscopy using antibodies to cytokeratins (a) and desmoplakin (b). N, nuclei. Bars are 20 µm long.

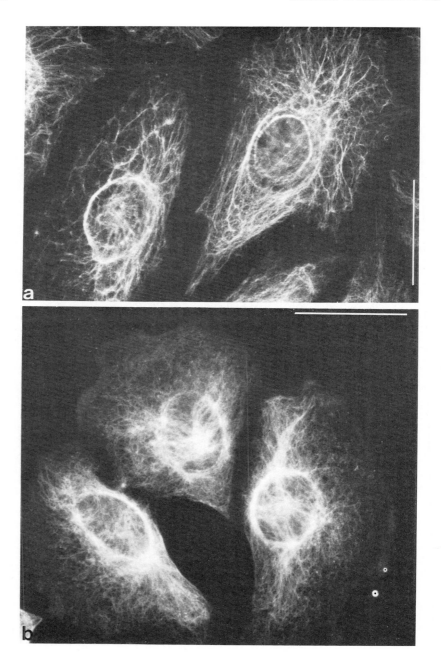

Fig. 5.   HeLa cells (ATCC-CCL2) prepared for immunofluorescence microscopy using antibodies to cytokeratins (a)

IV. POLYPEPTIDES OF INTERMEDIATE FILAMENTS OF CULTURED CELLS
     AS DETECTED BY GEL ELECTROPHORESIS

Gel electrophoretic comparisons of total cellular proteins with cytoskeletal polypeptides obtained by lysis and extraction of cultured cells and tissue samples in buffers containing detergents and high salt concentrations have shown, in
many cell types, that intermediate filament polypeptides represent major cell proteins (for reviews see Lazarides, 1980,
1982; Anderton, 1981; Bravo *et al*., 1982; Franke *et al*.,
1982c). This prominence of intermediate filament proteins is
also reflected in the corresponding populations of mRNA (for
examples see Fuchs and Green, 1979; Franke *et al*., 1980b;
O'Connor *et al*., 1981; Schiller *et al*., 1982). On two-
dimensional gel electrophoresis the various intermediate filament polypeptides (Table I) have characteristic coordinates,
helping in their identification, and they usually appear as a
series of isoelectric variants that primarily represent various degrees of phosphorylation (Sun and Green, 1978b; Gard *et
al*., 1979; Schiller *et al*., 1982; Steinert *et al*., 1982; for
review see Lazarides, 1982).

The identification of the specific type of intermediate
filament polypeptide present in the cytoskeleton of a given
nonepithelial cell is straightforward, but in cultures of epithelial and carcinoma cells some problems are presented (Figs.
7 and 8). Such epithelia-derived cells growing in culture may
continue to express certain cytokeratin polypeptides typical
of the tissue from which they have originated, but differences
of expression of certain cytokeratin polypeptides in cultured

(Fig. 5 continued) and vimentin (b) showing large amounts of
both types of intermediate-sized filaments that, however, are
distributed in different arrays. Bars are 30 μm long.

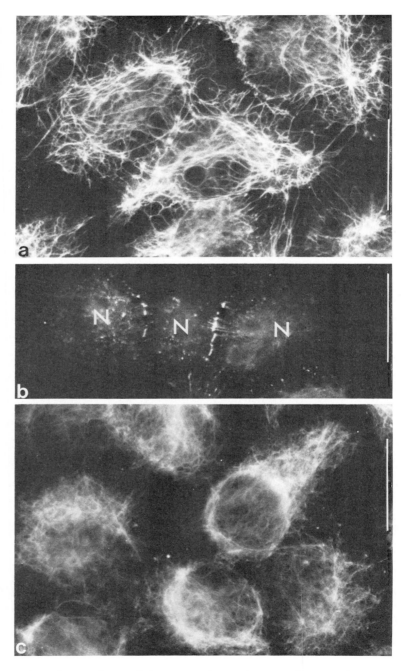

Fig. 6. Cultured human cells of the line designated "intestine 407" (ATCC-CCL6; assumed to be derived from embryonic

cells have been observed. Examples include cases of cessation of production of certain cytokeratins, such as the disappearance of some large and basic keratin polypeptides of epidermal cells (Sun and Green, 1978b; Fuchs and Green, 1978, 1979, 1980, 1981; Doran *et al.*, 1980; Wu and Rheinwald, 1981) as well as cells from mammary gland (Schmid *et al.*, 1983). In contrast, cytokeratin polypeptides have been found in certain cultured epithelial cells that have not been detected in the tissue of origin (e.g., see Figs. 7 and 8 and references just quoted). It is not clear whether these differences of cytokeratin composition reflect changes of expression or selection of certain cell types during culturing. In no case examined in detail, however, has a polypeptide of the cytokeratin family been found in cell cultures that does not occur in a tissue. In other words, cytokeratins expressed in cultured cells are not different from cytokeratins expressed *in situ*, but the polypeptide pattern characteristic of a specific epithelial tissue type may be lost. Some studies have indicated that contribution of factors present in the medium, such as vitamin A (Fuchs and Green, 1981) and certain hormones (Schmid *et al.*, 1982b), may influence the expression of cytokeratin polypeptide patterns (Fig. 8).

Nevertheless, there are examples of cells that produce exactly the same patterns of major cytokeratin polypeptides that are found in these cells when grown in the tissue. This

(Fig. 6 continued) intestine) shown by immunofluorescence microscopy using antibodies to cytokeratins (a), desmoplakin (b), and vimentin (c). Note coexpression of vimentin and cytokeratin filaments, as in HeLa cells. Detailed characterization of the cytokeratin polypeptide pattern of this cell has suggested that this cell line may be a morphological variant of HeLa cells, in agreement with the presence of chromosomal HeLa markers in this cell (American Type Culture Collection, Catalogue of Strains II, 2nd edition, 1979; Rockville, Maryland). Bars are 20 μm long.

TABLE I. Types of Intermediate Filaments Distinguished in Different Cells

Filaments containing	Subunit polypeptides (different types detected in one cell)	Molecular weight ($M_r \times 10^{-3}$)	Isoelectric pH (denatured molecules)	Occurrence
I. Cytokeratins	2–10	40–68	5.0–8.0	Epithelial and carcinoma cells
II. Vimentin	1	57	5.3	Nonepithelial cells, specifically mesenchymal cells, lens cells, some myogenic cells, sarcomas
III. Desmin	1	53	5.4	Muscle cells, excluding one type of vascular smooth muscle cell
IV. Glia filament protein (GFAP)	1	51	5.6	Astrocytes and some gliomas
V. Neurofilament protein	3	210, 160, 68	5.65, 5.28 5.25	Neuronal and pheochromocytoma cells
VI. Vimentin–desmin hybrid	2			Certain vascular smooth muscle cells; BHK-21 cell line
VII. Vimentin–GFAP hybrid	2			Astrocytes and some cultured human glioma cells

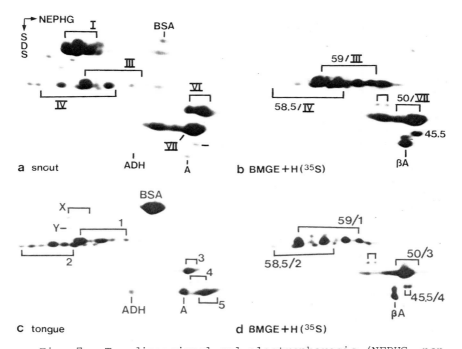

Fig. 7. Two-dimensional gel electrophoresis (NEPHG, non-equilibrium pH gradient electrophoresis in first dimension; SDS, direction of second-dimension gel electrophoresis in the presence of SDS) of cytoskeletal polypeptides from bovine snout (a) and tongue (c) in comparison with coelectrophoresed cyto-skeletal proteins from [^{35}S]methionine-labeled cells of a bo-vine epithelial cell line (BMGE + H cells; bovine mammary gland epithelial cells grown in culture medium to which vari-ous hormones have been added) (see Schmid et al., 1983). Comparison of autoradiofluorographs (b and d) with Coomassie Blue-stained gels (a and c) shows comigration of certain cyto-keratin polypeptides present in the cultured cells with those present in the tissues (for labeling and preparation see Franke et al., 1981c; Schmid et al., 1982b). All major components de-tected in the cultured cell line are identical in electrophore-tic migration to specific components present in the two tis-sues used for comparison (denoted by Roman and Arabic numerals). Cytokeratin polypeptides of BMGE cells are designated by molecu-lar weights ($M_r \times 10^{-3}$) such as 59, 58.5, 50, and 45.5 (bracket without number denotes a minor pair of cytokeratin polypeptide isoelectric variants identical to component A found in many simple epithelia; M_r 53,000, nearly isoelectric with BSA). Reference proteins used in coelectrophoresis are bovine serum albumin (BSA, M_r 68,000; isoelectric at pH 6.34), alcohol de-hydrogenase (ADH, M_r 43,500; isoelectric at pH 7.0), and

has been demonstrated for certain cultures of rat hepatocytes
and hepatoma cells (Franke *et al.*, 1981b) as well as for a
cell line (HT-29) from human colonic adenocarcinoma (Fig. 9a).
Clearly, one problem in comparing cytokeratin polypeptide patterns of cell cultures with those of their tissues of origin
is the cell type complexity of most epithelial tissues, and
only in rare cases is there an unequivocal correlation to only
one type of epithelial cell from which the cultured cell is
derived (for detailed discussion see Moll *et al.*, 1982b).

When comparing cytoskeletal polypeptide patterns from diverse cultured cell lines of human origin, profound differences
are obvious. Some epithelial cell lines do not synthesize
vimentin whereas others, such as HeLa cells, do (Fig. 9c).
Similar observations have been made with various animal cell
cultures (e.g., Fig. 8) (see Franke *et al.*, 1978a, 1979c,d,g,
1981b, 1982c; Summerhayes *et al.*, 1981; Virtanen *et al.*, 1981;
Osborn *et al.*, 1982). Some cell lines present rather simple
cytokeratin polypeptide patterns with two, three, or four cytokeratins (e.g., Fig. 9a-c), whereas other cell lines show
much more complex cytokeratin patterns (Fig. 9d presents the
example of the A-431 cell line). To date all examples of such
complex cytokeratin patterns have been found in cell cultures
derived from stratified squamous epithelia or squamous cell
carcinomas (see also Wu and Rheinwald, 1981; Moll *et al.*,
1982b).

HeLa cells have a very characteristic and unusual cytokeratin composition of four polypeptides (Numbers 7, 8, 17, and

(Fig. 7 continued) α-actin (A, M_r 42,000; isoelectric at pH
5.4). Residual β-actin (βA) is denoted in (b) and (d). Note
that some cytokeratins, such as components I and VI of epidermis (a) and components X, Y, and 5 of tongue (c) are not detected in the cultured cells. Note also synthesis of basic
cytokeratins of M_r 58,500 and 59,000 in this cell line (b and d).

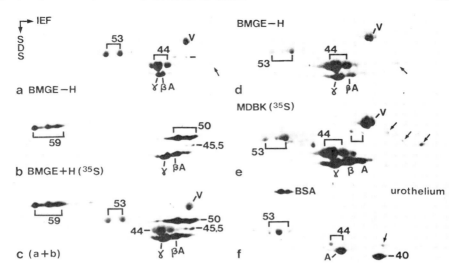

Fig. 8. Two-dimensional gel electrophoresis (IEF, isoelectric focusing in first dimension; SDS, direction of second-
dimension electrophoresis) of cytoskeletal polypeptides from
BMGE - H cells (a and d) and the hormone-treated cell line established in parallel, BMGE + H cells (b), as well as from MDBK
cells (e) and urothelium from cow's bladder (f; for details of
preparation see Schmid *et al.*, 1983). Comparison of coelectrophoresed cytoskeletal proteins from [35S]methionine-labeled
BMGE + H cells (b) with BMGE - H (a, Coomassie Blue staining)
shows different composition of cytoskeletons. Photographic
superposition of photograph (a) and fluorograph (b) of this gel
is shown in (c). Note absence of vimentin (V) in BMGE + H cells.
Coelectrophoresis of cytoskeletal proteins from BMGE - H cells
(d, Coomassie Blue staining) with [35S]methionine-labeled MDBK
cells (e, fluorograph) demonstrates identity of cytokeratins of
M_r 53,000 (53) and 44,000 (44) and of vimentin (V) in both
cells. In addition, a minor cytoskeletal polypeptide (bracket
below vimentin in e) is seen in MDBK cells. Arrows in (e) denote proteolytic degradation products from vimentin (see Gard
et al., 1979; Franke *et al.*, 1980b). Comparison of cytoskeletal polypeptides of these cultured cell lines with cytoskeletons from urothelium of cow's bladder (f) shows identical electrophoretic migration of components of M_r 53,000 and 44,000. A
predominant polypeptide of urothelium is the small cytokeratin
of M_r 40,000 (40), which is not detected in the three bovine
cell lines shown here. A basic urothelial cytokeratin is not
revealed with the focusing condition used here. Arrow in (a),
(d), and (f) denotes an unusual, very acidic cytoskeletal component of M_r 45,000 the significance of which is still unclear.
BSA, bovine serum albumin added; A, α-actin added; γA, βA,
endogenous γ- and β-actin.

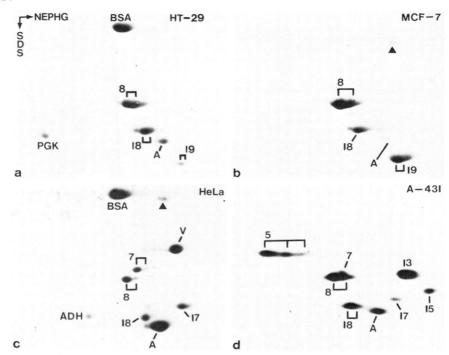

Fig. 9.   Differences of intermediate filament protein composition in different cultured human cell lines demonstrated by
two-dimensional gel electrophoresis (symbols as in Fig. 7; PGK,
phosphoglycerokinase, M_r 42,000; isoelectric at pH 7.4) of cytoskeletal polypeptides of various cultured human cell lines.
Cytokeratin polypeptides are designated by numbers (for catalogue see Fig. 11; Moll *et al.*, 1982b).   (a) HT-29 Cells (from
colonic adenocarcinoma; Fogh and Trempe, 1975) displaying a
very simple pattern of only three cytokeratins (Nos. 8, 18, and
19).   (b) MCF-7 Cells (from mammary adenocarcinoma; see Fig. 3)
showing the same cytokeratin polypeptides but with higher proportions of the very small and acidic cytokeratin No. 19.
(c) HeLa Cells (from cervical adenocarcinoma; see Fig. 5) showing four cytokeratin polypeptides only two of which (Nos. 8 and
18) are identical to those of HT-29 and MCF-7 cells.   (d) A-431
cells (from epidermoid carcinoma of vulva; see Fig. 4) showing
a remarkable complexity of cytokeratin polypeptides, including
a basic cytokeratin (No. 5).   Three minor cytokeratin polypeptides of these cells (Nos. 6, 14, and 16) (see Moll *et al.*,
1982b) are not detected at the protein concentration of this gel
loading.   Note presence of vimentin (V) in HeLa cells (c).   Ar-
rowheads denote a component of $\sim M_r$ 66,000 that is almost isoelectric with α-actin (A, added for reference) and is found as
a minor but consistent component of cytoskeletal preparations
from various tissues and cells.

18) present in almost stoichiometric amounts (Franke *et al.*, 1981c, 1982c; Bravo *et al.*, 1982; Moll *et al.*, 1982b). It has been somewhat surprising, therefore, to see that many of the cell lines kept by the American Type Culture Collection show exactly the same cytokeratin polypeptide pattern as HeLa cells (Fig. 10). We take this observation, along with the presence of chromosomal HeLa markers in these cell lines, as another independent indication of a contamination by HeLa cells during their history of culturing rather than the result of convergent expression of cytokeratin polypeptides during the establishment of these lines.

As a corollary of our studies of cytoskeletal polypeptide patterns in cultured cells, we present the scheme of Fig. 11, showing that so far 11 of 19 human cytokeratin filament-associated polypeptides have been detected in the various cultured cells. Whether or not the synthesis of the other cytokeratins is incompatible with cell proliferation *in vitro* remains to be examined. Clearly, different epithelial cell lines can be distinguished by their specific cytokeratin patterns, and in several cases these patterns can be correlated to those characteristic of the tissue of origin of these cultures. We also conclude that cell culturing does not result in the appearance of abortive or abnormal cytokeratin molecules but that cells growing *in vitro* produce cytokeratins that occur somewhere in the body.

V. EXPRESSION OF INTERMEDIATE FILAMENTS IN RELATION TO CELL DIFFERENTIATION IN EMBRYOGENESIS AND CARCINOGENESIS

Some functional roles and the regulation of assembly of other filamentous elements of the cytoskeleton, such as microfilaments and microtubules, are beginning to be understood

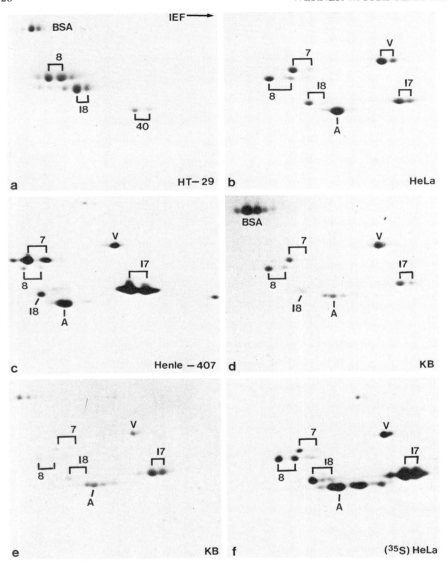

Fig. 10. Two-dimensional gel electrophoresis, using
isoelectric focusing (IEF) in first dimension, of cytoskeletal proteins from various human cell lines. (a) HT-29
Cells (40 is the smallest cytokeratin, i.e., No. 19),
(b) HeLa cells, (c) Henle intestine-407 cells (ATCC-CCL6),
(d) KB cells (ATCC-CCL17; assumed to be derived from oral epidermoid carcinoma). (e) and (f) Coelectrophoresis of cytoskeletal polypeptides from unlabeled KB cells (visualized by
Coomassie Blue staining in e) and [^{35}S]methionine-labeled

(Brinkley, 1982), but in the case of the intermediate filaments
the biological functions are still unknown. It is clear that
the various intermediate filament proteins are different by
various biochemical and immunological criteria, although they
share some amino acid sequence homologies (Osborn *et al.*, 1982)
and antigenic determinants (Pruss *et al.*, 1981), and that they
are expressed in relation to programs of cell differentiation
(for review see Franke *et al.*, 1982d). In mouse embryogenesis,
for example, no intermediate filaments have been detected until
the late morula stage and thereafter, in blastocysts, only in the
trophectodermal cells (Jackson *et al.*, 1980; Paulin *et al.*, 1980).

The first intermediate filaments recognized are cytokeratin filaments, which occur in the trophectoderm as well as in
embryonic ectoderm and proximal endoderm (Jackson *et al.*, 1980,
1981; Paulin *et al.*, 1980). These early embryonal cytokeratin
filaments are characterized by a very simple polypeptide pattern, predominantly cytokeratins A and D (equivalent to human
cytokeratins Nos. 8 and 18), which also occur in hepatocytes
of adult animals. The first appearance of vimentin filaments
appears to occur in the primary mesenchymal cells (Franke *et
al.*, 1982a). Myogenic differentiations characterized by production of desmin (e.g., Gard and Lazarides, 1980; Holtzer *et
al.*, 1982; Lazarides, 1982), neuronal differentiation characterized by the appearance of neurofilament proteins, and astro-

(Fig. 10 continued) authentic HeLa cells (f, autoradiofluoro-
graph). The same four characteristic cytokeratin polypeptides
(Nos. 7, 8, 17, and 18) found in HeLa, Henle intestine-407,
and KB cells have also been found in Chang liver cells (ATCC-
CCL13), NCTC-3075 cells (ATCC-CCL19.1) and HEp-2 cells (ATCC-
CCL23), suggesting that these cells are related, if not identical, to HeLa cells (for chromosomal HeLa markers in these cells
see American Type Culture Collection Catalogue of Strains II;
cf. Fig. 6). In some cultures of HeLa cells and NCTC-3075
cells an additional minor cytoskeletal component of $\sim M_r$ 40,000
has been detected that may be related to cytokeratin No. 19.

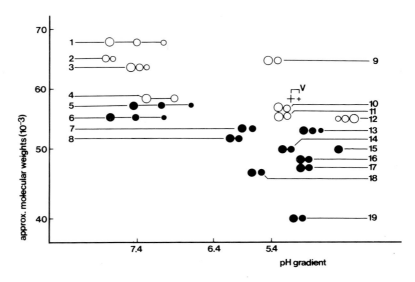

Fig. 11. Schematic diagram of human cytokeratin polypeptides arranged according to their separation by two-dimensional gel electrophoresis (for details see Moll *et al.*, 1982b). Of the 19 polypeptides described in various human tissues (circles and Arabic numerals), 11 cytokeratins (black circles) have so far been identified in cultured human cells, in which they are expressed in different patterns in different cell lines. V, Positions of vimentin and phosphorylated vimentin (+, +).

cyte differentiation with glial filaments, are all later events (Schnitzer *et al.*, 1981; Bignami *et al.*, 1982; Tapscott *et al.*, 1981; Shaw and Weber, 1982; see these for more references). The functional background of this precise programming of differential expression of the diverse intermediate filament proteins remains to be elucidated. Within the epithelia a further cytoskeletal differentiation occurs, resulting in epithelia type-specific patterns of cytokeratin expression. Moreover, it has been shown that even within the same epithelial organ, cytokeratins can be expressed differentially. In epidermis, for example, different keratin polypeptides are synthesized in different lateral domains (Moll *et al.*, 1982a) as well as in different layers (Fuchs and Green, 1980), and this is already recognized in embryonal skin formation (Banks-Schlegel, 1982). Again, the biological meaning of this differential synthesis of related polypeptides for the construction of the morphologically identical filament structure is not clear.

Examinations of tumors of various kinds have shown that these specificities of expression of types of intermediate filaments are not obscured or reversed during carcinogenesis. Thus intermediate filament proteins represent rather stable markers of differentiation the expression of which, in addition, does not seem to depend on the maintenance of cell-specific morphological differentiation. This stability of expression is important for the use of antibodies to these proteins as differentiation markers helping in classification of tumors. Stable expression of differentiation-related patterns of intermediate filament proteins is also frequently seen in cultured tumor cells (for references see Franke et al., 1979f,g, 1982c; Virtanen et al., 1981; Osborn et al., 1982), including various teratocarcinoma cells (Paulin et al., 1982). Although morphological changes of cell type-specific arrays of intermediate filaments can occur during the development of various tumors, notably "undifferentiated" forms, change of expression of the differentiation-specific type of intermediate filament protein is neither a necessary prerequisite nor a common consequence of cell transformation and carcinogenesis.

ACKNOWLEDGMENTS

We thank Mrs. Heiderose Kolb, Stefanie Winter, and Mr. Klaus Mähler (this institute) for expert technical assistance. We also acknowledge valuable discussions with Drs. Benjamin Geiger (Weizmann Institute of Sciences, Rehovot, Israel), Mary Osborn, and Klaus Weber (Max-Planck-Institut für Biophysikalische Chemie, Göttingen, FRG). The work has been supported in part by the Deutsche Forschungsgemeinschaft (Bonn-Bad Godesberg, FRG).

REFERENCES

Aaronson, R. P., and Blobel, G. (1975). *Proc. Natl. Acad.*
    Sci. USA 72, 1007-1011.
Anderton, B. H. (1981). *J. Muscle Res. Cell Motil. 2,* 141-166.
Banks-Schlegel, S. P. (1982). *J. Cell Biol. 93,* 551-559.
Bannasch, P., Zerban, H., Schmid, E., and Franke, W. W. (1980).
    Proc. Natl. Acad. Sci. USA 77, 4948-4952.
Battifora, H., Sun, T.-T., Bahu, R. M., and Rao, S. (1980).
    Hum. Pathol. 11, 635-641.
Bennett, G. S., Fellini, S. A., Croop, J. M., Otto, J. J.,
    Bryan, J., and Holtzer, H. (1978). *Proc. Natl. Acad.*
    Sci. USA 75, 4364-4368.
Bignami, A., Raju, T., and Dahl, D. (1982). *Dev. Biol. 91,*
    286-295.
Bowden, P. E., and Cunliffe, W. J. (1981). *Biochem. J. 199,*
    145-154.
Bravo, R., Small, J. V., Fey, S. J., Larsen, P. M., and Celis,
    J. E. (1982). *J. Mol. Biol. 154,* 121-143.
Brinkley, B. R. (1982). *Cold Spring Harbor Symp. Quant. Biol.*
    46, 1029-1040.
Cabral, F., Gottesman, M. M., Zimmerman, S. B., and Steinert,
    P. M. (1981). *J. Biol. Chem. 256,* 1428-1431.
Cohen, R. S., Blomberg, F., Berzins, K., and Siekevitz, P.
    (1977). *J. Cell Biol. 74,* 181-203.
Colaco, C. A. L. S., and Evans, W. H. (1981). *J. Cell Sci.*
    52, 313-325.
Cooke, P. (1976). *J. Cell Biol. 68,* 539-556.
Denk, H., Krepler, R., Lackinger, E., Artlieb, U., and Franke,
    W. W. (1982). *Lab. Invest. 46,* 584-596.
Doran, T. I., Vidrich, A., and Sun, T.-T. (1980). *Cell 22,*
    17-25.
Drochmans, P., Freudenstein, C., Wanson, J. C., Laurent, L.,
    Keenan, T. W., Stadler, J., Leloup, R., and Franke, W. W.
    (1978). *J. Cell Biol. 79,* 427-443.
Fabricant, R. N., Delarco, J. E., and Todaro, G. (1977).
    Proc. Natl. Acad. Sci. USA 74, 565-569.
Fogh, J., and Trempe, G. (1975). *In* "Human Tumor Cells *in*
    vitro" (J. Fogh, ed.), pp. 115-159. Plenum, New York and
    London.
Frank, E. D., Tuszynski, G. P., and Warren, L. (1982). *Exp.*
    Cell Res. 139, 235-247.
Franke, W. W., Schmid, E., Osborn, M., and Weber, K. (1978a).
    Proc. Natl. Acad. Sci. USA 75, 5034-5038.
Franke, W. W., Weber, K., Osborn, M., Schmid, E., and
    Freudenstein, C. (1978b). *Exp. Cell Res. 116,* 429-445.
Franke, W. W., Appelhans, B., Schmid, E., Osborn, M., and
    Weber, K. (1979a). *Eur. J. Cell Biol. 19,* 255-268.

Franke, W. W., Appelhans, B., Schmid, E., Osborn, M., and
    Weber, K. (1979b). *Differentiation (Berlin) 15,* 7-25.
Franke, W. W., Schmid, E., Breitkreutz, D., Lüder, M., Boukamp,
    P., Fusenig, N. E., Osborn, M., and Weber, K. (1979c).
    Differentiation (Berlin) 14, 35-50.
Franke, W. W., Schmid, E., Kartenbeck, J., Mayer, D., Hacker,
    H.-J., Bannasch, P., Osborn, M., Weber, K., Denk, H.,
    Wanson, J.-C., and Drochmans, P. (1979d). *Biol. Cell. 34,*
    99-110.
Franke, W. W., Schmid, E., Osborn, M., and Weber, K. (1979e).
    J. Cell Biol. 81, 570-580.
Franke, W. W., Schmid, E., Weber, K., and Osborn, M. (1979f).
    Exp. Cell Res. 118, 95-109.
Franke, W. W., Schmid, E., Winter, S., Osborn, M., and Weber,
    K. (1979g). *Exp. Cell Res. 123,* 25-46.
Franke, W. W., Schmid, E., Freudenstein, C., Appelhans, B.,
    Osborn, M., Weber, K., and Keenan, T. W. (1980a). *J. Cell
    Biol. 84,* 633-654.
Franke, W. W., Schmid, E., Vandekerckhove, J., and Weber, K.
    (1980b). *J. Cell Biol. 87,* 594-600.
Franke, W. W., Denk, H., Kalt, R., and Schmid, E. (1981a).
    Exp. Cell Res. 131, 299-318.
Franke, W. W., Mayer, D., Schmid, E., Denk, H., and Borenfreund,
    E. (1981b). *Exp. Cell Res. 134,* 345-365.
Franke, W. W., Schiller, D. L., Moll, R., Winter, S., Schmid, E.,
    Engelbrecht, I., Denk, H., Krepler, R., and Platzer, B.
    (1981c). *J. Mol. Biol. 153,* 933-959.
Franke, W. W., Schmid, E., Grund, C., Mueller, H., Engelbrecht,
    I., Moll, R., Stadler, J., and Jarasch, E.-D. (1981d).
    Differentiation (Berlin) 20, 217-241.
Franke, W. W., Winter, S., Grund, C., Schmid, E., Schiller, D.
    L., and Jarasch, E.-D. (1981e). *J. Cell Biol. 90,* 116-127.
Franke, W. W., Grund, C., Kuhn, C., Jackson, B. W., and Illmen-
    see, K. (1982a). *Differentiation (Berlin) 23,* 43-59.
Franke, W. W., Moll, R., Mueller, H., Schmid, E., Kuhn, C.,
    Krepler, R., Artlieb, U., and Denk, H. (1983). *Proc.
    Natl. Acad. Sci. USA 80,* 543-547.
Franke, W. W., Schmid, E., Grund, C., and Geiger, B. (1982b).
    Cell 30, 103-113.
Franke, W. W., Schmid, E., Schiller, D. L., Winter, S.,
    Jarasch, E.-D., Moll, R., Denk, H., Jackson, B., and
    Illmensee, K. (1982c). *Cold Spring Harbor Symp. Quant.
    Biol. 46,* 431-453.
Fuchs, E., and Green, H. (1978). *Cell 15,* 887-897.
Fuchs, E., and Green, H. (1979). *Cell 17,* 573-582.
Fuchs, E., and Green, H. (1980). *Cell 19,* 1033-1042.
Fuchs, E., and Green, H. (1981). *Cell 25,* 617-625.
Gabbiani, G., Schmid, E., Winter, S., Chaponnier, C.,

De Chastonay, C., Vandekerckhove, J., Weber, K., and Franke, W. W. (1981a). *Proc. Natl. Acad. Sci. USA 78,* 298-302.

Gabbiani, G., Kapanci, Y., Barrazone, P., and Franke, W. W. (1981b). *Am. J. Pathol. 104,* 206-216.

Gard, D. L., and Lazarides, E. (1980). *Cell 19,* 263-275.

Gard, D. L., Bell, P. B., and Lazarides, E. (1979). *Proc. Natl. Acad. Sci. USA 76,* 3894-3898.

Geiger, B. (1982). *Cold Spring Harbor Symp. Quant. Biol. 46,* 671-682.

Geiger, B., Schmid, E., and Franke, W. W. (1983). *Differentiation (Berlin) 23,* 189-205.

Geisler, N., and Weber, K. (1981). *J. Mol. Biol. 151,* 565-569.

Holtzer, H., Bennett, G. S., Tapscott, S. J., Croop, J. M., and Toyama, Y. (1982). *Cold Spring Harbor Symp. Quant. Biol. 46,* 317-339.

Huiatt, T. W., Robson, R. M., Arakawa, N., and Stromer, M. H. (1980). *J. Biol. Chem. 255,* 6981-6989.

Hynes, R. O., and Destree, A. T. (1978). *Cell 13,* 151-163.

Ishikawa, A., Bischoff, R., and Holtzer, H. (1968). *J. Cell Biol. 38,* 538-555.

Jackson, B. W., Grund, C., Schmid, E., Bürki, K., Franke, W. W., and Illmensee, K. (1980). *Differentiation (Berlin) 17,* 161-179.

Jackson, B. W., Grund, C., Franke, W. W., and Illmensee, K. (1981). *Differentiation (Berlin) 20,* 203-216.

Kubilus, J., Baden, H. P., and McGilvray, N. (1980). *J. Natl. Cancer Inst. (US) 65,* 869-875.

Lane, E. B. (1982). *J. Cell Biol. 92,* 665-673.

Lazarides, E. (1980). *Nature (London) 283,* 249-256.

Lazarides, E. (1982). *Annu. Rev. Biochem. 51,* 219-250.

Lee, L. D., Kubilus, J., and Baden, H. P. (1979). *Biochem. J. 177,* 187-196.

Milstone, L. M. (1981). *J. Cell Biol. 88,* 317-322.

Milstone, L. M., and McGuire, J. (1981). *J. Cell Biol. 88,* 312-316.

Moll, R., Franke, W. W., Volc-Platzer, B., and Krepler, R. (1982a). *J. Cell Biol. 95,* 285-295.

Moll, R., Franke, W. W., Schiller, D. L., Geiger, B., and Krepler, R. (1982b). *Cell 31,* 11-24.

O'Connor, C. M., Asai, D. J., Flytzanis, C. N., and Lazarides, E. (1981). *Mol. Cell. Biol. 1,* 303-309.

Osborn, M., Caselitz, J., and Weber, K. (1981a). *Differentiation (Berlin) 20,* 196-202.

Osborn, M., Ludwig-Festl, M., Weber, K., Bignami, A., Dahl, D., and Bayreuther, K. (1981b). *Differentiation (Berlin) 19,* 161-167.

Osborn, M., Geisler, N., Shaw, G., Sharp, G., and Weber, K. (1982). *Cold Spring Harbor Symp. Quant. Biol. 46,* 413-429.

Paetau, A., Virtanen, I., Stenman, S., Kurki, P., Linder, E.,
    Vaheri, A., Westermark, B., Dahl, D., and Haltia, M.
    (1979). *Acta Neuropathol.* 47, 71-74.
Paulin, D., Babinet, C., Weber, K., and Osborn, M. (1980).
    Exp. Cell Res. 130, 297-304.
Paulin, D., Jakob, H., Jacob, F., Weber, K., and Osborn, M.
    (1982). *Differentiation (Berlin)* 22, 90-99.
Pruss, R. M., Mirsky, R., Raff, M. C., Thorpe, R., Dowding,
    A. J., and Anderton, B. H. (1981). *Cell* 27, 419-428.
Quinlan, R. A., and Franke, W. W. (1982). *Proc. Natl. Acad.
    Sci. USA* 79, 3452-3456.
Quinlan, R. A., and Franke, W. W. (1983). *Eur. J. Biochem.* 132,
    477-484.
Ramaekers, F. C. S., Puts, J. J. G., Kant, A., Moesker, O.,
    Jap, P. H. K., and Vooijs, G. P. (1982). *Cold Spring
    Harbor Symp. Quant. Biol.* 46, 331-339.
Renner, W., Franke, W. W., Schmid, E., Geisler, N., Weber,
    K., and Mandelkow, E. (1981). *J. Mol. Biol.* 149, 285-
    306.
Rueger, D. C., Huston, J. S., Dahl, D., and Bignami, A. (1979).
    J. Mol. Biol. 135, 53-68.
Schiller, D. L., Franke, W. W., and Geiger, B. (1982). *EMBO
    J.* 1, 761-769.
Schlegel, R., Banks-Schlegel, S., McLeod, J. A., and Pinkus,
    G. S. (1980). *Am. J. Pathol.* 110, 41-49.
Schmid, E., Tapscott, S., Bennett, G. S., Croop, J., Fellini,
    S. A., Holtzer, H., and Franke, W. W. (1979). *Differen-
    tiation (Berlin)* 15, 27-40.
Schmid, E., Osborn, M., Rungger-Brändle, E., Gabbiani, G.,
    Weber, K., and Franke, W. W. (1982). *Exp. Cell Res.* 137,
    329-340.
Schmid, E., Schiller, D. L., Grund, C., Stadler, J., and
    Franke, W. W. (1983). *J. Cell Biol.* 96, 37-50.
Schnitzer, J., Franke, W. W., and Schachner, M. (1981). *J.
    Cell Biol.* 90, 435-447.
Sharp, G. A., Osborn, M., and Weber, K. (1982). *Exp. Cell
    Res.* 141, 385-395.
Shaw, G., and Weber, K. (1982). *Nature (London)* 298, 277-279.
Singer, S. J., Ball, E. H., Geiger, B., and Chen, W.-T. (1982).
    Cold Spring Harbor Quant. Biol. 46, 303-316.
Small, J. V., and Sobieszek, A. (1977). *J. Cell Sci.* 23, 243-
    268.
Soule, H. D., Vazquez, J., Long, A., Albert, S., and Brennan,
    M. (1973). *J. Natl. Cancer Inst. (US)* 51, 1409-1416.
Starger, J. M., Brown, W. E., Goldman, A. E., and Goldman, R.
    (1977). *J. Cell Biol.* 78, 93-109.
Steinert, P. M., Idler, W. W., and Zimmerman, S. B. (1976).
    J. Mol. Biol. 108, 547-567.

Steinert, P. M., Idler, W. W., Cabral, F., Gottesman, M. M.,
    and Goldman, R. D. (1981). *Proc. Natl. Acad. Sci. USA*
    78, 3692-3696.
Steinert, P. M., Wantz, M. L., and Idler, W. W. (1982). *Bio-
    chemistry 21,* 177-183.
Summerhayes, I. C., Cheng, Y.-S. E., Sun, T.-T., and Chen,
    L. B. (1981). *J. Cell Biol. 90,* 63-69.
Sun, T.-T., and Green, H. (1978a). *Cell 14,* 469-476.
Sun, T.-T., and Green, H. (1978b). *J. Biol. Chem. 253,* 2053-
    2060.
Sun, T.-T., Shih, C. H., and Green, H. (1979). *Proc. Natl.
    Acad. Sci. USA 76,* 2813-2817.
Tapscott, S. J., Bennett, G. S., Toyama, Y., Kleinbart, F.,
    and Holtzer, H. (1981). *Dev. Biol. 86,* 40-54.
Tuszynski, G. P., Frank, E. D., Damsky, C. H., Buck, C. A.,
    and Warren, L. (1979). *J. Biol. Chem. 254,* 6138-6143.
Virtanen, I., Lehto, V.-P., Lehtonen, E., Vartio, T., Stenman,
    S., Kurki, P., Wager, O., Small, J. V., Dahl, D., and
    Badley, R. A. (1981). *J. Cell Sci. 50,* 45-63.
Winter, S., Jarasch, E.-D., Schmid, E., Franke, W. W., and
    Denk, H. (1980). *Eur. J. Cell Biol. 22,* 371.
Wu, Y.-J., and Rheinwald, J. G. (1981). *Cell 25,* 627-635.
Yen, S.-H., and Fields, K. L. (1981). *J. Cell Biol. 88,* 115-
    126.

2

ION REGULATION AND THE CYTOSKELETON IN PRENEOPLASTIC AND NEOPLASTIC CELLS

Benjamin F. Trump, Irene K. Berezesky,
Patricia C. Phelps, and Andrew J. Saladino

Department of Pathology
University of Maryland School of Medicine
Baltimore, Maryland

I. INTRODUCTION

The past several years have seen the development of concepts and technology relating the chemical composition of cells to cellular structure and function. Although this simple statement sounds self-evident, it is a difficult one to establish in a rigorous manner, especially when one considers the current concept that diffusible ions (e.g., Na, Cl, Mg, Ca, K, and P) may play an important if not determining role in the reaction of cells to injury (Trump *et al.*, 1978, 1979a, 1980, 1981a,b, 1982a), in the present case to carcinogenic agents including promoters.

It is our concept that the understanding of cell injury is fundamental to the understanding of a variety of disease phenomena. The present chapter will discuss tumor promotion and carcinogenesis, although many of the arguments presented could apply to atherosclerosis and other disorders of growth and differentiation as well as to neoplasms.

Control of cellular metabolism, cell differentiation, and cell division plays a fundamental role in neoplasia. Currently, increasing evidence favors the concept that ion regulation plays an important if not decisive role in many cellular phenomena including tumor promotion. According to the ionic net theory developed by Rasmussen and Goodman (1977), all ion fluxes are interrelated and, with proper modulation, result in the development of "physiological triggers" or "second messengers" (Rasmussen, 1974). Such ions include Na^+, H^+, K^+, and Ca^{2+} and their corresponding anions. The activities of these ions may undergo individual or collective changes that may be reciprocal or identical, and they may stimulate, inhibit, or be permissive to many cell phenomena. Of particular interest to us are the potential interactions between membrane phenomena, cytoskeletal function, and ionic balance.

The phenomenon of tumor promotion is commonly regarded as a reversible event that alters the expression of genetic cellular information (Pitot, 1981). Examples of tumor-promoting compounds include hormones, drugs, natural products, and other agents that in themselves do not react directly with the genetic material but rather alter its expression through mechanisms that may involve cell membranes including receptors and/or other cytoplasmic or nuclear components. The definition of promoting agents is necessarily inexact at present. Pitot *et al.* (1981) have hypothesized that promoting agents may be grouped into specific and nonspecific classes. Specific agents would be those that bind to or interact with receptors or receptor-like molecules on or in target cells. Nonspecific promoters do not appear to act through such receptors but alter gene expression through as yet unknown mechanisms. An example would be iodoacetate (IAA) in the mouse skin (Gwynn and Salamon, 1953). It is of course entirely conceivable that both classes share one or more common mechanisms.

Slaga *et al.* (1982a) have subclassified promoters into first- and second-stage agents. First-stage promoters induce epidermal hyperplasia and increase the number of dark basal cells; examples of first-stage promoters include the Ca ionophore A23187. Second-stage promoters may or may not increase the number of dark basal keratinocytes; mezerein is the chief candidate as a model for second-stage promotion; 12-*O*-tetradecanoylphorbol 13-acetate (TPA) is a complete promoter. Both TPA and mezerein stimulate ornithine decarboxylase (ODC) activity and modify differentiation in Friend erythroleukemia cells or HL-60 human leukemic cells.

In this chapter we consider evidence that ion fluxes, specifically Na and Ca, are intimately involved in tumor promotion and altered phenotypic expression. We further develop a hypothesis that relates these ion shifts in tumor promotion to

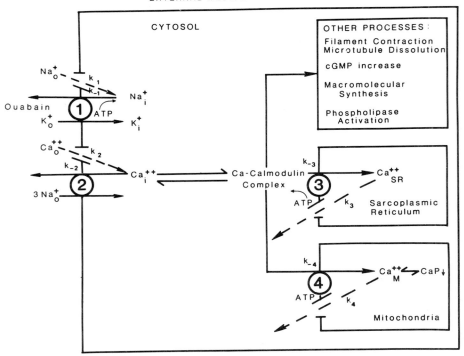

Fig. 1. Schematic illustration of Na and Ca regulation as
they occur in a typical cell. The model illustrates the principal routes of entry and exit of Na and Ca across the sarcolem-
ma, across the membrane of the endoplasmic reticulum, and across
the inner mitochondrial membrane. The k's refer to the rate co-
efficients for the Na and Ca movements. The ouabain-sensitive,
Na-K exchange pump ((1) in the diagram) is responsible for Na
extrusion and K accumulation. Calcium exits from the cell primarily via the Na-Ca exchange ((2) in the diagram) and is not
directly dependent on ATP, although in some cells, additional
ATP-driven Ca extrusion mechanisms (i.e., Ca^{2+}-ATPase) may occur. Ca sequestration by the ATP-driven Ca pump of the endoplasmic (or sarcoplasmic) reticulum is indicated by (3) in the
diagram, and the energy-dependent accumulation of Ca by the mitochondria is indicated by (4). Some of the important intracellular events that are modulated by $[Ca^{2+}]_i$, often through proteins such as calmodulin, are also indicated. For simplicity,
only the predominant pathways for Na and Ca movement are shown
in the diagram, although the k's actually refer to the total
movement of the respective ion species in the direction

those that occur in other forms of cell injury. Many of these
effects appear to involve modulation of the cytoskeleton, modifications of which are related to cellular ionic control and to
control of cyclic nucleotides.

II. ION REGULATION IN NORMAL AND INJURED CELLS

    This chapter does not attempt an exhaustive review of cur-
rent knowledge concerning ion regulation in normal cells; however, a few basic phenomena in this area need review to establish the premise of the investigation. It should also be borne
in mind by the reader that these phenomena are undergoing constant investigation and that in the immediate future new facts
concerning their normal regulation will be forthcoming.

    Na and Ca regulation, as they occur in a typical cell, are
shown schematically in Fig. 1. Intra- and extracellular ions
are in constant exchange through transplasmalemma diffusion, a
process that is complex, involves several mechanisms, and, in
many cases, may involve specific ionophorous channels including
specific proteins. Na and Ca both diffuse into the cell down
their respective concentration gradients. Preferential entry
channels appear to exist for both of these ions, with those for
Ca being of two types: neutral and electrically gated.
Specific blocking agents exist for Na and Ca, and many types
have been reviewed. Thus, Na tends to leak into the cell along
with Ca, whereas K and Mg tend to leak out. To maintain homeo-
stasis within the cell, mechanisms must exist that control
ionized Na and Ca at low levels while maintaining K and Mg at
high levels.

(Fig. 1 continued) indicated. Such ion regulation bears a very
important relationship to the structure and function of the cytoskeleton as described in the text.

Na and K appear to be regulated by membrane transport systems through the action of a specific protein, the Na^+, K^+, ouabain-sensitive ATPase, which extrudes Na and accumulates K in the presence of ATP. The significance of this vectorial transport system undoubtedly supersedes its effect on Na and K by also indirectly regulating Ca and, in some transporting epithelium, Cl secretion. Thus, through the phenomenon of Na–Ca exchange (Blaustein, 1974), Na as well as Ca accumulate within the cell if the (Na^+, K^+)-ATPase fails to operate. Any condition that lowers extracellular levels or raises intracellular levels of Na will favor the accumulation of Ca. It has also been suggested that changes in cytosolic Ca regulate epithelial Na transport (Taylor and Windhager, 1979). Any injury that results in increased leakage or decreased extrusion of Na will, at the same time, also favor the accumulation of Ca.

In the cytosol, Ca and possibly Na are also controlled by membrane transport systems in the organelles. Both mitochondria and endoplasmic reticulum (ER), especially in muscle, contain active transport systems for Ca that tend to sequester this cation in their respective organelles; both are energy dependent (Carafoli, 1982). Therefore, toxins that modify either of these organelles may modify Ca in the cytosol.

In the cytosol there are a variety of Ca-binding ligands, both organic and inorganic. An example is the protein calmodulin, which is not only an important Ca ligand but also an important Ca effector protein, mediating a number of Ca-related effects (Cheung, 1970, 1980, 1982a,b; Means and Dedman, 1980). Little appears to be known concerning Na-mediated effects in the cell, apart from its effects on Ca modulation.

A variety of factors both physiological and pathological can modify Na and Ca regulation in cells (Trump *et al.*, 1971, 1981b, 1982a). Energy deficiency (e.g., anoxia or metabolic

inhibitors) modifies the availability of ATP for (Na^+,K^+)-
ATPases and for Ca^{2+}-ATPases as well. This occurs immediately
when the ATP concentration is less than the K_m for these
ATPases and leads to increasing cytosol concentrations of Na,
Ca, and Cl, and thus usually to efflux of K. Energy deficiency also affects intracellular Ca-regulatory mechanisms, including both mitochondria and ER, and augments the increasing cytoplasmic Ca. In some cells, increased Na has the additional effect of fostering the efflux of Ca from mitochondria (Carafoli,
1982). A variety of conditions, including anoxia and chemical
toxins that inhibit respiration and/or glycolysis, are capable
of lowering the cellular ATP. Some such compounds, including
iodoacetic acid, an inhibitor of glycolytic ATP synthesis, are
known also to be promoters. However, it is not known what relationship, if any, the two phenomena have with each other.
There is also the possibility of genetic alteration of the mitochondrial Ca sequestration system, because a number of mutagens are capable of binding to mitochondrial DNA. This represents a theoretical possibility for some of the effects such
carcinogens have on ion regulation (Weinstein, 1981, 1982).

The other major category of conditions that modulate cell
ion regulation are those involving components of the cell membrane. A variety of chemical hormones and other compounds are
capable of such modification. The first category are those
agents that directly modify (Na^+,K^+)-ATPase. The best characterized of these are the cardiac glycosides, such as ouabain,
which specifically inhibit plasmalemmal (Na^+,K^+)-ATPase. This
rapidly leads to increased cellular Na and decreased K, and
consequent increased Ca, secondary to diminished Na-Ca exchange.
In many cells, because ouabain does not interfere with mitochondrial Ca uptake (Trump *et al.*, 1982a), this increased Ca
will be reflected by mitochondrial sequestration, which can
often be visualized by electron microscopy. Other mechanisms

include changes in the Na and/or Ca entry channels. This can
be specific (e.g., hormone binding to surface receptors) or
nonspecific, such as modification of membrane lipids with
surface-active agents or phospholipases, and modification of
membrane proteins by sulfhydryl-binding agents such as heavy
metals. In leukocytes, Ca entry is rapidly stimulated by phorbol esters, and Ca appears to represent an early mediator of
the effects of that compound in leukocyte activation (Weissmann,
1980; Hoffstein, 1980). The use of hydrophobic ionophores as
test compounds has greatly facilitated research in this area.
The Ca ionophore A23187 has been shown to be a first-stage promoter by Slaga *et al.* (1982b). A final type of membrane modification involves membrane lipid peroxidation. Many carcinogens, cocarcinogens, and promoters are metabolized to form or
incite the generation of reactive compounds and intermediates,
which include free radicals and various reactive oxygen
species (for review see McBrien and Slater, 1982). These reac-
tants are capable of initiating a number of cellular events,
including altered cell membrane ion permeability and modification of nucleic acids.

III. NORMAL CYTOSKELETON IN RELATION TO ION REGULATION

Some of the more notable functions of the cytoskeleton are
its involvement in cell shape and form, cell division, cell attachment, and cell motion. It is also involved in directing
the movement of intracellular proteins in activities such as
phagocytosis, autophagocytosis, and secretion, and in responding
to signals from the cell surface by regulating the movement of
extracellular membrane receptors for hormones, lectins, immunoglobulins, and xenobiotics, possibly including promoters.

The cytoskeleton is visualized as a network of three major classes of filament or fiber proteins: microtubules, microfilaments, and intermediate filaments. A fourth component, the microtrabecular lattice, may have integral association with the other three. All of these components may relate to cellular ionic regulation (see later). Because of the intimate relation of the cytoskeleton to cellular ionic regulation, this subject is reviewed in the following sections.

A. Microtubules

A microtubule is a cylindrical structure (20-25 nm in diameter) composed of polymers of the protein tubulin and consists of a circular array of 13 rows of dimers (protofilaments) that run parallel to its long axis. Microtubules are known to be in equilibrium with their tubulin dimer subunits, and appropriate agents are able to shift the equilibrium to either the direction of assembly or that of disassembly (Sloboda, 1980). Assembly involves both nucleation or initiation and elongation, and *in vitro* it requires the presence of Mg and GTP (guanosine triphosphate), ambient temperature, slightly acid or neutral pH, and the absence of excess Ca. Disassembly occurs in the cold (except for the stable class of microtubules in cilia, flagella, and brain), with antimitotic drugs, Ca, and increased hydrostatic pressure.

Microtubule-associated proteins (MAPs) (Murphy and Borisy, 1975; Sloboda *et al.*, 1975) are believed to be represented morphologically as fine projections on individual tubules, may function to stabilize or shift the microtubule-dimer equilibrium in the direction that favors assembly, and may assist in microtubule-microfilament interaction to form a continuous network *in vivo* (Griffith and Pollard, 1978).

Microtubules are able to polymerize (1 μm/min) or depolymerize rapidly. In interphase cells, they characteris-
tically extend from centrosomes in the perinuclear region
toward the cell periphery (Brinkley *et al.*, 1975; Weber *et al.*,
1975). During mitosis, the normal pattern is replaced by the
mitotic spindle. Microtubules do not appear to arise spontaneously, but grow from specific nucleating sites, the
microtubule organizing centers (MTOCs), which have been demonstrated to arise in the pericentriolar region (Brinkley *et al.*,
1975; Osborn and Weber, 1976; Frankel, 1976; Spiegelman *et al.*,
1979).

Microtubules are implicated in the movement of chromosomes during anaphase, which may be related to a polymerization-
depolymerization process, or to the interaction of microtubules
with microtubules or with other cytoplasmic proteins (Sloboda,
1980). There is also evidence that tubulin depolymerization
itself is sufficient stimulus for initiating DNA synthesis during the S phase of the cell cycle (Crossin and Carney, 1981).
The latter is of great interest in regard to Ca and cell division (see later).

B. Microfilaments

Microfilaments are basic structural proteins of all eukaryotic cells (Pollard and Weihing, 1974), and they contract on
interaction with myosin, Ca, and ATP. In nonmuscle cells, microfilaments include the major protein actin and its associated
proteins, α-actinin, filamin, tropomyosin, and myosin. Microfilaments are represented by double-stranded helices (6-8 nm in
diameter) and occur as asymmetric polymers having both a
"barbed" and a "pointed" end. Actin exists in a soluble, monomeric, globular form (G-actin), a polymerized fibrous form
(F-actin), and a paracrystalline form (P-actin; Harwell *et al.*,

1980). F-Actin and G-actin are in dynamic equilibrium; polymerization from G-actin to F-actin results by nucleation and elongation by the addition of monomers to the filament ends (when G-actin content is above a certain critical concentration; Oosawa and Asakura, 1975).

Villin, an actin-binding polypeptide found in chicken intestinal brush border epithelium, has been found to influence the polymerization of actin. In the presence of villin, the viscosity of prepolymerized F-actin is reduced and is correlated with the presence of very short actin filaments (Craig and Powell, 1980). Villin is also found to be Ca dependent and to be involved in modifying actin by attaching to its "barbed" end. Fragmin from Physarum (Hasegawa *et al.*, 1980) and capping protein (Isenberg *et al.*, 1980) also act to reduce actin viscosity. In addition, Ca-sensitive gelsolin (from macrophages) and a protein from *Acanthamoeba* affect the cross-linking of actin filaments to produce gelation (Yin and Stossel, 1979; Pollard, 1981).

The inhibitory effect of cytochalasin B is now known to be the result of a blocking of the addition of monomers to the "barbed" end of microfilaments (MacLean-Fletcher and Pollard, 1980) and apparently affects both the rate of polymerization and the interaction of microfilaments.

Microfilaments are often seen in high concentrations beneath the plasma membrane, and there is evidence that they are intimately associated with it (Pollard and Korn, 1973; Gabbiani *et al.*, 1975; Gruenstein *et al.*, 1975). Concentrations of microfilaments are seen in areas of active phagocytosis (Stossel and Hartwig, 1976; Berlin *et al.*, 1979), in areas of endocytosis (Albertini and Anderson, 1977), and in bundles attached to membranes of intestinal microvilli (Mooseker and Tilney, 1975).

Actin is seen in PtK_2 cells aligned parallel to microtubules of the mitotic spindle (Herman and Pollard, 1978;
Sanger *et al.,* 1979). Actin filaments remain intact in endothelial cells in the mitotic area throughout division and
could potentially be involved in redistribution of structural
proteins between daughter cells (Blose, 1979).

C. Intermediate Filaments

The term intermediate filament applies to a group of filaments that have a diameter of 7-11 nm. A number of filaments
with different biochemical structure and function but similar
morphology fall into this grouping. There are five known major
classes of intermediate filaments on the basis of the tissue of
origin, antigenic determinants, and subunit structure:
(1) keratin filaments found in epithelial cells that cross-
react with prekeratin antibodies, (2) desmin (or skeletin)
filaments found predominantly in muscle cells, (3) vimentin
filaments found in many normal and transformed cells, (4) neu-
rofilaments found in cells of neuronal origin, and (5) glial
filaments found in glial cells (Lazarides, 1982). In some
cases, a cell may contain two filament types, as is the case
with HeLa and PtK_2 cells, which have been shown to contain prekeratin and villin (Osborn *et al.*, 1980). All classes exhibit
extensive regions of amino acid divergence; however, they share
some common properties (Lazarides, 1982).

Keratin filaments are a common feature of most epithelial
cells (Sun and Green, 1978; Sun *et al.,* 1979) from diverse embryological origins including basal cells of the trachea,
bronchus, prostate, and cervix (Schlegel *et al.*, 1980). Keratin filaments are generally recognized to be extremely stable
and to play a role in structural support and cell shape, loco-
motion, and organelle transport. They are found widely

distributed throughout the cytoplasm areas and are also char-
acteristically seen in intimate contact with desmosomes and
hemidesmosome attachment sites (Weihing, 1979). Myoepithelial
cells from several different glands demonstrate extensive
keratin filament networks showing anchorage at desmosomes and
associations with contractile filaments (Franke *et al.,* 1980).
Ca is known to mediate transglutaminase and therefore to be
associated with the cross-linking of keratin proteins, and the
level of extracellular Ca in human skin and bronchial epithelium
is reported to affect the expression of keratin. Normal cells
grown in low-Ca medium exhibit very few tonofilaments, whereas
those grown in high-Ca medium (approximately 1 mM) show many
filaments (Hennings *et al.,* 1980; Lechner *et al.,* 1981; Yuspa
et al., 1981). Yuspa (1982) has extensively characterized the
response of mouse epidermal basal cells in culture to extracellular Ca concentration. Normal cells exhibit terminal differentiation with keratin formation in physiological concentrations of extracellular Ca (1.2-1.4 mM) but continue to divide
in low-Ca medium (0.02-0.09 mM). Neoplastic cells, in contrast,
do not respond to this stimulus and continue to divide even at
normal extracellular Ca levels. If normal cells are induced to
differentiate terminally with physiological Ca concentrations,
they tend to lose their ODC response to TPA.

D. Microtrabecular Lattice

     Porter and associates have provided strong evidence for
the existence of a fine filament meshwork called the microtrabecular lattice in the cytoplasmic ground substance of a number of cultured cells by means of high-voltage electron microscope study (Buckley, 1975; Wolosewick and Porter, 1979; Porter
and Tucker, 1981). The proposed model presents a three-
dimensional lattice network of interconnecting fine filaments

(3-6 nm in diameter) that extends throughout the cytoplasm and connects with the cell cortex. This extensive lattice supports or suspends the cytoplasmic organelles. A coating on the microtubules and microfilaments is coextensive with the lattice filaments, suggesting they are an integral part of the lattice. The lattice appears to link the individual cell components into a single structural and functional unit. This lattice may be important in holding microtubules and microfilaments in place in specialized cell extensions such as cilia and flagella.

Studies on pigment cell migration in the squirrel fish strongly suggest that the lattice is a dynamic meshwork capable of expanding and contracting for aggregation and dispersion of the granules. The granules are suspended in the microtrabeculae, and interconnected microtubules are implicated in providing guidance for granule movement (Byers and Porter, 1977; Luby and Porter, 1980). In addition, Ca appears to be required for granule translocation. Pigment granules in isolated denervated erythrophores do not aggregate spontaneously in the absence of external Ca. Aggregation is also impaired in the presence of compounds known to antagonize Ca influx into the cell. However, aggregation can be induced by the elevation of cytoplasmic Ca through the use of Ca ionophore A23187 (Luby-Phelps and Porter, 1982).

E. Calmodulin

Calmodulin has achieved major prominence since it was discovered to play an important role as a mediator of Ca regulation in a variety of cellular enzyme systems (Means and Dedman, 1980). Calmodulin is now known to bind Ca with high affinity and high specificity, and to form a calmodulin-Ca complex that in turn activates a number of Ca-dependent protein kinases. Calmodulin-Ca has specifically been shown to function in many cell activities such as cyclic nucleotide and glycogen metabolism, contractile processes, secretion, Ca metabolism, and activation of other Ca-dependent protein kinases, and to be a component of the mitotic spindle apparatus as well (Cheung, 1982a,b). In essence, calmodulin is the essential, ever-present participant in Ca-initiated cellular processes. Calmodulin has been purified (Dedman et al., 1977), and a monospecific antibody has been prepared against it (Dedman et al., 1978). The protein has been identified in cultured cells by indirect immunofluorescence (Welsh et al., 1978, 1979) and by immunohistochemistry in rat cerebellum (Lin et al., 1980). Welsh and colleagues (1979) demonstrated that calmodulin was a component of the mitotic apparatus in dividing PtK_2 and CHO cells, and suggested that it might play a physiological role in the process of chromosome movement. Ca and therefore presumably the calmodulin-Ca complex have been intimately associated with effecting changes in the cytoskeletal filament components.

IV.   IONIC REGULATION IN PRENEOPLASTIC AND NEOPLASTIC CELLS--
       RELATION TO PROMOTION

A.   Cell Division

The fertilization of an ovum by a sperm is a fundamental example of initiation of cell division. Much evidence has accumulated that the events occurring at the time of fertilization involve an influx of Na, an efflux of protons, an influx and intracellular redistribution of Ca, and, finally, cell division (Jaffe, 1980; Epel, 1980). These ionic events occur very rapidly. The increase in pH appears to be fundamental to the process, as Na influx can be replaced by ammonia-induced alkalinization of the extracellular fluid (Epel, 1980).

Alterations in pH, as in egg fertilization, have been related to cell division in a number of systems. For example, in
Physarum, Gerson and Burton (1977) observed that a high pH of
6.4 occurs at mitosis and a low pH of 5.8 at midinterphase.
The elevated pH is compatible with the influx of cations such
as Na. It is well known that elevations of pH increase the
sensitivity to Ca-mediated events. Thus, Na-H exchange may act
as a trigger involved in the initiation of mitosis.

It now appears that the initiating events for a number of
these phenomena may begin with membrane depolarization attendant
on Na influx (Gillies, 1981). At least in some systems, notably
fertilization, this is accompanied by a Na-proton exchange with
a wave of alkalinization within the cytosol. In a variety of
systems, increased pH facilitates the action of Ca whereas diminished pH appears to antagonize it. Little information is
available on cellular pH changes during tumor promotion in terms
of acute cell injury. We have observed in several cell types
that decreasing extracellular pH retards the course of acute
cell injury, whereas even slight increases in pH greatly augment
the response (Penttila and Trump, 1974, 1975a,b,c; Penttila *et
al.,* 1976). A number of tissue culture studies have related pH
and cell division (Eagle, 1973).

Ca influx may also involve an intracellular Ca redistribution. Although the source of intracellular Ca has not been
identified, calmodulin is probably an important mediator. The
alkalinization of the sperm also seems to promote actin polymerization, leading to the acrosome reaction.

Many studies suggest some relationship between Ca and cell
division (Boynton *et al.,* 1977; Swierenga *et al.,* 1980;
McGaughey and Jensen, 1980; Mikkelsen, 1978). Ca influx
has been associated with cell division and/or DNA synthesis
in a number of experimental systems, including fertilization
of marine eggs (Jaffe, 1980), mitotic activity of bone marrow,
liver, and thymus of the rat (Whitfield *et al.,* 1980), stimu-

lation of cell division in transformed skin epithelium (Yuspa
et al., 1981), hyperplasia and metaplasia in A23187-treated
hamster epithelium (Saladino *et al.*, 1982), cell division in
the moss funaria (Saunders and Hepler, 1982), A23187-treated
3T3 cells (Andersson and Norrby, 1977), and lectin treatment
of lymphocytes (Tsien *et al.*, 1982).

Tupper *et al.* (1982) observed that human lung fibroblasts
can be brought to a quiescent state by removal of serum from
the medium or by lowering of extracellular Ca. On return of
Ca or serum, cells leave G_1 and progress to S. Serum stimulation results in increased influx of a variety of materials including rubidium, 3-methylglucose, and α-aminoisobutyric acid.
Ca deprivation modifies the entry of the substances rapidly,
diminishing them when removed. In contrast, Ca stimulation of
Ca-deprived cells shows little increase in these transport systems, indicating that Ca and serum G_0 or G_1 block are not
equivalent and that the serum-induced changes do not appear
necessary. The sequence in which Ca or serum are presented
alters the ability to modulate the transport systems. If exposed to Ca prior to serum they possess a Ca modulation, but
when exposed to Ca in the absence of serum they do not.

However, increased levels of extracellular Ca and possibly
increased Ca influx can stimulate differentiation, sometimes
terminal differentiation, in a number of cell types including
cultured mouse skin basal cells (Yuspa *et al.*, 1981), cultured
human bronchial epithelium (Lechner *et al.*, 1981), and HL-60
cells (Gallagher *et al.*, 1979).

Changes in Na influx and/or changes in $[Na^+]$ have been associated with cell division in a number of systems (Pool *et al.*,
1981) including TPA-treated 3T3 cells (Dicker and Rozengurt,
1981), serum-treated 3T3 cells (Rozengurt and Mendoza, 1980),
vasopressin and serum-treated 3T3 cells (Rosengurt and Mendoza,
1980), fertilization of marine eggs (Epel, 1980), ouabain-
treated chick spinal cord (Cone, 1980), primary hepatocyte cul-

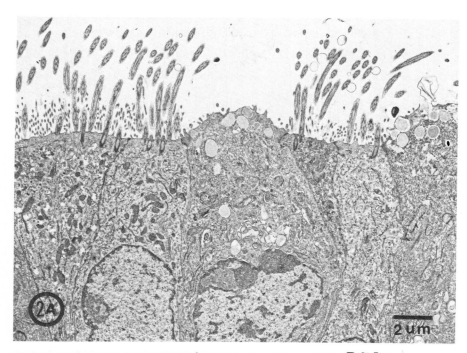

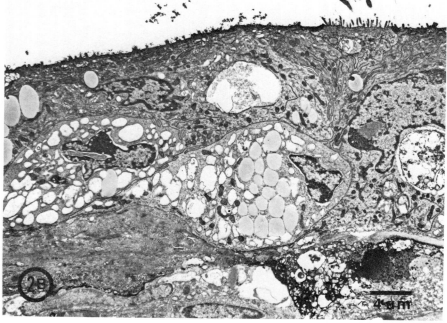

tures treated with insulin, glucagon, and epidermal growth factor (EGF) (Leffert and Koch, 1980), fibroblasts treated with amphotericin B (Kitagawa and Andoh, 1978), vaginal epithelium in
estrogen-treated rodents (Cameron and Smith, 1980), postnatal
uterine myocytes (Cameron and Smith, 1980), pre- versus postcon-
fluent 3T3 cells (Cameron and Smith, 1980), dividing versus
postmitotic enterocytes (Cameron et al., 1979), and mitotic Physarum cells (Jeter et al., 1979). In several cases these effects were inhibited, at least partially, by amiloride, a
blocker of Na entry channels (Leffert and Koch, 1980; Rozengurt
and Mendoza, 1980), and stimulated by veratridine (Cone, 1980).

The situation with ouabain is complex. Ouabain treatment
increases intracellular Na but lowers intracellular K. In one
study (Cone, 1980) it increased cell division, whereas in
others it decreased it. This might relate to differential effects on K in different cells. In many cells, K deficiency
rapidly leads to diminished protein synthesis (Lubin, 1967),
which could arrest cell division even in the presence of a positive signal.

B. Treatment of Cells with Ionophores for Ca or Na

1. *A23187*

Studies utilizing the carboxylic acid ionophore A23187
have materially contributed to our understanding of the various
roles of Ca in major physiological and pathophysiological
events at the cellular level. It was of interest to us, there-

Fig. 2. (A) Transmission electron micrograph (TEM) of control hamster tracheobronchial epithelium (HTBE) after 3 days in
culture in standard organ culture medium (OCM) showing ciliated,
mucous, intermediate, and basal cells. (B) TEM of HTBE in culture following 48 h continuous exposure to 10^{-5} M A23187. Note
the marked vacuolization and distension of the smooth ER, possibly suggesting sequestration of calcium.

fore, to ascertain what effects this compound might have with
continuous exposure to human and hamster tracheobronchial epithelium (TBE) in organ culture for periods of time varying
from several hours to several days.

Tracheal rings that had been incubated in organ culture
medium (OCM) for 3 to 14 days were treated with 10^{-3} to 10^{-7} *M*
A23187 plus DMSO (dimethyl sulfoxide), and with DMSO alone.
Following the treatment periods, rings were fixed for light,
scanning, and transmission electron microscopy to study morphology. Other rings from the same petri dishes were rapidly
quench-frozen, and 4-μm frozen sections were cut and freeze-
dried for X-ray microanalysis measurements. Also, immunofluorescent studies were performed on the hamster outgrowth
epithelium to study cytoskeletal changes.

Consistent with the findings of other investigators, high
levels of A23187 (10^{-3} *M*) were lethal to epithelium of the
hamster trachea within a short period of time (2-4 h), whereas
lower concentrations resulted in changes in the ER, Golgi (G),
mitochondria, lysosomes, and cellular secretory products
(Saladino *et al.,* 1982). The one ultrastructural feature that
predominated at all concentrations studied (10^{-4} to 10^{-7} *M*)
was fluid distension of the ER cisternae and G saccules (Fig.
2). This response appeared to occur first and was most pronounced in the deep cells of the tracheal mucosa. Ultimately,
all cells, including ciliated and mucus cells, showed ER-G
fluid distension. Hamster TBE incubated with low doses of
A23187 for periods of 24 to 48 h underwent characteristic
changes as seen by light and electron microscopy. These
changes involved cell size and shape, lateral membranes, and
smooth ER. The cytoplasm was markedly expanded by smooth
membrane-enclosed vesicles evenly distributed throughout the
cells, giving the appearance of marked hydropic alterations.

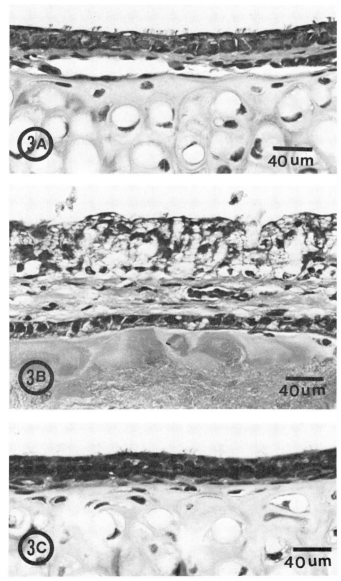

Fig. 3. (A) Light micrograph (LM) of control HTBE after
24 h in culture in standard OCM containing 5% bovine calf serum,
illustrating columnar epithelium with mucous and ciliated cells.
(B) LM of HTBE following 24 h exposure to 10^{-5} M A23187 in OCM
containing serum, illustrating enlarged and markedly vacuolated
columnar epithelium with loss of orientation and loss of cilia.
(C) LM of HTBE following 24 h exposure to 10^{-5} M A23187 in OCM
without serum. Note similarity to control HTBE in (A).

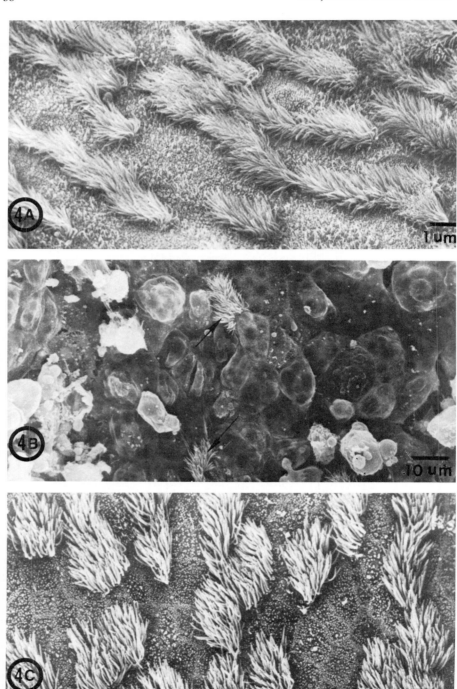

By several days and up to 1 week, epidermoid metaplasia with atypia was commonly seen.

At 10^{-5} M A23187, changes occurred rapidly and resulted in desquamation and denuding of the entire epithelial layer (Fig. 3). In this situation, the largest accumulations of fluid were seen at the basal portions of the columnar cells. These changes were enhanced in the presence of serum in the tissue culture medium (Fig. 4).

All concentrations resulted in variable changes related to other organelles, including nuclear chromatin alterations and mitochondrial swelling at high concentrations. These included increased numbers of lysosomes, discharge of mucus droplets, and condensation of mitochondrial matrices, with distension of some cristae at lower concentrations. Although a proliferative response appeared to occur at lower doses, it was not possible to determine whether this was directly related to stimulation of intracellular mechanics by Ca or simply secondary to cell injury and ensuing increased cell turnover.

In addition to morphological observations, hamster outgrowth epithelial cells were treated in the same manner to study cytoskeletal changes. These data are summarized in the following section.

Although our data are preliminary, changes observed in human trachea maintained in organ culture were identical to those seen in hamster trachea; however, the times of appearance

Fig. 4. (A) Scanning electron micrograph (SEM) of control HTBE after 24 h in culture in standard OCM with serum, illustrating ciliated cells with long microvilli and flattened mucous cells with short microvilli. (B) SEM of HTBE following 24 h exposure to 10^{-4} M A23187 in OCM containing serum. Note that the majority of the cell surface contains flattened desquamating cells. Only occasional ciliated cells with microvilli are present (arrow). (C) SEM of HTBE following 24 h exposure to 10^{-4} M A23187 in OCM without serum. Although some alterations exist, note the similarity to the control HTBE shown in (A).

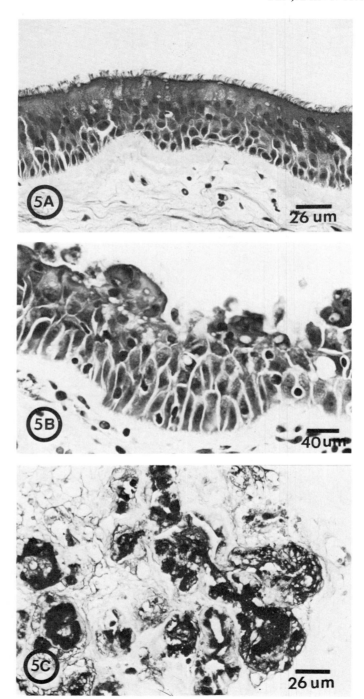

of responses were slightly different (Fig. 5). At 10^{-4} M, hydropic changes were noted at 24 h but not at 12 h. At 10^{-5} M, these changes were noted at 4 days but not at 2 days.

A23187 has provided some interesting findings in other tissues maintained *in vitro* that may pertain to the findings reported in our studies. For instance, at 19 μM, cultured rat hepatocytes are lethally injured within 1 h (Schanne et al., 1979). At 1 μM, over periods of 90 min to 4 h, this ionophore stimulated fluid secretion in isolated fly salivary glands (Prince et al., 1973), stimulated net chloride secretion in isolated dog tracheal mucosa (Al-Bazzaz and Jayaran, 1981), and inhibited baseline and hormone-dependent Na transport in toad bladder (Wiesmann et al., 1977). Interestingly, similar concentrations over periods of 24 to 72 h caused blast transformation and widespread mitoses among human peripheral lymphocytes (Jansen and Rasmussen, 1977; Luckasen et al., 1974) and 3T3 fibroblasts in tissue culture (Andersson and Norrby, 1977). These alterations were all shown to be Ca dependent.

The proliferative changes that are suggested in our studies need further evaluation. The hydropic changes involving the ER-G may relate to the movement of fluid as observed in the fly salivary gland. They may also relate to the survival of mucosal transport of chloride, as observed in the dog trachea. In this organ, it has been proposed that this may be the underlying mechanism for water flow to the luminal mucus

Fig. 5. (A) LM of human bronchus explant in culture in standard OCM with serum following 24 h exposure to 10% DMSO, illustrating pseudostratified tall columnar bronchial epithelium with ciliated and mucous cells. (B) LM of human bronchus explant in culture in standard OCM following 24 h exposure to 10^{-5} M A23187, illustrating desquamation, vacuolization, loss of cilia, and cytoplasmic blebbing (arrow). (C) LM of human bronchus explant in culture in standard OCM following 24 h exposure to 10^{-4} M A23187, illustrating completely degenerated epithelium with loss of orientation, marked vacuolization, and cell lysis.

carpet to enhance its fluidity and undersectional motion. The
Ca sequestration by the ER may also play a role in this phenomenon. The secretion of mucus droplets is quite similar to
that observed for pancreas, anterior pituitary, adrenal, and
mast cells.

2. *Amphotericin B*

To examine the hypothesis that an important early stimulus
for proliferation is Na influx, we also studied the effects of
amphotericin B (12 µg/ml) on hamster TBE *in vitro* (Trump *et al.*,
1982b). Amphotericin is a polyene antibiotic that reacts with
cholesterol in cell membranes and permits rapid redistribution
of cations. In normal extracellular fluid, this involves Na
and Cl influx, water influx, and K efflux. The great sensitivity of the ciliated cell to amphotericin is of interest. The
TBE secretes Cl^-, and some evidence suggests that this is a
function of the ciliated cell (Frizzell *et al.*, 1981).

In hamster TBE, we found that exposure to amphotericin B
was associated with rapid swelling of the ciliated cells, but
not mucous and basal cells, within 2 h (Fig. 6). In addition,
marked swelling of the cytosol occurred with dilated ER, condensation of mitochondria, and clumping of nuclear chromatin.
At later time intervals, the epithelium became metaplastic and
was several layers thick.

X-Ray microanalysis of treated explants revealed significant increases in Na, Cl, and Ca, and a decrease in K as compared to controls (Fig. 7). Examination of outgrowth epithelium, treated in a similar manner, revealed striking changes in
the cytoskeleton (see following section).

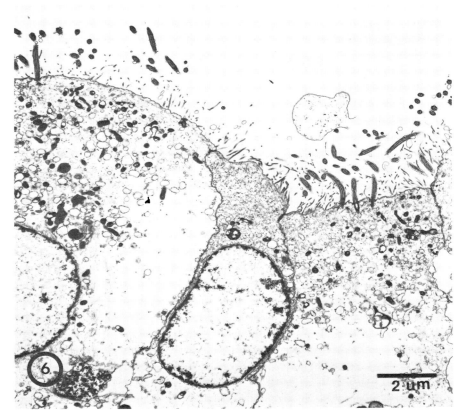

Fig. 6.   TEM of HTBE in culture following 2 h exposure to amphotericin B (12 µg/ml).   Note the marked swelling of the cytosol and the ER.   Mitochondria are condensed.   The nuclei show chromatin margination, and large blebs occur at the apical surfaces.   Note that the basal and mucous cells are not swollen.

C.   Neoplasia

Some years ago, Cone (1971) proposed that intracellular concentrations of Na should be greater in transformed cells than in normal cells.   Several groups of investigators have since then utilized X-ray microanalysis of frozen-dried tissues to begin examining this hypothesis.   This technique has the pronounced advantage of measuring intracellular elemental con-

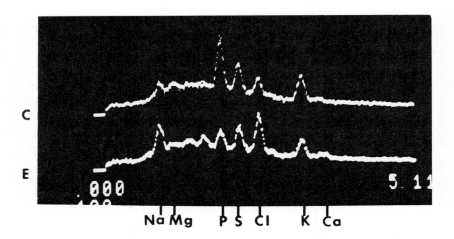

Fig. 7. Typical spectra obtained from X-ray microanalysis measurements over 4-μm freeze-dried cryosections of HTBE
in culture. C, Control; E, 2 h exposure to amphotericin B.
Note the increases in Na, Cl, and Ca, and the decrease in K
in the treated explants.

centrations for individual cells or even organelles, in contrast to other methods such as flame photometry or atomic absorption spectroscopy that by necessity look at average values
in tissues even if extracellular values can be estimated. The
latter, in itself, is a difficult problem.

X-Ray microanalysis measurements of Na in mouse mammary
tumor cells, H6 hepatoma in the mouse (Smith *et al.*, 1978),
Morris hepatoma in the rat, genitourinary tumors in humans
(Zs.-Nagy *et al.*, 1981), safrole-induced hepatic carcinomas
in the mouse (Trump *et al.*, 1979a), and mammary carcinomas including C3H in the mouse and 13762 NF in the rat (Cameron *et
al.*, 1980), neoplastic versus preneoplastic lesions in mice
(Smith *et al.*, 1981), have revealed increased concentrations
of Na. In our studies and in those of Cameron's group, the
possibility was carefully considered that acute injury by carcinogens or slightly ischemic areas in the neoplasms might in-

fluence these results (see earlier discussion on effects of
acute cell injury on ion concentrations) but concluded that
the results could not be thus explained. There was an interesting and unexplained increase in K in H6 and 777 hepatomas
studied by Cameron's group (Smith *et al.*, 1978) in contrast to
their studies on two mammary adenocarcinomas and our study on
safrole-induced mouse neoplasms.

In all of these studies, it is also necessary to consider
the possibility that increased electrolyte content might relate to increased water concentration with dissolved solutes
and might not reflect the true concentration range expressed
in mM/liter. Cameron has reviewed this problem, and if such
were the case, then it might be anticipated that each electrolyte would increase on an equimolar basis; however, such does
not appear to be the case (see earlier).

Both morphologic and chemical observations have suggested
that the water content of neoplastic cells is greater than
that of the normal counterparts (see review by Cone, 1974).
The same may well pertain to embryonic cells, at least from
the morphological standpoint. The application of nuclear mag-
netic resonance (NMR) techniques has yielded additional data
on this point. Damadian (1971) has noted that NMR relaxation
times of water protons in both Novikoff hepatoma and Walker
sarcoma were higher than their normal tissues of origin.
Beall *et al.* (1981) extended these findings to mammary tissues
and noted that neoplastic mammary cells had approximately
doubled relaxation times of water protons as compared to normal
or preneoplastic counterparts. Of course, the problem with
such studies is that the data are averaged over many cells.
However, utilizing these data in conjunction with the differential changes seen by X-ray microanalysis, it can be concluded
that changes in water per se do not explain these differences.

V.   CYTOSKELETAL CHANGES IN PRENEOPLASTIC AND NEOPLASTIC CELLS

In many pathological conditions (including neoplasia and
malignancy as well as cell transformation and other altered
physiological states), changes in the number, distribution,
arrangement, chemistry, and interrelationships of the cytoskeletal filament components have been reported. These changes
have been seen in a wide variety of tissues and cells by many
investigators using morphological, immunofluorescent, and immunohistochemical procedures at both the light and electron
microscopic level. Some of these findings for the various cytoskeletal filaments are reviewed here.

A.   Microtubules

Changes in the cellular pattern or distribution of microtubules and differences in numbers of microtubules or in total
tubulin content have been reported in studies of transformed
cells. Puck and co-workers experimented with dibutyryl-cAMP
on cultured hamster ovary cells and found that transformed
cells reverted to flattened, normal-appearing cells (Hsie *et
al.*, 1971; Puck *et al.*, 1972). They noted also that the effect of cAMP could be prevented by colcemid or cytochalasin B,
which led them to postulate that a microtubule-microfilament
system might be involved in cell transformation (Puck, 1977).
Studies on rat kidney cells transformed by virus revealed a
decreased number of cytoplasmic microtubules (Fonte and Porter,
1974). Brinkley *et al.* (1975) presented data showing that certain transformed cell lines were smaller, more polygonal in
shape, and contained shorter and more randomly dispersed tubules than normal cells. Edelman and Yahara (1976) made similar observations. However, others have reported that the microtubule networks of some transformed cells are the same as those

in normal cells (Osborn and Weber, 1977; Tucker *et al.*, 1978; DeMay *et al.*, 1978). Rubin and Warren (1979) concluded that normal cells have twice the number of microtubules as transformed cells. However, both cell populations were assayed and found to contain the same amount of total tubulin (monomeric and polymeric). Asch *et al.* (1979), in studies of normal, preneoplastic, and neoplastic mouse mammary epithelial cells, noted no significant differences in the microtubule or actin networks in the neoplastic cells.

Human breast carcinoma and normal cell lines were examined for cytoskeletal patterns by Brinkley *et al.* (1980). Three distinct carcinoma cell types were identified, and a definite relationship was noted between cell shape and cytoskeletal arrangement. However, it was concluded that no specific filament pattern or cell shape was characteristic of the malignant mammary cells. In our immunofluorescent studies on microtubules in primary outgrowth cells from normal and malignant human bronchial epithelium, we observed tubule pattern changes (Trump *et al.*, 1981d). In normal cells, the microtubules generally extended in relatively straight paths from the region of the nucleus toward the cell periphery (Fig. 8A). In contrast, the microtubules in the tumor cells extended in a more disorganized fashion and displayed a meshlike crisscrossing pattern (Fig. 8B). Also, the tumor cells appeared to have fewer microtubules than the normal cells. Another study from our laboratory on outgrowth cells from malignant human prostate epithelium revealed marked cell shape changes and microtubule patterns similar to those seen in human bronchus tumor cells (Trump *et al.*, 1981c) (Fig. 8C and D).

In vitro work on cells using agents known to cause microtubule depolymerization, such as cold and antimitotic drugs, commonly result in the formation of membrane blebs or buds that are often seen to detach from the cell surface. This type

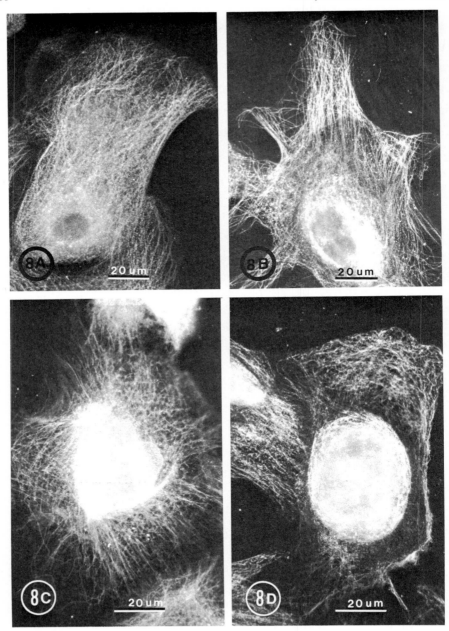

Fig. 8. Outgrowth cells from human lung explants stained
by indirect immunofluorescence with tubulin antibodies.
(A) Normal cell with straight microtubules radiating from the
nuclear region.   (B) Tumor cell with disorganized microtubules
displaying areas of crisscross patterns.   (C and D) Outgrowth

of surface change might correlate with changes demonstrated
in vivo in animal experiments. After cutting off the blood
supply in the rat kidney, large blebs appear at the luminal
surface of the proximal tubules that detach and ultimately oc-
clude the nephron and cause acute renal failure (Glaumann *et
al.*, 1977). The villus configurations and dome-shaped cell
changes seen in neoplastic cells of the prostate may also
represent bleblike formations resulting from microtubule depolymerization (Trump *et al.*, 1981c).

B. Microfilaments

Changes in microfilament density and arrangement in some
neoplastic cells under various conditions have been reported.
McNutt (1976), in an electron microscope study of invasive
basal cell carcinomas of the skin, observed an increase in
actin-like filaments at the advancing margin of tumors and a
decrease in hemidesmosomes. Gabbiani *et al.* (1976) described
increased numbers of contractile filaments in immunofluorescent
studies of frozen sections of carcinomas of the human skin,
oral cavity, and mammary gland. Later, Gabbiani and co-workers
showed that the changes in stainable actin in neoplastic and
regenerating cells represented polymerization changes rather
than total protein changes (G. Gabbiani, unpublished). An increase in the number of cytoplasmic microfilaments has also
been seen by immunofluorescence in experimental malignant tumors (Malech and Lentz, 1974), in hepatocytes during liver regeneration (Gabbiani and Ryan, 1974), and in aortic epithelial
cells during production of ·hypertension (Gabbiani *et al.*,
1975).

(Fig. 8 continued) cells from adenocarcinoma of human prostate
stained by indirect immunofluorescence with tubulin antibodies
illustrating different microtubule meshwork patterns.

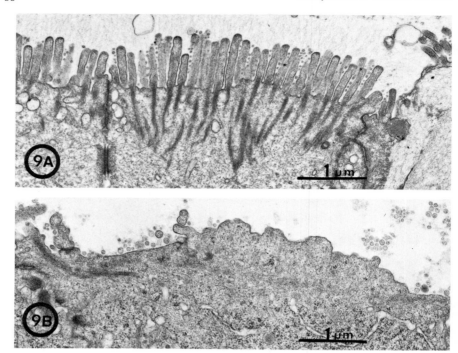

Fig. 9. (A) TEM of normal human colon cells at the terminal web region, illustrating relatively regular pattern of
dense-core microfilament elements extending from the microvilli
into the web. (B) TEM of the apex of adenocarcinoma cells exhibiting a disorganized web and the loss of microfilament
"rootlet" patterns.

In some studies on transformed cells, only minor differences have been noted. Pollack *et al.* (1975) observed minimal
numbers of actin cables in virus-transformed cells. Asch *et
al.* (1979) noted no actin changes in primary cultures of mouse
mammary tumors but did note a reduction in actin cables in one
of three clonal tumor cell lines.

Sufficient evidence has accumulated to suggest that there
is a correlation between changes in cell morphology and the
plasma membrane, and changes in the cytoskeletal complex. One
such example are the changes present in surgically removed tis-

sues from normal, premalignant, and malignant human colon as
studied by transmission and scanning electron microscopy
(Trump *et al.*, 1979d; Phelps *et al.*, 1979).   In adenomas and
tumors, there is an absence of the long, regular microvillae
seen normally.   They are replaced by scanty, short microvillae
or by pebbly and/or smooth surfaces.   The changes are most obvious between normal and tumor cells, with the latter being
highly irregular in size and shape and showing a haphazard
orientation.   Definite filament changes are noted in the apical terminal web region.   When comparing the normal cell (Fig.
9A) with the tumor cell (Fig. 9B), it is apparent that in the
tumor cell the normal uniform pattern of dense-core microfilament elements extending from the interior of microvillae into
the terminal web is missing.   Only intermittent bands of filament densities are seen just beneath the plasma membrane in
smooth-surfaced areas, whereas oblique-angled bands may be
present in regions displaying short or stubby microvillae.   The
most striking changes in the web area are the loss of a uniform
microfilament pattern, an increase in the number of junctional
complexes, and an increase in the number of tonofilament ag-
gregations.   Although specific changes are observed in tumor
cells, their significance regarding tumorigenicity is still
speculative.

C.   Intermediate Filaments

      Keratin filaments are classically found in great abundance
in the stratified squamous epithelium; however, they are also
found scattered throughout cells of other epithelia.   A number
of reports have presented evidence for significant changes in
the number of these filaments in neoplastic and malignant epithelia of internal organs.

Keratin filaments have been found in increased numbers in squamous cell carcinomas (Inoue and Dionne, 1977). Schlegal *et al.* (1980) have obtained positive staining for keratin by immunoperoxidase techniques in squamous cell carcinomas as well as in transitional cell tumors, but negative or minimal staining in mammary adenocarcinomas, undifferentiated lung carcinomas, and adenocarcinomas of the colon, kidney and prostate. The squamous metaplasia in prostate epithelium that results from the response to estrogen therapy is associated with abundant keratin filaments. McNutt (1976) found a decrease in hemidesmosomes in invasive basal cell carcinomas. In adenocarcinoma of human prostate, altered cell junctions and junctional-cytoskeletal relationships have also been observed (Trump *et al.*, 1981c).

In foci of epidermoid metaplasia found in many human pulmonary tumors, there is an increase in keratin filaments. Keratin proteins are conspicuously well developed in epidermoid carcinomas. In the many pulmonary tumors that show features of combined epidermoid and adenocarcinomas, tonofilament bundles and keratin proteins are also readily identified (McDowell *et al.*, 1978; Wilson *et al.*, 1981). The normal hamster trachea has little demonstrable keratin; however, during metaplasia elicited at the time of regenerative response following *in vivo* wounding, abundant keratin is demonstrated (Keenan, 1982).

As already noted, much evidence has accumulated regarding the effect of Ca on microtubule polymerization. In addition, Ca has also been shown to affect two gel-sol actin regulators such as villin (Craig and Powell, 1980) and gelsolin (Yin and Stossel, 1979). Low amounts of intracellular keratin in cultured human bronchus epithelia have also been correlated with low Ca medium concentrations and high keratin with high Ca concentrations.

As discussed already, in order to study the effects of altered ion regulation and the rapid membrane and cytoskeletal
changes that ensue, we performed a series of experiments in
which hamster TBE was exposed to the Ca ionophore A23187, and
the Na ionophore amphotericin B (Saladino *et al.*, 1982; Trump
et al., 1982b). The morphological and X-ray microanalysis observations have been discussed already.

Indirect immunofluorescence staining for actin of TBE exposed to A23187 (10^{-5} M) for 48 h revealed several pattern
changes from those seen in the normal (Fig. 10A), namely a compact, irregular net arrangement (Fig. 10B) and a loose circular
swirling arrangement of filaments around nuclei. Staining for
microtubules in these cells revealed scanty disintegrating tubules. After 2 h treatment with amphotericin B (12 µg/ml),
staining for actin showed fiber and fiber bundles with indistinct borders, suggesting that dissolution may have occurred
(Fig. 10C). Staining for tubulin revealed microtubules that
were no longer taut as in the normal (Fig. 11A) but were disorganized and "relaxed" in appearance (Fig. 11B). The changes
noted were attributed to the increased cellular Ca resulting
from treatment with the Na and Ca ionophores.

D.   Calmodulin

Nishida *et al.* (1979) reported that calmodulin caused an
inhibitory effect on microtubule assembly in the presence of
high (3 mM) ionic Ca. There is strong evidence that calmodulin
influences microtubule polymerization in a Ca concentration-
dependent manner (Schliwa *et al.*, 1981). Chafouleas *et al.*
(1981) have demonstrated that certain transformed mammalian
cells have twice the normal amount of intracellular calmodulin.
This apparently results from its increased synthesis relative
to its rate of degradation. Tubulin levels are unchanged, but

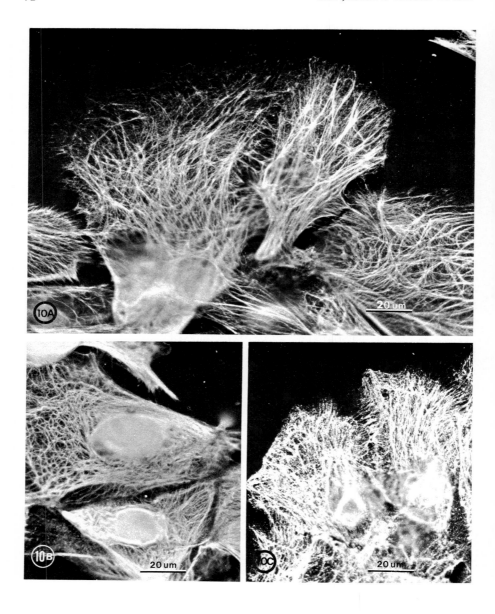

Fig. 10.   Indirect immunofluorescence staining for actin
on outgrowth cells from HTBE.   (A) Normal cell showing a complex
interwoven arrangement of actin cables and filaments.   (B) Cell
after 48 h exposure to 10^{-5} *M* A23187 showing a compact irregular

there is an increased calmodulin:tubulin ratio. Increased calmodulin may affect Ca-dependent microtubule polymerization and could possibly explain the differences seen by some investigators in microtubules in neoplastic and malignant cells. Criss and Kakiuchi (1982) observed a positive correlation between calmodulin content and hepatoma growth rates.

There is growing evidence that certain consistent cytoskeletal changes are seen in transformed cells and in pathological, neoplastic, and malignant tissues. These changes may well prove to be useful and valuable markers for distinguishing between normal, regenerative, premalignant, and malignant cells and epithelia.

VI. HYPOTHESIS AND SUMMARY

Figure 12 summarizes our hypothesis concerning the relationship between ion regulation, cell division, and tumor promotion. The diagram focuses on the relationship between Na, protons, and Ca. A variety of physiological and pathological stimuli are associated with transient or persistent elevations in intracellular Na that result in membrane depolarization. These include (1) conditions associated with inhibition of the (Na^+, K^+)-ATPase either specifically (e.g., with cardiac glycosides) or through energy deficiency and (2) conditions that increase Na entry either by specific interaction with receptors and/or Na entry channels, or nonspecifically by damaging the lipid and/or protein components of the membrane, for example membrane lipid peroxidation. Na entry blockers, such as amiloride, can retard Na entry presumably in either case.

(Fig. 10 continued) net arrangement. (C) Actin pattern in a cell following 2 h exposure to amphotericin B (12 µg/ml). Fibers exhibit indistinct "defective" borders.

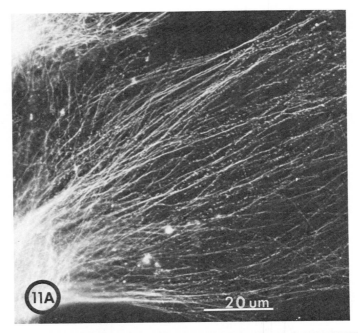

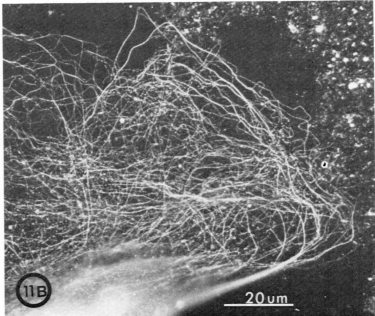

Fig. 11.   Indirect immunofluorescence staining for tubulin on HTBE outgrowth cells.   (A) Normal cell showing straight,

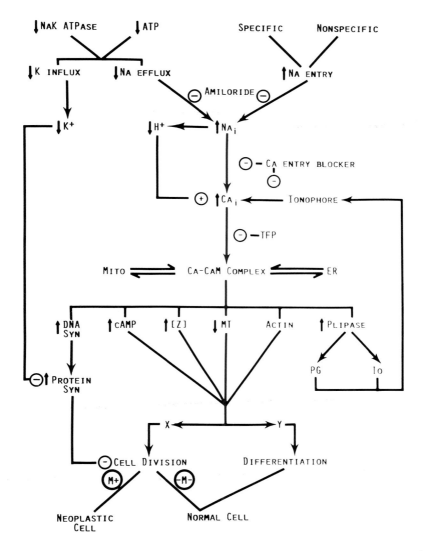

Fig. 12. Flowchart summarizing our hypothesis concerning the relationship between ion regulation, cell division, and tumor promotion. (See text for discussion and abbreviations used.)

(Fig. 11 continued) centrally radiating microtubules. (B) An example of the disorganized and "relaxed" microtubular pattern seen in cells after 2 h exposure to amphotericin B (12 μg/ml).

As mentioned in the text, a large number of conditions or substances associated with growth stimulation are associated with increased Na entry. Because of the importance of Na-Ca exchange in regulating Ca, increased Na concentration is followed by increased Ca concentration. Increased Na concentration is often associated with exchange for protons, simultaneously diminishing pH, which tends to sensitize regulatory mechanisms to increased levels of Ca. Ca entry can also be blocked with a number of compounds that specifically block Ca entry, such as Verapamil. The entry of Na can be bypassed by addition of Ca ionophores such as A23187 that directly permit entry of Ca across the cell membrane.

The increased Ca concentration interacts with calmodulin to activate a number of phenomena. Increased Ca-calmodulin (Ca-CaM) can be buffered by both mitochondria and ER, which have active sequestration systems that permit them to accumulate Ca in the presence of energy. In the presence of inhibitors of energy metabolism that decrease cellular ATP, these systems do not function and thus the situation appears to be accentuated. All the Ca-calmodulin-mediated actions can be potentially antagonized by inhibitors such as trifluoperazine (TFP). Ca-calmodulin complexes can activate a number of systems including cyclic nucleotide metabolism (e.g., cAMP), stimulate DNA synthesis, depolymerize microtubules (MT), modulate the interactions of actin, and activate phospholipase (Plipase).

These actions, as presently understood, are incomplete, and it must be inferred that other metabolites or substances (e.g., those labeled Z in the diagram) are also formed. The effects of such regulatory molecules appear to be highly dependent on cell type. In some cell types, the result is cell division, perhaps through other regulators (X), which in normal regeneration restores the normal cell; however, in initiated cells it may lead to preneoplastic and neoplastic stages. In some cells, other substances (labeled Y) apparently promote differentiation. Such is the case in skin and bronchial epithelium grown in Ca-containing serum containing media or in HL-60 cells. Note that K is permissive for increased protein synthesis and that K deficiency, which is caused by some agents that increase Na, may inhibit the process even in the presence of the other signals. Note also that activation of phospholipase leads to a variety of intermediates including the prostanoids (PG), some of which are also capable of forming Ca ionophores (Io), thus perpetuating the process. Prostaglandins themselves are putative promoters, and antiprostaglandins such as indomethacin may be antipromoters.

Furthermore, in many systems, both X and Y pathways may proceed simultaneously. For example, in phorbol ester treatment of the skin, there is both increased terminal differentiation to form keratinization and cell division. Neoplastic cells appear to differ from normal cells in their Ca requirements, and thus increased formation of the X metabolite may occur; in the case of noninitiated cells, this may lead to increased terminal differentiation and an increased population of that type, whereas in the case of initiated cells it leads to neoplasia. Therefore, it is evident that there is great interdependency of numerous cellular factors that ultimately determine the fate of a cell.

REFERENCES

Al-Bazzaz, F., and Jayaram, T. (1981). *Exp. Lung Res. 2,* 121-130.
Albertini, D. F., and Anderson, E. (1977). *J. Cell Biol. 73,* 111-127.
Andersson, R. G. G., and Norrby, K. (1977). *Virchows Arch. B* *23,* 185-194.

Asch, B. B., Medina, D., and Brinkley, B. R. (1979). *Cancer Res. 39,* 893-907.

Beall, P. T., Asch, B. B., Medina, D., and Hazlewood, C. (1981). *In* "The Transformed Cell" (I. L. Cameron and T. B. Pool, eds.), pp. 294-326. Academic Press, New York.

Berlin, R. D., Caron, J. M., and Oliver, J. M. (1979). *In* "Microtubules" (K. Roberts and J. S. Hyams, eds.), pp. 443-485. Academic Press, New York.

Blaustein, M. P. (1974). *Rev. Physiol. Biochem. Pharmacol. 70,* 33-82.

Blose, S. H. (1979). *Proc. Natl. Acad. Sci. USA 76,* 3372-3376.

Boynton, A. L., Whitfield, J. F., Isaacs, R. J., and Tremblay, R. G. (1977). *Cancer Res. 37,* 2657-2661.

Brinkley, B. R., Fuller, G. M., and Highfield, D. P. (1975). *Proc. Natl. Acad. Sci. USA 72,* 4981-4985.

Brinkley, B. R., Fistel, S. H., Marcum, J. M., and Pardue, R. L. (1980). *Int. Rev. Cytol. 63,* 59-95.

Buckley, I. K. (1975). *Tissue & Cell 7,* 51-72.

Byers, H. R., and Porter, K. R. (1977). *J. Cell Biol. 75,* 541-558.

Cameron, I. L., and Smith, N. K. R. (1980). *Scanning Electron Microsc. 2,* 463-474.

Cameron, I. L., Smith, N. K. R., and Pool, T. B. (1979). *J. Cell Biol. 80,* 444-450.

Cameron, I. L., Smith, N. K. R., Pool, T. B., and Sparks, R. L. (1980). *Cancer Res. 40,* 1493-1500.

Carafoli, E. (1982). *In* "Pathophysiology of Shock, Anoxia and Ischemia" (R. A. Cowley and B. F. Trump, eds.), pp. 95-111. Williams & Wilkins, Baltimore, Maryland and London.

Chafouleas, J. G., Pardue, R. L., Brinkley, B. R., Dedman, J. R., and Means, A. R. (1981). *Proc. Natl. Acad. Sci. USA 78,* 996-1000.

Cheung, W. Y. (1970). *Biochem. Biophys. Res. Commun. 33,* 533-538.

Cheung, W. Y. (1980). *Science (Washington, D.C.) 207,* 19-27.

Cheung, W. Y. (1982a). *Fed. Proc. Fed. Am. Soc. Exp. Biol. 41,* 2253-2256.

Cheung, W. Y. (1982b). *Sci. Am. 246,* 62-70.

Cone, C. D., Jr. (1971). *J. Theor. Biol. 30,* 151-181.

Cone, C. D., Jr. (1974). *Ann. N.Y. Acad. Sci. 238,* 420-435.

Cone, C. D., Jr. (1980). *Ann. N.Y. Acad. Sci. 339,* 115-131.

Craig, S. W., and Powell, L. D. (1980). *Cell 22,* 739-749.

Criss, W. E., and Kakiuchi, S. (1982). *Fed. Proc. Fed. Am. Soc. Exp. Biol. 41,* 2289-2291.

Crossin, K. L., and Carney, D. H. (1981). *Cell 23,* 61-71.

Damadian, R. (1971). *Science (Washington, D.C.) 171,* 1151-1153.

Dedman, J. R., Potter, J. D., Jackson, R. L., Johnson, J. D., and Means, A. R. (1977). *J. Biol. Chem. 252,* 8415-8422.

Dedman, J. R., Welsh, M. J., and Means, A. R. (1978). *J. Biol. Chem.* 253, 7515-7521.

DeMay, J., Moeremans, M., Guens, G., Nuydens, R., and DeBrabander, M. (1981). *Cell Biol. Int. Rep.* 5, 889-899.

Dicker, P., and Rozengurt, E. (1981). *Biochem. Biophys. Res. Commun.* 100, 433-441.

Eagle, H. (1973). *J. Cell. Physiol.* 82, 1-8.

Edelman, G. M., and Yahara, I. (1976). *Proc. Natl. Acad. Sci. USA* 73, 2047-2051.

Epel, D. (1980). *Ann. N.Y. Acad. Sci.* 339, 74-85.

Fonte, V., and Porter, K. (1974). 8th International Congress on Electron Microscopy, Vol. II, *Aust. Acad. Sci.* 334-335.

Franke, W. W., Schmid, F. E., Freudenstein, C., Appelhans, B., Osborn, M., Weber, K., and Keenan, T. W. (1980). *J. Cell Biol.* 84, 633-654.

Frankel, F. R. (1976). *Proc. Natl. Acad. Sci. USA* 73, 2798-2802.

Frizzell, R. A., Welsh, M. J., and Smith, P. L. (1981). *Ann. N.Y. Acad. Sci.* 372, 558-569.

Gabbiani, G., and Ryan, G. B. (1974). *J. Submicrosc. Cytol.* 6, 143-157.

Gabbiani, G., Badonnel, M. C., and Rona, G. M. (1975). *Lab. Invest.* 32, 227-234.

Gabbiani, G., Csank-Brassert, J., Schneeberger, J. C., Kapanci, Y., Trenchev, P., and Holborrow, E. (1976). *Am. J. Pathol.* 83, 457-474.

Gallagher, R., Collins, S., Trohillo, J., McRedie, K., Ahearn, M., Tsai, S., Metzgar, R., Aulukh, G., Ting, S., Metzgar, R., Aulakh, G., Ting, R., Ruscetti, F., and Gallo, R. (1979). *Blood* 54, 713-733.

Gerson, D. F., and Burton, A. C. (1977). *J. Cell. Physiol.* 91, 297-303.

Gillies, R. J. (1981). *In* "The Transformed Cell" (I. L. Cameron and T. B. Pool, eds.), pp. 236-267. Academic Press, New York.

Glaumann, B., Glaumann, H., Berezesky, I. K., and Trump, B. F. (1977). *Virchows Arch. B* 24, 1-18.

Griffith, L., and Pollard, T. (1978). *Biophys. J.* 21, 23a.

Gruenstein, E., Rich, A., and Weihing, R. R. (1975). *J. Cell Biol.* 64, 223-234.

Gwynn, R. H., and Salamon, N. H. (1953). *Br. J. Cancer* 7, 482-488.

Harwell, O. D., Sweeney, M. L., and Kirkpatrick, F. H. (1980). *J. Biol. Chem.* 255, 1210-1220.

Hasegawa, T., Takahashi, S., Hayashi, H., and Hatano, S. (1980). *Biochemistry* 19, 2677-2683.

Hennings, H., Michael, D., Cheng, C., Steinert, P., Holbrook, K., and Yuspa, S. H. (1980). *Cell* 19, 245-254.

Herman, I. M., and Pollard, T. D. (1978). *Exp. Cell Res. 114,*
    15.
Hoffstein, S. T. (1980). *In* "The Cell Biology of Inflammation"
    (G. Weissmann, ed.), pp. 387-430. Elsevier-North Holland,
    Amsterdam.
Hsie, A. W., Jones, C., and Puck, T. T. (1971). *Proc. Natl.*
    Acad. Sci. USA 68, 1648-1652.
Inoue, S., and Dionne, G. P. (1977). *Am. J. Pathol. 88,* 345-
    354.
Isenberg, G., Aebi, U., and Pollard, T. D. (1980). *Nature*
    (London) 288, 455-459.
Jaffe, L. F. (1980). *Ann. N.Y. Acad. Sci. 339,* 86-101.
Jansen, P., and Rasmussen, H. (1977). *Biochim. Biophys. Acta*
    468, 146-156.
Jeter, J. R., Jr., Smith, M. K. R., and Wille, J. J. (1979).
    J. Cell Biol. 83, 8a.
Keenan, K. P. (1982). Ph.D. Thesis, Univ. of Maryland School
    of Medicine, Baltimore.
Kitagawa, T., and Andoh, T. (1978). *Exp. Cell Res. 115,* 37-46.
Lazarides, E. (1982). *Annu. Rev. Biochem. 51,* 219-250.
Lechner, J. F., Haugen, A., Autrup, H., McClendon, I., Trump,
    B. F., and Harris, C. (1981). *Cancer Res. 41,* 2294-2304.
Leffert, H. L., and Koch, K. S. (1980). *Ann. N.Y. Acad. Sci.*
    339, 201-215.
Lin, C. T., Dedman, J. R., Brinkley, B. R., and Means, A. R.
    (1980). *J. Cell Biol. 85,* 473-480.
Lubin, H. (1967). *Nature (London) 213,* 451.
Luby, K. J., and Porter, K. R. (1980). *Cell 21,* 13-23.
Luby-Phelps, K., and Porter, K. R. (1982). *Cell 29,* 441-450.
Luckasen, J. R., White, J. G., and Kersey, J. H. (1974). *Proc.*
    Natl. Acad. Sci. USA 71, 5088-5090.
MacLean-Fletcher, S., and Pollard, T. D. (1980). *Cell 20,*
    329-341.
Malech, H. L., and Lentz, T. L. (1974). *J. Cell Biol. 60,*
    473-482.
McBrien, D. C. H., and Slater, T. F. (1982). "Free Radicals,
    Lipid Peroxidation, and Cancer." Academic Press, New
    York and London.
McDowell, E. M., McLaughlin, T. S., Merenyi, D. K., Kieffer,
    R. F., Harris, C. C., and Trump, B. F. (1978). *J. Natl.*
    Cancer Inst. (US) 61, 587-606.
McGaughey, C., and Jensen, J. L. (1980). *Res. Commun. Chem.*
    Pathol. Pharmacol. 27, 277-292.
McNutt, N. S. (1976). *Lab. Invest. 35,* 132-142.
Means, A. R., and Dedman, J. R. (1980). *Nature (London) 285,*
    73-77.
Mikkelsen, R. B. (1978). *Prog. Exp. Tumor Res. 22,* 123-150.
Mooseker, M. S., and Tilney, L. G. (1975). *J. Cell Biol. 67,*
    725-743.

Murphy, D. B., and Borisy, G. G. (1975). *Proc. Natl. Acad. Sci. USA 72*, 2696-2700.

Nishida, E., Kumagai, H., Ohtsuki, I., and Sakai, H. (1979). *J. Biochem. (Tokyo) 85*, 1257-1266.

Oosawa, F., and Asakura, S. (1976). "Thermodynamics of the Polymerization of Protein." Academic Press, New York.

Osborn, M., and Weber, K. (1976). *Proc. Natl. Acad. Sci. USA 73*, 867-871.

Osborn, M., and Weber, K. (1977). *Cell 12*, 561-571.

Osborn, M., Franke, W., and Weber, K. (1980). *Exp. Cell Res. 125*, 37-46.

Penttila, A., and Trump, B. F. (1974). *Science (Washington, D.C.) 185*, 277-278.

Penttila, A., and Trump, B. F. (1975a). *Lab. Invest. 32*, 690-695.

Penttila, A., and Trump, B. F. (1975b). *Virchows Arch. B 18*, 1-16.

Penttila, A., and Trump, B. F. (1975c). *Virchows Arch. B 18*, 17-34.

Penttila, A., Glaumann, H., and Trump, B. F. (1976). *Life Sci. 18*, 1419-1430.

Phelps, P. C., Toker, C., and Trump, B. F. (1979). *Scanning Electron Microsc. 3*, 1-14.

Pitot, H. C., Goldsworthy, T., and Moran, S. (1981). *J. Supramol. Struct. Cell. Biochem. 17*, 133-146.

Pollack, R., Osborne, M., and Weber, K. (1975). *Proc. Natl. Acad. Sci. USA 72*, 994-998.

Pollard, T. D. (1981). *J. Biol. Chem. 256*, 7666-7670.

Pollard, T. D., and Korn, E. D. (1973). *J. Biol. Chem. 248*, 448-450.

Pollard, T. D., and Weihing, R. R. (1974). *CRC Crit. Rev. Biochem. 2*, 1-65.

Pool, T. B., Cameron, I. L., Smith, N. K. R., and Sparks, R. L. (1981). *In* "The Transformed Cell" (I. L. Cameron and T. B. Pool, eds.), pp. 398-420. Academic Press, New York.

Porter, K. R., and Tucker, J. B. (1981). *Sci. Am. 244*, 57-67.

Prince, W. T., Rasmussen, H., and Berridge, M. J. (1973). *Biochim. Biophys. Acta 329*, 98-107.

Puck, T. T. (1977). *Proc. Natl. Acad. Sci. USA 74*, 4491-4495.

Puck, T. T., Waldren, C. A., and Hsie, A. W. (1972). *Proc. Natl. Acad. Sci. USA 69*, 1943-1947.

Rasmussen, H. (1974). *Hosp. Pract. 9*, 99-107.

Rasmussen, H., and Goodman, D. B. (1977). *Physiol. Rev. 57*, 422-509.

Rozengurt, E., and Mendoza, S. (1980). *Ann. N.Y. Acad. Sci. 339*, 175-190.

Rubin, R. W., and Warren, R. H. (1979). *J. Cell Biol. 82*, 103-113.

Saladino, A. J., Berezesky, I. K., Resau, J., and Trump, B. F. (1982). *Fed. Proc. Fed. Am. Soc. Exp. Biol. 41,* 740.

Sanger, J. W., Sanger, J. M., and Gwinn, J. (1979). *In* "Actin and the Mitotic Spindle in Cell Function" (F. A. Pepe, J. W. Sanger, and V. Nachmias, eds.), pp. 313-323. Academic Press, New York.

Saunders, M. J., and Hepler, P. K. (1982). *Science (Washington, D.C.) 217,* 943-945.

Schanne, F. A. X., Kane, A. B., Young, E. E., and Farber, J. L. (1979). *Science (Washington, D.C.) 206,* 700-702.

Schlegel, R., Banks-Schlegel, S., McLeoud, J., and Pinkus, G. (1980). *Am. J. Pathol. 101,* 41-50.

Schliwa, M., Eutenever, U., Bulinski, J. C., and Izant, J. H. (1981). *Proc. Natl. Acad. Sci. USA 78,* 1037-1041.

Slaga, T. J., Fischer, S. M., Weeks, C. E., Klein-Szanto, A. J. P., and Reiners, J. (1982a). *In* "Mechanisms of Chemical Carcinogenesis" (C. C. Harris and P. A. Cerutti, eds.), pp. 207-227. Liss, New York.

Slaga, T. J., Fischer, S. M., Weeks, C. E., Klein-Szanto, A. J. P., and Reiners, J. (1982b). *J. Cell. Biochem. 18,* 99-119.

Sloboda, R. D. (1980). *Am. Sci. 68,* 290-298.

Sloboda, R. D., Rudolph, S. A., Rosenbaum, J. L., and Greengard, P. (1975). *Proc. Natl. Acad. Sci. USA 72,* 177-181.

Smith, N. R., Sparks, R. L., Pool, T. B., and Cameron, I. L. (1978). *Cancer Res. 38,* 1952-1959.

Smith, N. K. R., Stabler, S. B., Cameron, I. L., and Medina, D. (1981). *Cancer Res. 41,* 3877-3880.

Spiegelman, B. M., Lopata, M. A., and Kirschner, M. W. (1979). *Cell 16,* 253-263.

Stossel, T. P., and Hartwig, J. H. (1976). *J. Cell Biol. 68,* 602-619.

Sun, T.-T., and Green, H. (1978). *Cell 14,* 469-476.

Sun, T.-T., Shih, C., and Green, H. (1979). *Proc. Natl. Acad. Sci. USA 76,* 2813-2817.

Swierenga, S. H. H., Whitfield, J. F., Boynton, A. L., McManus, J. P., Raxon, R. H., Sikorska, M., Tsang, B. K., and Walker, P. R. (1980). *Ann. N.Y. Acad. Sci. 349,* 294-311.

Taylor, A., and Windhager, E. E. (1979). *Am. J. Physiol. 236,* F505-F512.

Trump, B. F., Croker, B. P., Jr., and Mergner, W. J. (1971). *In* "Cell Membranes: Biological and Pathological Aspects" (G. W. Richter and D. G. Scarpelli, eds.), pp. 84-128. Williams & Wilkins, Baltimore.

Trump, B. F., Berezesky, I. K., Pendergrass, R. E., Chang, S. H., Bulger, R. E., and Mergner, W. J. (1978). *Scanning Electron Microsc. 2,* 1027-1039.

Trump, B. F., Berezesky, I. K., Chang, S. H., Pendergrass, R. E., and Mergner, W. J. (1979a). *Scanning Electron Microsc. 3,* 1-14.

Trump, B. F., Phelps, P. C., Shamsuddin, A. M., and Harris, C. C. (1979b). *Lab. Invest. 40,* 289.

Trump, B. F., Berezesky, I. K., Laiho, K. U., Osornia, A. R., Mergner, W. J., and Smith, M. W. (1980). *Scanning Electron Microsc. 2,* 437-462.

Trump, B. F., Berezesky, I. K., and Osornio-Vargas, A. R. (1981a). *In* "Cell Death" (I. D. Bowen and R. A. Lockshin, eds.), pp. 209-242. Chapman & Hall, London.

Trump, B. F., Berezesky, I. K., and Phelps, P. C. (1981b). *Scanning Electron Microsc. 2,* 435-545.

Trump, B. F., Heatfield, B. M., and Phelps, P. C. (1981c). *In* "The Prostatic Cell: Structure and Function, Part A: Morphologic, Secretory, and Biochemical Aspects" (G. P. Murphy, A. A. Sandberg, and J. P. Karr, eds.), pp. 25-53. Liss, New York.

Trump, B. F., Phelps, P. C., Brinkley, B. R., Resau, J. H., and Boone, L. B. (1981d). *J. Cell Biol. 91,* 332a.

Trump, B. F., Berezesky, I. K., and Cowley, R. A. (1982a). *In* "Pathophysiology of Shock, Anoxia and Ischemia" (R. A. Cowley and B. F. Trump, eds.), pp. 6-46. Williams & Wilkins, Baltimore.

Trump, B. F., Saladino, A. J., Berezesky, I. K., and Resau, J. H. (1982b). *Fed. Proc. Fed. Am. Soc. Exp. Biol. 41,* 491.

Tsien, R. Y., Pozzan, T., and Rink, T. J. (1982). *Nature (London) 295,* 68-71.

Tucker, R. W., Sanford, K. K., and Frankel, F. R. (1978). *Cell 13,* 629-642.

Tupper, J. T., Ryals, W. T., and Bodine, P. V. (1982). *J. Cell. Physiol. 110,* 29-34.

Weber, K., Bibring, T., and Osborn, M. (1975). *Exp. Cell Res. 95,* 111-120.

Weihing, R. R. (1979). *Methods Achiev. Exp. Pathol. 8,* 42-109.

Weinstein, I. B. (1981). *J. Supramol. Struct. Cell. Biochem. 17,* 99-120.

Weinstein, I. B. (1982). *In* "Mechanisms of Chemical Carcinogenesis" (C. C. Harris and P. A. Cerutti, eds.), pp. 107-128. Liss, New York.

Weissmann, G. (1980). *In* "Current Concepts" ( ), pp. 5-32. Upjohn, Kalamazoo, Michigan.

Welsh, M. J., Dedman, J. R., Brinkley, B. R., and Means, A. R. (1978). *Proc. Natl. Acad. Sci. USA 75,* 1867-1871.

Welsh, M. J., Dedman, J. R., Brinkley, B. R., and Means, A. R. (1979). *J. Cell Biol. 81,* 624-634.

Whitfield, J. F., Boynton, A. L., MacManus, J. P., Rixon, R. H., Sikorska, M., Tsang, B., and Walker, P. R. (1980). *Ann. N.Y. Acad. Sci. 339,* 216-240.

Wiesmann, W., Sinha, S., and Klahr, S. (1977). *J. Natl. Cancer Inst. (US) 59,* 418-425.

Wilson, T. S., McDowell, E. M., and Trump, B. F. (1981). *J. Cell Biol. 91,* 299a.

Wolosewick, J. J., and Porter, K. R. (1979). *J. Cell Biol. 82,*
    114-139.
Yin, H. L., and Stossel, T. P. (1979). *Nature (London) 281,*
    583-586.
Yuspa, S. H. (1982). *In* "Mechanisms of Chemical Carcinogene-
    sis" (C. C. Harris and P. A. Cerutti, eds.), pp. 169-181.
    Liss, New York.
Yuspa, S. H., Hennings, H., and Lichti, U. (1981). *J. Supramol.
    Struct. Cell Biochem. 17,* 245-257.
Zs.-Nagy, I., Lustyik, G., Sz.-Nagy, V., Zarandi, B., and
    Bertoni-Freddari, C. (1981). *J. Cell Biol. 90,* 769-777.

3

EXPRESSION OF KERATINS AND ENVELOPE PROTEINS IN NORMAL AND MALIGNANT HUMAN KERATINOCYTES AND MESOTHELIAL CELLS

James G. Rheinwald, Emily Germain, and Michael A. Beckett

Division of Cell Growth and Regulation
Dana-Farber Cancer Institute
Department of Physiology and Biophysics
Harvard Medical School
Boston, Massachusetts

I. INTRODUCTION

Neoplastic disease and carcinogenesis are frequently modeled in cell culture with the connective tissue fibroblast, using loss of ordered colony morphology, reduced serum requirement, and anchorage-independent growth as diagnostic and selective markers of malignant transformation. Studies of normal human epidermal keratinocytes, mesothelial cells, and squamous carcinoma cells have revealed great differences between fibroblasts and epithelial cells in the basic mechanisms that regulate their growth, both normally and after malignant transformation. We have analyzed 15 squamous cell carcinomas (SCCs) of the oral cavity and epidermis in culture and have found much phenotypic diversity, including a wide range of anchorage-independent growth ability among equally tumorigenic SCC lines. However, all SCCs can be readily distinguished from normal keratinizing epithelial cells and selected for in culture by a defect they possess in their terminal differentiation program leading to cornified envelope formation. This defect is associated with greatly reduced synthesis of the envelope precursor protein, involucrin. SCC cells also synthesize certain keratins that are not expressed by normal keratinocytes but are expressed by normal nonkeratinizing epithelial cell types, such as the mesothelial cell. Malignant transformation in the keratinocyte therefore appears to involve loss or diminution of keratinocyte-specific differentiated characteristics and expression of less specialized epithelial characters.

II.   GROWTH REGULATION AND DIFFERENTIATION IN CULTURED
      EPIDERMAL KERATINOCYTES

The epidermis is a stratified squamous epithelium that serves as a protective barrier to drying, abrasion, and infection. For clonal and long-term growth in culture, epidermal keratinocytes require a fibroblast feeder layer, hydrocortisone (HC), cholera toxin (which raises cAMP levels), a high adenine concentration, and epidermal growth factor (EGF) (Rheinwald and Green, 1975, 1977; Green, 1978; Peehl and Ham, 1980; Wu *et al.*, 1982; T. O'Connell and J. G. Rheinwald, unpublished). During exponential growth, some cells migrate laterally to expand the area of the colony, and some migrate upward and flatten out over the layer of dividing cells, remaining attached by desmosomes (stratification). The stratified cells no longer divide (Rheinwald and Green, 1975) but enlarge and covalently cross-link a large protein, involucrin, into a "cornified envelope" beneath the plasma membrane (Sun and Green, 1976; Rice and Green, 1979; Watt and Green, 1981). At the same time, they lose their selective membrane permeability function and die (Green, 1977).

EGF is a very important growth factor for keratinocytes (Rheinwald and Green, 1977). Rather than acting as a mitogen in the strictest sense of the word, EGF reduces the rate at which keratinocytes become committed to terminal differentiation. EGF not only aids the short-term growth of keratinocytes but also preserves their "stem" character, because their replicative life span is much longer in the presence of EGF (Rheinwald and Green, 1977). EGF does not have a similar effect on fibroblasts (Didinsky and Rheinwald, 1981) despite their high level of receptors and the demonstration that EGF can act as a mitogen for serum-starved fibroblasts (Carpenter and Cohen, 1979).

Irreversible commitment to differentiate followed by envelope formation can be triggered rapidly in normal epidermal keratinocytes by depriving them of anchorage. When cells growing in surface culture are suspended in semisolid medium for various lengths of time before being allowed to reattach to a suitable substratum, they irreversibly lose division potential with a $t_{1/2}$ of 3 to 5 h and develop cornified envelopes within several days thereafter (Rheinwald, 1979; Rheinwald and Beckett, 1980).

Cultured epidermal keratinocytes and oral epithelial cells synthesize a set of keratin proteins ("epidermal keratins") of

46, 50, 52, 56, and 58 kdaltons (Sun and Green, 1978; Fuchs
and Green, 1978). Some of these keratins plus a 67-kdalton and
a 56.5-kcalton keratin are synthesized by the epidermis *in vivo*.
If vitamin A is removed from the serum supplement of the culture
medium, epidermal keratinocytes synthesize the 67-kdalton keratin in culture, as well (Fuchs and Green, 1981).

III.   GROWTH REGULATION AND DIFFERENTIATION IN CULTURED
       MESOTHELIAL CELLS

    The mesothelium is a simple squamous epithelium that
covers the free surfaces, both visceral and parietal, of the
peritoneal, pericardial, and pleural cavities. In any of the
standard culture media plus fetal calf serum, mesothelial
cells grow very slowly and form a very flat, epithelioid
monolayer at saturation density, similar to their appearance
in vivo (Wu *et al*., 1982). The cells contain both keratin
and vimentin filaments in abundance, detectable by indirect
immunofluorescence (Connell and Rheinwald, 1983). When EGF
and hydrocortisone are added to the culture medium, mesothelial cells adopt a fibroblastoid morphology, divide
rapidly, lose their keratin, and overgrow to form dense multilayers of cells in parallel arrays, similar to the behavior of
connective tissue fibroblasts. At saturation density the cells
again begin to synthesize and accumulate keratin. When mesothelial cells that were growing rapidly in the presence of EGF
and hydrocortisone are deprived of EGF, they quickly flatten,
accumulate keratin, and stop dividing when they reach a single-
cell monolayer (Connell and Rheinwald, 1983).
    Two-dimensional gel analysis of the Triton-insoluble cyto-
skeletal proteins of cultured mesothelial cells reveals high
levels of vimentin and four other proteins (40, 44, 52, and 55

kdaltons) different in molecular size and/or charge from the epidermal keratins (Wu *et al.*, 1982). Immunoprecipitation tests and peptide mapping have shown that these proteins are keratins. Some or all of these mesothelial keratins are also expressed along with some or all of the epidermal keratins in cell type-specific patterns by simple and stratified, non-keratinizing epithelia in culture, including ovarian surface, mammary, bladder, esophageal, exocervical, and conjunctival epithelia (Wu *et al.*, 1982).

Mesothelial cells contain very low levels of involucrin--about 1% of the level found in keratinocytes (J. G. Rheinwald and R. H. Rice, unpublished). In contrast, fibroblasts contain no detectable involucrin (Rice and Green, 1979). Synthesis of involucrin may therefore be a character not only of cells that can undergo cornification, but of all epithelial cells. Cultured mesothelial cells never spontaneously cross-link their involucrin into cornified envelopes, but if a quiescent meso-thelial cell population is treated with a Ca^{2+} ionophore to activate the cross-linking enzyme transglutaminase (Rice and Green, 1979), about 5 to 10% of the cells form envelopes (J. G. Rheinwald, S. Rehwoldt, and M. A. Beckett, unpublished).

IV. SQUAMOUS CELL CARCINOMA IN THE CONTEXT OF NORMAL
    EPITHELIAL CELL BIOLOGY

Oral and epidermal squamous cell carcinomas (SCCs) can be cultured routinely from biopsies (Table I) and their growth and differentiation characteristics examined (Rheinwald and Beckett, 1980, 1981; Rheinwald, 1982). Comparison of 15 inde-pendent SCCs has yielded the following information about this tumor type: All are aneuploid, grow in culture as established lines, and form squamous cell carcinomas in an experimental

TABLE I.   Growth of Human SCCs in Primary Culture and as
           Established Lines

Fate in culture	Site of tumor		
	Epidermis	Oral cavity	Throat
Lost to contamination	4	1	5
No growth	1	3	8
"Normal" cells only	4	1	2
Abnormal cells, but senesce	1	0	2
Abnormal cells, grow as established line	2	10	3
Total cultured	12	15	20
Lines/uncontaminated cultures	2/8	10/14	3/15

[athymic (*nude*) mouse] host. With the exception of one line,
all remain unstratified during exponential growth in culture.
None requires EGF, HC, or cholera toxin for long-term or clonal
growth.   Their dependence on a fibroblast feeder layer varies
from complete independence to a requirement almost as stringent
as that exhibited by normal keratinocytes; most SCCs require
medium conditioned by 3T3 cells in order to grow optimally from
clonal plating densities.

Most SCCs are unable to form large, progressively growing
colonies in semisolid medium (Rheinwald and Beckett, 1981).
This appears to be the result of a residual tendency of SCC
cells to become committed to terminal differentiation when deprived of anchorage, even though this commitment and the consequent envelope formation occur at a much slower rate under
these conditions than they do in normal keratinocytes (Rheinwald and Beckett, 1980). In any event, anchorage-independent
growth is not an ideal selective or diagnostic marker for
malignant transformation in keratinocytes, because it excludes
many SCCs by its excessive stringency.

Most SCCs fail to form envelopes spontaneously during exponential growth in culture (Rheinwald and Beckett, 1980).

TABLE II.   Synthesis of Involucrin by Normal Human Epidermal
            Keratinocytes and SCCs in Culture[a]

Strain or line	Relative [35S]met or [3H]leu incorporation involucrin/total protein	Cells inducible to form envelopes (%)
Normal epidermal keratinocyte strain N	(100)	50
SCC-4	<0.15	≤0.2
SCC-4 *nu/nu* Tumor	6	--
SCC-13	1	12
SCC-15	2	22
SCC-9	(Detectable)	37
SCC-12B.2	0.7	4
SCC-12F.2	18	60

[a]*Near-confluent cultures growing as described in Rheinwald
and Beckett (1980) were labeled for 4-24 h with [3H]leucine or
[35S]methionine. Aqueous-soluble proteins were incubated with
an excess of anti-involucrin and the antigen-antibody complexes
precipitated with protein A-Sepharose. Total cell protein and
immunoprecipitated protein were separated by SDS-polyacrylamide
gel electrophoresis and labeled proteins revealed by autoradiography. Autoradiograms were scanned with a densitometer. The
area under the involucrin peak of the immunoprecipitated gel
lane was related to the total integrated area of the total cell
extract gel lane to determine the percentage of total protein
represented by involucrin. The percentage of involucrin in normal epidermal keratinocyte strain N protein was 0.7%. The table
shows levels relative to this in SCC cell lines.*

Quantitative immunoprecipitation experiments using a specific
antibody against involucrin (see Rice and Green, 1979) clearly
indicate that the level of involucrin synthesized by a cell
line is correlated with its ability to form a cornified envelope
(see also Watt and Green, 1981) and also suggest that involucrin
content and *in vitro* envelope inducibility are inversely proportional to tumorigenicity in the keratinocyte (Germain, 1981)
(Table II).   All SCC lines tested were found to synthesize less

than 1/50 the level of involucrin of normal keratinocytes during exponential growth in culture. This reduction appears to
be the result of a regulatory defect, because even a line that
synthesized no detectable involucrin in culture (SCC-4) synthesized detectable levels when growing as a tumor.

SCC-12 is an epidermal SCC line from which we identified
and isolated morphologically distinct subpopulations from
early-passage cultures. Two clones, SCC-12B.2 and SCC-12F.2,
were studied in detail (Germain, 1981). SCC-12B.2 had a long
survival half-life (16 h) in semisolid medium, a low degree of
cornified envelope inducibility during exponential growth (4%),
a low level of involucrin synthesis (0.7% of normal), and
formed progressively growing, well-differentiated tumors in
nude mice. SCC-12F.2 had a short survival half-life (4 h) in
semisolid medium, a high degree of envelope inducibility (60%),
a high level of involucrin synthesis (18% of normal), and did
not grow in *nude* mice. All other growth, differentiation, and
morphological characteristics of SCC-12F.2 fall within the same
range as all the other SCC lines. Comparison of the properties
of SCC-12F.2 with SCC-12B.2 and the other SCC lines leads us to
conclude that the reduction of involucrin synthesis and rate of
terminal differentiation is the limiting step for malignant
growth ability in the keratinocyte.

All SCCs in culture synthesize one or more of the mesothelial keratins at levels sufficiently high to be distinguishable from normal cultured keratinocytes by their gel patterns
(Wu *et al.*, 1982) (Table III). Examination of the keratins synthesized by keratinocytes cultured from biopsies of uninvolved
tissue near the primary lesions of three different patients with
oral or epidermal SCCs has identified no normal epithelial cell
from these tissues that synthesizes a keratin pattern identical
to that of any SCC line. All normal oral epithelial cell populations we have cultured synthesize no more than very low levels

TABLE III. Keratin Patterns of Normal and Malignant Keratinocytes in Culture

Cell line or strain	Mesothelial keratins				Epidermal keratins					
	40 kd	44 kd	52 kd	55 kd	46 kd	50 kd	52 kd	56 kd	58 kd	50 kd'
Normal epidermal keratinocyte	→±	→±	→±	→±	+++	+++	→±	+++	+++	→±
SCC-13		+	→±	→±	+++	+++	→±	+++	+++	
SCC-12	++	+	+	++	+++	+++	±	+++	+++	+−+
Normal oral epithelial cell	→±	→±	→±	→±	+++	+++	→±	+++	+++	
Normal ventral tongue (?)	+++	+	→±	++	+++	+++	+++	+++	+++	
SCC-25	±	±	+	±	++	+++	+−+	+++	+++	+−+
SCC-78		+	+		+++	+++		+++	+++	+−+
SCC-49		+	+		+++	+++		+++	+++	
SCC-9	+−+	+	+		+++	+++		+++	+++	
SCC-4		+	++	+±	+	+++		+++	+++	
SCC-15	+++	++	++		+++	+++	+−	+++	+++	
SCC-40		++	+++		+++	+++	++	+++	+++	+++
SCC-66		+	++		+++	+−	+++	+++	+++	

aSCC lines were derived as described in Rheinwald and Beckett (1981). SCC-12 and SCC-13 were cultured from SCCs of the epidermis. SCC-49 was cultured from an SCC of the tonsil. All other SCC lines were cultured from SCCs of the oral cavity. Normal cells were cultured as described in Wu et al. (1982). Cells were labeled with [35S]methionine, their keratins extracted and separated by two-dimensional gel electrophoresis, and detected by autoradiography. Keratins identified by molecular weight (e.g., 40 kd = 40 kdaltons) as described in Wu et al. (1982). 50 kd' is a keratin of similar sequence to, but more acidic than, the 50 kd epidermal keratin (see Wu et al., 1982). +++, High level; ++, moderate level ($\sim$1/3 as much as +++); +, low level ($\sim$1/10 as much as +++); ±, trace (≤1/50 as much as +++); blank, undetectable in normally loaded and exposed gels; →±, undetectable to trace amounts.

of the mesothelial keratins and the 52-kdalton epidermal keratin except for one fetal strain we have recently derived from
the underside of the tongue. This normal strain synthesizes
moderate to high levels of three of the mesothelial keratins
and the 52-kdalton epidermal keratin--a pattern that nevertheless is very different from that of any SCC. Most of the SCC
lines retain the normal tissue-specific, high-level expression
of the 46-, 50-, 56-, and 58-kdalton epidermal keratins, although three lines (SCC-4, SCC-40, and SCC-66) synthesize abnormal levels of one or more of the epidermal keratins (Wu *et
al.*, 1982). Electrophoretic analysis of the keratins synthesized by SCC-15 and SCC-66 while growing as tumors in *nude* mice
indicates that abnormal keratin expression is maintained *in
vivo* (Wu and Rheinwald, 1981; Y.-J. Wu and J. G. Rheinwald,
unpublished).

We have raised an antibody specific for the 40-kdalton
keratin (Wu and Rheinwald, 1981) and are currently determining
whether antibodies raised against other individual mesothelial
keratins are also specific enough to detect abnormal keratin
expression in single cultured cells and in tissue sections.
Such antibodies might prove to be useful immunohistopathologi-
cal reagents for the diagnosis of carcinoma in sectioned biopsies of the oral cavity and epidermis.

V.   CONCLUSIONS

Squamous cell carcinoma is very different from experimentally transformed fibroblasts with respect to characters relevant to detection *in vivo* and selective growth in culture.
These phenotypic differences between the transformed keratinocyte and transformed fibroblast suggest different genotypic alterations as well--a notion that is supported by the observation

that the SCC cell lines described here do not have DNA sequences that can transfect NIH 3T3 cells to a malignantly transformed state (Krontiris and Cooper, 1981; Shin *et al.*, 1981). Phenotypic alterations that consistently accompany keratinocyte transformation (as it occurs naturally in humans) are a reduced involucrin synthesis and rate of commitment to terminal envelope formation, and a change in the pattern of keratin synthesis. These alterations might result from a partial "dedifferentiation" from the very specialized function and stringent growth control of the normal keratinocyte to a state in which some characteristics of simpler epithelial cells, such as the mesothelial cell, become expressed.

REFERENCES

Carpenter, G., and Cohen, S. (1979). *Annu. Rev. Biochem. 48,* 193–216.
Connell, N. D., and Rheinwald, J. G. (1983). *Cell 34,* in press.
Didinsky, J. B., and Rheinwald, J. G. (1981). *J. Cell. Physiol. 109,* 171–179.
Fuchs, E., and Green, H. (1978). *Cell 15,* 887–897.
Fuchs, E., and Green, H. (1981). *Cell 25,* 617–625.
Germain, E. L. (1981). Honors Undergraduate Thesis, Harvard Univ., Cambridge, Massachusetts.
Green, H. (1977). *Cell 11,* 405–416.
Green, H. (1978). *Cell 15,* 801–811.
Krontiris, T. G., and Cooper, G. M. (1981). *Proc. Natl. Acad. Sci. USA 78,* 1181–1184.
Peehl, D., and Ham, R. (1980). *In Vitro 16,* 526–538.
Rheinwald, J. G. (1979). *Int. Rev. Cytol. (Suppl.) 10,* 25–33.
Rheinwald, J. G. (1982). *Natl. Cancer Inst. Monogr. 60,* 133–138.
Rheinwald, J. G., and Beckett, M. A. (1980). *Cell 22,* 629–632.
Rheinwald, J. G., and Beckett, M. A. (1981). *Cancer Res. 41,* 1657–1663.
Rheinwald, J. G., and Green, H. (1975). *Cell 6,* 331–344.
Rheinwald, J. G., and Green, H. (1977). *Nature (London) 265,* 421–424.
Rice, R. H., and Green, H. (1979). *Cell 18,* 681–694.

Shih, C., Padly, L. C., Murray, M., and Weinberg, R. A. (1981).
     Nature (London) 290, 261-264.
Sun, T.-T., and Green, H. (1976). *Cell 9,* 511-521.
Sun, T.-T., and Green, H. (1978). *J. Biol. Chem. 253,* 2053-
     2060.
Watt, F. M., and Green, H. (1981). *J. Cell Biol. 90,* 738-742.
Wu, Y.-Y., and Rheinwald, J. G. (1981). *Cell 25,* 627-635.
Wu, Y.-J., Parker, L. M., Binder, N. E., Beckett, M. A.,
     Sinard, J. G., Griffiths, C. T., and Rheinwald, J. G.
     (1982). *Cell 31,* 693-703.

4

DIFFERENTIATION AND THE CONTROL OF TUMORIGENICITY IN HUMAN CELL HYBRIDS

Eric J. Stanbridge, Barbara Fagg, and Channing J. Der

Department of Microbiology
College of Medicine
University of California
Irvine, California

I. INTRODUCTION

The technique of somatic cell hybridization (Harris and Watkins, 1965) has been extremely useful in studies of gene mapping (McKusick and Ruddle, 1977) and control of expression of differentiated functions (Davidson, 1974). The technique has also been applied to the study of the genetic analysis of

malignancy (Barski and Cornefert, 1962; Harris *et al.*, 1969;
Croce *et al.*, 1975a; Stanbridge, 1976; Sager and Kovac, 1978;
Kucherlapati and Shin, 1979), but until recently the interpretations of these analyses have been quite controversial. By
way of introduction to this controversy, a brief history is
presented.

Early investigators in this field (Barski and Cornefert,
1962; Scaletta and Ephrussi, 1965) isolated hybrid cells derived from the fusion of mouse cells of low malignant potential
with those of high malignant potential. The intraspecific
mouse cell hybrids derived from these fusions were as malignant
as the highly malignant parent, thereby leading to the interpretation that malignancy behaves as a dominant trait. Similar
conclusions were reached by others using polyoma-transformed
mouse cells as the malignant parent (Defendi *et al.*, 1967).
However, Harris, Klein, and their colleagues (Harris *et al.*,
1969; Harris, 1971; Wiener *et al.*, 1971, 1974), on the basis
of an extensive series of experiments, came to the opposite
conclusion. In their studies they showed that when highly
malignant mouse cells were fused with normal mouse embryo
cells or mouse cells of low malignant potential, the resulting
hybrids were transiently suppressed in their ability to form
tumors. Tumorigenic segregants appeared rapidly in these nontumorigenic populations. Analyses of the chromosome complements of the parental and hybrid cell populations indicated
that the tumorigenic segregants had lost substantial numbers
of chromosomes, including those originating from the normal
parent.

These findings have been confirmed by others (Stanbridge,
1976; Sager and Kovac, 1978; Kao and Hartz, 1977; Klinger,
1980), but there have been notable exceptions to this generalization (Croce *et al.*, 1975a; Aviles *et al.*, 1977). The major
drawback in all of these studies has been the chromosomal in-

stability of intraspecific rodent hybrid cells where a significant proportion of the total chromosome complement is rapidly lost. This rapidity of chromosome loss, in addition to making the initial premise of suppression of malignancy hard to evaluate, renders the identification of specific chromosome(s) that possibly control the expression of the tumorigenic phenotype an extremely arduous task.

In another approach interspecific human/rodent hybrids have been used in an attempt to identify the genetic elements regulating the control of expression of the tumorigenic phenotype (Croce *et al.*, 1975a; Jonasson and Harris, 1977; Kucherlapati and Shin, 1979). Here the situation is at least as controversial as with intraspecific rodent cell hybrids--different investigators working with the same cell combinations have again reached opposite conclusions. Jonasson and Harris (1977) found complete suppression of tumorigenicity in hybrids formed between mouse A9 cells and human fibroblasts, whereas Kucherlapati and Shin found no such suppression in their A9/human fibroblast hybrids (Kucherlapati and Shin, 1979). In another extensive study Croce and colleagues (Croce *et al.*, 1975a,b) showed that when SV40-transformed human fibroblasts are fused with normal mouse cells the tumorigenic phenotype continues to be expressed until the integrated SV40 genome is lost by chromosome segregation. Once again, the general rule in the foregoing studies is that chromosomes rapidly segregate from interspecific hybrids. However, other investigators have found that the tumorigenic phenotype of SV40-transformed cells is suppressed following fusions with normal cells (Gee and Harris, 1979; Howell and Sager, 1982; Weissmann and Stanbridge, 1983).

We have developed an intraspecies human hybrid cell system that eliminates the serious problem of chromosome instability (Stanbridge and Wilkinson, 1978; Stanbridge *et al.*, 1982b). The remainder of this chapter presents a brief description of

this system, emphasizing our findings on the role that differentiation plays in the control of tumorigenic expression in
these hybrid cells.

II.   HUMAN CELL HYBRIDS

Although we have examined several combinations of malig-
nant/normal human cell fusions (Stanbridge *et al.*, 1982b), we
will restrict most of our remarks to the HeLa/fibroblast and
HeLa/keratinocyte hybrids that have been studied most extensively.   In our initial studies we fused the D98/AH-2 clone of
HeLa (Szybalski *et al.*, 1962) with a series of different normal
human fibroblasts.   The hybrid clones that arose in HAT selective medium (Littlefield, 1964) all had essentially the same
morphology, which was intermediate between that of the HeLa
and fibroblast parental cells (Stanbridge and Wilkinson, 1978;
Der and Stanbridge, 1978).   At a later stage hybrids derived
from the fusion between HeLa and keratinocytes were isolated,
and these hybrid cells all had the morphology of epithelial-
like cells (Peehl and Stanbridge, 1981a).

III.   TUMORIGENIC POTENTIAL OF THE HeLa/FIBROBLAST HYBRIDS

The primary objective of our early studies was to determine whether the tumorigenic phenotype of the malignant HeLa
parent continued to be expressed in the HeLa/fibroblast hybrid
cell or became suppressed as a result of the introduction of
normal genetic material.   The use of appropriately immunosuppressed animals was obviously necessary for these tumorigenicity assays.   Mice in the studies were immunosuppressed in a
variety of ways, including (1) neonatally thymectomized and

antithymocyte serum treated, (2) adult thymectomized, whole-body irradiated, and bone marrow reconstituted (T^-B^+), and (3) congenitally athymic *nude* mice. In all cases the same result was obtained: Whereas 1×10^5 parental HeLa cells injected subcutaneously produced progressively growing tumors in 100% of animals, no tumors were found when as many as 1×10^8 hybrid cells were inoculated (Stanbridge and Wilkinson, 1978; Stanbridge and Ceredig, 1981).

Thus it would appear that tumorigenic potential is initially completely suppressed in these hybrids. However, possible artifacts could include immunological rejection of the hybrid cells by, for example, natural killer cell activity, a known complicating factor in *nude* mice in particular (Kiessling *et al.*, 1975). Also it might be possible that the human hybrid cells, like the rodent and interspecies human/rodent hybrids described previously, are chromosomally unstable and that the chromosomes responsible for malignant expression were rapidly lost from the hybrids in some nonrandom fashion. Both of these concerns were laid to rest when it was found that tumorigenic segregants arose from the nontumorigenic hybrids after prolonged time in culture. Extensive studies of the growth behavior of the hybrid cells in *nude* mice showed that immune rejection and natural killer cytotoxicity in particular (Stanbridge and Ceredig, 1981) played no role in the control of the tumor growth.

The most valuable aspect of the human hybrid cell system was revealed when chromosome analyses were performed on the nontumorigenic hybrids and the tumorigenic segregants derived from them. It was found that immediately following fusion most (but not all) hybrid clones had lost a few--less than 5%--chromosomes on the basis of the calculated sum of the modes of the parental HeLa and fibroblast populations. Following this early minor loss the chromosomal compositions of the hybrids

were extremely stable (Weissman and Stanbridge, 1980; Stanbridge
et al., 1981). Detailed chromosome analysis of paired nontumorigenic and tumorigenic HeLa/fibroblast hybrids showed that
the tumorigenic segregant populations differed only slightly
from their nontumorigenic counterparts with respect to chromosome number (Stanbridge *et al.*, 1981). Furthermore, the loss
of one copy of chromosomes 11 and 14, respectively, is correlated, with a high degree of statistical significance, with
the reexpression of tumorigenicity. The chromosome stability
of the hybrids provides us with the explanation why, in contrast to other hybrid cell systems, tumorigenic segregants appear only rarely in nontumorigenic human hybrid cell populations. The similarity in chromosomal makeup of the nontumorigenic and tumorigenic segregant hybrids also indicates that
these paired populations are both genotypically and phenotypically very similar. This similarity therefore allows one
to determine which phenotypic traits are specifically correlated with tumorigenic expression.

IV.   *IN VITRO* PHENOTYPIC CHARACTERISTICS OF HeLa/FIBROBLAST
      HYBRIDS

Two major factors prompted the comparative analysis of
nontumorigenic hybrids and their tumorigenic segregants. In
the first place, it is becoming increasingly clear from both
epidemiological (Armitage and Doll, 1954) and experimental
(Mondal *et al.*, 1976; Barrett and Ts'o, 1978) studies that the
progression of a normal cell to a frankly neoplastic one involves multiple steps. We consider, as will be apparent from
the following description, that the nontumorigenic hybrids be-
have as transformed cells in culture and are analogous to an
intermediate step in the progression of a normal cell to a neo-

plastic state in naturally occurring cancers. Furthermore, it has been shown that the process of neoplastic transformation is accompanied by a bewildering array of phenotypic changes in cultured cells. These changes include altered cellular morphology, loss of density-dependent inhibition of growth, reduced requirement for serum growth factors, enhanced proteolytic activity, altered metabolic rates, expression of new products and surface antigens, anchorage independence, and alterations in cytoskeletal and membrane architecture (reviewed in Nicolson, 1976). In the majority of cases these "markers of malignancy" have been identified on the basis of comparisons between the neoplastic cells and their normal progenitors. It appeared to be more useful to compare a tumorigenic cell with its transformed but nontumorigenic precursor in order to determine which phenotypic characteristics of the tumorigenic cells differ not only from the normal cells but also from the transformed precursor, and thereby specifically correlate with tumorigenic expression.

A summary of our findings is given in Table I. The details of these findings have been published elsewhere (Stanbridge and Wilkinson, 1978, 1980; Der and Stanbridge, 1978, 1980, 1981a,b; Stanbridge et al., 1981, 1982a). However, it is clear that many of the phenotypic traits examined are expressed in both nontumorigenic and tumorigenic segregant hybrid populations. Thus the expression of these "tumor-specific" markers may be necessary but is not sufficient for full tumorigenic expression. Those phenotypic traits that distinguish tumorigenic HeLa/fibroblast hybrids from their nontumorigenic hybrid counterparts include morphology, fibronectin distribution, and microfilament organization. All three phenotypic traits are completely reversible. Addition of low concentrations of dexamethasone or sodium butyrate to tumorigenic hybrid cells results in a phenotypic shift of these three traits to that corresponding to the

TABLE I. Summary of *In Vitro* Properties of Parental and Hybrid Human Cells

In Vitro phenotype	Parental cells		Nontumorigenic HeLa/fibroblast hybrids	Tumorigenic HeLa/fibroblast segregants[a]
	HeLa	Fibroblast		
Morphology	Epithelial	Fibroblastic	Intermediate	Epithelial[a]
Density-dependent inhibition of growth	No	Yes	No	No
Requirement for serum growth factors	Reduced	High	Reduced	Reduced
Lectin agglutination	+++	+/−	+++	+++
Anchorage-independent growth in soft agar and methyl cellulose	Yes	No	Yes	Yes
Fibronectin expression	None	High	Reduced (short, branched filaments)	Reduced (unbranched[a] stitch pattern)
Cytoskeleton				
Microtubules	Organized	Organized	Organized	Organized
Microfilaments	Poorly organized	Organized	Organized	Poorly organized[a]
Placental alkaline phosphatase	High	Low	High	High
Ganglioside analysis	Simple	Complex	Relatively complex	Relatively complex
α-hCG	Present	Absent	Absent	Present
75-kdalton Membrane phosphoprotein	Present	Absent	Absent	Present

[a] *Reversible properties—addition of dexamethasone or sodium butyrate induces a phenotypic shift to that of the nontumorigenic hybrid cells.*

nontumorigenic hybrids. Two tumor-associated markers have, however, been identified in HeLa/fibroblast hybrids. They are the expression of a 75-kdalton phosphoprotein in the membranes of parental HeLa cells and tumorigenic segregant hybrid cells (Der and Stanbridge, 1981b), and the expression of the α subunit of human chorionic gonadotropin (αhCG) in these tumorigenic cells (Stanbridge et al., 1982a). Neither phenotype is expressed in normal parental cells or nontumorigenic hybrids. The functional significance of these findings is as yet unclear.

One phenotype that does merit discussion here is that of anchorage-independent growth of cells in soft agar or methyl cellulose. It has repeatedly been documented (Freedman and Shin, 1974; Shin et al., 1975) that the ability of cells to grow in suspension in these milieus is correlated with tumorigenic expression. Although most of the studies have involved rodent cells, the dogma that anchorage-independent growth is synonymous with tumorigenicity has been extrapolated to other species, including human (Hamburger and Salmon, 1977). Our studies, which have been confirmed by others (Kahn and Shin, 1979; Klinger, 1980) indicate that this phenotype does not correlate specifically with tumorigenicity (although it may be a necessary alteration in the progression to malignancy in that many malignant cells express this trait), because transformed nontumorigenic cells grow perfectly well in suspension in agarose or methyl cellulose. Thus in human cells, this phenotypic trait may represent an early alteration in the progression from normalcy to malignancy. In fact, we have shown (Peehl and Stanbridge, 1981b) that normal human fibroblasts are capable of anchorage-independent growth in methyl cellulose under certain nutritional conditions. These findings illustrate the dangers of extrapolating from one mammalian system to another and underscore the necessity of working with human cells

in order to unravel the complexities of the human cancer phenotypes.

V.   THE ROLE OF DIFFERENTIATION IN THE CONTROL OF TUMORIGENIC
     EXPRESSION

One of the more intriguing aspects of our studies with the
human cell hybrids was the question why the nontumorigenic hybrids failed to form tumors in immunosuppressed mice when the
growth behavior of these cells in culture is almost identical
to that seen with the tumorigenic segregant hybrid populations.
We decided, therefore, to examine the growth behavior of paired
nontumorigenic and tumorigenic segregant HeLa/fibroblast hybrid
populations in congenitally athymic *nude* mice.

The hybrid cells were inoculated into separate subcutaneous sites, and the nodules that formed were removed at daily
intervals over a 2-week period (Stanbridge and Ceredig, 1981).
Examination of tissue sections of the nodules revealed remarkable similarities in the behavior of the two hybrid cell types
for the first 3-4 days postinoculation. Within 1 day after injection the majority of cells in the center of the nodule were
dead. However, in both cases the periphery of the nodule was
composed of healthy viable cells, and mitotic activity was apparent. The nodules formed by both nontumorigenic and tumorigenic segregant hybrid cells had the histological appearance
of undifferentiated carcinomas. However, by Day 4 there was a
dramatic decrease in mitotic activity in the nodules formed by
the nontumorigenic hybrids, whereas the tumorigenic segregant
cells continued their rapid proliferation for the entire period
of observation, forming large, progressive, undifferentiated
carcinomas. By Day 6-7 all mitotic activity had ceased in the
nodule formed by the nontumorigenic hybrid cells, and the cells

underwent a morphological alteration to a more fibroblastoid morphology (Fig. 1a). There was no evidence of lymphoid cell infiltration, and the nodules remained well vascularized. When these nodules were biopsied at various intervals up to 3 weeks post inoculation, nontumorigenic hybrid cells could be reestablished in culture from the biopsy material, indicating that no immunological rejection had taken place.

On the basis of these observations and others we postulated that the host animal presumably responds to the presence of inappropriately dividing foreign cells by inducing the release of growth-regulatory signals. The nontumorigenic hybrid cells receive and respond to these signals by terminating their mitotic activity, whereas the tumorigenic segregant hybrid cells (and the parental HeLa cells) either do not receive or certainly do not respond to these putative growth-regulatory signals. We have used the necessarily vague term of "signals" to describe the growth-regulatory events, because it is not clear at this time whether the factor(s) responsible for the cessation of proliferation of the hybrid cells in the *nude* mouse are derived from the host animal or are autoregulatory in nature and actually originate within the nontumorigenic hybrid cells themselves.

Whatever the origin of the growth-regulatory factor(s) is, they are quite specific in their effects on the human cell populations. Using genetically marked nontumorigenic and tumorigenic segregant hybrid cells, we have mixed the two cell populations together prior to inoculation into *nude* mice. In this case the nodules were excised at daily intervals, and the cells within the nodules were recovered and placed in selective media that discriminated between the two hybrid cell populations. Our results (Stanbridge and Ceredig, 1981) clearly showed that even when the two cell types were in intimate contact the nontumorigenic hybrids responded to growth-regulatory signals whereas the tumorigenic segregant cells did not.

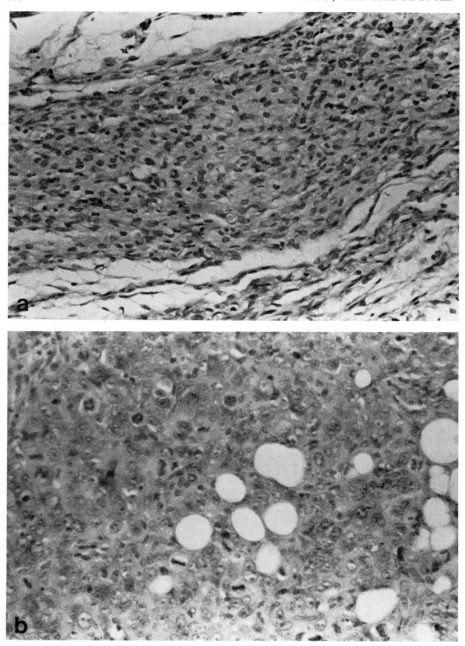

Fig. 1. Histological appearance of nontumorigenic and tumorigenic segregant hybrid cells in athymic *nude* mice.   (a) Six-
day nodule of a nontumorigenic HeLa/fibroblast hybrid.   Note the
lack of mitotic activity and the fibroblastoic morphology of the
quiescent cells.   (b) Eight-day nodule of a tumorigenic segregant
HeLa/fibroblastic hybrid.   The tissue has the appearance of an

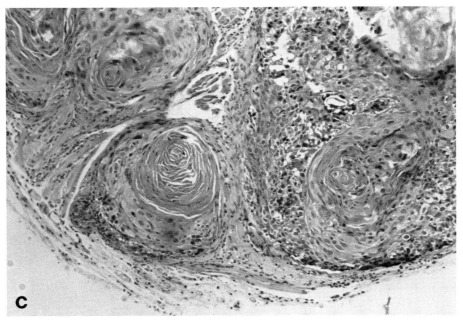

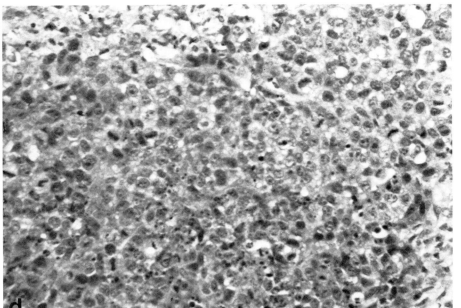

(Fig. 1 continued) undifferentiated carcinoma with high mitotic activity. (c) Four-week nodule of a nontumorigenic HeLa/keratinocyte hybrid. There are many elements of differentiation including horny pearl formation, karyopyknosis, and formation of mature keratin cysts. (d) Ten-day nodule of a tumorigenic segregant HeLa/keratinocyte hybrid. The tissue has the appearance of an undifferentiated carcinoma with high mitotic activity.

Further insight into the nature of the growth-regulatory events came when we examined the growth behavior of HeLa/keratinocyte hybrids in *nude* mice. These hybrid cells have morphological and growth properties in culture similar to that of the HeLa parent. When the cells are inoculated subcutaneously into *nude* mice, growth is completely suppressed, and no palpable nodules are formed or very small palpable nodules (1-2-mm diameter) appear. These nodules remain as small, hard lumps for months without progressing or regressing in size. Histological examination of these nodules revealed evidence of extensive differentiation. The tissue had the appearance of a moderate to highly differentiated squamous cell carcinoma (Fig. lc) with characteristic degenerating nuclei, keratohyalin granules, and keratin-filled cysts.

Because the nodules that arose in the *nude* mice have the histological appearance of moderately to highly differentiated squamous cell carcinomas it may be proposed that they represent benign tumors. However, an alternative possibility--and one that we subscribe to--is that these nodules represent a mimicry of squamous cell carcinoma and have taken on this appearance as a result of the activation of genes responsible for the differentiated phenotype of the keratinocyte parent. In this case the phenotypic "signature" of the normal parental cell is imposed on the hybrid cells when they are localized in the *nude* mouse. This possibility is all the more compelling when one recognizes that the HeLa parental cell line was probably derived from an adenocarcinoma of the cervix (Gey *et al.*, 1952; Jones *et al.*, 1971), which bears little or no resemblance to a differentiated squamous cell carcinoma. Furthermore, tumorigenic segregants of the HeLa/keratinocyte hybrids have been isolated that form undifferentiated anaplastic carcinomas in *nude* mice indistinguishable from those formed by the parental HeLa cells (Fig. ld).

VI. BIOCHEMICAL MARKERS OF DIFFERENTIATION IN HeLa/FIBROBLAST HYBRIDS

Our combined studies with HeLa/fibroblast and HeLa/keratinocyte hybrids have led us to speculate that the nontumorigenic phenotype of these hybrid cells is due to their ability to respond to regulatory signals that induce a cessation of mitotic activity followed by extensive differentiation. Although the HeLa/keratinocyte hybrids exhibit obvious morphological evidence of differentiation, there are no such distinctive morphological changes seen when HeLa/fibroblast hybrids are inoculated. These changes are more subtle and involve a cessation of mitotic activity with a concordant shift in morphology of the cells to a more fibroblastoid morphology (Stanbridge and Ceredig, 1981).

We have, however, identified the expression of several differentiation-specific products by the HeLa/fibroblast hybrids using the following experimental procedures. It quickly became clear that the nontumorigenic HeLa/fibroblast hybrids and their corresponding tumorigenic segregants had very similar chromosome complements and therefore were presumably genotypically and phenotypically similar. In an effort to distinguish possible phenotypic differences between the paired nontumorigenic and tumorigenic segregant hybrid cell populations, antisera were raised in rabbits to the two cell types using live cells as the immunogen. As expected (Table II), when the antisera were tested by immunofluorescence they reacted with the whole panel of cells, consisting of parental HeLa and fibroblast cell lines and the paired nontumorigenic and tumorigenic segregant hybrid cell populations. The antisera were then extensively cross-absorbed with the other cell type--that is, anti-nontumorigenic (NT) hybrid antiserum was absorbed with tumorigenic segregant (TS) hybrid cells, and anti-TS antiserum was absorbed with NT cells.

TABLE II. Identification of Differentiation-Specific Products Using Absorbed Antisera and Immunofluorescent Staining[a]

Antiserum[b]	Absorption with	Parental cells		Hybrid cell populations	
		HeLa	Fibroblast	NT HeLa/fibroblast	TS HeLa/fibroblast
Anti-TS	--	+	+	+	+
Anti-NT	--	+	+	+	+
Anti-TS	NT Cells	+[c]	-	-	+[c]
Anti-NT	TS Cells	-	+	-	-
Anti-NT[live]	NT Cells	-	+	-	-
Anti-NT[fixed]	NT Cells	-	-	-	-

[a] See text for experimental details.

[b] NT, Nontumorigenic HeLa/fibroblast hybrid cells; TS, tumorigenic segregant HeLa/fibroblast hybrid cells; NT[live], live cells used as the immunogen; NT[fixed], paraformaldehyde-fixed cells used as the immunogen.

[c] 75-kdalton phosphoglycoprotein.

When these absorbed antisera were tested, we made several interesting observations: The absorbed anti-TS antiserum reacted only against TS hybrid cells and parental HeLa cells. Further analysis of this absorbed antiserum, using radio-labeling techniques followed by immunoprecipitation and slab gel electrophoresis analysis, has shown that the antiserum recognizes a single 75-kdalton polypeptide that is a membrane glycophosphoprotein (Der and Stanbridge, 1981b). An extensive survey of various hybrid cell populations has indicated that this is a tumor-specific marker.

The absorbed anti-NT antiserum had an even more intriguing pattern of reactivity. When the absorbed antiserum was tested by immunofluorescence against NT hybrid cells (the immunogen), no reactivity was seen. This result indicated that the TS cells had absorbed out all the antibodies directed against the NT cells and suggested that all antigenic determinants (as recognized by the rabbit) expressed by NT cells are also ex-pressed by TS cells. Analysis by immunoprecipitation of radio-labeled cells also failed to show any NT-specific antigens (Fig. 2). The absorbed anti-NT antiserum, as expected, also failed to react with TS or parental HeLa cells (Table II). However, when this absorbed antiserum was tested against paren-tal fibroblasts, strong immunofluorescence was seen. This pre-sented us with somewhat of a paradox because the absorbed anti-NT antiserum did not react with the NT cells, which was the im-munogen, but did react with human fibroblasts, to which the rabbit had never been exposed. Furthermore, when the anti-NT antiserum was extensively absorbed with NT cells, the reactivi-ty toward the human fibroblasts persisted.

The key to this paradox lies in the nature of the immunogen. The NT hybrid cells used in the immunization protocol were live cells. It is our contention that these live cells were induced to differentiate rapidly in the rabbit--in a fashion analogous

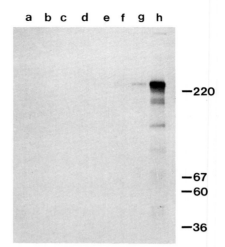

Fig. 2.   Identification of DS products using absorbed
antisera.   After iodination with ^{125}I, cells were solubilized
and immunoprecipitated with anti-NT$_{live}$ or anti-NT$_{fixed}$ antisera extensively absorbed with NT cells.   The immunoprecipitates
were then electrophoresed in SDS-polyacrylamide gels.   The
labeled cells were HeLa (lanes a and b), tumorigenic segregant
HeLa/fibroblast hybrids (lanes c and d), nontumorigenic
HeLa/fibroblast hybrids (lanes e and f), and human fibroblasts
(lanes g and h).   Lanes a, c, e, and g were immunoprecipitated
with absorbed anti-NT$_{fixed}$ antiserum, and lanes b, d, f, and h
were immunoprecipitated with absorbed anti-NT$_{live}$ antiserum.
See text (Section VI) for experimental details.

to that seen in the *nude* mouse--and that certain differentiation-specific (DS) products are rapidly expressed before the
rabbit begins to mount an immune response against the foreign
NT antigens.   The animal then proceeds to synthesize antibodies
directed against the spectrum of NT antigens, including the DS
products.   Because these DS products are not expressed by the
NT hybrid cells in culture, extensive absorption of the anti-NT
antiserum with NT cells does not remove antibodies directed
against the DS products.

Support for this contention was found when rabbits were
immunized with paraformaldehyde-fixed NT cells.   This fixation
procedure retains the immunogenicity of the cells, but of

course they are no longer able to differentiate. In this case extensive absorption of the anti-NT_{fixed} antiserum with either TS cells or NT cells removed all reactivity against the entire panel of parental and hybrid cells (Table II).

When the absorbed anti-NT_{live} antiserum was used to immunoprecipitate $[^{125}I]$- or $[^{35}S]$methionine-labeled cells, autoradiographic analysis of slab gels, in which the solubilized immunoprecipitates were electrophoresed, showed bands only in the lanes containing immunoprecipitates of fibroblast cells. Several bands were noted: two major bands corresponding to 220-240 and 135 kdaltons, respectively, and three or four minor bands (Fig. 2). These represent the profile of DS products.

The 220-240-kdalton band comigrates with fibronectin, a major cell surface glycoprotein of fibroblasts (Hynes, 1973). However, this DS product does not appear to be fibronectin. We have prepared a monoclonal antibody against this DS product (B. A. Fagg and E. J. Stanbridge, unpublished) and used it to evaluate the distribution of the 220-240-kdalton protein on fibroblast cells. As seen in Fig. 3, the distribution of this protein, as visualized by immunofluorescence, is quite distinct from the fibrillar pattern of fibronectin. Further characterization of these DS products is in progress.

The combined morphological evidence of differentiation in HeLa/keratinocyte hybrids and biochemical evidence of DS products in HeLa/fibroblast hybrids has led us to postulate that the reason nontumorigenic HeLa/normal cell hybrids fail to form tumors is that they come under the influence of growth-regulatory signals in the host animal that induce them to cease proliferating and undergo progressive differentiation, which, in the case of HeLa/keratinocytes, may result in terminal differentiation. Furthermore, the differentiating nontumorigenic hybrid cells take on the phenotypic "signature" of the *normal*

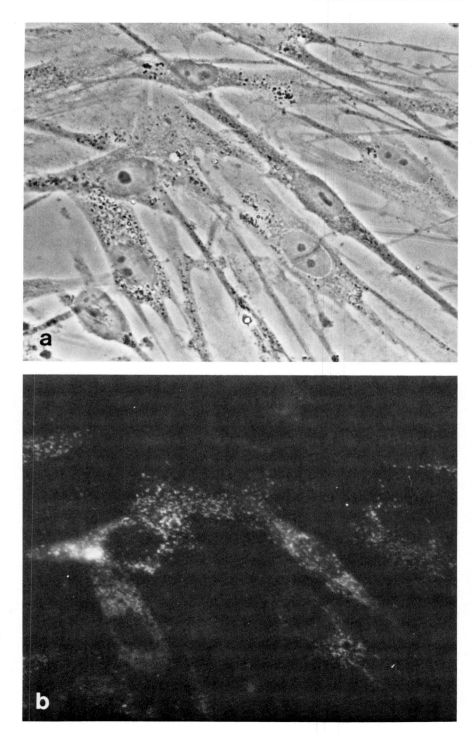

parental cell irrespective of the origin of the malignant parental cell. Tumorigenic parental or tumorigenic segregant hybrid cells, however, appear to have evaded this inducement to differentiate, either by not receiving or by not responding to the putative growth-regulatory signals.

We have encompassed our observations and speculations into a model system (Fig. 4) to explain the regulatory control of tumorigenic expression in human cell hybrids. This model states that normal cells in culture respond to autoregulatory signals and that they not only stop dividing when confluency is reached but, particularly in the case of keratinocytes, also terminally differentiate. These same normal cells also rapidly cease dividing and differentiate in *nude* athymic mice and other immunoincompetent animals. Nontumorigenic hybrids, in contrast, do not appear to exhibit division control, nor do they differentiate in culture. However, the capacity to respond to growth-regulatory and differentiation signals is maintained when the cells are inoculated into the host animal. The key difference between the nontumorigenic hybrids and their tumorigenic segregants is that the latter cells, as well as the malignant parental cells, appear not to respond to growth-regulatory or differentiation signals either in culture or in the intact animals.

Fig. 3. Distribution of 220-240-kdalton DS product on human fibroblasts. The DS product was visualized by paraformaldehyde fixation followed by reaction with mouse monoclonal antibody and rhodaminated rabbit anti-mouse immunoglobulin. (a) Phase contrast of normal human fibroblasts. (b) Same field as (a) showing rhodamine-stained DS product. The distribution is granular and predominantly perinuclear.

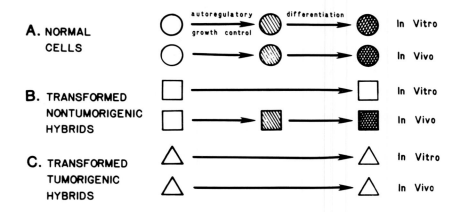

Fig. 4.   A model to explain the control of the tumorigenic phenotype in human cell hybrids.   See Section VI for
details.   Diagonal lines, nondividing cells; crosshatching,
differentiated cells.

VII.   CONCLUSIONS AND FUTURE PROSPECTS

This survey of our experiences with the use of somatic
cell hybrids in the analysis of malignancy in human cells illustrates some of the advantageous features of the system in
tackling this complex problem.   Human cell hybrids are chromosomally stable and thereby provide a system whereby one may
probe with confidence into the chromosomal control of expression of transformation and tumorigenicity, secure in the
knowledge that mass populations of cells may be propagated and
harvested for experimentation and yet still represent a homogeneous population.   This is a definite advantage over the
more unstable intraspecific rodent and interspecific human/ro-
dent systems previously described.

Using this system we have shown that (1) transformed and
tumorigenic phenotypes are under separate genetic control,
(2) nontumorigenic and tumorigenic segregant hybrid cells have

very similar phenotypes in culture, (3) tumor-specific antigens can be identified by comparing paired NT and TS populations, (4) reexpression of tumorigenicity is correlated with the loss of specific chromosomes, (5) control of tumor formation is due to differentiation-inducing signals, and (6) differentiation-specific products have been identified.

One major disadvantage of this intraspecific human hybrid cell system is that identification of those chromosomes controlling the expression of the transformed and tumorigenic phenotypes is very difficult; there are usually 95-100 chromosomes per metaphase spread to analyze by banding techniques. Furthermore, identification of the parental origin of a given chromosome in a parental cell is nearly impossible unless it is accompanied by some type of marker such as isoenzyme polymorphism or actual translocation of chromosome material. It would also appear that relatively few chromosomes, perhaps only 1 or 2, are involved in the control of tumorigenic expression. Therefore, fusion of a normal cell, containing 46 chromosomes, with a malignant cell in order to suppress tumorigenicity presumably involves considerable redundancy of transferred normal chromosomes.

Fortunately, technological advances have made it possible to transfer isolated chromosomes (McBride and Ozer, 1973; Fournier and Ruddle, 1977) and even isolated genes (Wigler et al., 1979; Mulligan and Berg, 1980) into recipient cells. Some of the exciting results include the possible transfer of human cancer genes via DNA transfection into mouse cells (Shih et al., 1979; Cooper et al., 1980). We are currently developing the technology whereby isolated, specific individual chromosomes may be transferred from a normal cell to a malignant cell and vice versa. Success in this approach will be followed, it is hoped, by the cloning of the discrete DNA sequences responsible for the expression and suppression of tumorigenic potential. Such technology will greatly accelerate our quest for the identification of those regulatory elements governing the neoplastic behavior of human cells.

ACKNOWLEDGMENTS

    These studies were supported by National Institute of Health grant CA-19401 and a gift from the Florence A. Clark Memorial Fund. Barbara Fagg was supported by a fellowship from the Cancer Research Institute. Eric J. Stanbridge is the recipient of National Institutes of Health Research Career Development Award CA-00271.

REFERENCES

Armitage, P., and Doll, R. (1954). *Br. J. Cancer 8,* 1-12.
Aviles, D., Jami, J., Rousset, J., and Ritz, E. (1977). *J. Natl. Cancer Inst. (US) 58,* 1391-1397.
Barrett, J. C., and Ts'o, P. O. (1978). *Proc. Natl. Acad. Sci. USA 75,* 3761-3765.
Barski, G., and Cornefert, F. (1962). *J. Natl. Cancer Inst. (US) 28,* 801-821.
Cooper, G. M., Okenquist, S., and Silverman, L. (1980). *Nature (London) 284,* 418-421.
Croce, C. M., Aden, D., and Koprowski, H. (1975a). *Proc. Natl. Acad. Sci. USA 72,* 1397-1400.
Croce, C. M., Aden, D., and Koprowski, H. (1975b). *Science (Washington, D.C.) 190,* 1200-1202.
Davidson, R. L. (1974). "Somatic Cell Hybridization." Raven, New York.
Defendi, V., Ephrussi, B., Koprowski, H., and Yoshida, M. C. (1967). *Proc. Natl. Acad. Sci. USA 57,* 299-305.
Der, C. J., and Stanbridge, E. J. (1978). *Cell 15,* 1241-1251.
Der, C. J., and Stanbridge, E. J. (1980). *Int. J. Cancer 26,* 451-459.
Der, C. J., and Stanbridge, E. J. (1981a). *J. Cell Sci. 52,* 151-166.
Der, C. J., and Stanbridge, E. J. (1981b). *Cell 26,* 429-438.
Fournier, R. E. K., and Ruddle, F. (1977). *Proc. Natl. Acad. Sci. USA 74,* 319-323.
Freedman, V. H., and Shin, S. (1974). *Cell 3,* 355-359.

Gee, C. J., and Harris, H. (1979). *J. Cell Sci. 36*, 223-240.

Gey, G. O., Coffman, W. D., and Kubicek, N. T. (1952). *Cancer Res. 12*, 264-265.

Hamburger, A. W., and Salmon, S. E. (1977). *Science (Washington, D.C.) 197*, 461-463.

Harris, H. (1971). *Proc. R. Soc. London Ser. B 179*, 1-20.

Harris, H., and Watkins, J. F. (1965). *Nature (London) 205*, 640-646.

Harris, H., Miller, O. J., Klein, G., Worst, P., and Tachibana, T. (1969). *Nature (London) 223*, 363-368.

Howell, N., and Sager, R. (1982). *Cytogenet. Cell Genet.*, in press.

Hynes, R. O. (1973). *Proc. Natl. Acad. Sci. USA 70*, 3170-3174.

Jonasson, J., and Harris, H. (1977). *J. Cell Sci. 24*, 255-263.

Jones, H. W., McKusick, V. A., Harper, P. S., and Wuu, K. D. (1971). *Obstet. Gynecol. (N.Y.) 38*, 945-949.

Kahn, P., and Shin, S. (1979). *J. Cell Biol. 82*, 1-16.

Kao, F., and Hartz, J. A. (1977). *J. Natl. Cancer Inst. (US) 59*, 409-413.

Kiessling, R., Klein, E., and Wigzell, H. (1975). *Eur. J. Immunol. 5*, 112-117.

Klinger, H. (1980). *Cytogenet. Cell Genet. 27*, 256-266.

Kucherlapati, R., and Shin, S. (1979). *Cell 16*, 639-648.

Littlefield, J. W. (1964). *Science (Washington, D.C.) 145*, 709-710.

McBride, O. W., and Ozer, H. L. (1973). *Proc. Natl. Acad. Sci. USA 70*, 1258-1262.

McKusick, V. A., and Ruddle, F. H. (1977). *Science (Washington, D.C.) 196*, 390-405.

Mondal, S., Brankow, D. W., and Heidelberger, C. (1976). *Cancer Res. 36*, 2254-2260.

Mulligan, R. C., and Berg, P. (1980). *Science (Washington, D.C.) 209*, 1422-1427.

Nicolson, G. L. (1976). *Biochim. Biophys. Acta 457*, 57-108.

Peehl, D. M., and Stanbridge, E. J. (1981a). *Int. J. Cancer 27*, 625-635.

Peehl, D. M., and Stanbridge, E. J. (1981b). *Proc. Natl. Acad. Sci. 78*, 3053-3057.

Peehl, D. M., and Stanbridge, E. J. (1982). *Int. J. Cancer 30*, 113-120.

Sager, R., and Kovac, P. E. (1978). *Somantic Cell Genet. 4*, 375-392.

Scaletta, L. J., and Ephrussi, B. (1965). *Nature (London) 205*, 1169-1171.

Shih, C., Shilo, B. Z., Goldbarb, M. P., Dannenberg, A., and Weinberg, R. A. (1979). *Proc. Natl. Acad. Sci. USA 76*, 5714-5718.

Shin, S., Freedman, V. J., Risser, R., and Pollack, R. (1975). *Proc. Natl. Acad. Sci. USA 72*, 4435-4439.

Stanbridge, E. J. (1976). *Nature (London) 260,* 17-20.

Stanbridge, E. J., and Ceredig, R. (1981). *Cancer Res. 41,* 573-580.

Stanbridge, E. J., and Wilkinson, J. (1978). *Proc. Natl. Acad. Sci. USA 75,* 1466-1469.

Stanbridge, E. J., and Wilkinson, J. (1980). *Int. J. Cancer 26,* 1-8.

Stanbridge, E. J., Flandermeyer, R. R., Daniels, D. W., Nelson-Rees, W. A. (1981). *Somatic Cell Genet. 7,* 699-712.

Stanbridge, E. J., Rosen, S. W., and Sussman, H. H. (1982a). *Proc. Natl. Acad. Sci. USA 79,* 6242-6245.

Stanbridge, E. J., Der, C. J., Doersen, C.-J., Nishimi, R. Y., Peehl, D. M., Weissman, B. E., and Wilkinson, J. (1982b). *Science (Washington, D.C.) 215,* 252-259.

Szybalski, W. S., Szybalska, E. H., and Ragni, G. (1962). *Cancer Inst. Monogr. 7,* 75-88.

Weissman, B. E., and Stanbridge, E. J. (1980). *Cytogenet. Cell Genet. 28,* 227-239.

Weissman, B. E., and Stanbridge, E. J. (1983). *J. Natl. Cancer Inst. (US),* in press.

Wiener, F., Klein, G., and Harris, H. (1971). *J. Cell Sci. 8,* 681-692.

Wiener, F., Klein, G., and Harris, H. (1974). *J. Cell Sci. 15,* 177-183.

Wigler, M. R., Sweet, R., Sim, G. K., Wold, B., Pellicer, A., Lacy, E., Maniatis, T., Silverstein, S., and Axel, R. (1979). *Cell 16,* 777-785.

5

GROWTH AND INVASIVENESS
OF PRIMARY HUMAN TUMOR EXPLANTS[1]

Emil Bogenmann and Peter A. Jones

Division of Hematology/Oncology
Childrens Hospital of Los Angeles
Los Angeles, California

[1]This work was supported by Grants R01-CA-29397 from the
National Cancer Institute and 83.828.0.80 from the Swiss
National Science Foundation.

I.   INTRODUCTION

The establishment of secondary tumor foci (metastasis) is ultimately responsible for the lethality of most malignancies. Metastasis involves the escape of tumor cells from the primary lesion via the blood system and/or lymphatics, extravasation from the circulation, invasion into normal tissues, and finally the growth of tumor cells (for review see Fidler *et al.*, 1978; Poste and Fidler, 1980). The mechanisms of invasion and metastasis have been studied extensively in animal model systems (Jones *et al.*, 1971; Sindelar *et al.*, 1975; Carr *et al.*, 1976; Dingemans *et al.*, 1978; Poste and Nicholson, 1980; Poste *et al.*, 1982). There are, however, many obstacles to the *in vivo* study of the biochemical and morphological events involved in the process of metastasis. Furthermore, substantial evidence has accumulated that primary neoplasms are composed of populations of tumor cells that are heterogeneous in regard to their invasive and metastatic potentials (Fidler, 1978; Poste and Fidler, 1980; Poste *et al.*, 1982). Tumor cell populations have been isolated by *in vivo* selection techniques from parental neoplasms that differ in their metastatic potentials (Fidler, 1973; Poste and Nicolson, 1980), and new *in vitro* approaches have led to the successful isolation of tumor cell subpopulations with enhanced tissue-invasive properties (Poste *et al.*, 1980).

The exact mechanisms by which tumor cells invade normal tissues are not known, but proteolytic enzymes such as plasminogen activator(s), cathepsins, and collagenolytic enzymes may be responsible for tissue breakdown and invasion (Liotta *et al.*, 1971, 1977; Reich, 1973; Poole, 1973). Several laboratories have studied the degradation of connective tissue proteins such as glycoproteins, glycosaminoglycans, elastin, and collagens by different tumor cells and normal cells. Basement membrane collagens can be degraded by tumor cell-associated collagenases (Liotta et al., 1971, 1977), whereas plasmin and trypsin digest fibronectin and laminin (Liotta et al., 1981).

Extracellular matrices elaborated in vitro by various connective tissue cells such as smooth muscle cells, endothelial cells, and fibroblasts have been used to study the role of tumor cell-associated proteases in the digestion of connective tissue proteins (Jones and DeClerck, 1980; Werb et al., 1980; Jones and Werb, 1980; Kramer et al., 1982). The invasive potentials of different tumor cells into whole tissues such as fragments of chick heart (Mareel et al., 1979), extracted hyaline cartilage (Pauli et al., 1981), chick chorioallantoic membrane (Hart and Fidler, 1978), human amnion (Russo et al., 1981; Siegal et al., 1982), and artificial blood vessels have also been investigated (Jones et al., 1981).

These experiments were carried out with established animal and human tumor cell lines, so that the relevance to tumor cell invasion as it occurs in vivo is questionable. We therefore decided to study the in vitro invasive potentials of primary pediatric tumors.

Considerable effort has been undertaken for several decades to grow human tumor cells in culture. Various culture techniques such as the use of clotted lymph (Harrison, 1907), cellulose sponge matrices (Leighton, 1954), reconstituted rat tail collagen (Ehrman and Gey, 1956), feeder layer cells (Puck and Marcus, 1955), agar cultures (McAllister and Reed, 1968; Hamburger and Salmon, 1977), and subendothelial matrices (Vlodavsky et al., 1980) have been developed in order to enhance the survival and growth of human neoplastic cells. None of the systems has been shown to be successful for the routine growth and maintenance of a high percentage of primary explants.

In the present study we present a new culture system using multilayers of cloned rat smooth muscle cells (SMC) or human

fibroblast cells, or their *in vitro* elaborated extracellular
matrices as biological substrates for the culture of primary
human neoplasms. More than 80% of the most common solid tumors
in childhood routinely survived or grew for 1 month or longer.
Only 2 of the 10 different neoplasms tested survived for longer
than 2 weeks when explanted onto tissue culture plastic. In
contrast, 9 of the 10 tumors survived on biological substrates.
It was found that all the neoplasms analyzed showed areas of
distinct cellular invasion into SMC or fibroblast multilayers
that corresponded with their *in vivo* pathological features.
Normal human kidney, however, was noninvasive when cultured on
human fibroblast tissue. The abilities of primary tumor explants to degrade connective tissue proteins was also investigated using biosynthetically labeled matrices.

II.   MATERIALS AND METHODS

A.   Preparation of Tumor Cell Suspensions from Human Material

     Needle biopsies or large pieces (1-2 cm cubes) were cut
from surgically excised human tumors and soaked in Dulbecco's
modified Eagle's medium (DMEM) (Grand Island Biological Co.,
Santa Clara, California), containing 5% fetal bovine serum
(FBS) (Irvine Scientific, Irvine, California), penicillin
(100 IU/ml) and streptomycin (100 µg/ml) (Grand Island Biological Co.), and 4 mM glutamine (Grand Island Biological Co.).
All further manipulations were done within 30 min in a laminar
flow hood. Tumor tissue was washed twice with prewarmed DMEM,
placed into 100-mm culture dishes (Falcon Plastics, Oxnard,
California), and minced with surgical blades into pieces
(1-3 mm cubes). Single cells and small cell clumps were
mechanically released from the tumor tissue and collected into
a 50-ml centrifuge tube. Fresh DMEM was added to the remaining

pieces, which were then gently pipetted to release additional
tumor cells.

Enzymatic treatment was used after the initial mechanical
treatment if the tumor tissue was very fibrous (some rhabdomyosarcomas, Wilms' tumors, or Ewing's sarcomas). Small tissue
pieces were incubated for 20 to 40 min in DMEM containing 0.25%
viokase (Viobin Corp., Monticello, Illinois) and 0.1% bacterial
collagenase (Sigma Type 1, St. Louis, Missouri).

Large pieces of tissue were separated from single cells
and small clumps of cells by a 1-g sedimentation after a mild
pipetting. The cell suspension was then centrifuged for 5 min
at 300 g and the pellet washed twice by centrifugation with
DMEM containing 5% FBS. The cell pellet was resuspended in
2 to 4 ml of DMEM layered over 5 ml of FBS and viable cells
separated from cellular debris by a low-speed centrifugation
(50 g) for 10 min. The final cell pellet was then resuspended
in culture medium containing DMEM supplemented with 10% human
serum, penicillin (100 IU/ml), streptomycin (100 μg/ml), and
4 mM glutamine and added to the various substrates.

B. Preparation of Cell Substrates

Rat smooth muscle cells (SMC) of the R22-Cl-D strain
(Jones *et al.*, 1979) and human fibroblast cells (T-1) obtained
from a skin biopsy were grown in Eagle's minimal essential
medium (MEM) (Grand Island Biological Co.) containing 10% FBS,
2% tryptose phosphate broth (Difco Inc., Detroit, Michigan),
penicillin (100 IU/ml), and streptomycin (100 μg/ml). SMC were
seeded into 16-mm multi-well plates (Costar, Cambridge, Massachusetts; 1 × 10^5/well) for extracellular matrix production.
The cultures received ascorbic acid (25 μg/ml) the following
day and daily thereafter, and were labeled with L-3,4[^{3}H]-
proline (0.33 μCi/mM, 24.9 Ci/mM, New England Nuclear, Boston,

Massachusetts) continuously for 12 days. Producer cells were
lysed as described previously (Jones and DeClerck, 1980) except
that 25 mM NH$_4$OH was used. The extracellular matrix remained
anchored to the bottom of the dish and was washed extensively
with distilled water and stored in water at 4°C.

Living SMC and fibroblast multilayers were obtained by
seeding R22-CL-D or T-1 cells (2 × 10^5/35-mm dish) under the
same conditions as described already, except that [^{3}H]proline
was not added to the cultures. Such cultures were used as
tumor cell substrates 2-4 weeks after seeding of the SMC. SMC
or T-1 multilayers were also established on nylon meshes
(100 μm mesh width). Meshes were first boiled in 0.1 M NaHCO$_3$
for 30 min, washed extensively with distilled water and auto-
claved for 30 min at 1 atm, cut into pieces (4 cm × 3 cm),
and inserted into 1.6-cm × 12.5-cm screw cap tubes (Falcon
Plastics). Feeder layer cells (10^7/tube) were added in 7 ml
of medium and the tubes rotated in a roller apparatus at 37°C
for at least 2 weeks. By this time, the cells covered the
nylon mesh completely. The cultures received ascorbic acid
(25 μg/ml) daily and the medium was changed twice a week. The
meshes were then cut into smaller pieces (1 cm × 1 cm) and
placed into 35-mm dishes with fresh medium.

Four small pieces of tumor tissue (1-3 mm cubes) were
placed onto each floating nylon mesh and incubated with 1 ml
of culture medium so that the explants grew at the air-medium
interface.

C. Monitoring the Cultures

Cultures were monitored daily with an inverted microscope
so that the viability of the cells could be followed by the increase in cell number, presence of mitotic figures, and lack of
gross cell death. The culture medium showed an increased acidi-

ty in cultures with highly metabolically active tumor cells as indicated by a color change in the phenol red indicator. The growth of tumor tissue was also assessed by examination of cross sections of fixed and embedded cultures, and the presence of mitotic figures served as a further criterion for cell growth.

D. Analysis of Degradation of Extracellular Matrix

The degradation of radioactively labeled SMC-derived extracellular matrix by tumor cells was followed by the appearance of radioactivity in the supernatant culture medium (Jones and DeClerck, 1980). Tumor cells were seeded onto matrices and the radioactivity in 100 μl samples of the supernatants determined prior to the medium change every third day. Values for radioactivity released in control cultures incubated without tumor cells have been subtracted from the data presented in this chapter. The values represent duplicates in which the variations were less than 10%.

E. Preparation of Human Serum

Donor blood (200 ml/donor) was obtained aseptically from a selected population of donors in the laboratory and coagulated individually in 50-ml glass tubes. The tubes were transferred to 4°C after 2-h incubation at 37°C and incubated overnight to complete coagulation. Serum was then pooled, centrifuged to separate residual blood cells, sterilized by filtration through 0.45-μm filters (Millipore Corp., Bedford, Massachusetts), and 50-ml aliquots stored at -80°C.

F. Light Microscopy

Cultures were washed with prewarmed DMEM, fixed with glutaraldehyde (2.4% in DMEM, pH 7.2) for 1 h at 4°C, and postfixed

with osmium tetroxide (1% OsO_4 in 0.1 M cacodylate buffer,
pH 7.2) for 1 h at 4°C. The specimens were dehydrated in a
series of ethanols and embedded in a mixture of epon and
araldite (1:1). Polymerization was carried out at 60°C for
2 days, and thick sections (2 μm) cut at right angles to the
surface and stained with azure II, methylene blue, and basic
fuchsin.

III.   RESULTS

A.   Childhood Neoplastic Material

    Neoplastic material obtained at surgery varied in size
from small fragments (several milligrams) to large pieces
(>10 g). Some tumors were very soft and easily dispersed,
whereas others were so fibrous that mechanical mincing was
not sufficient to disperse the material. The latter were
treated for periods of 20 to 40 min with collagenase-viokase
followed by a mild pipetting to dissociate the tumor specimens. No attempts were made to obtain single-cell suspensions,
and small cell clumps and isolated single cells were seeded
onto different substrates. Various culture mediums (MEM,
Ham's F12, Ham's F10, RPMI 1640, and DMEM) supplemented with
different amounts of FBS were tested for their abilities to
give the best survival of the tumor cells. Dulbecco's modified Eagle's medium (4.5 g/liter glucose) supplemented with
10% human serum gave the most consistent results and was used
for all further studies.

B.   Survival of Tumor Cell Explants on Different Substrates

    The effectiveness of the different cell substrates in sup-
porting the survival of primary tumor explants was investigated
in a series of 10 different tumors. Neoplastic cells survived

in only 2 of 10 tumors cultured on tissue culture plastic for
longer than 2 weeks. The remaining 8 tumors were overgrown by
presumably normal cells with a fibroblastic morphology. Tumor
cells were often flat and irregularly shaped, frequently bi-
nucleated, and containing cytoplasmic vacuoles, probably indicating an unfavorable culture environment. Cultures in which
substantial fibroblast growth occurred showed considerable cell
death, and cell detachment was evident.

In contrast, 9 of the 10 tumors survived and/or grew for
1 month or longer when cultured on biological substrates. Individual tumor cells or small cell clumps attached firmly to
the living SMC or their matrix, and these two substrates were
similar in promoting cell adhesion. Neoplastic cells were normally easily distinguishable from their substrates. Tumor cells
from medulloblastomas, neuroblastomas, and Ewing's sarcomas
attached to the SMC as spheroid-like aggregates of different
size, and cells stayed rounded up for several weeks (Fig. 1).
In contrast, epithelial-type tumors, such as yolk-sac carcinoma
cells and certain Wilms' tumor cells, formed tightly packed
islands on top of the SMC, and cell proliferation occurred at
the edges of such epithelial-like structures (Fig. 2).
Rhabdomyosarcoma cells, which spread out on biological substrates, were more difficult to identify, but spontaneous morphological differentiation into multinucleated myotubes was
detected in three of six cases (Fig. 3). Cellular differentiation could also routinely be seen with neuroblastoma cells,
which organized into aggregates from which extensive networks
of dendrites formed within the first week of culture (Fig. 4).

Explants seeded onto biological substrates could be maintained for several weeks, because both SMC and their matrices
stayed firmly anchored to the bottom of the dishes. Further
studies were therefore conducted with these biological substrates.

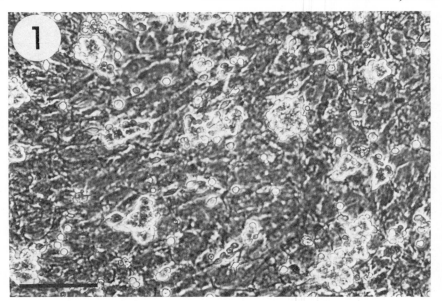

Fig. 1.   Phase contrast micrograph of a Ewing's sarcoma culture 2 weeks after seeding onto preformed SMC layers.   Tumor cells were mostly organized in spheroid-like aggregates, and few single neoplastic cells were present.   The SMC with associated extracellular matrix can be seen in the background (×400, bar is 50 μm long).

More than 80% of the 54 childhood tumors tested survived as long as 2 months when seeded onto biological substrates (Table I), and there were no differences between the efficiencies of these substrates in promoting survival.   However, certain medulloblastomas and neuroblastomas showed a preference for living feeder layer cells rather than their matrix.   Explants of Wilms' tumors were generally maintained for many weeks, and 13 of 17 tumors survived for longer than 3 weeks (Table II).   All neuroblastoma cultures survived for several weeks, but little cell division occurred, whereas medulloblastomas showed high survival rates and considerable cell multiplication (Table I).   Cells of osteogenic sarcomas and Ewing's sarcomas in general showed good survivals, and tumor cell

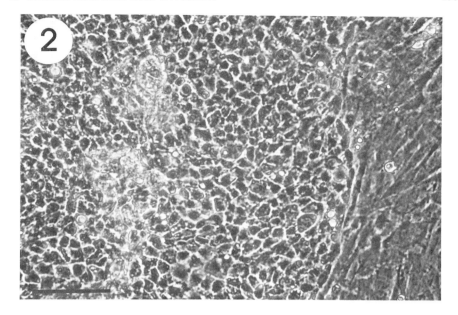

Fig. 2.   Phase contrast micrograph of a yolk-sac carcinoma culture 10 days after seeding onto SMC.   Tightly organized epithelial-like cells with cytoplasmic vacuoles can clearly be distinguished from the SMC layer (×400, bar is 50 µm long).

proliferation occurred, whereas only two of five rhabdomyosarcomas showed substantial cell multiplication.

C.   Invasiveness of Cultured Neoplasms into SMC and Fibroblast
     Cell Multilayers

Neoplasms cultured on SMC or fibroblast feeder layers were fixed for light microscopy to study the histopathology of the explants.   The invasion of tumor cells into preformed multilayers of SMC and fibroblast cells was also assessed and the data for four specimens summarized (Table II).

A cross section of a 5-week-old culture of an osteogenic sarcoma, in which tumor cell growth (mitotic figures) was observed, is shown in Fig. 5.   Tumor cells formed a densely organized tissue on top of the SMC multilayers, and an area in

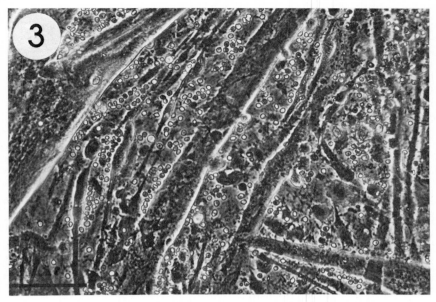

Fig. 3. Phase contrast micrograph of a rhabdomyosarcoma
culture grown on SMC. Numerous spontaneously differentiated
myotubes could be detected after 1 week of culture. The SMC
feeder layer and residual blood cells can be seen in the background (×400, bar is 50 μm long).

which invasion but not destruction of the SMC tissue occurred

can be identified. Analysis of the ability of these sarcoma

cells to degrade SMC-derived extracellular matrix proteins

showed that a significant amount of radioactivity was released

during the 9-day incubation period (Table II). In contrast,

almost complete destruction of the SMC multilayers occurred in

the medulloblastoma culture (Fig. 6). The histology of the

in vitro tissue was very similar to that of the tumor in the

patient (data not shown). This tumor, which was locally in-

vasive *in vivo*, showed tissue destruction *in vitro* as well as

degradation of connective tissue proteins (Table II).

The destruction of the SMC multilayers observed in Fig. 6

might have been due to atrophy of the SMC induced by oxygen

and/or medium depletion. To rule out this possibility, tumor

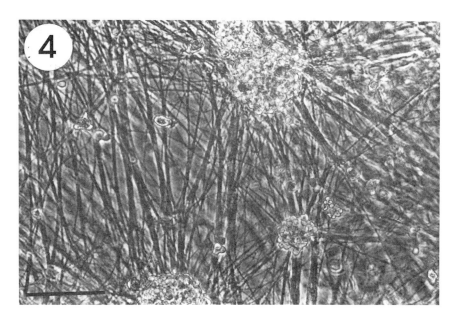

Fig. 4. Phase contrast micrograph of a neuroblastoma culture 1 week after initiation. Neoplastic cells were organized
in cell aggregates of different sizes, from which a network of
cellular extensions (dendrites) has spontaneously been formed
(×400, bar is 50 μm long).

TABLE I. Survival of Primary Neoplasms Cultured on SMC or
          Their Matrix in Long-Term Cultures[a]

Tumor class	Number of long-term survivors	Number tested
Renal tumor (Wilms')	13	17
Neuroblastoma	9	9
Brain tumor (medulloblastoma)	8	8
Ewing's sarcoma	5	7
Rhabdomyosarcoma	5	6
Osteogenic sarcoma	4	4
Carcinoma	3	3

[a]Explants of the indicated tumor types were cultured on
SMC or their extracellular matrix and scored for viability and
survival after 4 weeks in culture.

TABLE I.

Number	Tumor origin	Invasion in vivo[a]	Mitotic figures in vitro	Invasion in vitro[b]	Destruction of SMC/T-1 in vitro	Degration of matrix (%)	Cultured on
HTLA$_4$	Osteogenic sarcoma	+	+	+	-	7	SMC
HTLA$_3$	Medullo- blastoma	+	+	+	+	14	SMC
HTLA$_{44}$	Yolk-sac carcinoma	+	+	+	-	1	SMC/ Nylon mesh
HTLA$_{83}$	Wilms' tumor	+	+	+	+	No data	T-1/ Nylon mesh

[a]Analyzed by light microscopy on histological sections of the primary tumor from the patient.
[b]Determined by light and electron microscopy of tumor cells cultured on SMC.
[c]Percentage of radioactivity released from a radiolabeled SMC matrix after 9 days in culture.

5

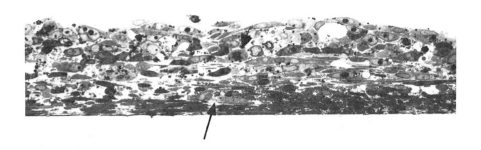

Fig. 5. Cross section of cells of an osteogenic sarcoma grown for 5 weeks on SMC multilayers. Tumor cells show prominent nuclei with large nucleoli and minimal cytoplasm. Mitotic figures (arrowhead) could be detected within the tumor tissue. The SMC was essentially intact; however, local invasion and disorganization of the SMC (arrow) was evident (×160, bar is 100 μm long).

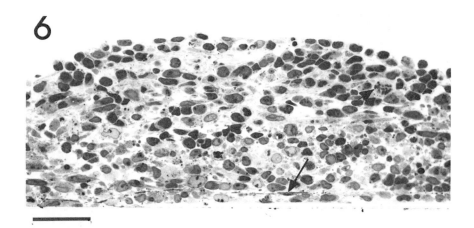

Fig. 6. Primary medulloblastoma culture after 5 weeks on SMC multilayers. Small sarcoma-type cells were organized into a loose tissue in which mitotic figures (arrowhead) could be detected. The SMC multilayer was essentially destroyed, and only a few elongated SMC (arrow) were still present (×160, bar is 100 μm long).

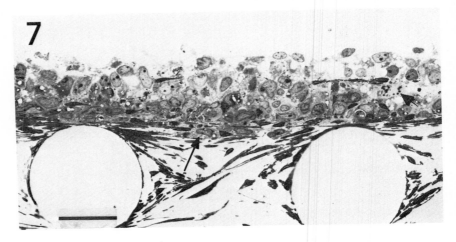

Fig. 7.   Cross section of yolk-sac carcinoma cells grown
for 5 weeks on a nylon raft previously covered with SMC multilayers.   Tumor cells showed large nuclei with prominent
nucleoli and numerous cytoplasmic vacuoles that were present
in the primary lesion *in vivo*.   Mitotic figures (arrowhead)
were present within the tissue.   The SMC multilayers were still
intact, although infiltrated by several tumor cells (arrow)
(×300, bar is 50 μm long).

explants were also cultured on floating nylon rafts (Sirica *et
al.*, 1979), which in the present study were previously coated
with either SMC or fibroblast cells.   Cells of a yolk-sac carcinoma and a Wilm's tumor were grown for different time periods
on such nylon meshes.   Cultured yolk-sac carcinoma cells, which
in thin sections showed well-differentiated desmosomes (data
not shown), also maintained characteristic cytoplasmic vacuoles
as seen in the patient.   It was interesting to note that these
tumor cells had invaded the SMC multilayers leaving the structure essentially intact (Fig. 7), whereas no significant SMC
matrix degradation by these tumor cells occurred (Table II).
This result indicated that cellular invasion can take place and
does not necessarily correlate with the capacity of tumor cells
to degrade connective tissue proteins.   In contrast, neoplastic
cells of a Wilm's tumor explanted on fibroblast multilayers

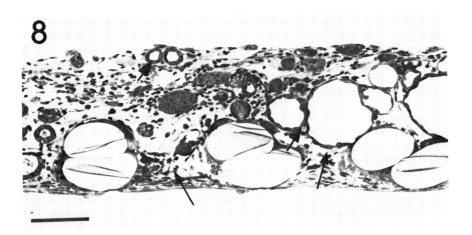

Fig. 8.   Light micrograph of a Wilms' tumor explanted onto a nylon mesh precovered with fibroblast multilayers.   Tumor tissue showed a high degree of histological variation.   Sarcoma-type cells that showed prominent tubular formation (differen-tiation) (arrowhead) could be detected.   The fibroblast multi-layers were successfully infiltrated by tumor cells and partly destroyed (arrow) (×160, bar is 100 µm long).

completely invaded and destroyed this structure within 10 days of culture (Fig. 8), whereas normal kidney cells after the same period of time did not show any sign of tissue invasion (data not shown).

Certain individual neoplasms explanted onto biological substrates could be maintained for several weeks with no evi-dent tumor cell proliferation.   It was therefore of special interest to study the invasive potentials of certain nongrowing tumors (neuroblastoma, Ewing's sarcoma) in order to demonstrate the general use of the culture system.   Histological analysis of quiescent explants grown for different time periods on SMC multilayers demonstrated that nonproliferating tumor cells were equally effective in invading and destroying the feeder layer tissue, indicating that cell multiplication was not a necessary criterion for tumor invasion.

IV.   DISCUSSION

Considerable efforts have been made to isolate and establish human neoplastic cell lines in order to study basic
biological properties of such tumor cells *in vitro* (McAllister
et al., 1975, 1977; Seeger *et al.*, 1977). However, the lack
of systems permitting the routine growth and survival of normal and neoplastic human cells has been a major hindrance to
such studies. Furthermore, a more satisfactory approach to
the study of the biology of human cells would be the use of
primary explants in which the strong selection pressures involved in the establishment of cell lines were avoided. In
the present study we present a new culture system in which
more than 80% of the solid pediatric neoplasms consistently
survived and/or grew in long-term cultures (more than 1 month).
Invasive properties of individual tumors cultured on SMC or
fibroblast multilayers were investigated morphologically and
quantitated biochemically.

Feeder layers have been used for some time to support
cell attachment and growth (Puck and Marcus, 1955). The SMC
and fibroblast cells used in the present investigation had the
added advantage that they produced, in the presence of ascorbic acid, a structure with several of the morphological and
biochemical features of a tissue (Jones *et al.*, 1979). These
tissues are composed of several layers of SMC or fibroblasts
embedded in the extensive extracellular matrix they had synthesized. The matrix produced by SMC contains glycoproteins,
elastin, and collagens (Jones *et al.*, 1979), whereas the
fibroblast-derived matrix is composed of glycoproteins linked
to an extensive collagen network. Several of these proteins
have been shown to increase the adhesion and growth of cultured
cells (Yamada *et al.*, 1976; Terranova *et al.*, 1980; Knox *et
al.*, 1982), and the use of a biologically synthesized mixture

of them may have provided a good substrate for primary neoplastic cells. Thus, the complex matrix, combined with the feeder layer function of the SMC or fibroblasts and human serum, may explain the high success rate of the present study.

The analysis of invasive potentials of primary human neoplasms extends our previous work with established cell lines (Jones *et al.*, 1981). Microscopic analysis of different cultured neoplasms explanted onto SMC or fibroblast multilayers demonstrated that tumor cells successfully invaded and destroyed such feeder layer tissues. The destruction of these multilayers was, however, not due to the atropy or oxygen depletion, because it was also noticed with tumor explants grown on floating nylon rafts. For comparison it was a general interest to note that fibroblast multilayers on nylon rafts did not show signs of invasion or destruction by normal kidney cells. Furthermore, the culture system demonstrated its usefulness, in that primary tumor explants could be maintained for several weeks in the absence of tumor cell proliferation, but neoplastic cells still invaded and destroyed the SMC and fibroblast multilayers. Clinical studies have shown that slowly growing tumors may be highly invasive and metastatic (Weinstein *et al.*, 1976).

The biochemical mechanisms by which neoplastic cells invade surrounding normal tissue are not understood, but proteolytic enzymes such as plasminogen activator(s), collagenase, elastase, and cathepsins have been implicated in this process (Liotta *et al.*, 1971; Ossowski *et al.*, 1973; Poole, 1973; Jones and DeClerck, 1980; Werb *et al.*, 1980). These proteases are capable of degrading connective tissue proteins in matrices elaborated *in vitro* (Jones and DeClerck, 1980; Werb *et al.*, 1980; Jones and Werb, 1980; Kramer *et al.*, 1982). In the present study we also found that primary human tumors can digest part of the substrates when seeded onto SMC or fibroblast matrices. However, simple correlations between the extent of invasion and matrix degradation could not be drawn, because some invasive cells (e.g., yolk-sac carcinoma) showed little if any ability to degrade matrix proteins.

The new *in vitro* system described may therefore be useful for the routine culture of primary human tumors for the study of their basic biological properties. Investigations of the production of hydrolytic enzymes and their role in tumor invasion as well as the growth and the differentiation potentials of primary neoplasms will give more detailed information on the phenomenon of cancer.

REFERENCES

Carr, I., McGinty, F., and Norris, P. (1976). *J. Pathol. 118,* 91-99.

Dingemans, K. P., Roos, E., Van Der Bergh, M. A., and Van De Pavert, I. V. (1978). *J. Natl. Cancer Inst. (US) 60,* 583-598.

Ehrmann, R. L., and Gey, G. O. (1956). *J. Natl. Cancer Inst. (US) 16,* 1375-1404.

Fidler, I. J. (1973). *Eur. J. Cancer 9,* 223-227.

Fidler, I. J. (1978). *Cancer Res. 38,* 2651-2660.

Fidler, I. J., Gersten, D. M., and Hart, I. R. (1978). *Adv. Cancer Res. 28,* 149-250.

Hamburger, A. W., and Salmon, S. E. (1977). *Science (Washington, D.C.) 197,* 461-463.

Harrison, R. G. (1907). *Proc. Soc. Exp. Biol. Med. 4,* 140.

Hart, I. R., and Fidler, I. J. (1978). *Cancer Res. 38,* 3218-3224.

Jones, D. S., Wallace, A. C., and Fraser, E. E. (1971). *J. Natl. Cancer Inst. (US) 46,* 493-504.

Jones, P. A., and Werb, Z. (1980). *J. Exp. Med. 152,* 1527-1536.

Jones, P. A., and DeClerck, Y. (1980). *Cancer Res. 40,* 3222-3227.

Jones, P. A., Scott-Burden, T., and Gevers, W. (1979). *Proc. Natl. Acad. Sci. USA 76,* 353-357.

Jones, P. A., Neustein, H. B., Gonzales, F., and Bogenmann, E. (1981). *Cancer Res. 41,* 4613-4620.

Knox, P., Wells, P., and Serafini-Francassini, A. (1982).
    Nature (London) 295, 614-615.
Kramer, R. H., Vogel, K. G., and Nicolson, G. L. (1982). *J.*
    Biol. Chem. 257, 2678-2686.
Leighton, J. (1954). *Tex. Rep. Biol. Med.* 12, 847.
Liotta, L. A., Shigeto, A., Robey, P. G., and Martin, G. R.
    (1971). *Proc. Natl. Acad. Sci. USA* 76, 2268-2272.
Liotta, L. A., Kleinerman, J., Catanzaro, P., and Rynbrandt, D.
    (1977). *J. Natl. Cancer Inst.* 58, 1427-1431.
Liotta, L. A., Goldfarb, R. H., Brundage, R., Siegal, G. P.,
    Terranova, K., and Garbisa, S. (1981). *Cancer Res.* 41,
    4629-4636.
Mareel, M., Kint, J., and Meyvisch, C. (1979). *Virchows Arch.*
    B 30, 95-111.
McAllister, R. M., and Reed, G. (1968). *Pediatr. Res. 2*,
    356-360.
McAllister, R. M., Nelson-Rees, W. A., Peer, M., Laug, W. E.,
    Isaacs, H., Gilden, R. V., Rongey, R. W., and Gardner,
    M. B. (1975). *Cancer (Philadelphia) 36*, 1804-1814.
McAllister, R. M., Gardner, M. B., and Greene, A. E. (1977).
    Cancer 27, 397-402.
Ossowski, L., Unkeless, J. C., Tobia, A., Quigley, J. P.,
    Rifkin, D. E., and Reich, E. (1973). *J. Exp. Med. 137*,
    112-126.
Pauli, B. U., Memoli, V. A., and Kuettner, K. E. (1981).
    Cancer Res. 41, 2084-2091.
Poole, A. R. (1973). *In* "Lysosomes in Biology and Pathology"
    (J. T. Dingle, ed.), Vol. 3, pp. 303-337. North-Holland,
    Amsterdam.
Poste, G., and Fidler, I. J. (1980). *Nature (London) 283*,
    139-146.
Poste, G., and Nicolson, G. L. (1980). *Proc. Natl. Acad. Sci.*
    USA 77, 399-403.
Poste, G., Doll, J., Hart, I. R., and Fidler, J. (1980).
    Cancer Res. 40, 1636-1644.
Poste, G., Doll, J., Brown, A. E., Tzeng, J., and Zeidman, I.
    (1982). *Cancer Res. 42*, 2770-2778.
Puck, T., and Marcus, P. I. (1955). *Proc. Natl. Acad. Sci.*
    USA 41, 432-437.
Reich, E. (1973). *Fed. Proc. Fed. Am. Soc. Exp. Biol. 32*,
    2174-2175.
Russo, R. G., Liotta, L. A., Thorgeirsson, U., Brundage, R.,
    and Schiffmann, E. (1981). *J. Cell Biol. 91*, 466-467.
Seeger, R. C., Rayner, S. A., Banerjee, A., Chung, H., Caug, W.
    E., Neustein, H. B., and Benedict, W. F. (1977). *Cancer*
    Res. 37, 1364-1371.
Siegal, G. P., Thorgeirsson, U. P., Russo, R. G., Wallace, D.
    M., Liotta, L. A., and Berger, S. L. (1982). *Proc. Natl.*
    Acad. Sci. USA 79, 4064-4068.

Sindelar, W. F., Tralka, T. S., and Ketcham, A. S. (1975).
    J. Surg. Res. 18, 137-161.
Sirica, A. E., Richards, W., Tsukada, Y., Sattler, C. A., and
    Pitot, H. (1979). Proc. Natl. Acad. Sci. USA 76,
    283-287.
Terranova, V. P., Rohrbach, D. R., and Martin, G. R. (1980).
    Cell 22, 719-726.
Vlodavsky, L., Lui, G. M., and Gospodarowicz, D. (1980).
    Cell 19, 607-616.
Weinstein, R. S., Merk, F. B., and Alroy, J. (1976). Adv.
    Cancer Res. 23, 23-89.
Werb, Z., Banda, M. J., and Jones, P. (1980). J. Exp. Med.
    152, 1340-1357.
Yamada, K. M., Yamada, S. S., and Pastan, I. (1976). Proc.
    Natl. Acad. Sci. USA 73, 1217-1221.

6

SPONTANEOUS CHANGES IN HUMAN CORPSE SKIN TRANSPLANTED TO *NUDE* MICE[1]

Niels Græm and Carl O. Povlsen

Pathological-Anatomical Institute
Kommunehospitalet
Copenhagen, Denmark

[1] *This study was supported by the Danish Cancer Society (M-55/80).*

I.   INTRODUCTION

The acceptance of heterografts by *nude* mice makes it possible to perform studies on intact human tissue that otherwise
would be impossible for ethical or technical reasons.   Thus
the system of human skin transplanted to *nude* mice first described by Rygaard (1973) may be a valuable tool in the study
of human skin carcinogenesis.   However, we have achieved con-
fusing results in an (unpublished) investigation of the acute
effects of topical application of certain carcinogenic and
promoting agents on the morphology and epidermal cell kinetics
of human corpse skin transplanted to *nude* mice, at least partly
because unforeseen alterations occurred spontaneously in the
skin after transplantation.   Because only one article (Duprez,
1979) has thus far systematically reported changes in normal
human skin transplanted to *nude* mice, we found it necessary to
perform a detailed study of the morphology and cell kinetics
in such grafts to define the basis for future investigations.

II.   MATERIALS AND METHODS

A.   Mice

We used 4- to 9-week-old male *nude* mice, representing the
first, third, and fourth cycles of a transfer of the *nu* gene
to the NC strain of inbred mice.   The animals were bred at
Pathological-Anatomical Institute, Kommunehospitalet, kept in
laminar flow benches, and caged separately on sterile wooden
granulate with free access to sterile food pellets and acidi-
fied chlorinated drinking water.

B. Grafting Technique

Skin was obtained from the front of the thighs of patients who had recently died in the hospital and who were submitted to autopsy. Patients with a clinical history or obvious signs of skin disease were omitted. The skin was washed for 10 min in sterile water and soap, shaved, and then greased with vaseline. With a hand-held dermatome set to a depth of 0.5 mm, skin pieces measuring approximately 10 × 5 cm were cut and placed with the dermis upward on sterile cork plates. From these pieces, 2 × 2-cm squares were cut and subsequently stored in phosphate-buffered saline containing penicillin G (0.5 IU/ml) and streptomycin (50 µg/ml) for up to 2 h until transplantation. The mice were anesthetized by an intraperitoneal injection of 0.5 ml propanidid (Epontol $^{®}$, Bayer AG, Federal Republic of Germany), whereupon a 2 × 2-cm square was excised from the mid-back skin and replaced by donor skin placed directly on the dorsal fascia. The grafts were fixed along the edges with the tissue adhesive Histoacryl $^{®}$ (Braun Melsungen, Federal Republic of Germany). Bandage was not applied. Samples of donor skin were prepared for histological examination using the same principles as the grafts (see follow section).

C. Experimental Groups

The study includes three series:

Group I. Skin from a 58-year-old man who died in hepatic coma caused by alcoholic cirrhosis was removed 12 h after death and was transplanted to 32 *nude* mice. Groups of 5 to 6 mice selected at random were killed 20, 40, 60, 81, and 104 days after the transplantation.

Group II. Skin from a 50-year-old man who died in hepatic coma caused by alcoholic cirrhosis was removed 18 h after death and was transplanted to 30 *nude* mice. Groups of 5 mice selected

at random were killed 10, 28, 43, and 99 days after the transplantation.

Group III. Skin from a 71-year old woman who died from
cerebral hemorrhage was removed 9 h after death and was transplanted to 31 *nude* mice. Groups of 7 mice selected at random
were killed 10, 31, and 94 days after the transplantation.

The donors were Caucasians, and the skin was in all cases
normal by microscopy (Fig. 1). Autolysis was indiscernible.
The dermis contained normal adnexal structures. Subcutaneous
components were not observed.

D. Morphological Observations

The mice were observed twice a week, and the appearance of
the grafts was noted. After the recipients had been killed by
neck extension, length and breadth of the grafts were measured.
After sacrifice, the grafts and surrounding 5 mm of mouse skin
were excised, divided along the median axis, and prepared for
histology. The material was mounted on Millipore filter ®
(Millipore Corp., Bedford, Massachusetts), fixed in formalin,
embedded in paraffin, and cut serially in 5-µm sections, which
were stained with hematoxylin-eosin, PAS, and a.m. van Gieson.
Toluidine blue, Perls' Prussian Blue, and Lillie's and
Verhoeff's methods were used for demonstration of, respectively,
metachromasia, iron, melanin, and elastin. The thickness of
the central portion of the grafts and of the donor material was
read in the microscope using a calibrated measuring eyepiece.

E. Autoradiography

An intraperitoneal injection of [^{3}H]thymidine in 0.5 ml
sterile water (100 µCi; specific activity 20 Ci/m*M*) was given
to the mice of groups I and III 1 h prior to sacrifice, which
took place in the period 10-12 A.M. Additional serial sections

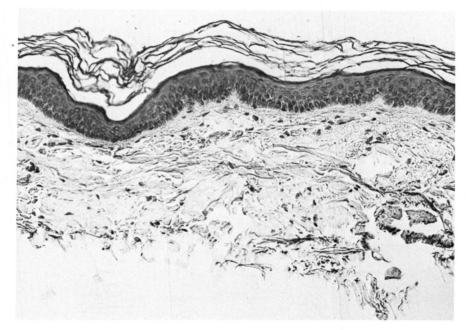

Fig. 1. Normal corpse split skin from the anterior femoral region. An arrector pili muscle is seen to the right (H&E, ×200).

of grafts from these groups were prepared by the following procedure: The deparaffinized slides were dipped in photographic emulsion under darkroom conditions (K-2, Ilford, England), diluted 1:1 by distilled water at 42°C, and thereupon dried in horizontal position at 20°C. After exposure at 4°C for 7 weeks the slides were developed and counterstained with hematoxylin-eosin. The labeling in nonulcerated central portions of the grafts was determined by counting epidermal cells containing five or more grains over the nuclei. Eight adjacent sections were counted by microscopy at a magnification of ×1000. Subsequently the sections were projected onto paper through a microscope, and tracings of the examined interfollicular epidermal surface were made. The length of the interfollicular epidermis was determined by analyzing the tracings with a calibrated

morphometric device (9874 A Digitizer, Hewlett-Packard, Greeley, Colorado). On an average, 5.20 mm were examined in each section Labeling index (LI) was calculated as the number of labeled cells per millimeter of interfollicular epidermis. The grafts of group II were additionally included in an ultrastructural study (to be described elsewhere). Therefore, the animals of this group were not injected with [^{3}H]thymidine in order to prevent possible cell damage due to self-irradiation (Aherne et al., 1977).

F. Autopsy

All mice, including those that died unexpectedly, were autopsied. Skin, lungs, heart, liver, spleen, and kidneys were removed and prepared for microscopy if not impossible because of autolysis. Mice that died naturally during the experimental period were not included in the graft study.

III. RESULTS

A. Fate of Mice

Table I shows that of the original 93 mice, 20 (21.5%) died unexpectedly before the scheduled histological graft study was carried out. Five mice were not sacrificed and were kept

TABLE I. Fate of *Nude* Mice in the Examination Period

	Number of mice			
Group	I	II	III	Total
Original stock	32	30	31	93
Dead during anesthesia	4	1	2	7
Naturally dead	0	8	5	13
Alive after end of experiment	1	1	3	5
Included in microscopic graft study	27	20	21	68

alive for further studies. Thus a total of 68 grafted mice
were included in the study of time-dependent changes distributed on 27, 20, and 21 grafts of group I, II, and III, respectively. Autopsy revealed no changes apart from visceral venous
stasis in the 7 mice that died during anesthesia. Hepatitis
and pneumonia, respectively, were the causes of death in 6 and
3 of the 13 mice that died naturally. In 4 cases autopsy
could not be performed because of cadaverosis. Autopsy was
normal in 52 of the mice included in the microscopic graft
study. In the remaining 16 mice, chronic pyelonephritis was
seen in 7, hepatitis in 6, and pneumonia in 4 cases. Additionally minor focal myocardial calcifications were seen in
2 mice.

B. Macroscopic Findings

The pattern of fine crossing lines and rhombic areas
characterizing human skin of the femoral region was retained
in the experimental periods, although it was partly obscured
in the middle of the periods by strong hyperkeratosis and subsequent scaling. The grafts were initially pale with a
yellowish hue, but turned faintly red in less than 2 weeks.
In the following period a gradually increasing brownish coloring was seen. This was by far most pronounced in group II, in
which all grafts had become heavily dark brown 6 weeks after
transplantation (Fig. 2A, B, and C).

The grafts shrank considerably and fairly equally in the
three experimental groups shortly after transplantation (Fig.
3), and at the end of the study ($\sim$ Day 100) the average graft
size was reduced to 1.2 cm^2 or 30% of the original 4.0 cm^2.
No grafts were rejected, but during the first month central
bulla formation was noted in 13 cases or 19.1%, equally distributed over the three groups. After 1 to 2 weeks the bullae
were followed by nonhealing ulcers.

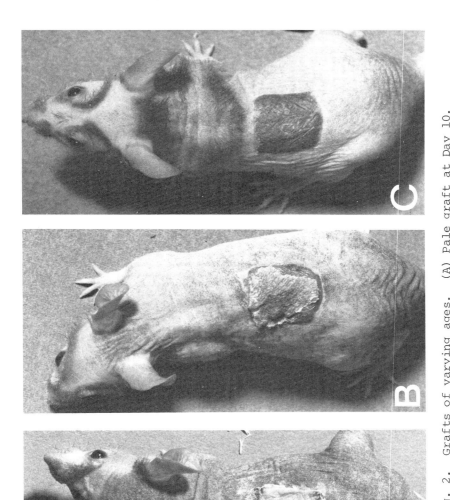

Fig. 2. Grafts of varying ages. (A) Pale graft at Day 10.
(B) Graft with scaling hyperkeratosis at Day 43. (C) Heavily
darkened graft at Day 99. Note slightly decreasing size with time.

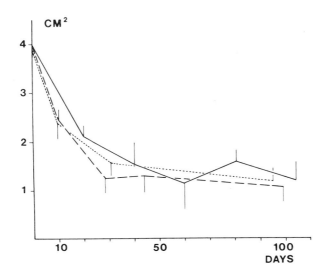

Fig. 3.   Mean and standard deviation of graft area size in groups I (solid line), II (long dashes), and III (short dashes), at varying graft age.

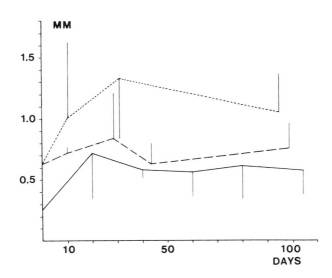

Fig. 4.   Mean and standard deviation of graft thickness in groups I, II, and III at varying graft age.   See Fig. 3 for identification of curves.

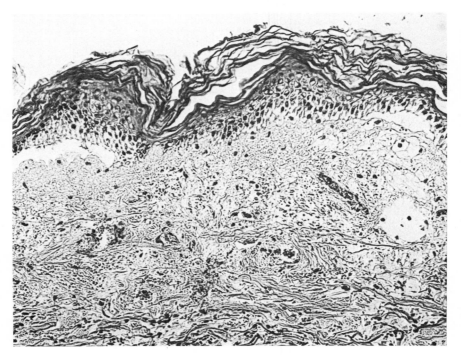

Fig. 5. Graft 10 days after the transplantation. In epidermis pronounced spongiosis and intracellular edema are present. Small vesicles are seen beneath the epidermis; in the dermis, severe edema is evident (H&E, ×200).

C. Microscopic Findings

The thickness of the skin increased shortly after transplantation to reach a maximum averaging 210% of the original values after 20 to 31 days (Fig. 4). Thereafter a slight decline was seen. Thus about Day 100, at the end of the experimental periods, the average graft thickness was 186% of the initial figure.

The grafts of the three experimental groups underwent a series of histological changes, some of which are illustrated in Figs. 5, 6, and 7 and summarized in Tables II, III, and IV. From the items listed in these tables it can be seen that the

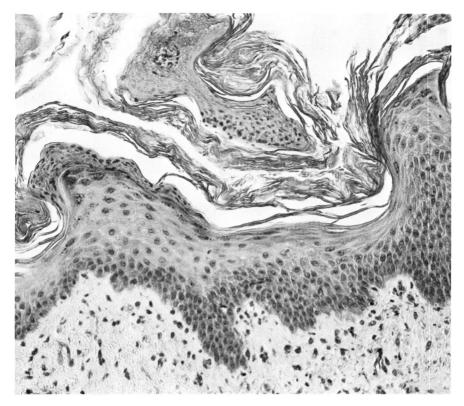

Fig. 6. Graft 31 days after the transplantation. The
epidermis is hyperplastic with marked acanthosis. The surface
is covered by parakeratinized scales (H&E, ×200).

skin of the three donors followed a general pattern, although
some diversity may be noted. Thus spongiosis, hydropic degeneration of basal cells, and bulla formation were dominating
features of the first experimental month, but were absent beyond
Day 40. The bullae, which contained fibrin and varying numbers
of neutrophil leukocytes, were subepidermal and covered by a
partially necrotic epidermis. Ulcers were not registered before Day 31. Irregular acanthosis, which was seen throughout
the experimental periods, reached a maximal frequency between
Day 31 and Day 43. It was by far most frequent in group III,

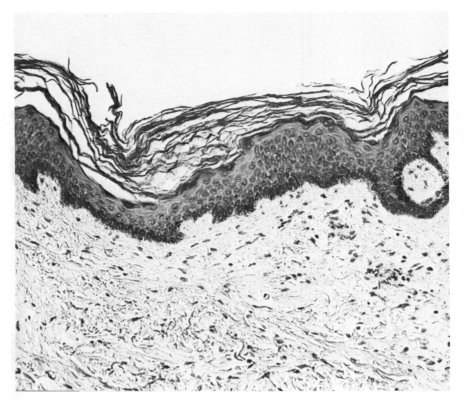

Fig. 7. Graft 99 days after the transplantation. The morphology of epidermis is normal except for slight hyperkeratosis and pronounced hyperpigmentation of the basal layer. The dermis is fibrotic (H&E, ×200).

in which all grafts had a thickened Malpighian layer at Day 31. The frequency of hyperkeratosis and concomitant focal parakeratosis had a similar distribution, with figures of 100% at Day 40, 28, and 31 in groups I, II, and III, respectively. Early in the study the parakeratotic areas were located in the deep part of the corneal layer, later on superficially. Increased melanin content of the basal layer was seen after Day 20 (group I) and was observed in 52.9% of the grafts at the end of the study.

TABLE II.   Histological Findings in the Grafts of Group I in
           Relation to Graft Age

Histological findings	Graft age (days)				
	20	40	60	81	104
Epidermal					
Spongiosis	6/6[a]	1/6	0/5	0/5	0/5
Hydropic degeneration					
of basal cells	6/6	4/6	0/5	0/5	0/5
Bullae	2/6	0/6	0/5	0/5	0/5
Ulcers	0/6	2/6	0/5	1/5	0/5
Irregular acanthosis	1/6	3/6	0/5	1/5	1/5
Hyperkeratosis with					
focal parakeratosis	5/6	6/6	2/5	3/5	1/5
Increased melanin	1/6	0/6	4/5	3/5	3/5
Dermal					
Edema and vascular					
dilation	6/6	4/6	0/5	0/5	0/5
Fibrosis	0/6	6/6	5/5	5/5	5/5
Melanophages	5/6	5/6	5/5	5/5	5/5

[a]The fractions indicate the number of grafts exhibiting
a particular finding in relation to the total grafts of a
given age. For example, of six grafts examined on Day 20,
all six exhibited spongiosis.

In the dermis, edema and pronounced dilation of arterio-
les, capillaries, and venules were seen in all grafts at Days
10 and 20. This vascular reaction, which was accompanied by
infiltration of neutrophils and macrophages and by extravasation of minor numbers of erythrocytes, gradually subsided as
fibrosis began. The fibrosis resulted in a reticular dermis
of thick hyaline bundles of collagen lying almost in parallel
to the surface and with a decreased number of vessels and fibroblasts. The upper dermis contained a varying number of
scattered melanophages and small amounts of hemosiderin after
Day 20.

Apart from extensive necrosis of keratinocytes seen in
relation to the previously mentioned initial bulla formation,

TABLE III.   Histological Findings in the Grafts of Group II in
             Relation to Graft Age

Histological findings	Graft age (days)			
	10	28	43	99
Epidermal				
Spongiosis	5/5[a]	0/5	0/5	0/5
Hydropic degeneration				
of basal cells	5/5	0/5	0/5	0/5
Bullae	1/5	2/5	0/5	0/5
Ulcers	0/5	0/5	0/5	1/5
Irregular acanthosis	0/5	3/5	4/5	3/5
Hyperkeratosis with				
focal parakeratosis	2/5	5/5	4/5	3/5
Increased melanin	0/5	5/5	5/5	2/5
Dermal				
Edema and vascular				
dilation	5/5	5/5	0/5	1/5
Fibrosis	0/5	5/5	5/5	5/5
Melanophages	0/5	5/5	5/5	5/5

[a]For explanation of fractions, see Table II.

single necrotic keratinocytes were seen scattered in the epidermis of all grafts throughout the study.   They appeared as
rounded eosinophilic PAS-positive bodies averaging 10 μm in
diameter.   Nuclear material was partially disintegrated or absent.   Adnexal structures were poorly preserved in the grafts
of group I, of which the donor material was relatively thin
(0.25 mm).   Thus only single arrector pili muscles were seen
in one graft beyond Day 20.   In the initially thicker (0.63 mm)
grafts of groups II and III the skin appendages except the
sebaceous glands were well preserved.   Thus at the end of the
study, hairs, arrector muscles, sweat glands, and sebaceous
glands were seen in, respectively, 58, 75, 33, and 0% of the
grafts.   The hair roots were often angulated, so that the
terminal portion ending in the bulb lay deeply in the dermis
paralleling the surface.

TABLE IV.   Histological Findings in the Grafts of Group III
            in Relation to Graft Age

	Graft age (days)		
Histological findings	10	31	94
Epidermal			
Spongiosis	7/7[a]	5/7	0/7
Hydropic degeneration of basal cells	7/7	0/7	0/7
Bullae	1/7	0/7	0/7
Ulcers	0/7	3/7	0/7
Irregular acanthosis	0/7	7/7	4/7
Hyperkeratosis with focal parakera-			
tosis	0/7	7/7	0/7
Increased melanin	0/7	0/7	4/7
Dermal			
Edema and vascular dilation	7/7	1/7	0/7
Fibrosis	0/7	7/7	7/7
Melanophages	0/7	4/7	7/7

[a]For explanation of fractions, see Table II.

A sharp line between human and murine tissue was observed
in the dermal zone. The human dermis contained coarse collagen
and few mast cells, whereas the murine dermis had delicate collagen fibres and was relatively rich in mast cells.   In the
majority of the specimens also a well-defined epidermal transitional zone was seen. As early as Day 10 the two epithelia
had fused and the two- to three-layered murine epidermis merged
into the four- to six-layered human epidermis through a zone of
20 to 30 μm.

D. Autoradiography

The results of the labeling index study are presented in
Table V, which makes it clear that the mean of LI in group III
was initially very low (0.15 counts/mm at Day 10) but increased
considerably at Day 31 (27.90 counts/mm) and became again rather
low (2.69 counts/mm) at Day 94.   Concerning group I quite

TABLE V.   Mean and Standard Deviation of Labeling Index (LI)
           in the Grafts in Relation to Graft Age

Group	Graft age (days)	Mean of LI (counts/mm)[a]
I	20	4.15 (134)
	40	6.21 (117)
	60	4.04 (62)
	81	3.72 (61)
	104	4.17 (31)
II	--	Not done
III	10	0.15 (220)
	31	27.90 (76)
	94	2.69 (36)

[a]*Standard deviation given as a percentage in parentheses.*

another pattern was observed, as a relatively high mean of LI
seen initially (4.15 counts/mm at Day 20) remained throughout
the experimental period.   It also appears that great variation
occurred even between grafts from the same donor and of equal
age.   However, the standard deviation decreased (expressed in
percentage of the mean) from 134 to 31% in group I and from
220 to 36% in group III during the study.

     Besides, the autoradiography specimens showed that the
labeling was restricted to the basal epidermal layer, except
for one graft in which additional single labeled cells occurred superficially in the spinous layer.   At Day 10 no labeling was seen over the nuclei of the epithelial cells of the
sweat glands and hair roots present in group III.   A heavy
labeling of these structures was seen at Day 31, whereas only
hair bulbs were labeled at Day 94.

IV. DISCUSSION

   Although great variation was seen even between skin grafts
from the same donor, certain features showed a general tendency
and illustrated the mechanisms of the graft healing. From a
practical point of view, the changes may be considered as early,
intermediate, and late-occurring, respectively, during the
first, second, and third months of the observation period.

A. Early Changes

   The same mechanisms that rule the healing of homografted
human split skin are reflected in the morphological changes in
the heterografted human skin of this investigation. Thus the
initial spongiosis and hydropic degeneration of basal cells reflected an early ischemic epidermal injury, which in 13 cases
(19.1%) additionally resulted in extensive epidermal necrosis
and formation of bullae and ulcers. Identical early changes
in human corpse split skin transplanted to *nude* mice have been
reported by Duprez (1979), who noted that the areas of epidermal
necrosis topographically corresponded to dermal hypovascularized
zones. In studies of human skin transplanted to *nude* mice,
Rygaard (1973, 1974) constantly found superficial necrosis at
the center of the grafts, probably because relatively thick
donor material was used. Cubie (1976) noticed that an intact
panniculus carnosus in the graft bed enabled vascularization
and healing, and prevented formation of central necrosis of
normal human split skin transplanted to *nude* mice. In the
present study blood circulation had been established in the
grafts at Day 10, possibly through a proliferation of new
vessels stimulated by epidermis, as reported by Ryan and Kurban
(1970) and Wolf and Harrison (1973) in their studies of injured and transplanted epidermis, respectively. The vessels

were dilated, and the concomitant dermal edema explains the
initial thickening of the grafts.

Although the murine and the human epithelia had already
fused along a well-defined zone before Day 10 after the transplantation, it cannot be excluded that murine keratinocytes
later on have invaded the human epidermis, particularly considering the epidermal damage and regeneration in the grafts.
In this investigation only the different morphology of the murine and human epidermis makes the human identity of the grafts
probable. However, other investigators have developed skin
marker systems for the *nude* mouse-human skin graft system.
Thus Brigaman (1980) has reported that markers of Y chromosomes
and of the ABH blood group are maintained in human epidermis
transplanted to *nude* mice for at least 2 months. These findings are supported by Haftek *et al*. (1981), who showed that a
distinct limit between human graft keratinocytes and those of
the *nude* mouse recipient was present for not less than 30 days
using an antiserum specifically binding to human keratin.

B.   Intermediate Changes

Acanthosis and hyperkeratosis with focal parakeratosis and
subsequent scaling observed macroscopically reached a maximal
frequency during the second month after transplantation in the
three experimental groups. Similar alterations have previously been described in human skin transplanted to *nude* mice.
Thus Krueger *et al*. (1975) observed sloughing crusts and parakeratosis 2 weeks after transplantation of involved and nonin-
volved psoriatic human skin to *nude* mice, and Haftek *et al*.
(1981) showed that acanthosis and thickening of the granular
layer occurred in normal human split skin maintained for over
20 days on *nude* mice. Such changes, which in principle are
identical to those seen in various types of dermatitis (exzema),

may be regarded as signs of a transient pronounced regeneration of the epidermis following the initial injury.

In this period another characteristic finding was a persistent brownish coloring of the grafts, which was determined partly by the presence of dermal melanophages and hemosiderin and partly by an increased melanin content of the basal epidermal layer. Similar pigmentary alterations have been noted by other investigators of human skin transplanted to *nude* mice (Reed and Manning, 1973; Duprez, 1979). The melanophages present in the dermis indicate previous damage to the epidermis, with necrosis of keratinocytes and melanocytes, and subsequent loss of melanin into the dermis, a phenomenon that is often encountered in microscopic specimens from cuteneous lesions with injury of the basal epidermal layer (e.g., lichen planus and lupus erythematosus). Whether the increased epidermal melanin in the same way represents a postinflammatory pigmentary alteration or in addition is a result of a murine hormonal stimulation, as proposed by Duprez (1979), is uncertain.

C. Late Changes

Except for the previously mentioned persistent hyperpigmentation of the basal layer, the epidermis gradually returned to normalcy during the third month after transplantation as irregular acanthosis and hyperkeratosis subsided. Pigmentary changes were also still present in dermis, but the initial edema was eventually followed by a strong fibrosis explaining the thickening and considerable shrinkage, which was also found by Yuspa *et al.* (1979) in their study of human foreskin transplanted to *nude* mice.

Long-term preservation of adnexal structures seems to be dependent on the initial graft thickness, as the grafts of 0.25 mm initial thickness (group I) preserved only single ar-

rector pili muscles, whereas hairs and sweat glands additionally were maintained in the 0.63-mm grafts (groups II and III).
This study confirms the finding of Duprez (1979) that sebaceous
glands are often destroyed.

D. Cell Kinetics

In the autoradiography study it was noted that the labeling indices of group I and III took different trends. Nevertheless it appears that the epithelial regeneration, as judged
by morphology, had temporal connection with the maxima of the
mean of the calculated labeling indices in the two groups.
This was by far most pronounced in group III, which showed a
distinct maximum at Day 31 and less marked in group I at Day
40, as the means of LI in this group only showed minor differences during the experimental period. The great variation in
LI even between grafts of equal age and origin was presumably
caused by differences in initial epidermal injury and subsequent regeneration, as it showed a falling tendency toward the
end of the experimental period, when the epidermal morphology
became less disturbed.

An important inference that can be drawn from these findings is that transplantation can trigger epidermal cell proliferation. Care should therefore be taken in future experiments
(e.g., carcinogenesis studies) comprising cell kinetic investigations of the human corpse skin-*nude* mouse model, in comparing
results from different donors and in choosing appropriate experimental periods.

E. Morbidity in the *Nude* Mouse Colony

The autopsy study confirms numerous other reports of a
high susceptibility to infectious agents of *nude* mice kept under semiconventional conditions. As in the study of Sharkey

(1978), the majority of natural deaths were caused by hepatitis and pneumonia. These diseases were also detected in the group of mice sacrificed in the graft study, as well as cases of chronic pyelonephritis and myocardial calcifications. The findings emphasize the necessity to keep the health of *nude* mouse colonies under close surveillance (e.g., by autopsy), as various diseases may be expected to influence experimental results.

V.   CONCLUSION

This study has shown that human corpse skin can be successfully transplanted to *nude* mice at least until 18 h postmortem. The morphology and epidermal cell kinetics of the grafts showed considerable temporal, intradonor, and interdonor variation. However, certain general features indicated that the grafts after an initial ischemic phase underwent epidermal proliferation and dermal fibrosis during the second month after transplantation. If these changes are taken into account, the human corpse skin-*nude* mouse model seems advantageous for studies of skin carcinogenesis as it permits long-term maintenance of large quantities of human skin of identical regional and genetic origin.

REFERENCES

Aherne, W. A., Camplejohn, R. S., and Wright, N. A. (1977).
     "An Introduction to Cell Population Kinetics." Arnold,
     London.
Briggaman, R. A. (1980). *Curr. Probl. Dermatol.* 10, 115-126.
Cubie, H. A. (1976). *Br. J. Dermatol.* 94, 659-665.
Duprez, A. (1979). *C.R. Hebd. Seances Acad. Sci. Ser. D 288,*
     1505-1508.

Haftek, M., Ortonne, J., Staquet, M., Viac, J., and Thivolet,
    J. (1981). *J. Invest. Dermatol.* *76*, 48-52.
Krueger, G. G., Manning, D. D., Malouf, J., and Ogden, B.
    (1975). *J. Invest. Dermatol.* *64*, 307-312.
Reed, N. D., and Manning, D. D. (1973). *Proc. Soc. Exp. Biol.*
    Med. *143*, 350-353.
Ryan, T. J., and Kurban, A. K. (1970). *Br. J. Dermatol.* *82*
    (Suppl. 5), 92-98.
Rygaard, J. (1973). "Thymus and Self. Immunobiology of the
    Mouse Mutant Nude." Wiley, London.
Rygaard, J. (1974). *Acta Pathol. Microbiol. Scand. Sect. A*
    82, 105-112.
Sharkey, F. E. (1978). *In* "The Nude Mouse in Experimental and
    Clinical Research" (J. Fogh and B. C. Giovanella, eds.),
    Vol. 1, pp. 75-93. Academic Press, New York.
Wolf, J. E., and Harrison, R. G. (1973). *J. Invest. Dermatol.*
    61, 130-141.
Yuspa, S. H., Viguera, C., and Nims, R. (1979). *Cancer Lett.*
    (Shannon, Irel.) *6*, 301-310.

II. Metabolism of Chemical Carcinogenesis, DNA Damage, and DNA Repair

7

METABOLISM OF CHEMICAL CARCINOGENS BY HUMAN TISSUES

Herman Autrup and Curtis C. Harris

Laboratory of Human Carcinogenesis
National Cancer Institute
Bethesda, Maryland

I. INTRODUCTION

Many chemical compounds and processes have been implicated in the induction of human cancer, and many more chemicals have been found to induce cancer in experimental animals (Report of an IARC Working Group, 1980). Because most of these chemical carcinogens require metabolic activation before they can exert their mutagenic and carcinogenic effects, it is obviously important to determine if human target tissues can metabolize these compounds into their ultimate carcinogenic forms. Furthermore, it is important to study the metabolic pathways of

potential chemical carcinogens in different human organs and
to compare them under identical experimental conditions with
the activation in animal tissues in which the compounds are
known to induce cancer. If the metabolic pathways are quantitatively and qualitatively similar, one might assume that the
compound is a potential human carcinogen for that particular
organ. Another important aspect of these studies is to elucidate the possible role of metabolism in relationship to the
organ specificity shown by many chemical carcinogens, and furthermore, whether the metabolic differences among individuals
could be partly responsible for the wide susceptibility seen in
the induction of some forms of human cancer (e.g., cigarette
smoking and lung cancer).

Early studies on carcinogen metabolism using human tissues were mostly done by measuring cytochrome P-450 and related
enzyme activity such as aryl hydrocarbon hydroxylase in subcellular fractions of human liver and lung. These cell-free
preparations were also used as activation systems for mutagenesis and transformation assays (Bartsch et al., 1980).
However, the development of improved culture conditions for
human tissues and cells (Harris et al., 1980) has made possible
the study of activation of chemical carcinogens in intact human target tissues, such as breast, bronchus, bladder, colon,
esophagus, endometrium, and skin (Autrup, 1982).

II.   MATERIALS AND METHODS

Normal-appearing human tissues were obtained at either
surgery or immediate autopsy, and kept at 4°C in L-15 medium
until cultured as explants (Trump et al., 1974; Harris et al.,
1980). These explants were cultured for 1 to 7 days before
treatment with radioactively labeled carcinogens at a nontoxic

dose, as determined by morphological criteria. After incubation for 24 h, the mucosa was scraped from the supporting tissues, and DNA was isolated for quantitation of the metabolic
activity as measured by level of binding of carcinogen to cellular DNA, and for qualitative analysis of carcinogen-DNA adducts (Harris et al., 1976b; Autrup et al., 1978b, 1979).
Binding of the carcinogens to cellular macromolecules represents only a minor part of the metabolic activity but is probably one of the most important parameters in relation to
chemical induction of cancer. Tissue culture media were analyzed for carcinogen metabolites excreted from cells and explants (Yang et al., 1977).

Culture of the tissues prior to incubation with carcinogens appears to be important for two reasons: (1) to minimize
the effect of any exogenous exposure to inducers of the mixed-
function oxidase (MFO) system, such as cigarette smoking and
drug therapy, and (2) to reverse the cellular ischemia observed
in most tissues immediately following surgery. Prior to culture the mitochondria and the endoplasmic reticulum are dilated
(Fig. 1A). This ischemic damage is reversed after a few hours
in culture (Barrett et al., 1977; Fig. 1B), which is accompanied by a significant increase in the cytochrome P-450-associated
enzyme activity (M. Khang and B. Trump, unpublished).

III. INTERSPECIES VARIATION

The metabolism of chemical carcinogens has been studied in
both explant and cell cultures of human target tissues and experimental animals (Table I). These compounds include polycyclic aromatic hydrocarbons such as benzo[a]pyrene (BP) and
7,12-dimethylbenz[a]anthracene (DMBA), cyclic and acyclic aliphatic N-nitrosamines, methylhydrazines, aromatic amines, and

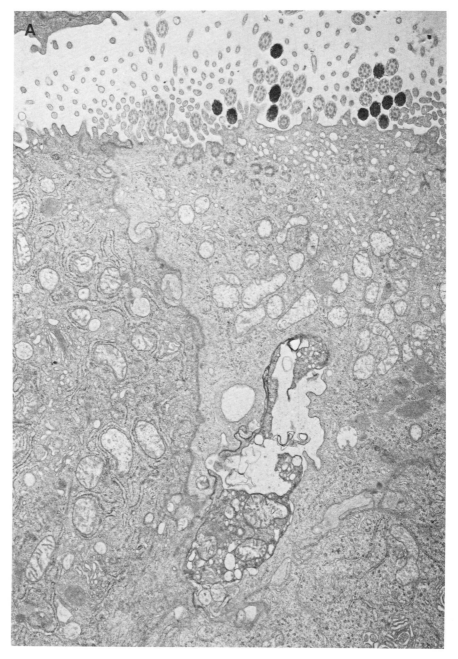

Fig. 1.   (A) Human bronchus epithelial cells obtained at
immediate autopsy (0 time).   Although mitochondria are somewhat
swollen, other organelles retain a normal appearance (×14,000).
(Courtesy of L. A. Barrett.)

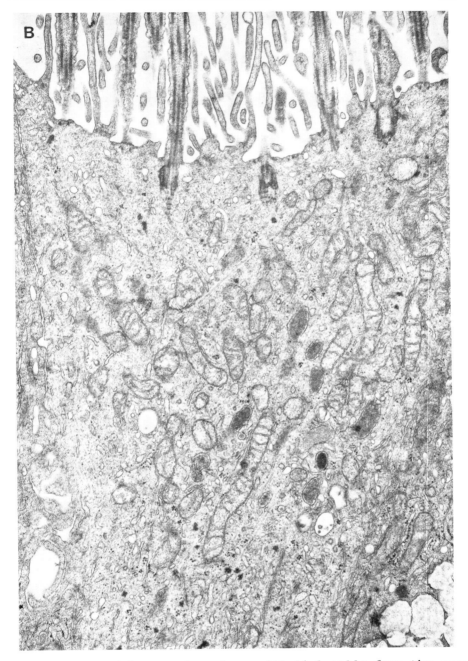

Fig. 1. (B) Human bronchus epithelial cells from the same case as shown in (A) following 4 days in organ culture. Note that the ultrastructure of the ciliated cell is well preserved (×14,000). (Courtesy of L. A. Barrett.)

TABLE I.   Metabolism of Benzo[a]pyrene by Cultured Human and
           Animal Tissues

Tissue	Human explant	Human cells	Experimental animals
Bladder	X[a]	X	Rat, monkey, dog, hamster
Breast	n.d.[b]	X	n.d.
Bronchus	X	X	Rat, mouse, hamster, dog
Colon	X	n.d.	Rat
Duodenum	X	n.d.	n.d.
Endometrium	X	n.d.	n.d.
Esophagus	X	X	Rat
Skin	n.d.	X	Mouse

[a]Carcinogen-DNA adducts formed.
[b]n.d., Not done.

a mycotoxin, aflotoxin B_1 (AFB) (Cohen et al., 1979; Harris
et al., 1976b, 1979; Autrup et al., 1978a,b, 1979, 1981,
1982; Stoner et al., 1978, 1982a,b; Dorman et al., 1981;
Lechner et al., 1981; Mass et al., 1981; Kuroki et al., 1982;
Moore et al., 1982). In addition, cultured explants of fetal
liver, stomach, and esophagus metabolized several of these
compounds (Table II; H. Autrup, unpublished). The metabolism
of BP, a ubiquitous chemical compound that induces cancer at
several sites in experimental animals, has been extensively
studied. A schematic representation of the major metabolic
pathways leading to the formation of the predominant carcinogen-
DNA adduct is shown in Fig. 2. At least three different enzymatic steps, two different cytochrome P-450-associated mixed-
function oxidases (MFO's) and an epoxide hydrolase (EH), are
involved in formation of the major adduct that is formed by
transaddition of (7R)-7,8-diol 9,10-epoxide BP (7R-BPDE I) to
the 2-amino group of guanine. Minor adducts have also been
identified (Autrup et al., 1980a). In addition, prostaglandin

TABLE II.   Carcinogen Metabolism in Cultured Fetal Human Tissues

| Carcinogen | Metabolism (pmol/10 mg DNA) | | |
	Esophagus	Liver	Stomach
Benzo[a]pyrene	9	25	55
Aflatoxin B_1	--[a]	31	n.d.
N-Nitrosodimethylamine	--	220	n.d.
N-Nitrosodiethylamine	2090	n.d.[b]	5085
N-Nitrosopyrrolidine	90	n.d.	710
N-Nitrosobenzylmethylamine	110	n.d.	490

[a]--, No detectable binding to DNA.
[b]n.d., Not done.

endoperoxidase synthetase can also mediate activation of
BP 7,8-diol into the ultimate carcinogen (Sivarajah et al.,
1981).   Competing metabolic reactions also take place, such as
formation of phenols, diols, and tetrols.   Furthermore, these
primary and secondary metabolites can be conjugated to form
sulfate esters, glucuronides, or glutathione conjugates.   The
rate difference between the pathway leading to BP-DNA adducts
and the competing pathways may reflect the risk of a particular
animal species or organ to the carcinogenic action of BP.

High-pressure liquid chromatography (HPLC) of enzymatically
hydrolyzed DNA (Jeffrey et al., 1977) revealed that the same
BP-DNA adducts are formed in the same organ from different animal species (Table III); repair rates of the various BP-DNA
adducts were also similar in human and hamster tracheobronchial
tissues after culturing the explants for an additional 24 h
without BP (Autrup et al., 1980a).   It has been suggested that
the adduct formed by further oxidation of 9-hydroxy-BP comigrates with the 7S-BPDE I-Gua adduct by the HPLC separation
(Chapter 8, this volume).   The adducts formed in rat trachea
were slightly different, in that approximately 20% of the adducts were formed between BPDE and adenine.   Similar observations were made by incubating BP with rat colon and esophagus,

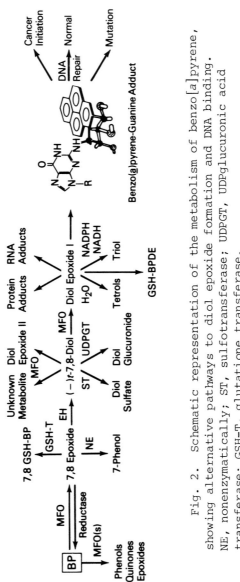

Fig. 2. Schematic representation of the metabolism of benzo[a]pyrene, showing alternative pathways to diol epoxide formation and DNA binding. NE, nonenzymatically; ST, sulfotransferase; UDPGT, UDPglucuronic acid transferase; GSH-T, glutatione transferase.

TABLE III. Benzo[a]pyrene–DNA Adducts Formed in Cultured Tissues[a]

Tissue	Unknown I	Unknown II	7S-BPDE I-Gua	7R-BPDE I-Gua	BPDE II-Gua	BPDE-Ade
			Adduct (%)			
Experimental animals (trachea)						
Hamster	--[b]	6	7	71	16	--
Rat (CD)	--	12	30	22	13	22
Mouse (DBA/2N)	--	3	4	83	10	--
Human						
Bronchus	9	8	21	56	7	--
Colon	--	10	5	62	13	4
Duodenum	--	22	10	52	12	4
Esophagus	--	28	7	59	6	--

[a]The adducts were analyzed as described by Jeffrey et al. (1977). The results are expressed as percentage of total identified adducts.
[b]--, Not detectable.

and with tracheal tissues from different strains of rats
(Autrup *et al.,* 1983a). When compared to results from studies
using cultured human bronchus, Syrian golden hamsters, a
species susceptible to the carcinogenic action of BP and in
which the induced tumors are morphologically similar to those
of human bronchial carcinoma, have both similar mean binding
level of BP to tracheal DNA and also a similar amount of metabolism as expressed in picomoles of metabolites per microgram
DNA. Furthermore, both human and hamster tracheobronchial
tissues were less efficient in conjugating the primary metabolites than tissues from species in which BP does not induce
bronchogenic carcinoma. Furthermore, no qualitative differences in the type of organic-soluble metabolites were observed.

A detailed comparative study on the metabolism of
N-nitrosamines has been made in human and rat esophagus (Autrup
and Stoner, 1982). This is of special interest, because
several *N*-nitrosamines induce esophageal cancer in the rats.
The level of metabolism in human and rat esophagus is the same
for symmetrical aliphatic *N*-nitrosamines, that is, *N*-nitrosodi-
methylamine (DMNA) and *N*-nitrosodiethylamine, but significantly
higher in the rat for cyclic and asymmetric *N*-nitrosamines, especially *N*-nitrosobenzylmethylamine (BMNA), an organospecific
carcinogen for the rat esophagus. Hecht *et al.* (1982) have
also reported that the metabolism of two tobacco-specific
N-nitrosamines, *N*-nitrosonornicotine and 4-(methylnitrosamino)-
1-(3-pyridyl)-1-butanone, was higher in rat esophagus than in
human. The first step in the metabolism of most *N*-nitrosamines
involves an α oxidation with the subsequent formation of an
alkylcarbonium ion that reacts with electronegative sites of
cellular macromolecules. In the case of BMNA, the major alkylation species was the methylcarbonium ion, as measured by using
BMNA labeled either in the methyl or in the benzyl group. The
major adducts were identified as O^6- and 7-methylguanine, with

TABLE IV.   Binding Level of Benzo[a]pyrene (BP) and Aflatoxin
            B_1 (AFB) to DNA in Explant Culture of Human Tissues[a]

Human tissue type	BP	AFB	Interindividual variation in BP metabolism
Bladder	6.4	1.7	55
Bronchus	1.0	0.5	75
Colon	0.3	0.1	150
Duodenum	0.6	0.4	50
Endometrium	0.1	n.d.	n.d.
Esophagus	0.7	0.4	99
Liver (fetal)	n.d.[b]	0.7	n.d.

[a]*Number of modifications per 10^6 nucleotides.*
[b]*n.d., Not done.*

a ratio of the two products of 0.12, a ratio similar to that
found with other methylating carcinogens in other organs
(Autrup and Stoner, 1982).   The preference for oxidation of the
methylene group was also supported by the observation of a 10-
fold higher level of benzaldehyde than formaldehyde and CO_2.
An even higher level of oxidation at the methylene group was
observed when rat esophageal subcellular fractions were used as
the activating system (Labuc and Archer, 1982).

IV.   ORGAN DIFFERENCES

The metabolism of BP and AFB has been studied in explant
cultures from several human organs (Harris *et al.*, 1976a, 1977b,
1979; Autrup *et al.*, 1979, 1982; Dorman *et al.*, 1981; Mass *et
al.*, 1981; Stoner *et al.*, 1982a,b).   The highest mean binding
level for both carcinogens was found in bladder (Table IV),
being six- and threefold, respectively, higher than values observed in bronchus.   Less difference was noted between the
other organs.   In most cases binding level of BP appears to be
greater than that of AFB in the same individual (Table V).

TABLE V. Comparison of DNA-Binding Levels of Benzo[a]pyrene (BP) and Aflatoxin B$_1$ (AFB) to DNA in Cultured Tissues from Immediate Autopsies[a]

Organ	BP			AFB			Binding of BP/AFB	Correlation coefficient
	Mean value	Range	No. of cases	Mean value	Range	No. of cases		
Bronchus	0.80	0.03-5.12	26	0.51	0.03-2.94	28	18/25	-0.20
Colon	0.26	<0.03-1.47	27	0.26	<0.03-1.47	24	14/22	-0.08
Duodenum	0.67	<0.03-1.86	10	0.73	<0.03-4.10	11	6/8	0.67
Esophagus	0.86	<0.03-3.33	11	0.35	<0.03 1.06	11	7/9	0.02

[a]Values given as number of modifications per 10^6 nucleotides.

A positive correlation has been found between the binding
of BP to DNA in human bronchus and colon/duodenum (Autrup *et*
al., 1982). Unfortunately, the numbers of patients are as yet
too few to indicate that if an individual is a high metabolizer
in one particular organ the same would be true for another organ
as well. Furthermore, our results indicate that this correlation will be valid only for that particular group of chemical
carcinogens, because different types of cytochrome *P*-450s may
be involved in the formation of the ultimate carcinogens; although a positive correlation has been found between the level
of binding of 7,12-DMBA and BP in human bronchus (Harris *et*
al., 1977b), and between BP and 1,2-dimethylhydrazine in human
colon (Autrup *et al.*, 1980b), no correlation has been found between BP and AFB (Table V), or BP and DMNA in either organ
(H. Autrup, unpublished).

The major BP-DNA adducts were identical in all the human
organs (Table III). A small variation in the relative distribution of the various adducts was observed in colon from
different individuals (Autrup *et al.*, 1978b). The adduct profiles were similar to the ones formed in the corresponding
cultured tissues from experimental animals. However, different
profiles were observed in both lung and liver after *in vivo* administration of [^{3}H]BP to rats (Boroujerdi *et al.*, 1981) and
when microsomal preparations were used as the activating system
(Pelkonen *et al.*, 1978).

The total metabolism of BP, as measured by pmol metabolites
per μg DNA, was highest in cultured bronchus followed by duodenum, esophagus, and colon. Some quantitative differences were
also observed in the distribution of BP metabolites released
into the culture media. The major organic-soluble metabolites
in most organs were tetrols and diols (Table VI). The higher
level of BP tetrols in bronchus and the slightly greater amount
of BP 7,8-diol in colon and duodenum may indicate that the

TABLE VI.   Metabolism of Benzo[a]pyrene to Organic-Soluble
            Metabolites Cultured by Human Tissues[a]

Major metabolites	Bronchus[b]	Bladder[c]	Colon[b]	Duodenum[b]	Esophagus[b]	Skin[c]
Tetrols	21	19	4	6	14	41
9,10-Diol	28	21	19	20	32	21
7,8-Diol	5	10	9	12	14	4
9-Hydroxy	4	3	2	3	2	6
3-Hydroxy	2	10	27	26	14	5

[a]*The ethyl acetate/acetone-extractable metabolites were
analyzed by HPLC as described by Yang et al. (1977), and the
results expressed as percentage of total organic-soluble metabolites.*
[b]*Autrup et al. (1982).*
[c]*Selkirk et al. (1982).*

latter organs have a smaller amount of the form of cytochrome
P-450 that is specific for conversion of BP diols to diol
epoxides (Gozuhara et al., 1982).   In addition, the higher
relative level of BP phenols in colon and duodenum suggest that
these organs are relatively deficient in the conjugation of the
BP phenols into glucuronides and sulfate esters.   The accumulation of BP phenols in gastrointestinal tissues may be important,
because these metabolites could be further metabolized into DNA-
binding species (Nordenskjold et al., 1978).   Sulfate esters
seem to be the predominant conjugated metabolites of BP in cultured normal human bronchus and colon, but a change in conjugation pattern to predominantly glucuronides occurs in tumorous
tissues (Cohen et al., 1983).   The BP metabolite profile in
cultured fetal human tissues appears to be more complex than
that in adult tissues.   An association between the total
amount of BP tetrols and diols and the level of binding to
DNA was observed in human bronchus (Autrup, 1982).

TABLE VII.   Metabolism of *N*-Nitrosamines by Cultured Adult Human Tissues[a]

N-Nitrosamine	Bronchus	Colon	Esophagus	Pancreatic duct
N-Nitrosodimethylamine	+	+	+	+
N-Nitrosodiethylamine	+	+	+	n.d.
N-Nitrosopyrrolidine	+	+	−	n.d.
N-Nitrosonornicotine	−	n.d.	−	n.d.
N-Dinitrosopiperazine	+	+	n.d.	n.d.
N-Nitrosopiperidine	+	−	−	n.d.
N-Nitrosobenzylmethyl-amine	n.d.[b]	n.d.	−	n.d.

[a]*References: Autrup et al. (1978b); Harris et al. (1977a, 1979).*
[b]*n.d., Not done.*

Although *N*-nitrosamines have not been proven to be causative agents in the induction of human cancer, these compounds are potent carcinogens in experimental animals and generally exhibit organotropic effects. Furthermore, Bartsch *et al.* (Chapter 34, this volume) have demonstrated that nitrosation of secondary amines occurs in humans. This class of compounds is also the only one so far to show marked organ differences in the metabolism into ultimate reactive species that react with cellular DNA (Table VII). This apparent lack of activation could be a quantitative difference in which the levels are too low to be detected. Although human bronchus can metabolize all of the *N*-nitrosamines tested to date, only the symmetrical aliphatic *N*-nitrosamines were activated by human esophagus to metabolites that bound to DNA. Human fetal liver and esophagus did not metabolize DMNA, whereas fetal stomach activated several *N*-nitrosamines to a higher extent than did cultured esophagus (H. Autrup, unpublished). DMNA has been reported to be metabolized by slices of human lung and liver (Montesano and Magee, 1970; den Engelse *et al.*, 1975), as

measured by the formation of $^{14}CO_2$, and by human *in vivo* by
the presence of 7- and O^6-methylguanines in DNA isolated from
a liver of a person who died of DMNA poisoning (Herron and
Shank, 1980), and by cultured pancreatic duct as shown by malignant transformation of explant cultures (Parsa *et al.*,
1981). Human liver microsomes are also able to convert
N-nitrosomorpholine and *N*-nitroso-*N*'-methylpiperazine into mutagenic metabolites (Sabadie *et al.*, 1980).

Activation of *N*-nitrosamines produces alkylcarbonium ions
that react predominantly at the 7- and O^6-positions of guanine
in DNA. Both of these reaction products were detected after
incubation of human tissues with DMNA. However, a significant
amount of radioactivity was associated with guanine and adenine,
as a result of the metabolic incorporation of C-1 fragments
produced by the metabolic activation of *N*-nitrosamines. One of
these products, formaldehyde, may contribute to the carcinogenic action of *N*-nitrosamines (Harris *et al.*, 1982b). Considerable amounts of radioactivity were also associated with
an early-eluting peak by HPLC of the hydrolyzed DNA. Chemical
analysis indicated that some of the early-eluting peak was due
to the alkylation of the phosphate groups in DNA (Autrup *et al.*,
1978a). The metabolism of *N*-nitrosopyrrolidine (NPy) can proceed through either α or β oxidations. The activation of NPy
was highest in human bronchus and colon, but a higher level of
activity was seen in the corresponding rat tissues. The anticipated ultimate carcinogenic form of NPy, 4-oxobutylcarbonium
ion, is formed by the α-oxidative pathway. Formation of this
reactive metabolite by human tissues has been established by the
detection of 4-hydroxybutanal after incubation of NPy with human
liver microsomes (Hecht *et al.*, 1979), and in the tissue culture
media after incubation of bladder cells or esophageal explants
with NPy (Autrup *et al.*, 1981; Autrup and Stoner, 1982). HPLC
analysis of hydrolyzed DNA after incubation of rat esophagus

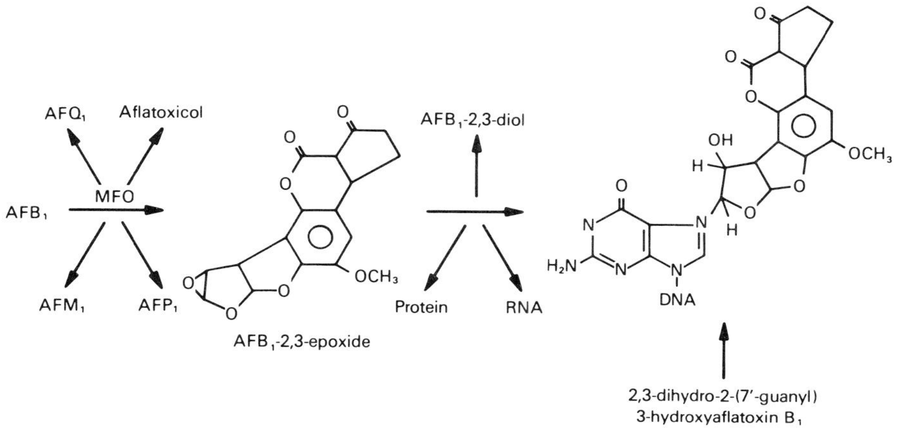

Fig. 3. Schematic representation of the metabolism of aflatoxin B_1.

explants with NPy revealed the presence of radioactivity associated with guanine and adenine, but the major proportion
eluted prior to these bases (H. Autrup, unpublished). The major NPy-DNA adduct has tentatively been suggested to be formed
by ring addition of the oxobutyl residue to guanine (Hecht *et
al*., 1982).

The metabolism of AFB to its ultimate carcinogenic form
is less complex than that of BP (Fig. 3); only one enzymatic
step is involved in the formation of AFB 2,3-oxide. There are
several competing pathways requiring different mixed-function
oxidases (MFOs), but most of these products retain the 2,3-
double bond and can potentially be converted to DNA-binding
metabolites. The major mixed-function oxidase responsible for
the formation of aflatoxin M_1 (AFM$_1$) is identical to the one
converting BP 7,8-diol to BP diol epoxide (Yoshizawa *et al*.,
1982), which may in part explain the lack of correlation between binding of levels of BP and AFB. The major AFB-DNA adduct (I) in cultured tissues was formed by the reaction of
AFB 2,3-oxide with the 7-position of guanine. Because of the

TABLE VIII.   Relative Distribution of Aflatoxin B_1-DNA Adducts
in Cultured Human and Rat Organs[a]

	Species	Initial peak	III	II	Diol	I	Ratio I:II
Bronchus	Human	4.1	8.7	33.6	n.d.[b]	41.3	1.23
	Rat	3.6	14.7	70.1	3.2	11.2	0.16
Esophagus	Human	1.3	16.2	70.0	1.2	7.0	0.10
	Rat	3.4	10.1	46.6	2.8	37.0	0.80
Colon	Human	73.0	16.8	7.1	n.d.	3.0	0.43
	Rat	3.4	14.5	63.4	4.1	14.4	0.23
Liver	Human	6.7	8.6	35.5	n.d.	47.8	1.35

[a]*Aflatoxin-DNA bases were separated by HPLC using a C-18
μ-Bondapak column by the method of Croy et al. (1978). See
text for more detailed explanation.*
[b]*n.d., Not done.*

instability of this adduct, another major peak (II) was detected in the HPLC analysis of acid-hydrolyzed DNA.   This product has been identified as 2,3-dihydro-2(N^5-formyl)-2',5',6'-
triamino-4'-oxo-N^5-pyrimidine-3-hydroxy AFB_1.   These major adducts were similar to the ones formed in rat liver *in vivo,* an
organ susceptible to the carcinogenic action of AFB (Croy *et
al.,* 1978).   The ratio between the relative amounts of adducts
I and II shows considerable difference among the various organs
(Table VIII) and may suggest an enzymatic pathway in addition
to the nonenzymatic pathway of ring opening in the modified
imidazole ring (Wang and Cerutti, 1980).   Such indications have
been found using human lung fibroblasts (Leadon *et al.,* 1981).

Human liver microsomes have been found to convert AFB into
metabolites mutagenic to *Salmonella typhimurium* TA 98 (Buening
et al., 1981).   An indirect proof for activation of AFB *in vivo*
in humans has been the detection of AFB-guanine (adduct I) in
the urine collected from individuals with a suspected exposure
to dietary AFB (Autrup *et al.,* 1983b).

TABLE IX. Benzo[a]pyrene Metabolism in Human Lung Tissue, Cells, and Microsomes[a]

Level of biological organization[b]	Early-eluting metabolites	Dihydrodiols			Phenols		Quinones
		9,10-	4,5-	7,8-	9-OH	3-OH	
Microsomes							
Lung[1]	--	12.0	2.7	6.1	18.4	33.9	26.8
Bronchial[2]	--	8.8	2.1	9.6	12.1	16.7	31.9
Cells							
Epithelial[3]	21.4	44.9	0.4	5.1	1.5	0.9	--
Fibroblast[3]	32.4	50.6	0.1	4.8	1.1	--	--
Explants							
Peripheral lung[4]	51.8	4.4	--	11.4	--	3.2	4.0
Bronchus[5]	36.2	21.2	3.9	4.4	4.1	2.4	11.5
Trachea[5]	21.4	28.4	3.9	4.9	4.1	2.4	26.4

[a]The results are expressed as percentage of total organic-soluble metabolites.
[b]References: [1]Sipal et al. (1979); [2]Autrup et al. (1983a); [3]Lechner et al. (1981); [4]Stoner et al. (1978); [5]Autrup et al. (1980a).
[c]--, Not detectable.

V.   INTERCELLULAR VARIATION

Because most human cancers are of epithelial origin, a
comparative study of metabolism of carcinogens in both epithelial and nontarget cells (e.g., fibroblasts) from the same
tissue is important. Using BP as the substrate, we did not
observe a major difference in the relative distribution of BP
metabolites in bronchial epithelial and fibroblast cells
(Table IX; Lechner et al., 1981), but the total metabolism is
threefold higher in the epithelial cells as measured by biochemical analysis (Lechner et al., 1981) and by autoradiography
of bronchial explants incubated with [^{3}H]BP (Harris et al.,
1976b). Similar results have also been found in mammary tissues (Stampfer et al., 1981) and between keratinocytes and skin
fibroblasts (Kuroki et al., 1982; Grunberger et al., Chapter 8,
this volume). In order to study the ability of different types
of epithelial cells to activate carcinogens, Harris et al.
(1976b) showed that when human bronchus explants were incubated
with [^{3}H]BP, a significantly higher number of grains was seen
in the ciliated cells than in basal and mucous cells. This
finding suggests that the ciliated cells have a higher level of
activating enzymes. However, the ultimate carcinogenic form of
BP, although chemically very unstable, can be transported from
one cell type to another as shown in the cell-mediated mutagenesis assay system (Hsu et al., 1978; Kuroki et al., 1982;
Gould et al., 1982). A similar transport could be anticipated
within the bronchial epithelium, so that the ultimate carcinogen
could be transported from the activating cell to the target cell
for carcinogenesis.

An important difference in the metabolic profiles of BP
was seen when subcellular systems were compared with intact
tissues. Phenols and quinones were the major metabolites produced by subcellular fractions, and no tetrols and only small

quantities of BP 9,10-diol were detected (Table IX). This
aberrant metabolic pattern and the different carcinogen-DNA
adduct profiles should be taken into consideration when subcellular systems are used for activation of carcinogens in mutation and transformation assays (Ashurst and Cohen, 1982;
Selkirk, 1977).

VI. INTERINDIVIDUAL VARIATION

   A wide interindividual variation in the ability to activate BP and other chemical carcinogens into DNA-binding species
has been observed in different organs. The magnitude in variation ranges from 50- to 150-fold (Table IV). This magnitude
of variation is similar to that observed in pharmacogenetic
studies of drug metabolism in humans. The distribution of the
binding level of BP to DNA appears to be unimodal with no detectable subpopulation being present (Harris et al., 1976a,
1982a; Autrup, 1982).

   Wide interindividual differences in the activities of the
enzymes involved in the metabolic conversion of polycyclic aromatic hydrocarbons have been reported in subcellular systems
(Harris et al., 1982a), including aryl hydrocarbon hydroxylase,
epoxide hydrolase, and glutathione transferase (Oesch et al.,
1980). This variation in enzyme activities may be a contributing factor to the greater variation seen in intact human
tissues. Other factors are the anatomical site of tissues and
patient history. In case of human respiratory tissue and esophagus, less than threefold variation was seen between explants
from the various anatomical segments (Autrup et al., 1980a;
Harris et al., 1979), whereas a greater difference was observed
in human colon with the highest level of activity in the sigmoid
colon (Autrup, 1981). The pathological state of the donor is

also associated with differences in BP binding to nontumorous
bronchi. Significantly higher values are found in bronchial
explants from individuals with primarily epidermoid differentiated cancer. Furthermore, a family history of cancer is
associated with higher binding values (C. C. Harris, unpublished). When the activity of aryl hydrocarbon hydroxylase
activity was compared in normal and cancerous lung tissues
from the same individual, lower activity was found in the cancerous tissue (Sabadie *et al.*, 1981).

VII. SUMMARY

The relationship between the interaction of carcinogens
with DNA and induction of cancer is generally unknown, and
furthermore, the quantitative relationship between carcinogen-
DNA modifications and the carcinogenic response is still poorly
understood. The extent and type of carcinogen-DNA modification
depends not only on the dose of carcinogen reaching the target
tissues, but also on the ability of the target organs to bio-
transform the carcinogen. Studies have shown that most human
tissues *in vitro* have the ability to convert potential carcinogenic compounds metabolically into their ultimate carcinogenic form. In addition, the metabolism in human tissues was
generally identical to that observed in animal tissues, in
which the compounds are carcinogenic; this result suggests that
the compound may be a potential human carcinogen. However,
quantitative differences exist between the different organs,
between species, and more interestingly between individuals.
Qualitative differences between organs and species were only
observed in the case of *N*-nitrosamines. Whether these metabolic differences may be responsible for the target specificity

in carcinogenesis and result in different susceptibility to
chemically induced cancer has as yet to be proven.

ACKNOWLEDGMENTS

We would like to thank our co-workers and collaborators,
Drs. Essigmann, Grafstrom, Jeffrey, Lechner, Stoner, Trump,
Weinstein, and Wogan for valuable contributions to the dif-
ferent projects. We would also like to thank Drs. Vahakangas
and Wilson for valuable criticism of the manuscript and
Ms. Richardson for typing the manuscript.

REFERENCES

Ashurst, S. W., and Cohen, G. M. (1982). *Carcinogenesis (N.Y.)*
    3, 267-273.
Autrup, H. (1981). *In* "Gastronintestinal Defense Mechanisms"
    (G. Mozsik, O. Hanninen, and T. Javor, eds.), pp. 385-404.
    Pergamon Press & Akademiai Kiado, Budapest.
Autrup, H. (1982). *Drug Metab. Rev. 13*, 603-646.
Autrup, H., and Stoner, G. D. (1982). *Cancer Res. 42*, 1307-
    1311.
Autrup, H., Harris, C. C., and Trump, B. F. (1978a). *Proc.
    Soc. Exp. Biol. Med. 159*, 111-115.
Autrup, H., Harris, C. C., Trump, B. F., and Jeffrey, A. M.
    (1978b). *Cancer Res. 38*, 3689-3696.
Autrup, H., Essigmann, J. M., Croy, R. G., Trump, B. F., Wogan,
    G. N., and Harris, C. C. (1979). *Cancer Res. 39*, 694-698.
Autrup, H., Wefald, F. C., Jeffrey, A. M., Tate, H., Schwartz,
    R. D., Trump, B. F., and Harris, C. C. (1980a). *Int. J.
    Cancer 25*, 293-300.
Autrup, H., Schwartz, R. D., Smith, L., Trump, B. F , and
    Harris, C. C. (1980b). *Carcinogenesis (N.Y.) 1*, 375-380.
Autrup, H., Grafstrom, R. G., Christensen, B., and Kieler, J.
    (1981). *Carcinogenesis (N.Y.) 2*, 763-768.
Autrup, H., Grafstrom, R. C., Brugh, M., Lechner, J., Haugen,
    A., Trump, B. F., and Harris, C. C. (1982). *Cancer Res.
    42*, 934-938.
Autrup, H., Grafstrom, R., and Harris, C. C. (1983a). *In*

"Organ and Species Specificity in Chemical Carcinogenesis"
(J. Rice, R. Langenbach, and S. Nesnow, eds.), pp. 473-495.
Plenum, New York.
Autrup, H., Bradley, K. O., Shamsuddin, A. K. M., Walehisi, J.,
and Wasunna, A. (1983b). *Carcinogenesis,* in press.
Barrett, L. A., McDowell, E. M., Harris, C. C., and Trump, B.
F. (1977). *Beitr. Pathol. 161,* 109-121.
Bartsch, H., Malaveille, C., Camus, A.-M., Marbel-Planche, G.,
Grun, G., Hautefeville, A., Sabadie, N., Barbin, A.,
Kuroki, T., Drevon, C., Piccoli, C., and Montesano, R.
(1980). *Mutat. Res. 76,* 1-50.
Boroujerdi, M., Kung, H.-C., Wilson, A. G. E., and Anderson,
M. W. (1981). *Cancer Res. 41,* 951-957.
Buening, M. K., Chang, R. L., Huang, M.-T., Fortner, J. G.,
Wood, A. W., and Conney, A. H. (1981). *Cancer Res. 41,*
67-72.
Cohen, G. M., Mehta, R., and Meredith-Brown, M. (1979). *Int.
J. Cancer 24,* 129-133.
Cohen, G. M., Grafstrom, R. C., Gibby, E. M., Smith, L., Autrup,
H., and Harris, C. C. (1983). *Cancer Res. 43,* 1312-1315.
Croy, R. G., Essigmann, J. M., Reinhold, V. N., and Wogan,
G. N. (1978). *Proc. Natl. Acad. Sci. USA 75,* 1745-1749.
den Engelse, L., Gebbink, M., and Emmelot, P. (1975). *Chem.
Biol. Interact. 11,* 535-544.
Dorman, B. H., Genta, V. M., Mass, M. J., and Kaufman, D. G.
(1981). *Cancer Res. 41,* 2718-2722.
Gould, M. N., Cathers, L. E., and Moore, C. J. (1982). *Cancer
Res. 42,* 4619-4624.
Gozukara, E. M., Guengerich, F. P., Miller, H., and Gelboin,
H. V. (1982). *Carcinogenesis (N.Y.) 3,* 129-134.
Harris, C. C., Autrup, H., Connor, R., Barrett, L. A.,
McDowell, E. M., and Trump, B. F. (1976a). *Science
(Washington, D.C.) 194,* 1067-1069.
Harris, C. C., Frank, A. L., van Haaften, C., Kaufman, D. G.,
Connor, R., Jackson, F. E., Barrett, L. A., McDowell, E.
M., and Trump, B. F. (1976b). *Cancer Res. 36,* 1011-1018.
Harris, C. C., Autrup, H., Stoner, G. D., McDowell, E. M.,
Trump, B. F., and Schafer, P. (1977a). *J. Natl. Cancer
Inst. (US) 59,* 1401-1406.
Harris, C. C., Autrup, H., Stoner, G., Yang, S. K., Leutz, J.
C., Gelboin, H. V., Selkirk, J. K., Connor, R. J.,
Barrett, L. A., Jones, R. T., McDowell, E. M., and Trump,
B. F. (1977b). *Cancer Res. 37,* 3349-3355.
Harris, C. C., Autrup, H., Stoner, G. D., Trump, B. F., Hillman,
E., Schafer, P. W., and Jeffrey, A. M. (1979). *Cancer
Res. 39,* 4401-4406.
Harris, C. C., Trump, B. F., and Stoner, G. D. (eds.) (1980).
"Methods in Cell Biology," Academic Press, N.Y., Vol. 21A,B

Harris, C. C., Trump, B. F., Grafstrom, R. G., and Autrup, H. (1982a). *J. Cell. Biochem. 18*, 285-294.

Harris, C. C., Grafstrom, R. C., Lechner, J. F., and Autrup, H. (1982b). *In* "Nitrosamines and Human Cancer" (P. N. Magee, ed.), pp. 121-140. Cold Spring Harbor Lab., Cold Spring Harbor, New York.

Hecht, S. S., Chen, C.-H. B., McCoy, C. D., and Hoffman, D. (1979). *Cancer Lett. (Shannon, Irel.) 8*, 35-41.

Hecht, S. S., Castonguay, A., Chung, F. L., and Hoffman, D. (1982). *In* "The Possible Role Nitrosamines in Human Cancer" (P. Magee, ed.), pp. 103-120. Cold Spring Harbor Lab., Cold Spring Harbor, New York.

Herron, D. C., and Shank, R. C. (1980). *Cancer Res. 40*, 3116-3117.

Hsu, I.-C., Stoner, G. D., Autrup, H., Trump, B. F., Selkirk, J. K., and Harris, C. C. (1978). *Proc. Natl. Acad. Sci. USA 75*, 2003-2007.

IARC Working Group (1980). *Cancer Res. 40*, 1-12.

Jeffrey, A. M., Weinstein, I. B., Jennette, K. W., Grzeskowiak, K., Nakanishi, K., Harvey, R. G., Autrup, H., and Harris, C. (1977). *Nature (London) 269*, 348-350.

Kuroki, T., Hosomi, J., Munakata, K., Ohizuka, T., Terauchi, M., and Nemoto, N. (1982). *Cancer Res. 42*, 1859-1865.

Labuc, G. E., and Archer, M. C. (1982). *Cancer Res. 42*, 3181-3186.

Leadon, S. A., Tyrrell, R. M., and Cerutti, P. A. (1981). *Cancer Res. 41*, 5125-5129.

Lechner, J. F., Haugen, A., Autrup, H., McClendon, I. A., Trump, B. F., and Harris, C. C. (1981). *Cancer Res. 41*, 2294-2303.

Mass, M. J., Rodgers, N. T., and Kaufman, D. G. (1981). *Chem. Biol. Interact. 33*, 195-205.

Montesano, R., and Magee, P. N. (1970). *Nature (London) 228*, 173-174.

Moore, B. P., Hicks, R. M., Knowles, M. A., and Redgrave, S. (1982). *Cancer Res. 42*, 642-648.

Nordenskjold, M., Soderhall, S., Moldeus, P., and Jernstrom, B. (1978). *Biochem. Biophys. Res. Commun. 85*, 1535-1541.

Oesch, F., Schmassmann, H., Ohnhaus, E., Althaus, U., and Lorenz, J. (1980). *Carcinogenesis (N.Y.) 1*, 827-835.

Parsa, I., Marsh, W. H., Sutton, A. L., and Butt, K. M. H. (1981). *Am. J. Pathol. 102*, 403-411.

Pelkonen, O., Boobis, A. R., Yagi, H., Jerina, D. M., and Nebert, D. W. (1978). *Mol. Pharmacol. 14*, 306-322.

Sabadie, N., Malaveille, C., Camus, A.-M., and Bartsch, H. (1980). *Cancer Res. 40*, 119-126.

Sabadie, N., Richter-Reichhelm, H. B., Saracci, R., Mohr, V., and Bartsch, H. (1981). *Int. J. Cancer 27*, 417-426.

Selkirk, J. K. (1977). *Nature (London) 270,* 604-607.
Selkirk, J. K., Nikbakht, A., and Stoner, G. (1983). *Cancer Lett. (Shannon, Irel.) 18,* 11-19.
Sipal, Z., Ahlenius, T., Bergstrand, A., Rodriguez, L., and Jakobsson, S. W. (1979). *Xenobiotica 9,* 633-645.
Sivarajah, K., Lasker, J. M., and Eling, T. E. (1981). *Cancer Res. 41,* 1834-1839.
Stampfer, M. R., Bartholomew, J. C., Smith, H. S., and Barkley, J. C. (1981). *Proc. Natl. Acad. Sci. 78,* 6251-6255.
Stoner, G. D., Harris, C. C., Autrup, H., Trump, B. F., Kingsbury, E. W., and Myers, G. A. (1978). *Lab. Invest. 38,* 685-692.
Stoner, G. D., Daniel, F. B., Schenck, K. M., Schut, H. A. J., Goldblatt, P. J., and Sandwisch, D. W. (1982a). *Carcinogenesis (N.Y.) 3,* 195-202.
Stoner, G. D., Daniel, F. B., Schenck, K. M., Schut, H. A. J., Sandwisch, D. W., and Gohara, A. F. (1982b). *Carcinogenesis (N.Y.) 3,* 1345-1348.
Trump, B., McDowell, E., Barrett, L., Frank, A., and Harris, C. (1974). *In* "Experimental Lung Cancer" (E. Karbe and J. J. Park, eds.), pp. 548-558. Springer-Verlag, Berlin.
Wang, V., and Cerutti, P. A. (1980). *Cancer Res. 40,* 2904-2909.
Yang, S. K., Roller, P. P., and Gelboin, H. V. (1977). *Biochemistry 16,* 3680-3686.
Yoshizawa, H., Uchimaru, R., Kamataki, T., Kato, R., and Ueno, Y. (1982). *Cancer Res. 42,* 1120-1124.

8

METABOLISM AND DNA BINDING OF CARCINOGENS IN CULTURED HUMAN EPIDERMAL CELLS[1]

Dezider Grunberger and Gail Theall

Department of Biochemistry and Public Health
Institute of Cancer Research
Columbia University
New York, New York

Magdalene Eisinger

Memorial Sloan-Kettering Cancer Center
New York, New York

[1]*This investigation was supported by PHS Grants CA 21111
and CA 31696 from the National Institutes of Health, DHHS to
D. G., EPA Grant No. CR 807282 to G. T., and PCM 7911783 from
the National Science Foundation to M. E.*

I. INTRODUCTION

During the 1970s many new experimental systems were developed to study the mechanism of carcinogenesis *in vitro*
(see review in Weinstein, 1981). Because a high level of
variation exists in the response to carcinogens among different species, tissues, and cell types, it is problematic to
extrapolate data obtained in animal systems to situation in
humans.

Advances in the maintenance and growth of human tissues
in culture have made it possible to study the mechanism of
carcinogenesis directly. Because the majority of human cancers arise in epithelial tissues (Higginson and Muir, 1973),
cultured human epithelial cells are the most promising systems
to study metabolic pathways of chemical carcinogens, interactions with cellular macromolecules, repair, and interindividual
variations in these processes. Metabolism of chemical carcinogens and binding to DNA have been explored extensively in cultured human tissues and cells. Benzo[a]pyrene (BP), the most
widely distributed carcinogen in our environment, was studied
in several human organs including lung (Autrup *et al.*, 1978),
bronchus (Jeffrey *et al.*, 1977; Harris *et al.*, 1976a,b), pancreatic duct (Harris *et al.*, 1977), mammary gland (Grover *et
al.*, 1980; Stampfer *et al.*, 1981), endometrium (Mass *et al.*,
1981), colon (Autrup *et al.*, 1977, 1978), esophagus (Harris
et al., 1979), monocytes (Lake *et al.*, 1977), and epidermal
keratinocytes (Parkinson and Newbold, 1980; Kuroki *et al.*,
1980; Theall *et al.*, 1981).

It has been shown that BP is converted into several metabolites but especially into the 7,8-diol 9,10-epoxides, which
are involved in binding to DNA and probably in the initiation
of carcinogenesis (Gelboin, 1980).

Because skin is one of the tissues most extensively exposed to environmental carcinogens, we have chosen to work
with human epidermal keratinocytes and melanocytes. Interindividual variations in the metabolism of BP and the extent of
DNA modification were explored by using several identically
grown primary keratinocyte cultures. For the elucidation of
the mechanisms involved in tissue specificity exhibited by
different carcinogens, a potent hepatocarcinogen, N-2-acetyl-
aminofluorene (AAF), to which the skin is not sensitive, has
been used. Some of these results were published previously
(Theall *et al.*, 1981).

II.   MATERIALS AND METHODS

A. Growth of Keratinocytes and Melanocytes in Culture

Human keratinocytes were isolated from breast skin specimens obtained from surgery for breast reduction or cadaver
skin shavings. The tissue culture method for growth of keratinocytes was similar to the procedure described previously
by Eisinger *et al.* (1979). Human melanocytes were isolated
from circumcised foreskins of newborns. The method for the
growth of melanocytes was similar to that previously described
by Eisinger and Marko (1982). The cells were grown in Eagle's
minimal essential medium containing nonessential amino acids,
2 mM L-glutamine, phorbol 12-myristate 13-acetate (10 ng/ml)
in dimethyl sulfoxide, 10 nM cholera toxin, and 5% fetal bovine serum (pH 7.2). Pure cultures of melanocytes were obtained by immune rosetting, using a mouse monoclonal antibody,
R_{24}, which recognizes an antigen on melanocytes but not on
fibroblasts or epidermal cells, and protein A conjugated human
red blood cells. Melanocytes so rosetted were separated from

nonrosetted cells on discontinuous Percoll gradients described
by Marko *et al.* (1982).

B. Analysis of BP Metabolites

The methods used were essentially described by Theall *et*
al. (1981). The media from cells treated with different concentrations of $[^3H]$BP (40-65 Ci/mmol), as indicated in Section
III, were extracted with ethyl acetate three times, evaporated
to dryness, dissolved in methanol, and analyzed by HPLC using
a Waters µBondapac C_{18} column, and developed by a linear gradient of 40 to 100% methanol in water. Fractions were assayed
by scintillation counting.

C. DNA Binding and Adduct Analysis

The cells treated with $[^3H]$BP or $[^3H]$*N*-hydroxy-AAF (590
mCi/m*M*) or $[^3H]$*N*-acetoxy-AAF (450 mCi/m*M*) were digested with
0.1% sodium dodecylsulfate, 10 m*M* Tris-HCl (pH 7.9), 10 m*M*
EDTA, and 200 µg/ml proteinase K for 2 h at 37°C. DNA was
isolated by phenol extraction and ethanol precipitation as
described by Theall *et al.* (1981). Binding levels were determined by quantitation of DNA by UV spectroscopy and BP bound
by radioactivity.

For the characterization of the carcinogen-deoxynucleo-
side adducts, the enzymatically hydrolyzed DNA was chromatographed on a Sephadex LH-20 column using a stepwise elution of
water and 80% methanol. Fractions from the methanol region
combined with the markers were separated by high-pressure
liquid chromatography (HPCL) using a 35-60% nonlinear methanol-
water gradient at 50°C at 1 ml/min flow rate over 100 min.

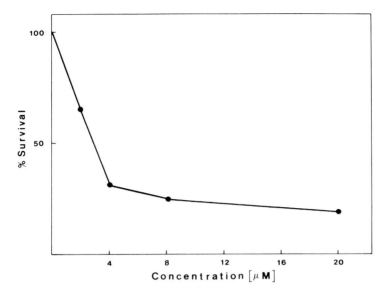

Fig. 1. Number of viable human epidermal keratinocytes 5 days after a 24-h incubation with different doses of BP. From Theall *et al.* (1981).

III. RESULTS

A. Toxicity of BP to Keratinocytes

The effect of BP on the human epidermal keratinocytes was explored on 2-week-old cultures that were composed predominantly of basal cells and a minor population of keratinizing cells. After 24 h of incubation with increasing doses of BP, the cultures did not show noticeable cytotoxic changes when viewed by light microscopy. However, when cells after 24-h treatment with BP were allowed to grow for an additional 5 days and the numbers of viable cells were counted, it was found that in 2 μM BP 65%, and in 20 μM BP only 18% of the cells survived (Fig. 1).

B.   Correlation between BP Metabolism and DNA Binding in
     Keratinocytes

The key factor in the initiation stage of carcinogenesis
is the metabolic activation of carcinogens to electrophiles
that bind covalently to cellular macromolecules, especially to
DNA (Miller and Miller, 1981).   Therefore, it was desirable to
find out the effect of metabolism of BP on the level of DNA
modification in cultured human epidermal keratinocytes.
Fifteen-day-old primary cultures in an exponential stage of
growth were exposed to a nontoxic level of BP.   The media from
tissue-cultured cells were removed 6, 18, 28, and 48 h after
addition of 1.3 μM [^{3}H]BP and analyzed for the presence of BP
metabolites.   The cells were used for determination of the
level of DNA modification.

Figure 2 relates DNA binding and the levels of BP and its
metabolites as a function of the incubation time.   The concentration of BP decreases steadily with time, and by 28 h, only
5% of the BP is not metabolized.   The BP is converted into
water-soluble and ethyl acetate-extractable metabolites.   As
the concentration of BP decreases, the level of water-soluble
products increases.   The ethyl acetate metabolites, however,
reach a peak level of 18 h and begin to decrease slightly with
increased incubation time.   This, presumably, is a result of
their further detoxification.   Concomitantly, the binding of
BP residues to DNA increases linearly during the first 28 h to
a maximal level of 9.1×10^{-6} mol BP/mol DNA.   This level is
retained through 48 h.

A detailed analysis of the total ethyl acetate metabolites
presented in Fig. 2 was performed by HPLC.   Figure 3 shows the
elution profiles of the ethyl acetate metabolites corresponding
to 6-, 18-, and 48-h incubations of culture with 1.3 μM BP.
The metabolites have been identified as 7,8,9,10-tetrahydro-

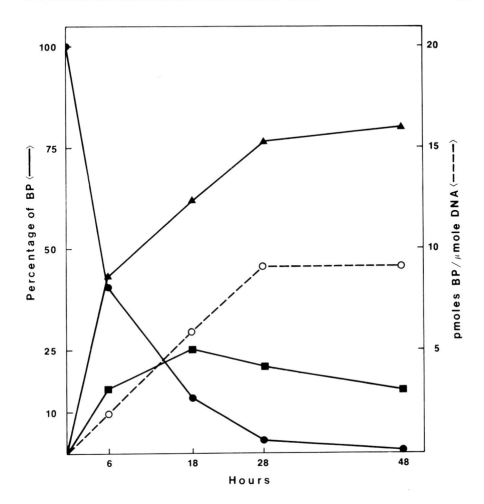

Fig. 2.   The correlation of BP metabolism and DNA binding with incubation time.   The levels of water-soluble metabolites (▲——▲), ethyl acetate-extractable metabolites (■——■), and BP (●——●) are expressed as the percentage of the initial dose of 1.3 μ*M* [³H]BP.   The total BP-DNA binding levels (O---O) are expressed as pmol BP bound/μmol DNA.   From Theall *et al*. (1981).

benzo[*a*]pyrene (tetraol), *trans*-9,10-dihydro-9,10-dihydroxy-
benzo[*a*]pyrene (9,10-diol), *trans*-7,8-dihydro-7,8-dihydroxy-
benzo[*a*]pyrene (7,8-diol), quinones, and phenols.   A series of

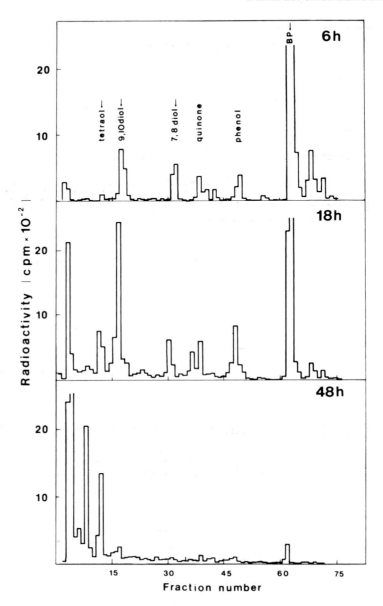

Fig. 3.   HPLC profiles of ethyl acetate-extracted BP
metabolites.   Keratinocytes were incubated with 1.3 μ*M* BP for
6 h, 18 h, and 48 h.   The arrows indicate the positions of the
UV markers.   From Theall *et al.* (1981).

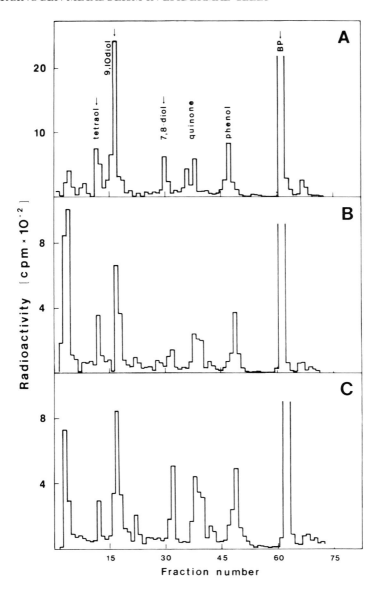

Fig. 4. HPLC profiles of ethyl acetate-extracted metabolites from various cultures. Culture A was incubated 18 h
with 1.3 μM BP; culture B, 21 h with 1.2 μM BP; and culture C,
24 h with 1.2 μM BP. From Theall et al. (1981).

peaks eluting in the initial fractions have not been identified. The quinones and phenols of BP are mixtures that are
not resolved in this chromatographic system. As can be seen
in Fig. 3, by 6 h a substantial amount of 9,10-diol and 7,8-
diol have been formed. At 18 h, there is more 9,10-diol and
tetraol, and only a slightly elevated level of 7,8-diol. The
ratio of 7,8-diol to 9,10-diol is twofold lower than at 6 h.
At 48 h, the only ethyl acetate metabolites remaining are
tetraols, triols, and a substantial level of unidentified
polar products.

C.   Interindividual Variation in BP Metabolism and DNA
     Binding in Keratinocytes

     The investigation of the possible interindividual varia-
tions in ethyl acetate-extractable metabolites of BP was performed with several different primary cultures. Cultures A
and C were derived from skin of various areas of two males,
68 and 85 years old, 3-4 h postmortem. Culture B was taken
from surgically removed breast skin of a middle-aged woman.
Figure 4 represents HPLC profiles of BP metabolites from these
cultures. All three cultures generated essentially similar
metabolites. However, there were differences in the relative
levels of individual metabolites, especially that of 9,10-diol
to 7,8-diol.

     A detailed analysis of the DNA adducts was also performed
on the three different cultures. The DNA was hydrolyzed and
chromatographed on an LH-20 Sephadex column (not shown). The
methanol eluant contained 60% of the BP-bound DNA in each culture. Figure 5 shows the HPLC profiles of these methanol elution products. When culture A was incubated with BP for various
lengths of time and at various doses, qualitatively, the same
elution profile was observed (Fig. 5A). The predominant adduct

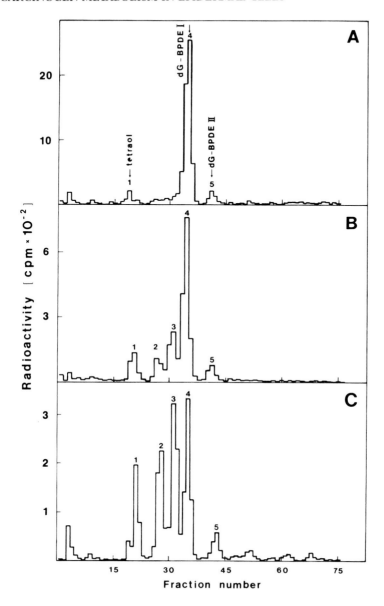

Fig. 5. HPLC profiles of DNA digests eluted in the methanol region of LH-20 Sephadex from cultures A, B, and C. From Theall *et al.* (1981).

(peak 4) is identified as the BPDE I (7,8-diol 9,10-epoxide BP) bound to deoxyguanosine (dG) at the N^2 position (dG-BPDE I). This adduct has been seen in human bronchial and colon explants, lung cells (Jeffrey *et al.*, 1977), and human mammary cells. However, when cultures derived from various sources were used, differences were detected not only in the types of DNA adducts formed but also in the relative levels of the adducts. Figure 5B and C are the HPLC profiles from cultures B and C, respectively. Peak 1 elutes in the region of the BP-tetraol marker. Peak 2 is in the general position that a BPDE-deoxycytosine adduct would be expected; however, identification cannot be made without proper markers. Peak 3 coelutes with a marker thought to be an adduct of deoxyguanosine and 9-hydroxy-4,5-oxide BP seen extensively in microsomal systems. Because the structure of this adduct has not yet been determined, complete characterization of the product is required. Peak 5 coelutes with dG-BPDE II marker.

D. Metabolism of BP by Melanocytes

Only 5–7% of the total number of cells in human epidermis is made up of melanocytes. In addition to being a minor cell population of epidermis, they also replicate relatively slowly in comparison with keratinocytes or fibroblasts. Therefore, previous attempts to culture melanocytes have been frustrated by the overgrowth of fibroblasts and keratinocytes, which has prevented subculturing and long-term studies. We have now found that by using phorbol ester we can select for melanocytes, and a combination of phorbol ester and cholera toxin enhances the rate of melanocyte proliferation. Availability of melanocyte cultures and major interest in transformation of melanocytes into melanomas has led us to investigate the ability of melanocytes and melanomas to metabolize BP.

TABLE I. Percentage of ^{3}H Radioactivity in Metabolism of
          Benzo[a]pyrene by Human Cells in Culture[a]

Cell culture	Incubation time (h)	Water extract	Ethyl acetate extract	Non-metabolized BP
Keratinocytes	18	62	38	13
	48	80	20	0.4
Melanocytes	18	2.5	97.5	96
Melanomas HO1	18	6	94	94
	48	12	88	84

[a]*Keratinocytes (∿3 × 10^6 cells), melanocytes (∿7 × 10^5 cells), and melanomas (∿3 × 10^6 cells) were incubated in the presence of 1.2 μM [^{3}H]benzo[a]pyrene for 18 or 48 h as indicated. The medium was extracted three times with ethyl-acetate. The ethyl acetate extracts were analyzed by HPLC. The initial radioactivity of BP in the experiments was 100%.*

Table I compares metabolism of BP by human keratinocytes, melanocytes, and melanomas grown in culture. It is evident that keratinocytes in 48 h metabolize BP almost completely. In contrast, melanocytes and melanoma cells grown in the presence of the same concentration of BP (1.2 μM) did not metabolize BP. In the ethyl acetate extract of the medium, the remaining nonmetabolized BP has been detected by HPLC (not shown). The only difference between keratinocytes and melanocyte cultures was that the keratinocytes were primary cultures and the melanocyte and melanoma cells were passaged about 20 times. It was not possible to collect sufficient amounts of melanocytes in an earlier passage. Therefore, it remains to be determined whether the lack of BP metabolism by melanocytes is due to the absence of the P-450 system in these cells or whether, during the cell passaging, the metabolizing enzymes were lost.

E.   Binding of *N*-Hydroxy- and *N*-Acetoxy-*N*-2-acetylamino-
     fluorene to DNA of Keratinocytes

There is evidence that tissue specificities of chemical carcinogens result from differences in the metabolism of these compounds (J. A. Miller, 1970; E. C. Miller, 1978). Therefore, it was of interest to find out whether *N*-2-acetylaminofluorene (AAF), a potent liver but not skin carcinogen, can be activated by keratinocytes into electrophilic, ultimate carcinogenic form that binds to DNA.

It was shown that, in the first stage of metabolism, AAF is *N*-oxidized by liver microsomal enzymes to *N*-hydroxy-AAF (*N*-OH-AAF) (Miller *et al*., 1961). This "proximate" carcinogen derivative is not reactive per se but is converted into the "ultimate" carcinogenic form either by sulfotransferase to sulfate (King and Phillips, 1968; DeBaun *et al*., 1970) or by *N,O*-Acetyltransferase to yield *N*-acetoxy-2-aminofluorene (AF) (King, 1974; Bartsch *et al*., 1972). Both the acetylated and deacetylated esters bind primarily to C-8 of dG residues in DNA (Kriek *et al*., 1967; Kriek, 1969, 1972). A lower level of binding of AAF residues also occurs at the N^2 of dG residues in DNA (Westra *et al*., 1976).

To find out whether human keratinocytes are capable of activating *N*-OH-AAF into an electrophilic form that binds to DNA, we incubated keratinocytes with [^{3}H]*N*-OH-AAF. Figure 6 illustrates that in human keratinocytes there is a very low binding of [^{3}H]*N*-OH-AAF to DNA. It implies that these cells possess a very low level of the enzymatic system to convert *N*-OH-AAF into an "ultimate" carcinogenic form that modifies DNA. Therefore, we incubated keratinocytes with [^{3}H]*N*-acetoxy-AAF, the ultimate electrophilic derivative of AAF, and measured its binding to DNA. Figure 6 shows that *N*-acetoxy-AAF (*N*-OAc-AAF), in contrast to *N*-OH-AAF, binds intensively to DNA.

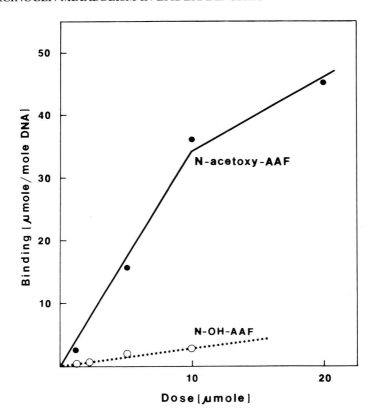

Fig. 6. Binding of [³H]*N*-OH-AAF (O···O) and [³H]*N*-acetoxy-AAF (●——●) to DNA. Keratinocytes were incubated with *N*-OH-AAF for 6 h or with *N*-OAc-AAF for 1 h.

Because binding of *N*-OAc-AAF to DNA can yield different guanosine adducts, we have hydrolyzed DNA enzymatically and characterized the modified nucleosides by HPLC. Figure 7 shows that the majority of adducts are the deacetylated AAF residue bound to C-8 of dG (C-8-dG-AF). A minor adduct cochromatographed with the C-8-dG-AAF marker, but no adduct appeared in the position of the N^2-dG-AAF marker. Some radioactivity was detected in the fractions where the imidazole ring opened product of C-8-dG-AF adduct is located (Kriek and Westra, 1980)

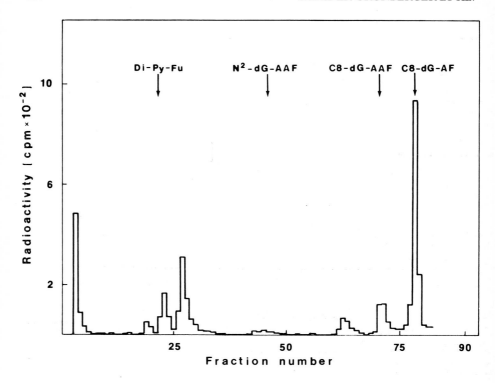

Fig. 7. HPLC profile of DNA digest of keratinocytes
treated with *N*-OAc-AAF for 3.5 h.

(Di-Py-FU). Similarly, a high level of deacetylated G adduct
was detected by Poirier *et al.* (1980) when mouse epidermal
cells were exposed to *N*-OAc-AAF.

IV. DISCUSSION

The main question posed in this study was whether there
is a correlation in human keratinocytes between metabolism of
a carcinogen and DNA adduct formation on one hand and sensitivity to a carcinogen on the other hand. Our results show
that human keratinocytes are capable of metabolizing BP at a

substantial rate. Cultures derived from several different individuals and incubated with BP under similar conditions converted BP into the same metabolites at comparable levels.
Although interindividual differences in the ratios of metabolites were observed, the variance was no greater than the
range of the ratios seen in one culture. This result is not
in complete agreement with Kuroki et al. (1980), who observed
significantly different metabolic abilities of three primary
cultures. This disparity could be the result of different
tissue culture conditions or different doses of BP, as well
as different sources of the primary cultures used. The results
of Parkinson and Newbold (1980), observing no more than a two-
to threefold difference in the metabolism of BP in keratinocytes from six patients, are more in accord with our observations.

The cultures tested show similar metabolic activity by HPLC analysis, some differences are observed in DNA
adduct formation. However, the major adduct observed in all
human epidermal cell cultures is dG-BPDE I. The dG-BPDE II
adduct is a minor contributor to overall DNA binding. The relationship of dG-BPDE I to dG-BPDE II adducts remained constant
as the exposure time and BP dose was altered.

The appearance of peak 3 in Fig. 5B and C could represent
an adduct formed by binding of 9-hydroxy-4,5-oxide BP to deoxyguanosine residues. Although there have been reports that BP
binds DNA via an epoxidation of 9-hydroxy-BP (King et al.,
1976) to yield a 9-hydroxy-4,5-oxide BP-dG adduct, the structural characterization of this product has not been determined
yet.

There are several possible explanations for the difference
in DNA adduct formation among various cultures. Epoxide hydrolase, an essential enzyme in the cytochrome P-450 enzyme system, has been shown by Guentner and Oesch (1981) to have an

important role in DNA adduct formation *in vitro*. High levels
of epoxide hydrolase favor binding of 7,8-diol products to DNA,
whereas low levels of the enzyme result in the preferential
formation of 9-hydroxy-benzo[a]pyrene-DNA adducts. Thus, the
observed interindividual variation in BP-DNA adduct formation
can be the result of different levels of epoxide hydrolase activity in different cultures much as it was observed in human
fibroblasts (Oesch *et al.*, 1980). Another reason for the
variation in DNA adducts could be an altered ability of the
cells to detoxify the BP metabolites by formation of glucuro-
nide, glutathione, sulfate, or other conjugates (Nemoto *et al.*,
1978a,b; Cooper *et al.*, 1980). A twofold variation in
glutathione *S*-transferase activity in human fibroblasts has
been observed (Oesch *et al.*, 1980). It has also been demonstrated that cellular nucleophiles can selectively affect
binding of BP metabolites to DNA (Guenther *et al.*, 1980).
Thus differences in detoxification enzymes and potential interindividual variations in cellular nucleophiles may result in
different DNA adduct formation by the selective removal of BP
metabolites. Further it implies that quantitative relationships between mechanisms of activation and detoxification may
have a primary role in the determination of the interindividual
variation in DNA adduct formation.

However, melanocytes did not metabolize BP. Although BP
has been shown to be a potent inducer of epidermal cell tumors
in vivo, it has never been shown to induce melanomas. Therefore, it would appear that melanocytes might be naturally lacking the enzymes necessary for BP metabolism. However, further
experiments on early cultures of melanocytes should be performed to confirm these notions. In contrast to BP, human
keratinocytes were not able to convert *N*-OH-AAF, which has not
been shown to be an initiator of skin cancer, to the ultimate
carcinogenic form and to modify DNA. Because the activation

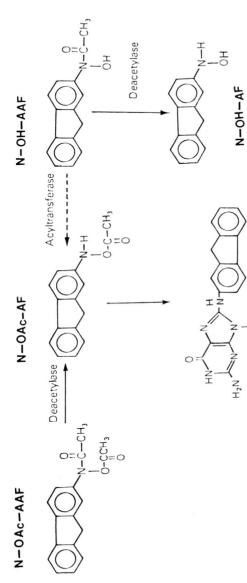

Fig. 8. The scheme of possible metabolic pathways of *N*-2-acetylamino-fluorene derivatives. Broken arrow indicates nonfunctional pathway in kera-tinocytes.

of *N*-OH-AAF in the liver mainly involves sulfotransferase and
N,*O*-acetyltransferase enzymes (King and Phillips, 1968; King,
1974), it implies that keratinocytes lack these enzymes.
However, when the ultimate carcinogen *N*-OAc-AAF was incubated
with keratinocytes, significant binding to DNA occurred. Because most of the DNA adducts were formed with the deacetylated
derivative of AAF, it appears that human keratinocytes contain
a very active deacetylase but not *N*,*O*-acetyltransferase system.
If keratinocytes had an active transferase it would catalyze
the conversion of *N*-OH-AAF into electrophilic *N*-OAc-AF that
would bind to DNA. Formation of C-8-dG-AF adduct after incubation of keratinocytes with *N*-OAc-AAF, however, can be the result of action of deacetylase that catalyzes the removal of the
acetyl group from *N*-OAc-AAF to form the highly electrophilic
N-OAc-AF that binds to DNA. The scheme of these reactions is
shown in Fig. 8.

Taken together, our results demonstrate in human keratinocytes a relatively good correlation between activation, DNA
binding, and sensitivity to a carcinogen. Better understanding
of these processes in other tissues by different carcinogens
should help to explain the variability in the induction of tumors by chemical carcinogens in humans.

REFERENCES

Autrup, H., Harris, C. C., Stoner, G. D., Jesudason, M. L.,
    and Trump, B. F. (1977). *J. Natl. Cancer Inst. (US) 59*,
    351-354.
Autrup, H., Harris, C. C., Stoner, G. D., Selkirk, J. K.,
    Schafer, P. W., and Trump, B. F. (1978a). *Lab. Invest.
    38*, 217-224.
Autrup, H., Harris, C. C., Trump, B. F., and Jeffrey, A. M.
    (1978b). *Cancer Res. 38*, 3689-3696.
Bartsch, H., Dworkin, M., Miller, J. A., and Miller, E. C.
    (1972). *Biochim. Biophys. Acta 286*, 272-298.

Cooper, C. S., Hewer, A., Ribeiro, O., Grover, P. L., and
Sims, P. (1980). *Carcinogenesis (N.Y.) 1*, 1075-1080.
DeBaun, J. R., Miller, E. C., and Miller, J. A. (1970).
Cancer Res. 30, 577-595.
Eisinger, M., and Marko, O. (1982). *Proc. Natl. Acad. Sci.
USA 79*, 2018-2022.
Eisinger, M., Lee, J. S., Hefton, J. M., Darzynkiewicz, Z.,
Chiao, J. W., and deHarven, E. (1979). *Proc. Natl. Acad.
Sci. USA 76*, 5340-5344.
Gelboin, V. H. (1980). *Physiol. Rev. 60*, 1107-1166.
Grover, P. L., MacNicoll, A. D., Sims, P., Easty, G. C., and
Neville, A. M. (1980). *Int. J. Cancer 26*, 467-475.
Guenther, T. M., and Oesch, F. (1981). *Cancer Lett. (Shannon,
Irel.) 11*, 178-183.
Guenther, T. M., Jernstrom, B., and Orrenius, S. (1980).
Carcinogenesis (N.Y.) 1, 407-418.
Harris, C. C., Autrup, H., Connor, R., Barrett, L. A.,
McDowell, E. M., and Trump, B. F. (1976a). *Science
(Washington, D.C.) 194*, 1067-1069.
Harris, C. C., Frank, A. L., van Haaften, C., Kaufman, D. G.,
Connor, R., Jackson, F., Barrett, L. A., McDowell, E. M.,
and Trump, B. F. (1976b). *Cancer Res. 36*, 1011-1018.
Harris, C. C., Autrup, H., Stoner, G., Yang, S. K., Lentz,
J. C., Gelboin, H. V., Selkirk, J. K., Connor, R. J.,
Barrett, L. A., Jones, R. T., McDowell, E. M., and Trump,
B. F. (1977). *Cancer Res. 37*, 3349-3355.
Harris, C. C., Autrup, H., Stoner, G. D., Trump, B. F.,
Hillman, E., Schafer, P. W., and Jeffrey, A. M. (1979).
Cancer Res. 39, 4401-4406.
Higginson, J., and Muir, C. (1973). *In* "Cancer Medicine"
(J. Holland and E. Frei, eds.), pp. 241-306. Lea &
Febiger, Philadelphia, Pennsylvania.
Jeffrey, A. M., Weinstein, I. B., Jennette, K. W.,
Grzeskowiak, K., Nakanishi, K., Harvey, R. G., Autrup, H.,
and Harris, C. (1977). *Nature (London) 269*, 348-350.
King, C. M. (1974). *Cancer Res. 34*, 1503-1515.
King, C. M., and Phillips, B. (1968). *Science (Washington,
D.C.) 159*, 1351-1353.
King, H. W. S., Thompson, M. H., and Brookes, P. (1976).
Int. J. Cancer 17, 270-274.
Kriek, E. (1969). *Chem. Biol. Interact. 1*, 3-17.
Kriek, E. (1972). *Cancer Res. 32*, 2042-2048.
Kriek, E., and Westra, J. G. (1980). *Carcinogenesis (N.Y.) 1*,
459-468.
Kriek, E., Miller, J. A., Juhl, U., and Miller, E. C. (1967).
Biochemistry 6, 177-182.
Kuroki, T., Nemoto, N., and Kitano, Y. (1980). *Carcinogenesis
(N.Y.) 1*, 559-565.

Lake, R. L., Pezzutti, M. R., Kropko, M. L., Freeman, A. E.,
    and Igel, H. J. (1977). *Cancer Res.* 37, 2530-2537.
Marko, O., Houghton, A., and Eisinger, M. (1983). *Exp. Cell
    Res.*, in press.
Mass, M. J., Rodgers, N. T., and Kaufman, D. G. (1981). *Chem.
    Biol. Interact.* 33, 195-205.
Miller, E. C. (1978). *Cancer Res.* 38, 1479-1496.
Miller, E. C., and Miller, J. A. (1981). *Cancer (Philadelphia)*
    47, 2327-2345.
Miller, E. C., Miller, J. A., and Hartmann, H. A. (1961).
    Cancer Res. 21, 815-824.
Miller, J. A. (1970). *Cancer Res.* 30, 559-576.
Nemoto, N., Herakawa, T., and Takayama, S. (1978a). *Chem.
    Biol. Interact.* 22, 1-14.
Nemoto, N., Takayama, S., and Gelboin, H. (1978b). *Chem. Biol.
    Interact.* 23, 19-30.
Oesch, F., Tegtmayer, F., Kohl, F. V., Rudiger, H., and Glatt,
    H. R. (1980). *Carcinogenesis (N.Y.)* 1, 305-309.
Parkinson, E. K., and Newbold, R. F. (1980). *Int. J. Cancer*
    26, 289-299.
Poirier, M. C., Williams, G. M., and Yuspa, S. H. (1980).
    Mol. Pharmacol. 18, 581-587.
Stampfer, M. R., Bartholomew, J. C., Smith, H., and Bartley,
    J. C. (1981). *Proc. Natl. Acad. Sci. USA* 78, 6251-6255.
Stoner, G. D., Harris, C. C., Autrup, H., Trump, B. F.,
    Kingsbury, E. W., and Myers, G. A. (1978). *Lab. Invest.*
    38, 685-692.
Theall, G., Eisinger, M., and Grunberger, D. (1981). *Carcino-
    genesis (N.Y.)* 2, 581-587.
Weinstein, I. B. (1981). *J. Supramol. Struct. Cell. Biochem.*
    17, 99-120.
Westra, J. G., Kriek, E., and Hittenhausen, H. (1976). *Chem.
    Biol. Interact.* 15, 149-164.

9

CELLULAR RESPONSES TO DAMAGE IN DNA[1]

Thomas C. Brown, Paul A. Amstad,
Hugo J. Niggli, and Peter A. Cerutti

Department of Carcinogenesis
Swiss Institute of Experimental Cancer Research
Epalinges, Switzerland

I.   INTRODUCTION

Many carcinogens react with DNA to form covalent adducts. Such lesions are cytotoxic and mutagenic, and they may represent causative factors in malignant transformation. It is therefore of interest to characterize cellular responses that act to modulate the effects of carcinogen-DNA adducts. Most

[1]*Original work described in this chapter was supported by Grant No. 3'305.78 from the Swiss National Science Foundation and a grant from the Swiss Association of Cigarette Manufacturers.*

mammalian cells possess the capability to excise DNA lesions.
Excision repair has been shown to reduce both the toxic and
the mutagenic effects of damage (Maher *et al.*, 1979), and human patients with diseases whose characteristics include defective excision repair are prone to the development of malignancies in tissues that are exposed to carcinogens (Setlow
et al., 1977). Despite the intervention of excision repair,
however, often a substantial fraction of carcinogen-DNA
lesions persists over several cell generations (Cerutti, 1982).
As reported in this chapter, the knowledge of lesion excisa-
bility and persistence does not always suffice to explain the
biological effects of a carcinogen. This is well documented
by confluent-holding (CH) experiments.

In CH experiments cultured cells are maintained in confluence until DNA replication has ceased. Under these conditions cells are generally arrested in the G_1 phase of the
cell cycle (Pardee *et al.*, 1978). Following exposure to a
carcinogen, the cultures are held in confluence for various
times and then subcultured. According to the rationale for
CH experiments, the deleterious effects of DNA damage are
expressed when cells undergo DNA replication using a damaged
template. Cell proliferation *in vivo* is an important factor
in tumorigenesis (Cayama *et al.*, 1978), and cell division *in
vitro* is a prerequisite for the formation of foci of transformed cells (Borek and Sachs, 1968; Kakunaga, 1975). As a
rule, CH results in a partial recovery from the toxic (Wang
and Cerutti, 1980a; Maher and McCormick, 1982) and transforming (Kakunaga, 1975; Ikenaga and Kakunaga, 1977) effects of
DNA damage. Undoubtedly DNA repair processes active during
the holding period play a role in reversing the effects of carcinogen treatment (Maher *et al.*, 1979; Weichselbaum *et al.*,
1979). As illustrated here, however, in some instances the
situation is more complex.

This chapter discusses three sets of experiments that address different aspects of cellular responses to DNA damage. First we describe experiments demonstrating that structurally similar cyclobutane-type pyrimidine photodimers in the DNA of normal human fibroblasts are excised at different rates. We then turn to experiments that characterize the role of chromatin structure in modulating both the formation and the subsequent excision of bulky carcinogen-DNA adducts. Finally, we review CH experiments indicating that the toxic and transforming effects of carcinogens are not always attributable to the concentration of carcinogen-DNA adducts in cellular DNA at the time cells are released from confluence.

II. EXCISABILITY OF STRUCTURALLY SIMILAR CYCLOBUTANE-TYPE PHOTODIMERS

Ultraviolet light in the range of 280 to 320 nm is the component of solar radiation most likely responsible for sunlight-induced skin cancer (Urbach, 1975). The most abundant photoproducts introduced into cellular DNA by light of these wavelengths are cyclobutane-type pyrimidine photodimers, although many other types of lesions are formed. Dimers have been implicated as causative agents of lethality and mutagenesis in human cells and of human skin cancer.

Experiments designed to measure the rates of excision of different cyclobutane-type dimers rely on a newly developed chromatography protocol that allows resolution and determination of low levels of thymine-thymine (TT) dimers and cytosine-thymine (CT) dimers in cellular DNA (Niggli and Cerutti, 1983). Cells are prelabeled with [3H] thymidine, irradiated, and incubated in medium for various periods to allow excision repair to occur. DNA is isolated from

the cells and hydrolyzed in formic acid. This hydrolysis
results in the deamination of some of the cytosine and all CT
dimers to uracil and UT dimers. The hydrolysate is chromatographed on high-pressure liquid chromatography (HPLC)
μBondapak C_{18}, and two peaks are collected, one containing
mostly TT dimers and the other containing mostly uracil and
UT dimers. These samples are pooled and reduced with $NaBH_4$
under conditions that convert UT and TT dimers, but not uracil
and thymine, to ring-open derivatives. The reduced sample,
when rechromatographed, yields two well-resolved peaks of TT
and UT dimers. The radioactivity in these peaks, internally
controlled for losses in manipulation by the presence of
$[^{14}C]$TT and $[^{14}C]$UT dimer standards, serves as a measure of
the concentrations of TT and CT dimers in cellular DNA.

Irradiation of normal human fibroblasts (CRL1221) or ex-
cision-defective human fibroblasts, xeroderma pigmentosum
complementation group A (XPA) (strain XP12BE, CRL1223), with
light at 313 nm produced dimers at rates of 2.06 $CT/10^8$ daltons
per kJm^{-2} and 1.66 $TT/10^8$ daltons per kJm^{-2}. Normal fibroblasts exposed to 10 kJm^{-2} of 313-nm light rapidly excised dimers from cellular DNA. Excision of CT dimers was much more
rapid than excision of TT dimers. After 8 h of postirradiation
incubation, normal cells removed 66% of the CT dimers initially
present, compared to 30% of the TT dimers. Neither CT dimers
nor TT dimers were excised by XPA cells during this time
(Niggli and Cerutti, 1983).

The observation that CT dimers are excised more rapidly
than are TT dimers is intriguing in view of the structural
similarity of these two lesions. Both are *cis-syn* cyclobutane
dimers and would be expected to produce similar structural dis-
tortions in DNA. It has been suggested that CT dimers may be
more biologically significant than TT dimers because cytosine
in dimer form is prone to spontaneous deamination to form

uracil (Wacker, 1963; Freeman *et al.*, 1965; Setlow, 1974; Hariharan and Johns, 1968). Photorepair of CT dimers would therefore leave, in some instances, a uracil residue potentially capable of mispairing, whereas photorepair of TT dimers would restore the integrity of the DNA. Although uracil can be removed from the DNA of mammalian cells by the action of a glycosylase (Caradonna and Cheng, 1980; Krokan and Wittwer, 1981), preferential repair of CT dimers would avoid the occurrence of secondary mutagenic lesions.

III. EFFECTS OF THE NUCLEOSOMAL STRUCTURE OF CHROMATIN
      ON THE FORMATION AND PROCESSING OF DNA LESIONS

Carcinogens that form bulky lesions in DNA usually damage nucleosomal linker DNA more readily than they do core DNA (Niggli and Cerutti, 1982; Cerutti *et al.*, 1981). Relative lesion concentrations for linker versus core DNA range from twofold for 7-bromomethylbenz[a]anthracene (Oleson *et al.*, 1979), four- to sixfold for *N*-acetoxyacetylaminofluorene (AAAF·) (Metzger *et al.*, 1977; Kaneko and Cerutti, 1980) and $7\beta,8\alpha$-dihydroxy-$9\alpha,10\alpha$-epoxy-7,8,9,10-tetrahydrobenzo[a]pyrene (BPDE I) (Jahn and Litman, 1979; Feldman *et al.*, 1980; Kaneko and Cerutti, 1982), 10- to 12-fold for aflatoxin B_1 (AFB_1) (Leadon *et al.*, in press) to linker being damaged exclusively by trimethylpsoralen plus light (Cech and Pardue, 1977; Wiesenhahn *et al.*, 1977). In general, damage is removed from linker DNA more efficiently than from core DNA. Thus, adducts in core DNA account for a major proportion of persistent lesions (Cerutti, 1982). An exception to this rule is BPDE I (Kaneko and Cerutti, 1982), whose adducts are excised from core DNA almost as rapidly as from linker, indicating that core DNA is accessible to excision repair processes. It is not known why core DNA reacts less readily with carcinogens, but protection of the DNA is not due to an ability of histone proteins to act as electrophile scavengers, because histones are modified only at very low levels (MacLeod *et al.*, 1981).

The high reactivity of carcinogens toward linker relative to core DNA may result in hypermodification of actively transcribed DNA. Direct visualization of transcribed chromatin (Igo-Kemenes *et al.*, 1982), as well as nuclease sensitivity studies (Elgin, 1981), suggest that transcribed regions of DNA contain fewer nucleosomes than do nontranscribed regions of the same length. Although nucleosome-free chromatin may not be free of protein, its sensitivity to exogenous nuclease suggests it may resemble linker DNA in its structure and therefore its reactivity. DNA fractions enriched for transcribed sequences are more extensively modified than is bulk DNA of benzo[a]pyrene-treated human cells (Arrand and Murray, 1982), although it is not clear whether hypermodification results from an unusual chromatin structure or from the location of such sequences in the nucleus.

Experimental evidence that nucleosome-free regions of transcribed DNA are especially prone to attack by carcinogens can be found in a study showing that AAAF preferentially modifies a control region of intracellular SV40 (Beard *et al.*, 1981). Monolayers of monkey kidney cell line BSC-1 were infected with SV40 and exposed to [^{3}H]AAAF during the late phase of viral infection. Viral DNA was purified and cleaved with restriction enzymes. Fragments were separated by electrophoresis on agarose and the proportion of radioactivity in each fragment was compared to its guanine content (over 95% of AAAF-DNA adducts occur at guanine residues). One fragment containing sequences governing the transcription of viral late genes was labeled to a specific activity 1.5-2 times higher than was expected from its guanine content. The radioactivities of all other fragments were proportional to their guanine content. No hypermodified fragments were observed when free viral DNA was treated with AAAF. The hypermodified fragment of SV40 corresponds to a region that is nucleosome free in 20 to 25% of isolated viral chromosomes (Saragosti *et al.*, 1980; Jakobovits *et al.*, 1980). Thus a nucleosome-depleted region of viral DNA similar in structure to nucleosome-depleted regions of transcribed cellular chromatin was particularly susceptible to modification by AAAF. It is not yet known whether adducts are preferentially excised from this control region.

Hypermodification of transcribed DNA by carcinogens could have important consequences. Not only would essential genes sustain high mutation rates, but lesions that inhibit transcription (Sauerbier and Hercules, 1978) could produce temporary modulation of gene expression. Reports that damage at certain sites can prevent interaction between DNA sequences and proteins that regulate the transcription of specific genes (Siebenlist *et al.*, 1980; Ptashne *et al.*, 1980; Simpson, 1980) reinforce the notion that the expression of genes crucial to cell behavior may be affected in a fraction of damaged cells.

IV.   CONFLUENT HOLDING

AFB_1 and benzo[a]pyrene (BP) are both procarcinogens that must be converted metabolically to electrophilic, ultimate carcinogens in order to react with DNA and to exhibit mutagenic and carcinogenic activity (e.g., see Miller and Miller, 1981). Low-passage mouse embryo fibroblast 10T1/2 cells are able to metabolize both of these carcinogens to reactive forms (Brown *et al.*, 1979; Wang and Cerutti, 1980a). 10T1/2 Cells are widely used in quantitative studies of *in vitro* malignant transformation. For CH experiments, with AFB_1, 10T1/2 cells at passage

10-11 were treated with various amounts of AFB_1. Previous studies have shown that the best abundant (90%) lesion, 2,3-dihydro-
2-(N^7-guanyl)-3-hydroxy-AFB_1 (AFB_1-N^7-Gua) is in part excised
by cellular repair mechanisms (Leadon *et al.*, 1981) but mostly
undergoes spontaneous degradation (Wang and Cerutti, 1980b) to
form unmodified guanine, aguanidinic sites and the secondary
adduct 2,3-dihydro-2-(N^5-formyl-2',5',6'-triamino-4'-oxo-N^5-
pyrimidyl)-3-hydroxy-AFB_1 (AFB_1-triamino-Py), which persists
in the DNA (Wang and Cerutti, 1980a; Leadon *et al.*, 1981). The
composition of AFB_1 adducts in 10T1/2 cells could be varied,
therefore, by incubating cells with a constant concentration of
AFB_1 for different times, with different concentrations of AFB_1
for the same amount of time, and by allowing AFB_1-treated cells
to rest in confluence for different lengths of time. The
colony-forming ability of treated cells decreased exponentially
with increased total AFB_1 adduct density at the time of subculture regardless of the treatment protocol that was used
(Leadon *et al.*, in press). In these experiments the toxicity
of AFB_1 was completely attributable to the presence of well-
characterized adducts in cellular DNA. It is concluded that
all covalent AFB_1-DNA adducts possessed comparable killing efficiencies.

In contrast, 10T1/2 cells released from confluency at
various times after treatment with AFB_1 formed foci of transformed cells with frequencies unrelated to the density of AFB_1
adducts at the time of subculturing (Amstad *et al.*, 1983).
Treatment of cells with 0.3 μM AFB_1 for 16 h produced five to
eight AFB_1 adducts per 10^6 bases in cellular DNA. After 15 h
of confluent holding, half of the total adducts initially produced had disappeared from the DNA, and the concentration of
the major adduct, AFB_1-N^7-Gua, was reduced to 50 and 25% of the
initial value after 13 h and 40 h at confluence, respectively.
The concentration of AFB_1-triamino-Py increased twofold over a

period of 16 h at confluence and remained essentially unchanged
from this value at 40 h. The frequency with which subcultured
cells formed transformed foci (mostly foci of type II) increased from 0.073 foci per dish immediately after treatment to
0.128 foci per dish after 16 h at confluence, but decreased to
0.062 foci per dish after 40 h at confluence. The increased
transformation frequency at 16 h contrasts with the reduced total AFB_1 adduct density at this time and is correlated only with
the increase in concentration of the AFB_1-triamino-Py adduct.
The decreased transformation frequency at 40 h, however, is at
variance with the persistence of this secondary adduct. These
data implicate cellular responses that modulate the efficiency
with which AFB_1 adducts in DNA can cause malignant transformation.

In separate experiments (P. A. Amstad and P. A. Cerutti,
unpublished), confluent cultures of 10T1/2 cells were exposed
either to the procarcinogen BP or to BPDE I, which represents
the electrophilic metabolite most responsible for the production of covalent adducts in DNA. Concentrations of BP and
BPDE I were chosen to produce 8-11 adducts per 10^6 bases, and,
with the exception of an additional minor adduct produced by
BP, the two chemicals produced the same types of lesions and in
similar proportions. The minor adduct formed only by BP represented about 14% of the total adducts and may correspond to
N^2-(7β,8α,9α-trihydroxy-7,8,9,10-tetrahydrobenzo[a]pyrene-10-
yl)deoxyguanosine (BPDE II-dG). Cells treated with either carcinogen removed adducts from their DNA at about the same rate.
The concentration of each type of adduct decreased 30-40% after
30 h and decreased 70% after 80 h at confluence.

Despite the similarity in the rate of adduct removal,
cells responded to the toxicity of BP and BPDE I in different
ways. Cells treated with BPDE I and held in confluence for
various times up to 30 h exhibited a gradual increase in colony-

forming ability relative to values for cells subcultured immediately after treatment. Thus, covalent BPDE I-DNA adducts
account for a major part of the cytotoxicity of BPDE I.
Colony-forming ability did not increase further, however, for
cells held in confluence for longer than 30 h, despite the
disappearance of an additional proportion of lesions from cellular DNA. This result indicates that toxicity is not absolutely correlated with the persistence of these lesions. Cells
exposed to the procarcinogen BP display a gradual fourfold decrease in colony-forming ability as they are held in confluence
for 30 h. No subsequent recovery from this depressed value is
observed for cells held in confluence for as long as 80 h after
exposure despite the disappearance of most of the BP-DNA adducts. Thus, some factor other than the density of covalent
BP-DNA adducts plays a crucial role in the cytotoxicity of BP.

The higher toxicity of BP relative to BPDE I may be due to
its ability to damage cells via indirect action, through the
generation of active oxygen species. BP may form active oxygen
by stimulating the arachidonic acid cascade (Levine, 1981;
Cerutti *et al.*, 1983). Hydroperoxides of arachidonic acid can
release active oxygen as they decay to more stable compounds
(Egan *et al.*, 1976; Rahimtula and O'Brien, 1976; Sugioka and
Nakano, 1976). In addition, BP is metabolized to 1,6-, 3,6-,
and 6,12-quinones that can generate active oxygen by participation in redox cycles (Lesko *et al.*, 1982). Indeed, human lung
cells treated with BP exhibit thymine base damage characteristic of that formed by OH radicals (Cerutti and Remsen, 1977; Ide
et al., in press). Attack of the thymine methyl group by HO·
is nearly 20-fold more frequent in treated cells than are adducts formed by the covalent attachment of BP to DNA. Indirect
damage either in DNA or in other cellular targets is thus induced in abundance by BP and may be the governing factor in its
toxicity. Fewer, if any active oxygen species would be produced

in those cells treated with BPDE I, not only because very low concentrations of this reactive metabolite were used, but also because BPDE I rapidly hydrolyzes in aqueous solution or reacts with cellular components to derivatives that are not metabolized in the same way that the parent hydrocarbon BP is.

We conclude that the biological effects of carcinogens are not always wholly attributable to the concentration of covalent adducts present in cellular DNA. For example, the toxicity of benzo[a]pyrene may depend more on DNA damage (and damage to non-DNA targets) introduced indirectly through the production of active oxygen species than on the presence of bulky BP-DNA lesions. Similarly, the ability of AFB_1 to induce transformation in 10T1/2 cells was found to be affected by factors other than the concentration of AFB_1-DNA adducts.

REFERENCES

Amstad, P. A., Wang, T. V., and Cerutti, P. A. (1983). *J. Natl. Cancer Inst. (U.S.)* 70, 135-139.
Arrand, J. E., and Murray, A. M. (1982). *Nucleic Acids Res.* 10, 1547-1555.
Beard, P., Kaneko, M., and Cerutti, P. (1981). *Nature (London)* 291, 84-85.
Borek, C., and Sachs, L. (1968). *Proc. Natl. Acad. Sci. USA* 59, 83-85.
Brown, H. S., Jeffrey, A. M., and Weinstein, I. B. (1979). *Cancer Res.* 39, 1673-1677.
Caradonna, S., and Cheng, Y. (1980). *J. Biol. Chem.* 255, 2293-2300.
Cayama, E., Tsuda, J., Sarma, D., and Farber, E. (1978). *Nature (London)* 275, 60-62.
Cech, T., and Pardue, M. (1977). *Cell* 11, 631-640.
Cerutti, P. A. (1982). *In* "Mechanisms of Chemical Carcinogenesis" (C. C. Harris and P. A. Cerutti, eds.), pp. 419-427. Liss, New York.
Cerutti, P., and Remsen, J. (1977). *In* "DNA Repair Processes" (W. Nichols and D. Murphy, eds.), pp. 147-166. Miami Symp. Specialists, Miami, Florida.

Cerutti, P. A., Kaneko, M., and Beard, P. (1981). *In* "Chromosome Damage and Repair" (E. Seeberg and K. Kleppe, eds.), pp. 55-69. Plenum, New York.

Cerutti, P., Emerit, I., and Amstad, P. (1983). *In* "Genes and Proteins in Oncogenesis" (H. Vogel and I. B. Weinstein, eds.), pp. 55-69. Academic Press, New York.

Egan, R., Paxton, J., and Kuehl, F. A. (1976). *J. Biol. Chem.* *251*, 7329-7335.

Elgin, S. C. R. (1981). *Cell 27*, 413-415.

Feldman, G., Remsen, J., Wang, T. V., and Cerutti, P. A. (1980). *Biochemistry 19*, 1095-1101.

Freeman, K. B., Hariharan, P. V., and Johns, H. E. (1965). *J. Mol. Biol. 13*, 833-848.

Hariharan, P. V., and Johns, H. E. (1968). *Photochem. Photobiol. 8*, 11-22.

Ide, M.-L., Kaneko, M., and Cerutti, P. (1983). *In* "Protective Agents in Human and Experimental Cancer" (D. McBrien and T. Slater, eds.), Academic Press, New York, in press.

Igo-Kemenes, T., Hörz, W., and Zachau, H. (1982). *Annu. Rev. Biochem. 51*, 89-121.

Ikenaga, M., and Kakunaga, T. (1977). *Cancer Res. 37*, 3672-3678.

Jahn, C., and Litman, G. (1979). *Biochemistry 18*, 1442-1449.

Jakobovits, E., Bratosin, S., and Aloni, Y. (1980). *Nature (London) 285*, 263-265.

Kakunaga, T. (1975). *Cancer Res. 35*, 1637-1642.

Kaneko, M., and Cerutti, P. A. (1980). *Cancer Res. 40*, 4313-4319.

Kaneko, M., and Cerutti, P. A. (1982). *Chem. Biol. Interact. 38*, 261-274.

Krokan, H., and Wittwer, C. (1981). *Nucleic Acids Res. 9*, 2599-2613.

Leadon, S. A., Tyrrell, R. M., and Cerutti, P. A. (1981). *Cancer Res. 41*, 5125-5129.

Leadon, S., Amstad, P., and Cerutti, P. (1983). *Use Hum. Cells Assess Risk Phys. Chem. Agents* (A. Castillani, ed.), Plenum Press, London, in press.

Lesko, S., Ts'O, P., Jang, S.-U., and Cheng, R. (1982). *In* "Free Radicals, Lipid Peroxidation and Cancer" (D. McBrien and T. Slater, eds.), pp. 401-414. Academic Press, New York.

Levine, L. (1981). *Adv. Cancer Res. 35*, 49-79.

MacLeod, M. C., Kootstra, A., Mansfield, B. K., Slaga, T. J., and Selkirk, J. K. (1981). *Cancer Res. 41*, 4080-4086.

Maher, V. M., and McCormick, J. J. (1982). *In* "Mechanisms of Chemical Carcinogenesis" (C. C. Harris and P. A. Cerutti, eds.), pp. 429-439. Liss, New York.

Maher, V. M., Dorney, D. J., Mendrala, A. L., Konze-Thomas, B., and McCormick, J. J. (1979). *Mutat. Res. 62*, 311-323.

Metzger, G., Wilhelm, F., and Wilhelm, M. (1977). *Biochem. Biophys. Res. Commun. 75*, 703-710.

Miller, E. C., and Miller, J. A. (1981). *Cancer (Philadelphia) 47*, 1055-1064.

Niggli, H. J., and Cerutti, P. A. (1982). *Biochem. Biophys. Res. Commun. 105*, 1215-1223.

Niggli, H. J., and Cerutti, P. A. (1983). *Biochemistry 22*, 1390-1395.

Oleson, F., Mitchell, B., Dipple, A., and Lieberman, M. (1979). *Nucleic Acids Res. 7*, 1343-1361.

Pardee, A. B., Dubrow, R., Hamlin, J. L., and Kletzien, R. F. (1978). *Annu. Rev. Biochem. 47*, 715-750.

Ptashne, M., Jeffrey, A., Johnson, A. D., Maurer, R., Meyer, B. J., Pabo, C. O., Roberts, T. M., and Sauer, R. T. (1980). *Cell 19*, 1-11.

Rahimtula, A., and O'Brien, P. J. (1976). *Biochem. Biophys. Res. Commun. 70*, 893-899.

Saragosti, S., Moyne, G., and Yaniv, M. (1980). *Cell 20*, 65-75.

Sauerbier, W., and Hercules, K. (1978). *Annu. Rev. Genet. 12*, 329-363.

Setlow, R. B. (1974). *Proc. Natl. Acad. Sci. USA 71*, 3363-3366.

Setlow, R. B., Ahmed, F. E., and Grist, E. (1977). *In* "Origins of Human Cancer" (H. H. Hiatt, J. D. Watson, and J. A. Winsten, eds.), Book B, pp. 889-902. Cold Spring Harbor Lab., Cold Spring Harbor, New York.

Siebenlist, U., Simpson, R. B., and Gilbert, W. (1980). *Cell 20*, 269-281.

Simpson, R. B. (1980). *Nucleic Acids Res. 8*, 759-766.

Sugioka, K., and Nakano, M. (1976). *Biochim. Biophys. Acta 423*, 203-216.

Urbach, F. (1975). *In* "Climatic Impact Assessment Program" (D. S. Nachtwey, ed.), Part I, pp. 19-25. Dept. Transportation, Washington, D.C.

Wacker, A. (1963). *Prog. Nucleic Acid Res. 1*, 369-399.

Wang, T. V., and Cerutti, P. A. (1980a). *Cancer Res. 40*, 2904-2909.

Wang, T. V., and Cerutti, P. A. (1980b). *Biochemistry 19*, 1692-1698.

Weichselbaum, R., Nove, J., and Little, J. (1979). *Nature (London) 271*, 261-262.

Wiesenhahn, G., Hyde, J., and Hearst, J. (1977). *Biochemistry 16*, 925-932.

10

VARIATIONS IN DNA REPAIR AMONG HUMANS

Richard B. Setlow

Biology Department
Brookhaven National Laboratory[1]
Upton, New York

I.   INTRODUCTION

A.   DNA Repair and Disease

The roles of DNA repair in human disease have been reviewed extensively (Setlow, 1978; Arlett and Lehmann, 1978;

---

[1]*Brookhaven National Laboratory is operated by Associated
Universities for the Department of Energy.*

Copyright © 1983 by Academic Press, Inc.
All rights of reproduction in any form reserved.
ISBN 0-12-327660-8

Friedberg *et al.*, 1979; Paterson, 1979; Kraemer, 1981), the
field of DNA repair has been summarized in a number of workshops
and review articles (Hanawalt and Setlow, 1975; Hanawalt *et al.*,
1978, 1979; Roberts, 1978; Lindahl, 1982), and the techniques
used to measure DNA repair are given in a laboratory manual
(Friedberg and Hanawalt, 1981). The following conditions are
known (or at least suspected) to involve such DNA repair deficiencies: xeroderma pigmentosum (XP), ataxia telangiectasia
(AT), Fanconi's anemia, Bloom's syndrome, and Huntington's
disease (HD) (Scudiero *et al.*, 1981).

   The identification of thymine dimers in DNA as the most
common and important UV lesion led rapidly to the discovery
of dimer excision repair in the DNA of bacteria. The relevance of such observations to humans was established when
Cleaver (1968) showed that cells from individuals with XP--a
syndrome in which the individuals are very prone to sunlight-
induced skin cancer--were defective in unscheduled DNA synthesis (UDS). Because UDS has been shown, when tested, to represent the polymerization step in excision repair, Cleaver's
observations connected a defect in such repair with a high
risk of cancer from an environmental agent. The UV in sunlight is known to cause many damages to cellular DNA. The
connection was greatly strengthened when it was shown that XP
cells were defective in the excision repair of pyrimidine dimers (Setlow *et al.*, 1969). Such observations represented
direct experimental evidence that damage to DNA is potentially
carcinogenic and that the potential depends strongly on DNA
repair systems. For example, the probability of an XP individual developing skin cancer (nonmelanoma and melanoma) is
10^3- to 10^4-fold greater than that of the average white person
of comparable age (Kraemer, 1981). DNA repair mechanisms (excision, photoreactivation, and postreplication repair) work to
reduce the effective dose to normal individuals by a factor

estimated between 7 and 20 compared to the average XP individual (Setlow, 1980). XP cells are not absolutely defective in DNA repair. For example, the magnitude of the excision repair defects measured directly (Cleaver and Bootsma, 1975; Ahmed and Setlow, 1979a,b) or by cytotoxicity of UV for fibroblasts (Andrews et al., 1978) depends on the complementation group and ranges from about 40 to 95%. Thus what seem to be small differences in DNA repair from the normal may have very large biological effects. The big biological amplification of repair defects may result from the fact that the DNA damage produced by UV is tremendous compared to that experienced by the cells of the body when exposed to ambient chemicals in the environment (Setlow, 1982). Cairns (1980) concluded, from the absence of internal cancers among XP individuals, that environmental chemicals that mimic UV and that produce lesions that are repaired by the same general type of system as is UV damage are not significant environmental carcinogens. A similar conclusion can be reached from the analysis of Feinberg and Coffey (1982).

The connection between defective DNA repair and skin cancer in XP has led to the search for other repair-deficient diseases, and indeed others have been found (see earlier). However, it is only for XP that the etiological agent is known. It should not be inferred from the simplistic description just given that the molecular mechanisms and the controls of excision repair in mammalian cells are well understood. They are not. For example, there are no ready explanations for the existence of large numbers of complementation groups of XP (Cleaver and and Bootsma, 1975). Nevertheless, the lack of ready explanations is not surprising, because the details of excision repair in bacteria are just beginning to be worked out satisfactorily.

B.   Nucleotide Excision Repair

Effective excision repair for pyrimidine dimers involves
the coordinated action of a number of steps, including an endonuclease attack near a dimer, an exonuclease attack to remove the dimer and/or adjacent bases, a repolymerization using
the opposite polynucleotide strand as a template, and finally,
ligation of the reconstructed DNA. The same general sequence
of steps as that elucidated for pyrimidine dimers is also observed for a number of chemicals that mimic UV radiation. In
human cells such chemicals and UV give rise to what is termed
long-patch repair (Regan and Setlow, 1974). Long-patch repair
is associated with nucleotide excision because in the process
of repair such units are removed from one strand of the DNA
duplex. Almost all the steps just outlined are used as
measures of such repair, for example, (1) the loss of products
from DNA measured directly or by the loss of endonuclease-
sensitive sites, (2) the appearance and disappearance of strand
breaks in DNA during the process of repair by alkaline sucrose
gradient sedimentation or by alkaline elution, and (3) the repolymerization step by UDS or by repair replication or by the
photolysis of BrdUrd incorporated during repair (Friedberg and
Hanawalt, 1981).

C.   Base Excision Repair and Dealkylation

A second type of repair, called base excision repair,
does not involve an initial attack on the polynucleotide chain
but removes by glycosylase action only the base from the polynucleotide. The resulting apurinic site in the DNA may be restored to its normal configuration in several ways, including
direct replacement of a purine or subsequent endonuclease attack. A special case of base excision would be the direct dealkylation of an alkylated base. Such repair works on

O^6-alkylguanine--presumptive mutagenic and carcinogenic lesions (Singer, 1979)--in *E. coli* (Olsson and Lindahl, 1980), mouse liver (Bogden *et al.*, 1981), rat liver (Mehta *et al.*, 1981), and human lymphocytes and fibroblasts (Waldstein *et al.*, 1982a,b). Repair by dealkylation would not be detected by any of the methods just outlined except one that determines directly the loss of products. In particular, repair would not be detected by the appearance and disappearance of strand breaks, by UDS, or by repair replication.

The interest in the dealkylation pathway arises because many cell lines from human tumors or virus-transformed cell lines are deficient in the removal of methyl groups from O^6-methylguanine (O^6MeGua) (Day *et al.*, 1980; Sklar and Strauss, 1981), leading to the classification of cells as either Mer$^-$ or Mer$^+$. Mer$^-$ Cells are killed more readily and show appreciably more SCEs than Mer$^+$ cells after treatment with *N*-methyl-*N'*-nitro-*N*-nitrosoguanidine (MNNG) (see Section II,C). A past complication in the interpretation of the pathways of DNA repair was a report that XP cells were unable to repair O^6-alkylguanine residues (Goth-Goldstein, 1977). However, such a failure seems to have been the result of the fact that the cells used for the assay were transformed ones. Untransformed XP cells are probably Mer$^+$ (Day *et al.*, 1980; Waldstein *et al.*, 1982b). In contrast, studies of the cytotoxicity of alkylating agents toward untransformed XP fibroblast strains (Simon *et al.*, 1981) indicate that although, in comparison to normal strains, they are not sensitive to MNNG (a methylating agent), they are sensitive to ENNG (an ethylating agent).

The difference between the Mer$^+$ and Mer$^-$ phenotypes of mammalian cells in culture does not seem to lie in the constitutive amounts of acceptor protein per cell but in the ability of Mer$^+$ cells to adapt to treatment with low levels of MNNG by making more acceptor protein (Waldstein *et al.*, 1982b). Cells that are phenotypically Mer⁻ do not adapt readily, and their repair system is easily saturated by treatment with low doses of alkylating agents, because the reaction of the acceptor protein with the alkylated DNA is a stoichiometric one (Waldstein *et al.*, 1982a).

D. Effects of X Irradiation on Normal and AT Cells

On the average, agents that produce base damage in the form of alkylation or small changes in conformation, as distinguished from the large ones arising from interactions with agents such as benzo[a]pyrene, give rise to small repair patches. Such patches are, on the average, only a few nucleotides in normal human cells, compared to the long patches of approximately 100 nucleotides found in UV-irradiated cells. It is not clear how much of the small-patch observation arises from an average including zero patch from dealkylation or direct insertion of a purine into an apurinic site. BrUra-Photolysis experiments measure only the incorporation of pyrimidines and, in most cases, UDS and repair replication use pyrimidines as the precursors; such an apurinic insertion would not be measured. From the point of view of patch sizes, ionizing radiation damage falls into the short-patch category, although at long times after irradiation some long-patch component is detectable (Setlow *et al.*, 1976). However, the molecular nature of the lesions responsible for such repair patches is not known, even though endonucleases are known that act on DNA damaged by ionizing radiation (Paterson, 1978). Such endonucleases can be used as reagents to detect the presence of the repair of damage even though the precise type of damage is not known, and can only be described by the general phrase "base damage."

After X irradiation of normal cells with doses in the range of hundreds of rads, or after treatment with low doses of bleomycin (a DNA strand breaker), there is an immediate decrease in the rate of DNA synthesis that is associated with the failure to initiate new clusters of replicons. These data imply that there is some supraorganization of DNA so as to control the initiation of such clusters. DNA synthesis returns to normal rates within periods of the order of hours. X Irradiation or bleomycin treatment of AT cells does not result in an immediate decrease in DNA synthesis, indicating that the inhibition of initiations in these cells is much more resistant than in normal ones (Painter and Young, 1980; Cramer and Painter, 1981). One interpretation of such data is that the failure to inhibit DNA synthesis in AT cells means that replication will take place more readily on a damaged template, and therefore, the chance of a lethal event will be increased. However, AT cells have been found to be hypomutable (Arlett and Lehmann, 1978). Thus on the surface it looks as if lethal and mutagenic events are quite separate, and by inference, lethal and carcinogenic events are not necessarily related.

It is of interest that the UV irradiation of normal human fibroblasts just before the beginning of the S phase results in a high yield of transformants compared to the number obtained by radiation in early G_1 phase (Maher et al., 1982). Moreover, there is a high yield of mutation when the irradiation is carried out just before the beginning of the S phase (Konze-Thomas et al., 1982). However, there is little difference between the cytotoxicity of UV delivered at different times in the cell cycle. Hence transformation and mutation but not lethal events are "fixed" in S. Nevertheless, the lethal events are subject to excision repair because XP cells are much more sensitive than normal to the transforming, mutagenic, and cytotoxic effects of UV. These data therefore indicate that the lethal event for cells in culture is not DNA synthesis. It was hypothesized by Konze-Thomas *et al.* (1982) that the lethal events were the synthesis of defective RNA and hence aberrant proteins following UV irradiation (Kantor *et al.*, 1977).

Data on X-irradiated lymphoblastoid cell lines (Houldsworth and Lavin, 1980) are similar to those obtained on fibroblasts. Moreover, they indicate that the failure to inhibit DNA synthesis in AT cells is associated with a failure of radiation to stimulate the synthesis of poly(ADPribose) (Edwards and Taylor, 1980). Synthesis of this polymer has been associated with the introduction of single-strand nicks into DNA, but nicks are certainly introduced into the DNA of AT cells by X rays and the repair rate of single-strand breaks in such cells is equivalent to that of normal (Vincent *et al.*, 1975; Taylor *et al.*, 1975). Perhaps there is a special kind or locale of breaks that is important for poly(ADPribose) synthesis and for the inhibition of initiation.

E. Contradictory Observations

At present there are contradictory data for the sensitivity of AT cells to MNNG; some experimenters say they are more sensitive than normal cells (Scudiero, 1980), whereas others indicate that they are not (Jaspers *et al.*, 1982). The contradiction may have to do with the concentration of NAD in the medium (Jaspers *et al.*, 1982), low values giving high sensitivity. HD fibroblasts obtained from United States sources are sensitive to X rays, but HD cells from Great Britain are not (Bridges, 1981). The explanation for this anomaly is not known, but such findings should make one cautious about interpretations of similar data such as the sensitivity of HD cells to MNNG.

II.   VARIATIONS IN REPAIR IN THE "NORMAL" POPULATION

The definition of normal value is complicated by three variances: (1) that of repeat values for a particular cell culture, (2) that for independent cell cultures obtained from the same person at different times, and (3) that between cultures obtained from different normal individuals. Most of the data on normal variances come from investigations attempting to correlate age, life-style, or abnormal conditions with DNA repair (e.g., UDS in human leukocytes), or cell survival after treatment with radiations or chemicals. If each of the variances mentioned were normally distributed, the resulting distribution would not be Gaussian. However, as the experiments cited here indicate, many of the distributions are close to normal ones.

A number of investigations have attempted to correlate various human conditions with UDS in human lymphocytes treated with radiations or chemicals. For example, DNA repair after UV irradiation is less in individuals with actinic keratoses than in normal individuals (Abo-Darub et al., 1978) and there is less DNA repair following UV irradiation in the lymphocytes of patients with recurrent herpes simplex infection (Fanta et al., 1978). Madden et al. (1979) showed that leukocytes of smokers and drug addicts had less unscheduled synthesis after UV treatment than did controls. The usefulness of radiation and its good dosimetry as a repair probe is indicated by the studies of Pero et al. (1976), who concluded that after AAAF treatment there was more repair in lymphocytes from individuals with high blood pressure than from those with average blood pressure. But the higher amount of repair seemed to have resulted from more damage, and there seemed to be equal amounts of repair per unit damage. Lambert et al. (1979) showed that there is an association, although a weak one, between repair in leukocytes

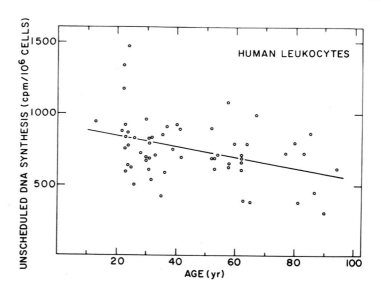

Fig. 1. Unscheduled DNA synthesis after UV irradiation of human leukocytes plotted versus age of the donor. In these experiments, scheduled DNA synthesis was inhibited by hydroxyurea. Data from Lambert *et al.* (1979).

after UV irradiation *in vitro* and age of the donor, with older people having less repair. The striking thing about most of these studies is not so much the correlations with the characteristics of the individuals, but the large variation--several-fold--among presumably normal individuals in the populations investigated.

A.   UV Damage

Most of the measurements on repair following UV damage have been made by UDS, and, for human leukocytes, most of the measurements of UDS use scintillation counting to determine the radioactivity incorporated per microgram of DNA or per cell. Such measurements, although easy to make, would not detect a heterogeneous population of cells that include both repairing and non-repairing ones, or populations containing several different cell

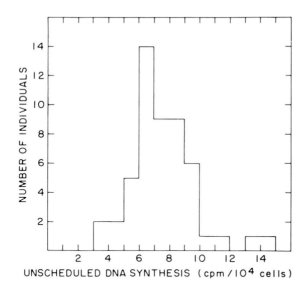

Fig. 2. The number of individuals whose leukocytes exposed to UV give the amount of unscheduled DNA synthesis shown on the abscissa. These are the same data shown in Fig. 1.

types each of which has a different level of repair. Heterogeneous populations have been detected in late-passage fibroblasts (Hart and Setlow, 1976). Nevertheless, UDS measurements by scintillation counting rather than by autoradiography are reasonably reproducible. Typical results from Lambert *et al.* (1979) are shown in Fig. 1. There is a decrease in UDS with age of the donor, although the decrease is not particularly large. However, as pointed out already, the interesting aspect of the data is the wide variance observed for individuals of equivalent ages.

The data in Fig. 1 may be lumped together and presented as a distribution curve plotting the number of individuals with a given level of UDS versus UDS as shown in Fig. 2. The extremes of this distribution range over almost a factor of 4.5, with a range from the mean of close to a factor of two. If one called

the upper end of this distribution the normal value, the lower
end of the distribution would be described as repair deficient
and, in terms of repair, would correspond to a mild case of
xeroderma pigmentosum. The repair capacity for UV damage--a
long-patch system--increases markedly after stimulation of
lymphocytes (Scudiero et al., 1976), and it is conceivable
that some of the differences reported for the unstimulated
white cells shown in Figs. 1 and 2 could arise from differences
in the fractions of cycling cells in peripheral lymphocytes.

A second approach to the problem of variation in normal
repair used fibroblast cultures and estimated the amount of
repair by permitting repair to take place in the presence of
BrdUrd. The incorporated analog sensitizes the repaired DNA
to long-wavelength UV light (Regan and Setlow, 1974), and the
photolysis of the repaired regions permits one to estimate
both the patch size and the numbers of repaired regions. The
measure of repair in such studies is not the incorporated
radioactivity per cell but the number of single-strand breaks
introduced into the repaired DNA by the photolytic radiation.
The breaks are easily enumerated by sedimentation in alkali.
Figure 3 shows a distribution curve giving the change in the
reciprocal of weight-average molecular weight ($1/M_w$) as a result of photolytic treatment for both normal and XP fibroblast
cultures. In this group of cell strains there is a clear separation between XP and normal individuals, and there is a wide
distribution in the range of normal values. The repeatability
of this assay has a standard deviation of approximately 10%.
Hence the width of the normal distribution reflects the differences between cell strains rather than errors in the experimental assay.

A summary of three experiments carried out to measure the
distribution of UV repair among cell cultures is shown in
Table I. The width of the distribution for fibroblasts is

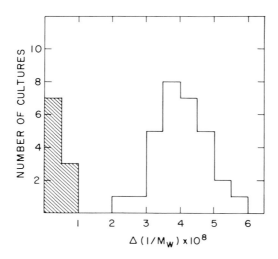

Fig. 3. The number of fibroblast cultures from normal (□) or XP (▨) individuals that when exposed to UV (20 J/m^2) and permitted to repair in BrdUrd give the number of breaks per dalton, $\Delta(1/M_w)$, shown on the abscissa as a result of exposure to a large photolytic dose of 313-nm radiation. In such experiments, the value on the abscissa is proportional to the number of repaired sites in the DNA. Data from Regan and Setlow (unpublished).

TABLE I.   Variations in UV-Induced Excision Repair among Cell Cultures from Apparently Normally Repairing Individuals[a]

Number of cultures	Method	Standard deviation (%)	Reference
30 Fibroblast	BrUra Photolysis	17	Setlow and Regan (unpublished)
40 Leukocyte	UDS	26	Lambert *et al.* (1979)
90 Leukocyte	UDS	∿50	Madden *et al.* (1979)
38 Leukocyte[b] (heroin addicts)	UDS	100	Madden *et al.* (1979)

[a]*Data from experiments shown in Figs. 2 and 3 or similar experiments.*
[b]*Average UDS was 0.3 of normal.*

appreciably narrower than those for leukocytes. This difference is not a direct result of the UDS measurement, because
the amount of UDS in exposed fibroblast cultures is just as
expected from the number of pyrimidine dimers removed per cell
and the patch size (Ahmed and Setlow, 1979a).

B. X-Ray Damage

    X Rays kill cells in culture, but because the lesion or
lesions responsible for the cytotoxic effect of X rays is not
known, there is no good molecular measure for the repair of
X-ray damage. For example, AT cells are sensitive to X rays,
but all AT cell strains are not defective in the various
measures of DNA repair such as repair replication or failure
to remove endonuclease-sensitive sites (Paterson and Smith,
1979). Hence the only reliable measure that can be used at
present is cytotoxicity. If the logarithm of the fraction of
cells surviving and able to make colonies is plotted versus
dose, there will be an appreciable portion of the dose-response
curve that is a straight line and that may be characterized by
a value D_0, the dose necessary to reduce survival to 0.37.
For this portion of the curve, D_0 is the dose necessary to give
an average of one lethal hit. There have been three extensive
surveys of the values of D_0 for a number of fibroblast strains
obtained for normal and AT individuals (Arlett and Harcourt,
1980; Weichselbaum et al., 1980; Cox and Masson, 1980). The
data from these three surveys are shown in Fig. 4.

    There is a clear separation between the sensitivities of
AT cell strains and normal cell strains in all the surveys, and
they all show a rather wide distribution of normal sensitivities, although the widths of the distributions seem to differ
from one survey to another. Moreover, the maximum of the distribution for normal individuals is at different values of D_0

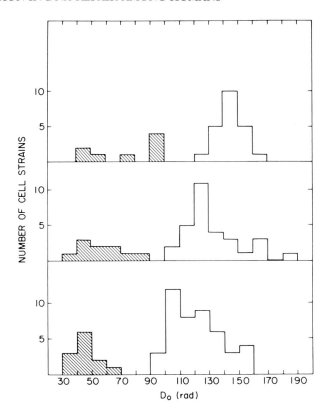

Fig. 4. The effect of ionizing radiation on fibroblast strains is shown for three surveys (normal, ■ ; AT, ▧) in which the number of fibroblast strains with a given D_0 is plotted versus D_0. Data are from (top) Weichselbaum et al. (1980); (middle) Arlett and Harcourt (1980); (bottom) Cox and Masson (1980).

for the three surveys. It is improbable that these differences arise from dosimetry, and one must ascribe the differences to the use of different cell strains or different methods of handling the cells. Arlett and Harcourt and Cox and Masson used similar techniques for measuring cell survival, and Arlett and Harcourt and Weichselbaum et al. made measurements on, presumably, some of the same cell strains. The two groups of investigators obtained similar D_0 values for the strains investi-

gated in common. Hence, the reasons for the differences between the distributions shown in Fig. 4 are not known. Some
of the differences may arise because even repeat biopsies give
different D_0 values (Arlett and Harcourt, 1980), although the
few cases investigated seem to give a somewhat narrower distribution than shown in Fig. 4.

The difference in radiosensitivity between AT and normal
cells can account for the high radiation sensitivity of AT individuals. However, the difference cannot account directly for
the higher cancer incidence among them, because the spectrum of
cancer in AT individuals is quite different from that observed
in the irradiated survivors of the atomic bomb attacks on Japan
(Paterson and Smith, 1979). Thus there is no direct connection
between cancer proneness and radiation sensitivity.

C. Alkylation Damage

The cytotoxic effects of an alkylating agent such as MNNG
on fibroblasts may be measured in terms similar to those used
for X rays, namely the concentration giving a survival of 0.37
on the exponential part of the dose-response curve. This type
of analysis gave rise to the characterization of cells as Mer$^+$
and Mer$^-$. Such cells differ not in their constitutive levels
of methyl acceptor protein but in their ability to adapt to
small doses of MNNG (Waldstein et al., 1982b). Regardless of
the explanation for enhanced cytotoxicity to alkylating agents,
the values of D_0 are good measures of sensitivity. A priori
one would expect distribution curves of such values to show
larger variances than the D_0 values for radiation sensitivities, because not only is chemical dosimetry inherently more
variable than physical dosimetry, but compounds such as MNNG
need activation before they can react with DNA, and
nitrosamines--commonly used carcinogenic alkylating agents--

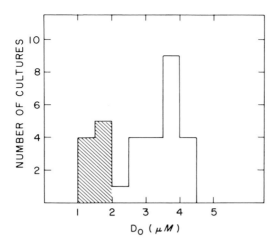

Fig. 5. The distribution for the number of fibroblast strains as a function of the dose D_0 of MNNG necessary to give a survival of 0.37 on the exponential part of the survival curve for 5 HD patients (▨) and 13 normal (▫) individuals. Data from Scudiero et al. (1981).

need enzymatic activation before they can react with macromolecules. Typical distribution curves are shown in Fig. 5 (Scudiero et al., 1981). These data show a clean separation in sensitivity between fibroblasts of American patients with HD and normal fibroblasts. There may be an uncertainty about this clean separation, however, because HD fibroblasts obtained from English patients do not show enhanced sensitivity to γ rays, whereas those from American patients do (Bridges, 1981).

The cytotoxic alkylating product has not been well identified, but there are good indications in E. coli that it may be N-3-methyladenine or N-3-methylguanine (Karran et al., 1982; Evensen and Seeberg, 1982). In contrast, there are good data indicating that the mutagenic lesion is O^6MeGua, and indeed Mer⁻ cells, defective in the removal of this product, are more sensitive to its cytotoxic action and show appreciably

less host cell reactivation of treated mammalian viruses (Day
et al., 1980). Thus one might infer that a good measure of
DNA repair of O^6MeGua in cells would be the rate of loss of
this product from the DNA of cells treated with radioactive
MNNG. This assay is not an ideal one, because in order to at-
tain acceptable sensitivity large numbers of cells (approximately 10^8) are needed, and concentrations of MNNG high enough
to saturate the stoichiometric methyl-accepting proteins in
the cell are used. This assay really measures adaptation and
not the constitutive level of acceptor protein for O^6MeGua.
Hence it is easier and more precise to measure directly the
amounts of acceptor proteins in extracts of cells by reacting
the extracts with exogenous DNA containing radioactive O^6MeGua.
Either the loss of O^6MeGua from DNA can be measured by high-
performance liquid chromatography, or the transfer of radioactive methyl groups from DNA to protein can be determined directly. Both assays give the same answer (Waldstein *et al.*,
1982c). An assay can be carried out on 100 to 300 µg of protein representing approximately 2×10^6 cells. A measurement
of the number of cells used to make the cell extract and the
number of O^6MeGua gives the number of acceptor sites per cell.
Such assays have been done on extracts of unstimulated and
stimulated human lymphocytes. They show a wide variation
among the apparently normal human population (Fig. 6). A summary of the values obtained for a number of different types of
mammalian cells is shown in Table II. It is obvious that the
variation among lymphocytes is much greater than that observed
in fibroblast-like lines and fibroblast strains.

To deplete the O^6MeGua acceptor sites per cell by exposure
to MNNG would require concentrations greater than 0.5 µ*M*. Such
concentrations of alkylating agents are not met in real life,
although they are used extensively in laboratory experiments,
in which it is the ability of cells to adapt that determines

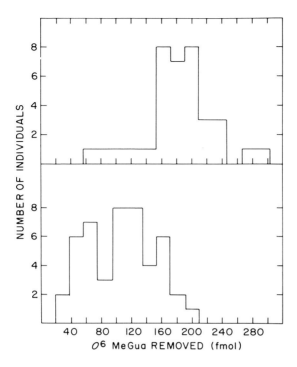

Fig. 6. The relation between the number of individuals and the activity of extracts of lymphocytes able to remove the indicated amount of O^6MeGua from exogenous DNA. Stimulated lymphocytes (top) were tested at 46 h after stimulation. Unstimulated lymphocytes (bottom) were tested immediately after isolation. Data from Waldstein *et al.* (1982a).

the response. Hence it is the constitutive level of acceptor sites that is important for the environmental exposure of people. The association, if any, between the big spread in values obtained for acceptor activities in lymphocytes and other parameters such as life-style or genetic background, has not yet been made.

TABLE II. Constitutive Levels of O^6-Methylguanine Acceptor
          Sites per Cell × 10^{-3} [a]

Cell type	Mer cell type	Average	Range
4 Human fibroblast strains	Mer[+]	121	110-133
3 Human tumor lines	Mer[+]	138	119-175
3 Human tumor lines	Mer[-]	124	114-130
2 SV40-transformed human lines	Mer[-]	118	107-128
2 Chinese hamster lines	Mer[-]	102	94-111
53 Normal human T lymphocytes	--	60	14-110
4 Normal human B lymphocytes	--	22	20-23
6 Chronic lymphocytic leukemia B lymphocytes	--	150	86-193

[a]Data from Waldstein et al. (1982a,b,d).

III. CONCLUSIONS

   There are wide variations in the abilities of human cells
to repair damage to their DNA, measured either by direct biochemical or biophysical means, or by cytotoxicity. The variations for particular tissues in DNA repair among the normal
population seem to be significantly greater than experimental
error. Nevertheless, we are not clear about four points.

   1. The tissue dependence may well be a factor. Lymphocytes and fibroblasts of XP or AT show similar deficits in repair (Cleaver and Bootsma, 1975; Paterson and Smith, 1979).
However, there is a significant difference between the repair
capability for UV damage by normal neural tissue and fibroblasts
(Gibson and D'Ambrosio, 1982).

   2. We know nothing about genetic factors that might influence what seems to be the variation among the normal population.

3.   Life-style factors could be important in modulating the levels of DNA repair (e.g., see Madden *et al.*, 1979).

4.   Do any of the variations in DNA repair among apparently normal individuals have prognostic value? Are people on the low side more prone to disease than people on the high side of the repair distribution? Can one interpolate between the effects of severe repair deficiencies, as in XP and AT, and the average normal population to predict the effects of the variations in the normal population?

A fruitful analysis of the last three factors just mentioned can only be made if the variations described are real in the sense that they do not reflect errors in the repair measurements themselves or variations in the growth of cells in culture. Such factors must be evaluated thoroughly before the variations in DNA repair can be taken seriously as possible prognostic indicators. Nevertheless, there may be strong deterministic factors--variations in normal levels of DNA repair-- not just stochastic ones in carcinogenesis.

REFERENCES

Abo-Darub, J. M., Mackie, R., and Pitts, J. D. (1978). *Bull. Cancer 65*, 357-362.
Ahmed, F. E., and Setlow, R. B. (1979a). *Cancer Res. 39*, 471-479.
Ahmed, F. E., and Setlow, R. B. (1979b). *Photochem. Photobiol. 29*, 983-989.
Andrews, A. D., Barrett, S. F., and Robbins, J. H. (1978). *Proc. Natl. Acad. Sci. USA 75*, 1984-1988.
Arlett, C. F., and Harcourt, S. (1980). *Cancer Res. 40*, 926-932.
Arlett, C. F., and Lehmann, A. R. (1978). *Annu. Rev. Genet. 12*, 95-111.
Bogden, J. M., Eastman, A., and Bresnick, E. (1981). *Nucleic Acids Res. 9*, 3089-3103.
Bridges, B. A. (1981). *Proc. R. Soc. London Ser. B 212*, 263-278.

Cairns, J. (1980). *Nature (London)* *289,* 353–357.

Cleaver, J. E. (1968). *Nature (London)* *218,* 652–656.

Cleaver, J. E., and Bootsma, D. (1975). *Annu. Rev. Genet.* *9,* 19–38.

Cox, R., and Masson, W. K. (1980). *Int. J. Radiat. Biol.* *38,* 575–576.

Cramer, P., and Painter, R. B. (1981). *Nature (London)* *291,* 671–672.

Day, R. S., III, Ziolkowski, C. H. J., Scudiero, D. A., Meyer, S. A., Lubiniecki, A. S., Girardi, A. J., Galloway, S. M., and Bynum, G. D. (1980). *Nature (London)* *288,* 724–727.

Edwards, M. J., and Taylor, A. M. R. (1980). *Nature (London)* *287,* 745–747.

Evensen, G., and Seeberg, E. (1982). *Nature (London)* *296,* 773–775.

Fanta, D., Topaloglou, A., and Altman, H. (1978). *Bull. Cancer* *65,* 341–346.

Feinberg, A. P., and Coffey, D. S. (1982). *Cancer Res.* *42,* 3252–3254.

Friedberg, E. C., and Hanawalt, P. C. (eds.) (1981). "DNA Repair, a Laboratory Manual of Research Procedures." Dekker, New York.

Friedberg, E. C., Ehmann, U. K., and Williams, J. I. (1979). *Adv. Radiat. Biol.* *8,* 85–174.

Gibson, R. E., and D'Ambrosio, S. M. (1982). *Photochem. Photobiol.* *35,* 181–185.

Goth-Goldstein, R. (1977). *Nature (London)* *267,* 81–82.

Hanawalt, P. C., and Setlow, R. B. (eds.) (1975). "Molecular Mechanisms for Repair of DNA." Plenum, New York.

Hanawalt, P. C., Friedberg, E. C., and Fox, C. F. (eds.) (1978). "DNA Repair Mechanisms." Academic Press, New York.

Hanawalt, P. C., Cooper, P. K., Ganesan, A. K., and Smith, C. A. (1979). *Annu. Rev. Biochem.* *48,* 783–836.

Hart, R. W., and Setlow, R. B. (1976). *Mech. Ageing Dev.* *5,* 67–77.

Houldsworth, J., and Lavin, M. F. (1980). *Nucleic Acids Res.* *8,* 3709–3720.

Jaspers, N. G. J., deWit, J., Regulsiki, M. R., and Bootsma, D. (1982). *Cancer Res.* *42,* 335–341.

Kantor, G. J., Warner, C., and Hull, D. R. (1977). *Photochem. Photobiol.* *25,* 483–489.

Karran, P., Hjelmgren, T., and Lindahl, T. (1982). *Nature (London)* *296,* 770–773.

Konze-Thomas, B., Hazard, R. M., Maher, V. M., and McCormick, J. J. (1982). *Mutat. Res.* *94,* 421–434.

Kraemer, K. H. (1981). *Prog. Dermatol.* *15,* 1–6.

Lambert, B., Ringborg, U., and Skoog, L. (1979). *Cancer Res.* *39,* 2792–2795.

Lindahl, T. (1982). *Annu. Rev. Biochem. 51*, 61-87.

Madden, J. J., Falek, A., Shafer, D. A., and Glick, J. H. (1979). *Proc. Natl. Acad. Sci. USA 76*, 5769-5773.

Maher, V. M., Rowan, L. A., Silinskas, K. C., Kateley, S. A., and McCormick, J. J. (1982). *Proc. Natl. Acad. Sci. USA 79*, 2613-2617.

Mehta, J. R., Ludlum, D. B., Renard, A., and Verly, W. G. (1981). *Proc. Natl. Acad. Sci. USA 78*, 6766-6770.

Olsson, M., and Lindahl, T. (1980). *J. Biol. Chem. 255*, 10569-10571.

Painter, R. B., and Young, B. R. (1980). *Proc. Natl. Acad. Sci. USA 77*, 7315-7317.

Paterson, M. C. (1978). *Adv. Radiat. Biol. 7*, 1-53.

Paterson, M. C. (1979). *In* "Carcinogens: Identification and Mechanisms of Action" (A. C. Griffin and C. R. Shaw, eds.), pp. 251-276. Raven, New York.

Paterson, M. C., and Smith, P. J. (1979). *Annu. Rev. Genet. 13*, 291-318.

Pero, R. W., Bryngelsson, C., Mitelman, F., Thulin, T., and Norden, A. (1976). *Proc. Natl. Acad. Sci. USA 73*, 2496-2500.

Regan, J. D., and Setlow, R. B. (1974). *Cancer Res. 34*, 3318-3825.

Roberts, J. J. (1978). *Adv. Radiat. Biol. 7*, 211-436.

Scudiero, D. A. (1980). *Cancer Res. 40*, 984-990.

Scudiero, D. A., Norrin, A., Karran, P., and Strauss, B. (1976). *Cancer Res. 36*, 1397-1403.

Scudiero, D. A., Meyer, S. A., Clatterbuck, B. E., Tarone, R. E., and Robbins, J. H. (1981). *Proc. Natl. Acad. Sci. USA 78*, 6451-6455.

Setlow, R. B. (1978). *Nature (London) 271*, 713-717.

Setlow, R. B. (1980). *Arch. Toxicol.* Suppl. 3, 217-228.

Setlow, R. B. (1982). *Natl. Cancer Inst. Monogr. 60*, 249-255.

Setlow, R. B., Regan, J. D., German, J., and Carrier, W. L. (1969). *Proc. Natl. Acad. Sci. USA 64*, 1034-1041.

Setlow, R. B., Faulcon, F. M., and Regan, J. D. (1976). *Int. J. Radiat. Biol. 29*, 125-136.

Simon, L., Hazard, R. M., Maher, V. M., and McCormick, J. J. (1981). *Carcinogenesis (Oxford) 2*, 567-570.

Singer, B. (1979). *J. Natl. Cancer Inst. (U.S.) 62*, 1329-1338.

Sklar, R., and Strauss, B. (1981). *Nature (London) 289*, 417-420.

Taylor, A. M. R., Harnden, D. G., Arlett, C. F., Harcourt, S. A., Lehmann, A. R., Stevens, S., and Bridges, B. A. (1975). *Nature (London) 258*, 427-429.

Vincent, R. A., Sheridan, R. B., and Huang, P. C. (1975). *Mutat. Res. 33*, 357-366.

Waldstein, E. A., Cao, E.-H., Bender, M. A., and Setlow, R. B. (1982a). *Mutat. Res. 95*, 405-416.

Waldstein, E. A., Cao, E.-H., and Setlow, R. B. (1982b). *Proc.
        Natl. Acad. Sci. USA 79,* 5117-5121.
Waldstein, E. A., Cao, E.-H., and Setlow, R. B. (1982c). *Anal.
        Biochem. 126,* 268-272.
Waldstein, E. A., Cao, E.-H., Miller, M. E., Cronkite, E. P.,
        and Setlow, R. B. (1982d). *Proc. Natl. Acad. Sci. USA 79,*
        4786-4790.
Weichselbaum, R. R., Nove, J., and Little, J. J. (1980).
        Cancer Res. 40, 920-925.

11

REGULATION OF DNA REPAIR IN HUMAN CELLS

Michael A. Sirover and Pawan K. Gupta

Fels Research Institute and the Department of Pharmacology
Temple University School of Medicine
Philadelphia, Pennsylvania

I. INTRODUCTION

Although environmental agents implicated as causative factors in human carcinogenesis bind to diverse cellular macromolecules, their interaction with cellular DNA is thought to be of critical significance. DNA modification by chemical carcinogens increases the infidelity of DNA synthesis (Sirover and Loeb, 1974, 1976) and alters transcriptional specificity, which could result in the inappropriate expression of dormant genes. Thus, DNA repair pathways may have evolved as a defense mechanism to eliminate such hazards by enzymatically removing these perturbations of DNA structure and by restoring the correct genetic information contained in the nucleotide sequences in cellular DNA (Hanawalt et al., 1979; Lindahl, 1982). Two major DNA repair pathways have been identified. (1) Nucleotide excision repair is responsible for the removal of pyrimidine dimers and other bulky lesions from DNA. For thymine dimers, the initial incision in human cells is thought to be an endonucleolytic cleavage 5' to the dimer. Subsequent exonuclease digestion would result in the removal of an oligonucleotide segment containing the modified nucleotide. (2) Base excision repair is responsible for the removal of small alkylated bases or spontaneous base alterations in DNA. The initial incision is the cleavage of the base-sugar glycosyl linkage by a DNA glycosylase, resulting in the removal of the modified base and the production of either an apurinic or an apyrimidinic site in DNA. Several DNA glycosylases have been identified to date in human cells; each appears to recognize a specific lesion in DNA. The uracil DNA glycosylase functions to remove uracil residues from DNA. Uracil can arise in DNA either by the mutagenic deamination of cytosine (spontaneously or after exposure to DNA-damaging agents) or by the incorporation of deoxyuridine 5'-monophosphate during DNA synthesis.

We have been concerned with the mechanisms through which human cells regulate the expression of excision repair genes. As cell proliferation is an a priori requirement for carcinogenesis, the regulation of DNA repair within the defined pattern of gene expression observed during cell proliferation (Baserga, 1976; Pardee et al., 1978) may be of significance. Some evidence has been obtained to indicate that there is a specificity with respect to increased gene expression during cell growth. Although many enzymes involved in nucleic acid metabolism and DNA replication are induced during proliferation, the activities of a number of such enzymes are not enhanced during cell growth and division (Loeb et al., 1970; Champoux et al., 1978). Thus there is an implied significance in the specific induction of singular enzymes and pathways.

We have posed a number of questions with respect to regulatory mechanisms of DNA repair in human cells. First, do human cells increase the activity of individual DNA repair enzymes as quiescent cells are stimulated to proliferate? Such an induction would occur in the absence of exogenous damage as a normal regulatory event during cell proliferation. Second, does the induction of DNA repair enzymes in the absence of exogenous damage correlate with an enhanced capacity of the cell to repair DNA when exposed to DNA-damaging agents whose lesions are repaired by that pathway? In particular, the temporal relationship between the stimulation of DNA repair and the induction of DNA replication may be of special significance. The supposition is that repair is ineffective if it occurs after replication. Third, what are the cellular consequences if there are defects in regulatory mechanisms of DNA repair during cellular proliferation? Can we correlate specific perturbations in the modulation of excision repair genes with cellular hypersensitivity to specific types of DNA damage?

This chapter describes the studies in which we have attempted to answer these questions. Our primary approach has been to examine the regulation of DNA repair in human fibroblasts synchronized by serum depletion and then stimulated to proliferate by the readdition of serum. The use of synchronized cells permits not only an examination of the enhancement of DNA repair during cell growth but also a determination of the temporal sequence with which DNA repair is regulated with respect to the induction of DNA replication. Using this system we have examined (1) the induction of the base excision repair enzyme uracil DNA glycosylase in the absence of exogenous DNA damage as a normal regulatory event during cell proliferation; (2) the enhancement of nucleotide excision repair and base excision repair during cell proliferation in WI-38 normal diploid human fibroblasts; and (3) whether cells from cancer-prone individuals might be characterized by defects in regulatory mechanisms of DNA repair. Our results suggest that normal human cells regulate excision repair genes in a defined temporal sequence with respect to the induction of DNA replication such that DNA repair is stimulated prior to DNA synthesis. Further, our results suggest that defects in regulatory mechanisms of DNA repair in cells from cancer-prone individuals could provide a molecular mechanism to explain their hypersensitivity to specific chemical carcinogens.

II. MATERIALS AND METHODS

A. Uracil DNA Glycosylase Assay

The uracil DNA glycosylase may be measured by quantitating the release of [^{3}H]uracil from uracil-containing DNA. The template preparation and the basic parameters of the glycosylase assay are depected in Fig. 1. As all DNA polymerases that have

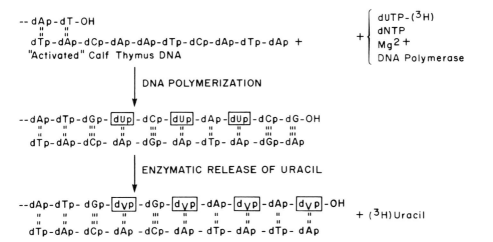

Fig. 1. Uracil DNA glycosylase assay. The uracil DNA glycosylase is assayed by quantitating the release of [3H]uracil into ethanol-soluble supernatants. A typical reaction is performed as a total volume of 100 µl and contains 100 mM Tris-HCl (pH 8.0), 5 mM dithiothreitol, 10 mM k_2EDTA, 1-5 µg of uracil containing DNA (100-2000 cpm/pmol). Reactions are performed for 30 min at 37°C and terminated by the sequential addition of 300 µl of cold ethanol, 100 µl of heat-denatured DNA (1 mg/ml), and 60 µl of 2 M NaCl. After a minimum of 60 min at -20°C, the mixture is centrifuged at 2300 g for 10 min. An aliquot of the supernatant (200 µl) is removed and radioactivity released determined by liquid scintillation spectroscopy.

been characterized to date will utilize deoxyuridine triphosphate (dUTP) in lieu of deoxythymidine triphosphate (dTTP), uracil containing DNA of high specific activity (10,000-50,000 dpm/pmol) can be prepared in an *in vitro* DNA polymerase reaction substituting [3H]dUTP for dTTP as a precursor. The activity of the uracil DNA glycosylase can then be examined by quantitating the release of [3H]uracil into ethanol-soluble supernatants using the purified DNA as a substrate. The specificity of the assay was verified by (1) determining that the 3H radioactivity released was [3H]uracil by co-chromatography with authentic uracil, and (2) using DNA substrates labeled in other bases and

demonstrating that, under our reaction conditions, no other
base is released from DNA.

B. Quantitation of DNA Repair

1. *Unscheduled DNA Synthesis as a Measure of DNA Repair*

The incorporation of [^{3}H]thymidine into DNA during the inhibition of semiconservative DNA synthesis by hydroxyurea (HU)
has been used to measure DNA repair and has been termed unscheduled DNA synthesis (UDS). Using this procedure, DNA repair has been investigated in mammalian cells after irradiation
or after exposure to environmental agents. For our studies,
human cells were synchronized by serum depletion, then stimulated to proliferate by the readdition of serum. At various
intervals after serum stimulation, cells were incubated with
10 mM HU for 30 min to inhibit semiconservative DNA synthesis.
Nucleotide excision repair was quantitated by exposing cells
to UV light at 254 nm. Before UV irradiation, media were removed and cultures were washed with Hank's balanced salt solution. After irradiation the media were returned, and the cells
were incubated with [^{3}H]thymidine for 120 min prior to collection. In parallel, base excision repair was measured using
methylmethane sulfonate (MMS) as a DNA-damaging agent. MMS
was added directly to cells preincubated with 10 mM HU. Cells
were pulsed 15 min later with [^{3}H]thymidine, and incubations
were continued for 120 min. Control cultures were treated simultaneously in an identical fashion but were not exposed to UV
light or treated with MMS. Unscheduled DNA synthesis was quantitated by the incorporation of [^{3}H]thymidine into acid-
precipitable material as measured by liquid scintillation spectroscopy. Repair activity was calculated as the difference between the values of [^{3}H]thymidine incorporation in the presence
of hydroxyurea after exposure to DNA-damaging agents and

[^{3}H]thymidine incorporation in cells incubated with 10 mM HU but not exposed to the agent.

2. Repair Replication as a Measure of DNA Repair

The distinction between conservative and semiconservative DNA synthesis has been utilized to investigate DNA repair using bromodeoxyuridine, a thymidine analog. The substitution of bromodeoxyuridine for thymidine results in DNA that sediments at a higher density in isopycnic gradients as compared to un-substituted DNA. Thus one may isolate parental DNA and determine [^{3}H]thymidine incorporation into parental DNA as a measure of DNA repair (Pettijohn and Hanawalt, 1964). Repair replication is determined in the absence of hydroxyurea. At various intervals after cell stimulation, 1×10^7 cells are preincubated for 60 min in media containing 5 µg/ml bromodeoxy-uridine, then exposed either to UV light at 254 nm (20 J/m^2) or to 2 mM MMS. Cells are then incubated with [^{3}H]thymidine for 120 min in the presence of 5 µg/ml bromodeoxyuridine. Repli-cated and unreplicated (parental) DNA are separated by equi-librium density centrifugation through neutral and alkaline cesium chloride. The specific activity in parental DNA is determined and used as a measure of DNA repair.

III.   RESULTS AND DISCUSSION

A.   Induction of the Uracil DNA Glycosylase During Cell
     Proliferation

The capacity of normal human cells to regulate the uracil DNA glycosylase during cell proliferation was examined using WI-38 normal diploid human fibroblasts (Gupta and Sirover, 1980). WI-38 cells were synchronized by serum depletion, then stimu-lated to proliferate by the readdition of serum. The induction

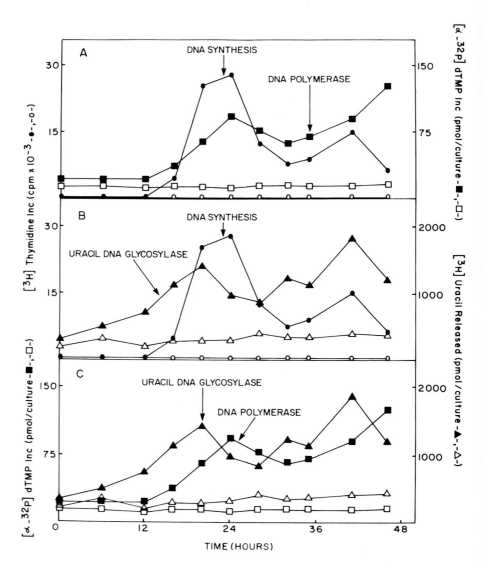

Fig. 2.   Induction of the uracil DNA glycosylase (▲) in
normal human cells.   Reaction conditions for the uracil DNA
glycosylase were described in the legend to Fig. 1.   DNA polymerase activity (■) was examined using "activated" calf thymus
DNA as a substrate; DNA replication (●) was quantitated by the
incorporation of [3H]thymidine for 30 min at the indicated intervals.   (From Gupta and Sirover, 1980, reprinted by permission
of the publisher.)

of cell proliferation was monitored by quantitating the stimulation of DNA synthesis as $[^3H]$ thymidine incorporation into
DNA and by measuring the induction of DNA polymerase in an *in
vitro* assay. As shown in Fig. 2A, DNA synthesis and DNA polymerase were induced by serum stimulation of quiescent cultures.
DNA synthesis was maximal in cultures pulsed with $[^3H]$ thymidine
at 20 to 24 h after serum addition. DNA synthesis then decreased and was restimulated for a second round of DNA replication. Using the identical cultures, the induction of DNA polymerase was also monitored. DNA polymerase activity was also
enhanced during cell proliferation. Polymerase activity was
maximal 20-24 h after cell stimulation, declined, and was restimulated for the second round of DNA synthesis. There was no
increase in basal levels of DNA polymerase or in DNA synthesis
in cells kept in low serum for the identical intervals. The
coordinate stimulation of this DNA-replicative enzyme with the
induction of DNA replication is in agreement with previous
studies using serum stimulation of mammalian cells to examine
the regulation of DNA polymerase during cell proliferation
(Craig *et al.*, 1975).

  The induction of the uracil DNA glycosylase was examined
in parallel cultures. As shown in Fig. 2B, the uracil DNA glycosylase was also enhanced during cell proliferation. Glycosylase activity reached its maximum at 20 h after cell stimulation; it then declined and was restimulated during the second
round of DNA replication. At 24 h, the interval in which DNA
polymerase and DNA replication was maximal, the uracil DNA glycosylase activity was diminished. At 14 h after serum addition,
the interval at which the glycosylase was induced to 50% of its
maximum, there was no enhancement of either DNA replication or
DNA polymerase. Furthermore, there was no increase in glycosylase activity in cultures kept in low serum and examined in
parallel.

Although these results suggested that the uracil DNA glycosylase was enhanced prior to DNA replication, the experiments
represented in Figs. 2A and B were performed in parallel. Thus,
to verify this temporal sequence, the induction of the uracil
DNA glycosylase and the stimulation of DNA polymerase were examined using the identical cell-free extracts to quantitate
each activity. The results of this second experiment are shown
in Fig. 2C. The uracil DNA glycosylase and DNA polymerase were
both enhanced during cell proliferation. However, the uracil
DNA glycosylase was induced prior to DNA polymerase and declined
when DNA polymerase was maximal. It should be noted that there
is not a quantum separation between glycosylase stimulation and
the induction of DNA polymerase; rather it appears as if there
was a temporal frameshift such that the pattern of glycosylase
induction was continually several hours ahead of that observed
for DNA polymerase and for DNA replication. In the absence of
any added serum, there was no increase in the basal levels of
either enzyme.

These results demonstrate that the uracil DNA glycosylase
was induced during cell proliferation in the absence of exogenous damage and that the temporal sequence of glycosylase induction was such that this repair enzyme was induced prior to
the induction of DNA replication or the induction of DNA polymerase.

Specificity of Glycosylase Induction

The specificity of glycosylase induction was examined by
quantitating the specific activities of individual glycosylase
species during cell proliferation (Gupta and Sirover, 1981b).
In particular, Anderson and Friedberg (1980) had reported that
human KB cells contain a nuclear and a mitochondrial uracil DNA
glycosylase. Thus it was of interest to examine whether the
glycosylase induction observed in cell-free extracts represented

an increase in both glycosylase species or whether there was a specificity in the induction such that only one of the species was enhanced.

In these studies we compared the specific activity of the glycosylase species at 0 h to that at 20 h after serum addition, which was the interval at which the glycosylase was induced to its maximum. In cell-free extracts, there was a 2.3-fold increase in enzyme activity at 20 h as compared to that measured at 0 h. Similarly, the specific activity of the nuclear enzyme was increased 2.6-fold at 20 h. However, there was no increase in the specific activity of the mitochondrial enzyme measured at 20 h after serum addition. Thus the increase in glycosylase activity as measured in cell-free extracts (Fig. 2B, C) is due to an increase in the nuclear species. These results suggest that quiescent human cells do not simply increase the activity of all DNA repair enzymes when they are induced to proliferate. Instead, there may be a specificity of repair regulation such that only certain repair activities are induced during cell stimulation.

B.   Regulation of DNA Repair in Normal Human Cells

1.   *Sequential Stimulation of Nucleotide Excision and Base Excision Repair*

To investigate the regulation of DNA repair during cell proliferation in normal human cells, unscheduled DNA synthesis after exposure to diverse DNA-damaging agents was measured in WI-38 cells as they were stimulated to proliferate (Gupta and Sirover, 1980, 1981a). The regulation of nucleotide excision repair was examined using UV irradiation at 254 nm as a DNA-damaging agent; base excision repair was examined after exposure to 2 mM methylmethane sulfonate (MMS). Each agent produces characteristic lesions in DNA, several of which can be excised

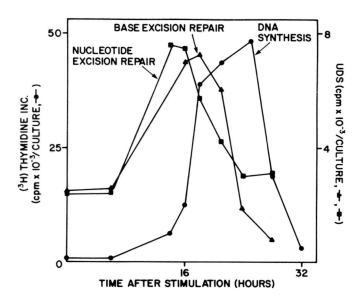

Fig. 3.   Regulation of DNA repair in normal human cells.
Nucleotide excision repair (■) and base excision repair (▲)
were quantitated as unscheduled DNA synthesis in the presence of 10 mM hydroxyurea. All experiments were performed
in parallel. UDS is expressed as the difference in incorporation in cells damaged with either UV light or MMS, and cells
were treated in parallel except for the addition of the DNA-
damaging agent.

by the nucleotide excision pathway or the base excision repair

pathway, respectively. WI-38 cells were synchronized by serum

depletion, then stimulated to proliferate by the readdition of

serum. At various intervals after serum addition, unscheduled

DNA synthesis was quantitated in cells exposed in parallel to

either 20 J/m^2 UV light or 2 mM MMS.

As defined by these criteria, both nucleotide excision re-

pair and base excision repair were enhanced in synchronous WI-38

cells during cell proliferation. As shown in Fig. 3, un-

scheduled DNA synthesis after UV irradiation was maximal in cul-

tures irradiated at 14 h after serum addition. At 14 h, nucleotide excision repair was increased threefold as compared to the amount of repair observed at 0 h. UDS after UV irradiation was decreased in cultures irradiated at later intervals and returned to basal levels during S phase. No stimulation of nucleotide excision repair was observed in cultures kept in low serum at any interval examined.

The modulation of base excision repair after MMS exposure and the induction of DNA replication were examined in parallel cultures. UDS after exposure to MMS was maximal in cultures exposed to this chemical mutagen at 18 h after cell stimulation. At 18 h, base excision repair was increased 3.1-fold as compared to the amount of repair observed at 0 h. Further, UDS after MMS exposure then declined at later intervals and was diminished in S phase. At maximal levels of nucleotide excision repair (14 h after serum stimulation), base excision repair had increased to 86% of the levels observed at 18 h. DNA replication had increased to 13% of its maximum. At maximal levels of base excision repair (18 h after serum addition), nucleotide excision repair had decreased to 74% of the level observed at 14 h. Both excision repair pathways were diminished at 25 h, which was the time in which DNA replication was maximally induced. Further, this temporal sequence of stimulation could be observed when UDS was measured at hourly intervals between 10 and 20 h after cell stimulation. These results suggest not only that DNA repair pathways are regulated during cell proliferation, but that there is a defined temporal sequence of regulation such that nucleotide excision repair is enhanced prior to the stimulation of base excision repair, which is stimulated prior to the induction of DNA replication.

To examine whether nucleotide excision repair of structurally distinct lesions may be coordinately regulated during cell proliferation, UDS after exposure to UV light or after exposure to N-acetoxy-acetylaminofluorene (N-AcO-AAF) were measured

in parallel in WI-38 cells (Gupta and Sirover, 1981a).
N-Acetoxy-acetylaminofluorene produces several lesions in DNA;
the primary adducts are formed on guanine and are thought to
be repaired by the nucleotide excision repair pathway. UDS
after DNA damage increased in cultures UV-irradiated with
20 J/m^2 or exposed to 15 μM N-AcO-AAF at 12 h after cell stimulation and reached a twofold enhancement in cells exposed at
15 h after serum addition. Both repair capacities decreased
thereafter and then were diminished during DNA replication.
These results suggest that there is a temporal coordination in
the regulation of the enzyme(s) within the nucleotide excision
repair pathway responsible for the removal of these structurally
dissimilar lesions.

    To examine whether base excision repair of structurally
distinct lesions may be coordinately regulated during cell proliferation, UDS after exposure to sodium bisulfite or to methylmethane sulfonate (MMS) was measured in parallel in WI-38 cells
(Gupta and Sirover, 1980). Exposure of cells to sodium bisulfite results in cytosine deamination to uracil (Hayatsu, 1977).
Thus, the repair of this DNA damage would be initiated by the
uracil DNA glycosylase. UDS after DNA damage increased in cultures exposed to methylmethane sulfonate or to sodium bisulfite
at 14 h after stimulation and reached a maximum in cultures exposed at 18 h after serum addition. The temporal sequences of
the increase in repair capacity caused by exposure to either
agent was coordinate. Both increased to a maximal level at 18 h
and then diminished. Furthermore, both repair capacities were
enhanced prior to the induction of DNA replication and were decreased when DNA replication was maximal. Thus these results
suggest that there is a distinct pattern of gene regulation such
that the entire base excision repair pathway is coordinately enhanced during cell proliferation.

TABLE I.   Enhancement of Repair Replication in Synchronous
            WI-38 Fibroblasts

Agent	DNA Repair pathway	Time after stimulation (h)	DNA (cpm/μg)	Fold increase
Ultraviolet light	Nucleotide excision	0	58	1.0
		15	240	4.1
		18	133	2.3
		21	32	0.6
Methyl-methane sulfonate	Base excision	0	7	1.0
		18	16	2.3
		22	13	1.9

*2. Repair Replication as a Measure of the Regulation of DNA
    Repair*

The results described in the previous section demonstrate
that WI-38 cells enhance their capacity to perform unscheduled
DNA synthesis during cell proliferation. UDS in the presence
of 10 mM hydroxyurea is one of several techniques used to quantitate DNA repair. We thus examined whether similar regulatory
mechanisms of DNA repair could be observed by another standard
technique routinely used to quantitate DNA repair. In particular, the regulation of nucleotide excision repair and base excision repair during cell proliferation was examined using repair replication into parental DNA in the absence of HU to
measure repair capacity (Pettijohn and Hanawalt, 1964). The
stimulation of repair replication after UV irradiation was
used to quantitate nucleotide excision repair; enhancement
after MMS exposure was used to quantitate base excision repair.
As shown in Table I, repair replication increased during cell
proliferation using either agent to damage DNA. For nucleotide
excision repair after UV irradiation, repair replication increased fourfold, reaching this peak level at 15 h after serum
addition. For base excision repair after MMS exposure, repair

TABLE II. Regulation of DNA Repair During Mammalian Cell Proliferation[a]

System	Method of stimulation	DNA Repair activity	Cell cycle stimulation (fold increase)	DNA Polymerase stimulation (fold increase)
Human lymphocytes	Phytohemagglutinin	Uracil DNA glycosylase	10.0	30.3
WI-38 Human fibroblasts	Serum	Uracil DNA glycosylase	8.4	6.3
Rat liver	Partial hepatectomy	Uracil DNA glycosylase	2.2	2.7
		3-Methyladenine DNA glycosylase	2.9	2.7
BHK Fibroblasts	Exponential growth	Uracil DNA glycosylase	9.5	8.4
		3-Methyladenine DNA glycosylase	4.5	8.4

[a]In each system the identical sample was used to measure each enzymatic activity.

replication increased twofold reaching this maximum enhancement at 18 h after cell stimulation. The temporal sequence of enhancement and the magnitude of enhancement of repair replication during cell proliferation were identical to what was observed using UDS as a measure of DNA repair.

C. Regulation of DNA Repair in Mammalian Cells during Cell Proliferation

1. *Comparative Induction of DNA Repair and DNA-Replicative Enzymes*

The observation that normal human cells regulate DNA repair during cell proliferation suggested that this regulation of gene expression might be characteristic of most eukaryotic cells. To address this question, the induction of DNA glycosylases was examined in a variety of cell types using diverse mitogenic stimuli. In particular, the extent of glycosylase induction was compared to that observed for DNA polymerase using the identical cell-free extracts to quantitate both activities (Sirover, 1979; Gupta and Sirover, 1980, 1981; Gombar *et al.*, 1981).

As shown in Table II, the uracil DNA glycosylase and the 3-methyladenine (3-MeA) DNA glycosylase were induced during cell proliferation. Furthermore, the extent of glycosylase induction was comparable to that observed for DNA polymerase. The only exception was that of human peripheral lymphocytes stimulated by phytohemagglutinin. In that instance the uracil DNA glycosylase was induced 10-fold whereas DNA polymerase was increased 30-fold. The 3-methyladenine DNA glycosylase was also induced in regenerating rat liver and in BHK cells during exponential growth. Furthermore, the extent of the 3-MeA DNA glycosylase induction was comparable to both that of the uracil DNA glycosylase and that of DNA polymerase in each system.

Glycosylase induction occurred in the absence of exogenous damage in each system. Thus, in each mammalian cell system, the uracil DNA glycosylase and the 3-MeA DNA glycosylase were induced as part of the normal pattern of gene regulation during cell proliferation. In addition, the induction of the 3-MeA DNA glycosylase demonstrated that the induction of the uracil DNA glycosylase is not unique but is representative of the increase in activity of a number of DNA repair enzymes as a function of cell proliferation (Duker and Grant, 1980; Pegg *et al.*, 1981).

2. *Kinetic Analysis of Adduct Excision in Quiescent versus Proliferating Cells*

The capacity of mammalian cells to regulate DNA repair pathways actively during cell proliferation suggests that kinetic differences may exist in the excision rates of DNA adducts as a function of cell growth. The supposition is that there should be an inverse relationship between the capacity to repair as related to cell proliferation and the half-life of specific DNA adducts. This relationship can be examined by quantitating the $t_{1/2}$ of specific DNA adducts in quiescent and proliferating cells treated in parallel with the same dose of a DNA-damaging agent. Friedlos and Roberts (1978) demonstrated that the $t_{1/2}$ of 7-bromomethylbenz[a]anthracene adducts in quiescent Chinese hamster cells was greater than 80 h. The half-life of such adducts was 20 h in proliferating cells. Fravel and Roberts (1979) observed that the $t_{1/2}$ of *cis*-diamminedichloroplatinum(II) adducts was 96 h in quiescent Chinese hamster cells but was 3.4-fold less in proliferating cells $(t_{1/2}$ of 28 h). Using *N*-AcO-AAF to damage normal human fibroblasts, Kaneko and Cerutti (1980) reported that the $t_{1/2}$ of *N*-AcO-AAF adducts in nuclear DNA was 24 h in quiescent cells. In contrast, the $t_{1/2}$ in proliferating cells was

6.7 h. Thus these adducts were excised at a 2.3-fold greater rate in proliferating cells. These results suggest that increases in the levels of relevant DNA repair enzymes and pathways during cell proliferation is directly reflected in increased rates of adduct excision in proliferating cells.

IV. ABERRANT REGULATION OF DNA REPAIR IN CELLS FROM CANCER-PRONE INDIVIDUALS

A series of human genetic syndromes have been identified in which the afflicted individuals are characterized, in part, by significant increases in rates of neoplasia. Examination of several of these disorders revealed that they could be characterized at the cellular level by hypersensitivity to a specific DNA-damaging agent (Setlow, 1978; Arlett and Lehmann, 1978; Friedberg et al., 1979). The supposition is that these individual hypersensitivities result from specific perturbations in some DNA repair capacity. Although the cellular deficiencies of cells from these individuals have been studied in detail, the molecular mechanisms that underlie these deficiencies remain unknown. Accordingly, we have started to examine whether cells from these individuals might be characterized by unique alterations in regulatory mechanisms of DNA repair during cell proliferation.

A. Regulation of DNA Repair in Xeroderma Pigmentosum Cells

Xeroderma pigmentosum is an autosomal recessive syndrome characterized, in part, by pronounced increases in rates of skin cancer. At the cellular level xeroderma pigmentosum (XP) cells exhibit defects in the removal of pyrimidine dimers and other lesions excised by the nucleotide excision repair pathway. It has been demonstrated that several complementation groups

TABLE III. Aberrant Regulation of DNA Repair in Cells from Cancer-Prone Individuals

Cell type	Proficiency	Deficiency	Regulation of DNA repair during cell proliferation[a]		
			Nucleotide excision	Base excision	Uracil DNA glycosylase
Normal human cells	Nucleotide, base excision	--	3.0, 14, 25	3.1, 18, 25	5.0, 20, 25
Xeroderma pigmentosum[b]	Base excision (MMS)	Nucleotide excision (UV light)			
XP-A			0, --, 24[c]	5.3, 20, 24	3.5, 14, 24
XP-C			0, --, 22[c]	2.7, 14, 22	2.7, 18, 22
XP-D			0, --, 24[c]	2.8, 18, 24	5.8, 14, 24
Ataxia telangiectasia	Nucleotide excision; base excision	Inhibition of DNA synthesis after DNA damage?	5.2, 16, 24	11.6, 20, 24	11, 20, 24

[a]The first number in each series is the fold increase in the respective repair capacity as compared to the level of that repair capacity observed at 0 h; the second number in each series is the time interval (hours) after serum stimulation at which the maximal increase in that repair capacity was observed; the third number in each series is the time interval after serum stimulation at which DNA replication was maximally enhanced in that experiment.

[b]Complementation groups A, C, and D as shown.

[c]No enhancement of nucleotide excision repair was observed at any interval during cell proliferation.

exist within this syndrome (Kraemer *et al.*, 1975). We have thus examined the regulation of DNA repair in three of these complementation groups (A, C, and D) to determine whether any regulatory defects observed are restricted to that group per se or whether all of the complementation groups may share a common deficiency.

As summarized in Table III, XP-A, XP-C, and XP-D skin fibroblasts failed to enhance nucleotide excision repair after UV irradiation at any interval during cell proliferation. This failure of gene expression was observed using a UV dose of either 5 J/m^2 or 20 J/m^2 to damage DNA. However, all three complementation groups regulated normally both base excision repair after MMS exposure and the induction of the uracil DNA glycosylase after serum stimulation. The fold increases in both repair capacities were equivalent to those observed in WI-38 cells. Furthermore, each repair capacity was enhanced prior to the induction of DNA replication. In addition, their inability to regulate nucleotide excision repair normally during cell proliferation could be observed using either UDS or repair replication to quantitate DNA repair.

B. Regulation of DNA Repair in Ataxia Telangiectasia Cells

Ataxia telangiectasia (AT; Louis-Bar syndrome) is an autosomal recessive syndrome characterized, in part, by a pronounced increase in rates of lymphoreticular neoplasms. AT cells are proficient in nucleotide excision repair after UV irradiation and are proficient in base excision repair after MMS exposure. However, they are sensitive to ionizing radiation. Painter and Young (1980) have suggested that the defect in AT cells may not relate to a specific DNA repair defect per se. Instead, the defect in AT cells may reside in their inability to inhibit DNA replication after DNA damage to allow

DNA repair to occur before DNA replication past the modified
nucleotides.   The regulation of DNA repair was determined in
AT cells to examine the specificity of aberrations in regulatory mechanisms of DNA repair observed in xeroderma pigmentosum
cells.

As shown in Table III, AT cells regulated both nucleotide
excision repair and base excision repair during cell proliferation.   Nucleotide excision repair was increased 5.2-fold at 16 h
and was decreased prior to the induction of DNA replication.
Similarly, base excision repair was increased 11.6-fold with a
temporal sequence comparable to that observed in WI-38 cells.
Furthermore, AT cells normally regulated the induction of the
uracil DNA glycosylase as they were stimulated to proliferate.
Glycosylase induction was maximal at 20 h after serum addition
and decreased at intervals at which DNA replication reached its
peak enhancement.   Thus the normal sensitivity of AT cells to
UV irradiation and to MMS exposure is reflected in normal regulatory mechanisms of DNA repair during cell proliferation.
The specificity of defects in regulatory mechanisms of DNA repair is reemphasized by the normal regulation of these excision
repair pathways as contrasted with the sensitivity of AT cells
to ionizing irradiation.

V.   SUMMARY AND PERSPECTIVES

Numerous studies have documented that quiescent human cells
possess measurable levels of DNA repair.   However, the same
studies also demonstrate that DNA repair in quiescent cells is
usually not complete, with a large amount of residual damage
remaining in the DNA.   In most instances, the level of DNA damage that remained represented greater than 50% of the initial
DNA modification(s).   During cell proliferation, these modifi-

cations could present a block to DNA synthesis that might be cytotoxic. Alternatively, these DNA lesions might be miscopied during DNA replication, which could be either a mutagenic or a carcinogenic event, or both.

Our results suggest that human cells seek to eliminate these potential dangers by active regulation of DNA repair pathways as quiescent cells are stimulated to proliferate. In particular, using three separate criteria to measure DNA repair, we have demonstrated that WI-38 normal human diploid fibroblasts increase the activity of the nucleotide excision repair pathway and the base excision repair pathway during cell proliferation. The use of synchronous cells permitted an analysis of the temporal sequence with which DNA repair was regulated with respect to the induction of DNA replication. This analysis suggested that both excision repair pathways are enhanced prior to the induction of DNA replication. We suggest that this temporal sequence of DNA repair followed by DNA replication might function as a protective mechanism designed to reduce mutagenesis or carcinogenesis by prescreening DNA prior to DNA replication. The supposition is that this sequence of gene expression would result in the removal of critical lesions prior to DNA replication and thus ensure the fidelity of DNA replication. Our studies with other eukaryotic cells suggests that similar regulation occurs in most eukaryotic species when quiescent cells are stimulated to proliferate.

We have also started to examine whether cells from cancer-prone individuals might be characterized by specific aberrations in regulatory mechanisms of DNA repair. In this instance, the expectation is that one might relate such regulatory defects to the unique cellular sensitivities characteristic of each of these human syndromes. Our results with xeroderma pigmentosum cells and ataxia telangiectasia cells suggest the feasibility of this approach. In particular, xeroderma pigmentosum cells

fail to enhance nucleotide excision repair during cell proliferation, whereas ataxia telangiectasia fibroblasts normally
regulate DNA repair with respect to the induction of DNA replication. These results are indicative of alterations at the
molecular level that may be causally related to the cellular
hypersensitivities of afflicted individuals. Using the protocols we have described, one may now investigate whether other
human genetic disorders predisposing to malignancy may be
characterized by specific defects in regulatory mechanisms of
DNA repair.

Our studies on the regulation of DNA repair have essentially been concerned with cellular and biochemical responses
during cell proliferation. One needs now to use the tools of
molecular biology to examine this regulation at the genomic
level. In particular, this approach is required for an understanding of the normal regulation of DNA repair and its alteration in XP cells. In XP cells, it is necessary to know whether
the failure to induce nucleotide excision repair in several
complementation groups is related to a common failure to synthesize a specific gene product. Alternatively, sequence alterations may have occurred in different genes each of whose
products is required for nucleotide excision repair (Gruenert
and Cleaver, 1981; Cleaver, 1982). In either instance it may
be possible to delineate molecular events that occur during the
regulation of DNA repair in normal human cells and to define
the specific alterations in these molecular events that have
occurred in cancer-prone individuals.

ACKNOWLEDGMENTS

This study was supported by grants from the National Institutes of Health (CA-29414) and by the National Science Foun-

dation (PCM-8118176), by grants to the Fels Research Institute from the National Institutes of Health (CA-122227) and from the American Cancer Society (IN-88J).

REFERENCES

Anderson, C. T. M., and Friedberg, E. C. (1980). *Nucleic Acids Res. 8,* 875-888.
Arlett, C. F., and Lehmann, A. R. (1978). *Annu. Rev. Genet. 12,* 95-115.
Baserga, R. (1976). "Multiplication and Division in Mammalian Cells." Dekker, New York.
Champoux, J. J., Young, L. S., and Been, L. S. (1978). *Cold Spring Harbor Symp. Quant. Biol. 43,* 53-59.
Cleaver, J. E. (1982). *Cancer Res. 42,* 860-863.
Craig, R. K., Costello, P. A., and Keir, H. M. (1975). *Biochem. J. 145,* 233-240.
Duker, N. J., and Grant, C. L. (1980). *Exp. Cell Res. 125,* 493-497.
Fravel, H. N. A., and Roberts, J. J. (1979). *Cancer Res. 39,* 1793-1797.
Friedberg, E. C., Ehmann, U. K., and Williams, J. I. (1979). *Adv. Radiat. Biol. 8,* 86-174.
Friedlos, F., and Roberts, J. J. (1978). *Nucleic Acids Res. 5,* 4795-4803.
Gombar, C. T., Katz, E. J., Magee, P. N., and Sirover, M. A. (1981). *Carcinogenesis (N.Y.) 2,* 595-599.
Gruenert, D. C., and Cleaver, J. E. (1981). *Chem. Biol. Interact. 33,* 163-177.
Gupta, P. K., and Sirover, M. A. (1980). *Mutat. Res. 72,* 273-284.
Gupta, P. K., and Sirover, M. A. (1981a). *Chem. Biol. Interact. 36,* 19-31.
Gupta, P. K., and Sirover, M. A. (1981b). *Cancer Res. 41,* 3133-3136.
Hanawalt, P. C., Cooper, P. K., Ganesan, A. K., and Smith, C. A. (1979). *Annu. Rev. Biochem. 48,* 783-836.
Hayatsu, H. (1977). *J. Mol. Biol. 115,* 19-31.
Kaneko, M., and Cerutti, P. A. (1980). *Cancer Res. 40,* 4313-4319.
Kraemer, K. H., Coon, H. G., Petinga, R. A., Barrett, S. F., Rahe, A. E., and Robbins, J. H. (1975). *Proc. Natl. Acad. Sci. USA 72,* 59-63.
Lindahl, T. (1982). *Annu. Rev. Biochem. 51,* 61-87.

Loeb, L. J., Ewald, J. L., and Agarwal, S. S. (1970). *Cancer Res. 30*, 2514-2520.

Painter, R. B., and Young, B. R. (1980). *Proc. Natl. Acad. Sci. USA 77*, 7315-7317.

Pardee, A. B., Dubrow, R., Hamlin, J. L., and Kletzien, R. F. (1978). *Annu. Rev. Biochem. 47*, 715-750.

Pegg, A. E., Perry, W., and Bennett, R. A. (1981). *Biochem. J. 197*, 195-201.

Pettijohn, D. E., and Hanawalt, P. C. (1964). *J. Mol. Biol. 8*, 170-174.

Setlow, R. B. (1978). *Nature (London) 271*, 713-717.

Sirover, M. A. (1979). *Cancer Res. 39*, 2090-2095.

Sirover, M. A., and Loeb, L. A. (1974). *Nature (London) 252*, 414-416.

Sirover, M. A., and Loeb, L. A. (1976). *Cancer Res. 36*, 516-523.

12

ULTRAVIOLET LIGHT-INDUCED SEQUENCE-SPECIFIC DNA DAMAGE AND MUTAGENESIS

Kwok Ming Lo, Douglas E. Brash, William A. Franklin, Judith A. Lippke, and William A. Haseltine

Laboratory of Biochemical Pharmacology
Dana-Farber Cancer Institute
Boston, Massachusetts

I.   INTRODUCTION

Damage to DNA may have several biological consequences. Extensive DNA damage sometimes results in cell death. Some lethal damage may be repaired with no obvious consequence or may result in permanent phenotypic or genotypic alterations.

Most potent mutagens are agents that damage DNA, as are many of the powerful carcinogens. One suspects that such car-

cinogens initiate the cancer process via permanent alterations
in DNA structure. However, in no case has this supposition
been proven. It is known that the tumor cell phenotype is
heritable; the cancer cells give rise to cancer cells upon division. This elementary observation establishes only the
property of phenotypic stability, a stability that may be
achieved via alterations in regulatory networks as well as by
rearrangements or changes in the structure of DNA.

The uncertainty as to the fundamental character of the
initiated tumor cell reflects ignorance of the events that
follow DNA insult. Such events may be traced, provided one
has in hand knowledge of (1) the relevant DNA alterations,
(2) the enzymes that process such lesions, (3) regulatory
pathways that respond to DNA damage, and (4) the genetic
mechanisms that regulate cellular response to DNA damage.
The challenging task that lies ahead is to map this difficult
terrain and to provide detail to areas that are now blank.

Toward this end, we have initiated a series of experiments designed to trace the consequences of UV irradiation.
Ultraviolet light was selected for these studies as we believed that the chemistry of the biologically relevant lesion
was known.

DNA efficiently absorbs UV light in the range of 240 to
300 nm. Although solar radiation below 300 nm drops sharply
as a result of absorption by atmospheric constituents, enough
radiation reaches the surface to produce substantial damage to
the DNA of human skin. Short-term effects (sunburn), as well
as long-term effects (skin cancer and premature aging phenomena), can be attributed, at least in part, to such damage.

The chemical consequences of absorption of UV light by
DNA have been explored by a number of workers. Progress up to
1976 is summarized in S. Y. Wang's book (1976). Most of the
UV light work has been done at a wavelength of 254 nm, very

near the absorption maximum of DNA. However, it has been suggested that wavelengths between 350 and 400 nm may also result
in significant biological effects (Hanawalt *et al.*, 1979).

Chemical analysis of irradiated DNA nucleosides and free
bases have revealed a plethora of products. The major products
observed in the DNA are the cyclobutane pyrimidine dimers
T⟨ ⟩T, T⟨ ⟩C, C⟨ ⟩T, C⟨ ⟩C formed between adjacent pyrimidines
(Wang, 1976). Other significant photoproducts include photo-
hydrates of the pyrimidines and a product formed between
thymine and cytosine that Wang called Thy(6-4)Pyo (Wang,
1976).

Attention has been centered on the role of cyclobutane
pyrimidine dimers. Physical and genetic evidence suggests that
these lesions do contribute substantially to the biological
consequences of UV exposure (Hanawalt *et al.*, 1979; Freidberg
et al., 1979). At low UV fluences, cyclobutane dimers, particularly T⟨ ⟩T, predominate as the major chemical lesion. Prokaryotic and eukaryotic cells deficient in the ability to remove pyrimidine dimers from DNA are much more sensitive to the
lethal and mutagenic effects of UV light than are their normal
counterparts.

The lethal effects of UV light can be largely overcome by
exposure of cells to high doses of visible light. This photoreactivation phenomenon is mediated by enzymes, which have been
characterized in some bacteria and in yeast, that directly reverse the formation of pyrimidine dimers. Ultraviolet light-
induced mutations can, for the most part, also be reversed by
photoreactivation activities, although certain exceptions have
been reported (Witkin, 1966a,b, 1976).

These arguments seemed sufficiently persuasive that we began to study the physiology of pyrimidine dimer lesions in human DNA. Our intent was to apply advances in recombinant DNA
technology and sequencing to repair of such lesions. Our

previous studies using defined fragments of DNA as substrates
for the repair activities of the pyrimidine dimer specific endonucleases of *M. luteus* and phage T4 had convinced us of the
value of this approach (Haseltine *et al.*, 1980; Gordon and
Haseltine, 1980). Biochemical events at individual nucleotide
sequences can be monitored using this approach. The surprising
nature of the conclusions from this work, that both the
M. luteus and T4 enzymes possess pyrimidine dimer *N*-glycosylase,
and not simple endonuclease activity, was initially deduced
from analysis of individual scission products using such
methods (Haseltine *et al.*, 1980; Gordon and Haseltine, 1980).

II. DISTRIBUTION OF UV-INDUCED DAMAGE IN DEFINED DNA SEQUENCE

        The initial question addressed was whether the distribu-
tion of pyrimidine dimer damage within a defined sequence is
the same upon irradiation of naked DNA as it is upon irradiation of intact cells. A positive answer would permit a broad
extrapolation of DNA damage obtained by *in vitro* irradiation of
DNA samples.
        The spectrum of DNA damage in the alphoid sequence of DNA
was analyzed. The α sequence is a tandemly repeated 342 base
pair-long sequence that comprises about 1% of the human DNA
(Lippke *et al.*, 1981). It can be purified from the bulk of
cellular DNA by cleavage by the restriction enzyme *Eco*RI. The
strategy of our experiments was to purify total cellular DNA
from both untreated and irradiated human cell lines in culture.
Experiments were done using DNA cleaved with *Eco*RI. A 342-base
long DNA fragment was separated by centrifugation from the bulk
of cellular DNA. The DNA was labeled with radioactive phospho-
rus at the termini and subsequently cleaved with the enzyme
*Eco*RI*. Such cleavage produced a 90 base pair-long fragment

labeled at one end. This fragment was purified by gel electrophoresis (Lippke *et al.*, 1981).

Application of the Maxam-Gilbert DNA-sequencing technique
(Maxam and Gilbert, 1980) to α fragments prepared in this manner yielded homogeneous sequences. The location of the pyrimidine dimers within the α sequence was determined by cleavage
of the DNA with an excess of the *M. luteus* UV-specific endonuclease. Under the conditions used, cleavage is quantitative
at all four dimer sites. Treatment of irradiated DNA resulted
in cleavage at sites of adjacent pyrimidines. No such breaks
were observed in unirradiated DNA samples so treated (Fig. 1).
The extent of dimer formation was measured at each site by determination of the amount of radioactivity in each scission
product. There was no significant difference in the relative
distribution of dimers formed under the two conditions. However, the effective dose of UV irradiation received by cellular
DNA was about one-half that received by naked DNA--most likely
a result of shielding of the nuclear DNA by cellular constituents.

The experiment recorded in Fig. 1 presented a surprising
result. To ensure quantitative cleavage at dimer sites (the
AP endonuclease activity of some enzyme preparations is low),
DNA treated with the *M. luteus* enzyme was also treated with
hot alkali (0.1 *N* NaOH, 90°C, 15 min). Such treatment of irradiated DNA resulted in the formation of new scission products.
The alkali-induced scission products were also evident in DNA
samples that had not been treated with the *M. luteus* enzyme.
Moreover, the scission events did not occur at the *M. luteus*
enzyme-induced breaks.

The relative distribution of alkali-labile sites was similar in DNA irradiated before or after extraction, again with a
twofold reduction in apparent dose for irradiation of cells.

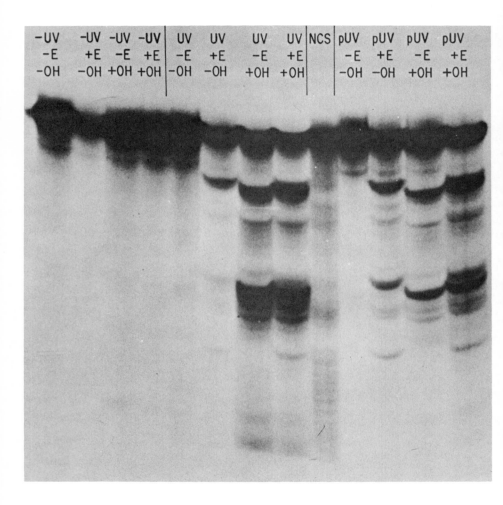

-UV	-UV	-UV	-UV	UV	UV	UV	UV	NCS	pUV	pUV	pUV	pUV
-E	+E	-E	+E	-E	+E	-E	+E		-E	+E	-E	+E
-OH	-OH	+OH	+OH	-OH	-OH	+OH	+OH		-OH	-OH	+OH	+OH

Fig. 1.   Comparison of UV light-induced damage to the α sequence irradiated as naked DNA or as cellular DNA.   The 342 base pair-long α-DNA fragment of human DNA was prepared from HeLa cells before (lanes 1-9) or after (lanes 10-13) irradiation with 5000 J/m^2 of UV light.   The DNA was labeled at the 3' termini in reactions that included [α-^{32}P]dATP and [α-^{32}P]TTP and the Klenow fragment of *E. coli* DNA polymerase I.   The DNA was digested with the restriction endonuclease *Eco*RI* and a 92-base pair fragment separated from other labeled DNA fragments by electrophoresis on a nondenaturing polyacrylamide gel. The DNA was treated as described previously prior to layering

These experiments answered our initial question. Within a defined sequence, the distribution of pyrimidine dimer damage is much the same *in vivo* as it is in the cellular environment. The results also revealed a new type of UV-induced lesion detected at sites of alkaline lability. The unusual dose response of this lesion suggested that the chemistry was substantially different from that of cyclobutane dimers, as a photosteady state was not achieved for such lesions at high UV fluences.

Determination of the quantitative yield of alkali-labile sites in UV-irradiated DNA revealed striking differences in the rate of formation of such lesions, dependent on sequence. At some sequences, the alkali-labile sites were produced at a frequency greater than that of nearby T< >T dimers, even at UV fluences of 15 to 50 J/m^2. At other sequences the rate of formation as a function of dose was 20- to 40-fold lower. Large differences in the rate of formation of T< >T dimers were not observed (Fig. 2) (Brash and Haseltine, 1982).

The high frequency of formation at some sites suggested the alkali-labile lesions might account for some of the observed effects of UV light. In particular, we speculated that

(Fig. 1 continued) on a urea-containing 8% polyacrylamide gel. The sequence of the unirradiated (-UV) DNA fragment determined by the chemical DNA-sequencing reactions is indicated. (lanes 1-4) DNA prepared from unirradiated cells, (lane 1) untreated, (lane 2) treated with *M. luteus* pyrimidine dimer endonuclease (E), (lane 3) and (lane 4) treated with 1 *M* piperidine (OH) at 90°C for 20 min, treated with *M. luteus* pyrimidine dimer endonuclease followed by treatment with 1 *M* piperidine at 90°C for 20 min. (lanes 5-8) DNA extracted from unirradiated cells, exposed to 5000 J/m^2, and then subjected to the same four treatments in the same order prior to layering as described for lanes 1-4. (lanes 10-13) DNA purified from cells exposed to 5000 J/m^2 treated as described for DNA of lanes 1-4 prior to layering. (lane 9) DNA purified from unirradiated cells with neocarzinostatin (NCS).

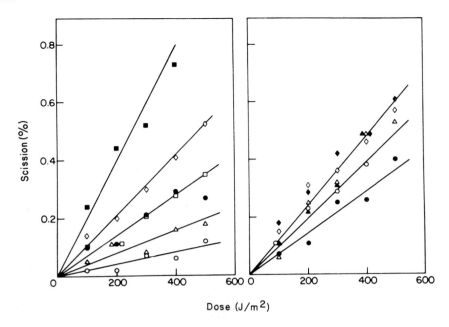

Dose (J/m²)

Fig. 2. Dose-response curve of UV-induced (6-4) lesions and cyclobutane pyrimidine dimers at several sites in the *lacI* gene. Plasmic pMCI containing the *lacI* gene was 3' end-labeled at the bp 565 *Bst*EII or bp 770 *Sau*3AI site. DNA Was irradiated with 500 J/m² of UV light (254 nm), incubated with piperidine to cause strand scission at (6-4) sites, or with *M. luteus* UV endonuclease to incise at cyclobutane-type pyrimidine dimers, and analyzed on 8% urea-containing polyacrylamide gels. Bands were cut from the polyacrylamide gels and analyzed by Cerenkov counting; the data were corrected for multiple cuts within the same DNA fragment, and the percentage of initial molecules carrying scissions at a particular site was computed. (A) (6-4) Lesions at CC dinucleotides 627 (O), 671 (△), and 676 (□), and at TC dinucleotides 665 (●), 684 (◇), and 689 (■). (B) Cyclobutane pyrimidine dimers at CT dinucleotides 661 (●) and 691 (△), and at TT dinucleotides 637 (O), 655 (◇), 709 (▲), and 673 (◆).

the sites of frequent formation of alkali-induced lesions might correspond to UV-induced mutagenic hotspots.

III.   CORRELATION OF UV-INDUCED BASE DAMAGE AND MUTATION
       FREQUENCY

    To test this hypothesis, we measured the distribution of
both pyrimidine dimer and alkali-labile lesions in a segment
of the *lacI* gene of *E. coli*. Miller and colleagues had previously measured the relative distribution of UV-induced missense
and chain-terminating mutations in this gene (Coulondre and
Miller, 1977a,b). The precise nucleotide changes for a collection of about 700 independently isolated chain-terminating mutations was obtained by elegant genetic methods. A dose of
about 100 J/m^2 was used by Miller *et al.* to induce the mutants.
Our measurements of relative damage frequency were done at a
dose of 500 J/m^2. However, the dose response for both pyrimidine dimers and alkali-labile lesions was linear within this
range (Brash and Haseltine, 1982).

    The extent of pyrimidine dimer damage and alkali-labile
lesions formed at mutation sites within a segment of the *lacI*
DNA sequence is summarized in Table I.

    Can one conclude from these data that the alkali-labile
lesions are premutagenic? In favor of this hypothesis is the
observation that hotspots for the formation of alkali-labile
lesions are also hotspots for UV-induced mutations. Figure 3
illustrates the observed proportionality between the relative
rate of formation of alkali-labile lesions and mutation frequency. Such a correlation cannot be made with cyclobutane pyrimidine dimers. In particular, no chain-terminating hotspots
occur at TT sequences, although these comprise a major set of
the most reactive sites for UV-induced DNA damage.

    In contrast, the selection for nonsense mutations probably
has biased the results. Transition mutations at TT and CT
sequences cannot be scored in this selection. This is particularly serious as all UV-induced mutations that arise at high

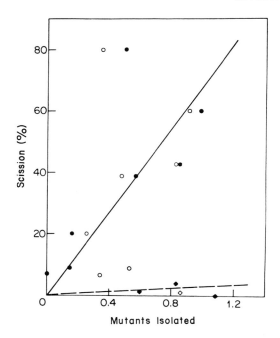

Fig. 3.   Dependence of site-specific incidence of nonsense
mutation on site-specific base damage incidence: (6-4) lesions
(● , ◆) and cyclobutane pyrimidine dimers (O, ◇) at C → T substitution sites (—) and at C → A substitution sites (--).
Site A23 is an apparent exception.

frequency and that yield chain-terminating codons are transi-

tions.   Moreover, at any given TC and CC sequences, the rates

of formation of dimers generally correlates with the rate of

formation of the alkali-labile lesions--where the rate of one

is high, so is the rate of the other.   At such sites, mutation

frequency correlates as well with dimer damage as it does with

the alkali-sensitive lesion.

Four sites in the region of the *lacI* gene examined repre-

sent pronounced exceptions to this observation.   At these sites,

the rate of formation of the alkali-labile lesion is much lower

than that of the dimers.   In both cases, the mutation frequency

is low, favoring the hypothesis that the alkali-labile lesions

are premutagenic.

TABLE I. Distribution of UV-Induced Base Damage in the *lacI* Gene

Dinucleotide	Site of label	Sequence	(6-4) Product (%)	Dimer (%)	Mutants	Substitution	Nonsense site number
TC	652	<u>TC</u>	0.86	0.82	43	C → T	O24
	658	T<u>TC</u>	0.49	0.36	80	C → T	A23
	672	T<u>TC</u>C	0.60	0.86	1	C → A	O25
	678	T<u>TC</u>C	0.83	--	4	C → A	O26
	689	C<u>TC</u>C	0.57	0.48	39	C → T	U6
	706	TTT<u>TC</u>	0.98	0.91	60	C → T	O27
	732	CCC<u>TC</u>	1.08	--	0	C → A	A25
CC	418	<u>CC</u>*	0.01	0.35	7	C → T	A15
	484	<u>CC</u>	0.16	0.25	20	C → T	A16
	688	CT<u>CC</u>	0.15	0.53	9	C → T	A24
TT	636	T<u>TT</u>	0.08	2.08	1	T → A	Y4

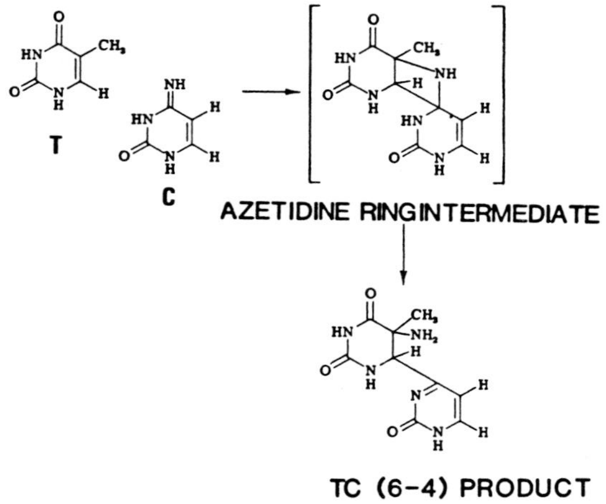

TC (6-4) PRODUCT

Fig. 4. Proposed mechanism for the formation of the thymine-cytosine (6-4) UV-induced photoproduct [TC (6-4) product]. The product is formed via an azetidine ring intermediate as shown.

IV.   CHEMICAL STRUCTURE OF THE UV-INDUCED ALKALI-LABILE LESIONS

The possibility that the alkali-labile lesions might be premutagenic led us to investigate the chemical structure of the damage. Relevant to such analysis is the sequence specificity of these lesions. The DNA scissions always occur at the 3' position of adjacent pyrimidines. High-frequency events occur at TC and CC sequences exclusively. Low-frequency events arise at TT, and also at some TC and CC sequences. These observations indicate that there is a chemical polarity to the lesions at bipyrimidine sites, and that 3'-cytosines are potentially more reactive than are 3'-thymines.

The observation that the highest frequency of events occurred at TC sequences raised the possibility that the lesion that gave rise to sites of alkali lability was the same as the one that produced the precursor of the product Thy(6-4)Pyo

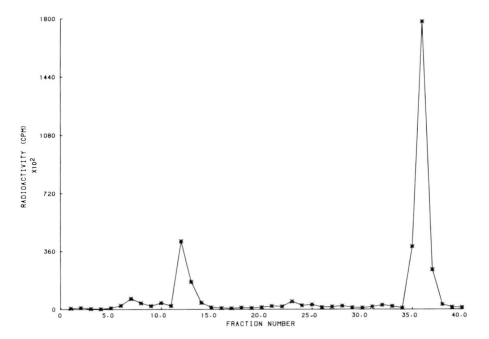

Fig. 5. Formation of the TC (6-4) product as the major photoproduct upon UV irradiation of the dinucleotide dTpdC. The dinucleotide dTpdC was 5' labeled with ^{32}P and was exposed to a total UV dose of 50,000 J/m[2]. The exposed sample was then injected onto a reverse-phase column and separated by HPLC. Fractions were collected and were counted by Cerenkov counting. The figure is a plot of a radiochromatogram of the irradiated dinucleotide [^{32}P]dTpdC. Four major peaks are seen in this separation. The first peak, at fraction 7, represents the solvent front; the second large peak at fraction 12 is the TC (6-4) product; the small peak at fraction 23 is the T( )C cyclobutane dimer; the large peak at fraction 37 is the radiolabeled dinucleotide.

identified by Wang and co-workers upon acid hydrolysis of UV-irradiated DNA. The structure of this compound and postulated intermediates is shown in Fig. 4. The compound is red shifted in absorbance relative to nucleosides and is fluorescent.

To study the chemistry of potential precursor lesions, we used a series of pyrimidine dinucleotides as model compounds.

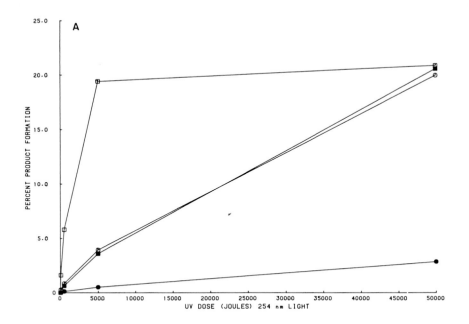

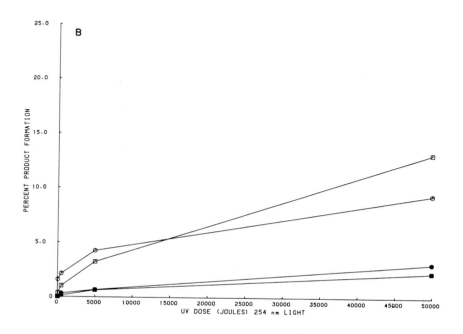

A major product of irradiation of all four pyrimidine dinucleotides was found to have a maximum UV absorbance between 310 and
320 nm and was fluorescent. These fluorescent photoproducts
were readily separated from their parent dinucleotides by the
use of reverse-phase high-pressure liquid chromatography (HPLC).
Irradiation of the dinucleotide dTpdC with a high dose of UV
light resulted in the formation of a fluorescent product in substantial yield (Fig. 5). The relative ratio of formation of
the two photoproducts for all four nucleotides is shown in
Fig. 6. Only for the case of T( )T is the rate of formation of
the dimer higher than it is for the fluorescent compounds.
These unusual compounds form the major UV photoproducts, even
at low UV doses, for the other three dinucleotides.

The fluorescent compounds obtained upon UV irradiation of
the dinucleotides were subjected to acid hydrolysis with tri-
fluoroacetic acid. The acid-hydrolyzed TC product was found
to be identical to the product Thy(6-4)Pyo, as it had identical
UV absorption and fluorescence spectra. The product also co-
eluted with an authentic sample of Thy(6-4)Pyo on reverse-phase
and anion-exchange HPLC separations.

If these compounds are the precursors of the alkali-labile
lesions, they should be unstable under conditions of hot alkali. Treatment of all four compounds with hot alkali resulted
in a rapid loss of the original compound and formation of a

Fig. 6. UV Dose responses for the formation of UV-induced
photoproducts. Radiolabeled dinucleotides were exposed to UV
doses ranging from 50 to 50,000 J/m^2 and were separated by
reverse-phase HPLC. The percentage photoproduct formation at
each dose was determined by dividing the amount of ^{32}P radioactivity contained in the photoproduct fraction by the total radioactivity of the photoproduct and parent radiolabeled dinucleotide, multiplied by 100. (A) Dose response for the formation of dimers and (6-4) products in *pdTpdC and *pdTpdT.
(B) Dose response for the formation of dimers and (6-4) products in *pdCpdC and *pdCpdT.

compound that migrated as if it were much more polar on the
reverse-phase column. The original fluorescent products were
unaffected by treatment with either bacterial alkaline phosphatase or the 3'-phosphatase activity of polynucleotide kinase.
Such treatment of the alkali-treated compounds resulted in a
shift in the elution profile. From these observations, we conclude that the precursors to the alkali-labile lesions are the
(6-4) class of photoproducts. Therefore, we call these precursor products UV-induced pyrimidine-pyrimidone (6-4) photoproducts [abbreviated (6-4) products]. We suspect that the
structure of these compounds is that pictured in Fig. 4.

V.   STRUCTURAL BASES FOR SEQUENCE PREFERENCE OF FORMATION OF
     THE (6-4) LESION

     Comparison of the relative rates of formation of the (6-4)
products at different pyrimidine-pyrimidine sites in DNA and in
dinucleotides presented a puzzling problem. The ratio of (6-4)
products formed in dinucleotides were comparable to one another.
However, in DNA no such products were observed at CT sequences,
and the rate of formation of these products at TT sequences was
much lower than that at most TC and CC sites. One difference
between dinucleotides and DNA is the extent of rotational freedom permitted the bases. To address the effect of structural
constraints, we analyzed the spatial relationship of dipyrimi-
dine sequences in the B form of DNA. The reaction distances
for formation of the postulated intermediate for the (6-4) products are only favorable if the 4 position of the 3'-pyrimidine
participates in the exocyclic reactions. This consideration
should determine the polarity of the reaction.
     Consideration of the geometry of base stacking does not
explain the discrepancy between the results for TC and TT in

DNA with respect to those obtained with dinucleotides. For example, the difference cannot be due to a rate difference in the formation of oxetane versus azetidine ring intermediates, as (6-4) products form readily in TT dinucleotides. We suggest that the exclusion of T in the 3' position of (6-4) products is due to interference by the 5-methyl group of the 3'-pyrimidine and to the additional degrees of rotational freedom in dinucleotides as compared to polynucleotides. This could explain why such products form at a high rate in dinucleotides but not in DNA. Consistent with the hypothesis of steric hindrance by 5-methyl groups is the observation that no alkali-labile lesions arise at the sequence C-5-methyl-C in the *lacI* gene, although C( )C dimers were formed at a high rate at the same site (Brash and Haseltine, 1982).

We conclude that the unusual sequence specificity observed in the (6-4) lesion is best explained by two parameters: (1) The structure of B DNA and (2) the interference of formation of the reactive intermediate by 5-methyl groups of the 3' base.

If the (6-4) products are premutagenic, it is expected that UV-induced mutations will arise at a much higher frequency at TC than at CT sequences. Hutchinson and co-workers at Yale have found a dramatic preference for mutations at TC as compared to CT sequences in UV-induced missense mutations in the *cI* gene of phage λ. Such a preference is not expected for cyclobutane dimers, as both TT and CT sequences are equally reactive for formation of such compounds. In the same collection of missense mutations, it was also noted that there was a strong preference for transition mutations at the 3' position of pyrimidines at potential dimer sites. A 5' to 3' polarity is anticipated from the structure of the (6-4) lesion--provided that one assumes that the structure of the DNA lesion is informative for the mutational specificity.

The experiments just presented raised a clear possibility that the (6-4) lesion is premutagenic. However, before a firm conclusion can be reached, the physiology of such lesions must be examined. As mentioned previously, it is known that the major repair functions of both bacteria and mammalian cells exert profound influences on both the lethal and mutagenic effects of UV light. Therefore, the ability of these repair pathways to excise (6-4) lesions must be studied. Furthermore, photoreactivation with visible light is known to reverse most of the lethal and mutagenic effects of sunlight damage. The effect of photoreactivation on (6-4) lesions must therefore be investigated as well.

VI. SUMMARY

Methods for analysis of the sequence-specific DNA damage by carcinogens and antitumor agents are presented. The methods developed are applicable to a study of DNA damage as it occurs in DNA sequences within intact human cells.

The example of UV light is given. UV Light creates both cyclobutane dimers and (6-4) products at adjacent pyrimidine sites. The mutational specificity of UV light in both the *lacI* gene of *E. coli* and the *cI* gene of phage λ is better explained by the assumption that the (6-4) lesion, rather than the cyclobutane dimer, is the major premutagenic damage, at least for mutations of the base substitution type.

REFERENCES

Brash, D. E., and Haseltine, W. A. (1982). *Nature (London)*
    298, 189-192.
Coulondre, C., and Miller, J. H. (1977). *J. Mol. Biol. 117*,
    525-567.

Coulondre, C., and Miller, J. H. (1977b). *J. Mol. Biol. 117,* 577-606.

Freidberg, E. C., Ehmann, U. K., and Williams, J. I. (1979). *Adv. Radiat. Biol. 8,* 86-173.

Gordon, L. K., and Haseltine, W. A. (1980). *J. Biol. Chem.* 255, 12047-12050.

Hanawalt, P. C., Cooper, P. K., and Smith, C. A. (1979). *Annu. Rev. Biochem. 48,* 783-836.

Haseltine, W. A., Gordon, L. K., Lindan, C. P., Grafstrom, R. H., Shaper, N. L., and Grossman, L. (1980). *Nature (London) 285,* 643-641.

Lippke, J. A., Gordon, L. K., Brash, D. E., and Haseltine, W. A. (1981). *Proc. Natl. Acad. Sci. USA 78,* 3388-3392.

Maxam, A. M., and Gilbert, W. (1980). *Methods Enzymol. 65,* 499-560.

Wang, S. Y. (ed.) (1976). "Photochemistry and Photobiology of Nucleic Acids," Vol. 1, Academic Press, New York.

Witkin, E. M. (1966a). *Radiat. Res. 6* (Suppl), 30-47.

Witkin, E. M. (1966b). *Science (Washington, D.C.) 152,* 1345-1353.

Witkin, E. M. (1976). *Bacteriol. Rev. 40,* 869-907.

III. Tumor Promotion

13

NEW TUMOR PROMOTERS: DIHYDROTELEOCIDIN B, TELEOCIDIN, LYNGBYATOXIN A, APLYSIATOXIN, AND DEBROMOAPLYSIATOXIN

Hirota Fujiki, Masami Suganuma, and Takashi Sugimura

National Cancer Center Research Institute
Tokyo 104, Japan

Richard E. Moore

Department of Chemistry
University of Hawaii
Honolulu, Hawaii

I. INTRODUCTION

The process of human carcinogenesis is very complicated. The two-step concept of chemical carcinogenesis, which explains the formation of tumors as a result of two different

Copyright © 1983 by Academic Press, Inc.
All rights of reproduction in any form reserved.
ISBN 0-12-327660-8

processes, initiation and promotion, is very attractive
(Berenblum, 1941), and initiation and promotion were shown to
be at least two qualitatively different processes. However,
the situation has now become more complicated because of the
possible existence of three steps. This possibility is supported by the finding that second application of a carcinogen
(initiator) after the first initiation and then promotion induced a higher incidence of carcinomas *in vivo* mouse systems
(S. H. Yuspa, personal communication), and by reports that initiation, promotion, and propagation are involved in chemical
carcinogenesis (Boutwell, 1964; Hecker, 1978).

The two-step concept was based on animal experiments in
which cancer was initiated with 7,12-dimethylbenz[a]anthracene
(DMBA) and promoted with croton oil (Berenblum, 1941; Mottram,
1944). The most active principle of croton oil (seed oil) was
isolated from *Croton tiglium* L. (Euphorbiaceae) and identified
as 12-*O*-tetradecanoylphorbol 13-acetate (TPA) (Hecker, 1967;
Van Duuren, 1969). Since 1960, TPA has been widely used in
in vivo and *in vitro* systems as the only available potent tumor
promoter. Because cancer can be explained by the two-step concept in experimental carcinogenesis, it seemed worthwhile to
pay attention to the important role of tumor promoters in human
carcinogenesis also.

Therefore, we tried to find new tumor promoters other than
TPA in our environment. To screen for new tumor promoters, we
developed a convenient short-term method consisting of three
tests (Fujiki *et al.*, 1981a; Sugimura, 1982a). The first test
is on irritation of mouse ear, the second on induction of ornithine decarboxylase (ODC) in the skin of the back of mice,
and the third on adhesion of human promyelocytic leukemia cells
(HL-60). After this three-step screening test, we finally carried out *in vivo* animal experiments with a two-step protocol.
With this three-step screening test and *in vivo* carcinogenesis

experiments we found two new classes of tumor promoters. These
were indole alkaloids and polyacetates, which are structurally
unrelated to phorbol esters (Fujiki *et al.*, 1981b, 1982a,b;
Fujiki and Sugimura, 1982; Sugimura, 1982a). The indole alkaloids included dihydroteleocidin B, teleocidin, and lyngbyatoxin A; the polyacetates included aplysiatoxin and debromoaplysiatoxin.

Dihydroteleocidin B, which was supplied by Dr. M. Takashima, is a hydrogenated derivative of one isomer of teleocidin B
(Takashima *et al.*, 1962). Teleocidin, which is a mixture of
teleocidin A and teleocidin B, was isolated from mycelia of
Streptomyces mediocidicus (Takashima and Sakai, 1960). Lyngbyatoxin A was isolated from the blue-green alga *Lyngbya majuscula*
(Cardellina *et al.*, 1979). Aplysiatoxin and debromoaplysiatoxin
were isolated from another variety of *L. majuscula* in Hawaii and
in Okinawa, Japan (Mynderse *et al.*, 1977; Moore, 1982; H. Fujiki, M. Suganuma, and T. Sugimura, unpublished). Before we found
these five compounds in heterogeneous sources, we had tested almost 300 specimens from various sources. These specimens were
not chosen at random; in their selection, we paid special attention to irritants, analogs of irritants, and information on out-
breaks of swimmer's itch. In fact, several pieces of important
information from different scientific fields were used in
selecting suitable specimens for tests, as one of the authors
has described (Sugimura, 1982b). These compounds were all subjected to our three-step screening test. This nonrandom
screening approach led to the discovery of several new tumor
promoters.

The tumor-promoting activities of these five compounds are
summarized in Table I. Dihydroteleocidin B, teleocidin, lyngbyatoxin A, and aplysiatoxin showed strong tumor-promoting activity on mouse skin, like TPA. In contrast, debromoaplysiatoxin, a debrominated form of aplysiatoxin, was only a weak

TABLE I. Effects of Various Tumor Promoters

Parameter	TPA	Dihydro-teleocidin	Teleocidin	Lyngbya-toxin A	Aplysia-toxin	Debromo-aplysiatoxin
Irritant test ID_{50}^{24} (nmol/ear)	0.016	0.017	0.008	0.011	0.005	0.005
Induction of ODC (nmol CO_2/5.0 μg compound)	1.45	1.55	1.89	2.05	2.15	2.05
Adhesion of HL-60 cells ED_{50} (ng/ml)	1.5	0.3	4.0	7.0	2.0	180
Phagocytosis of HL-60 cells ED_{30} (ng/ml)	2.5	1.4	3.6	2.5	1.7	100
Aggregation of NL-3 cells ED_{50} (ng/ml)	11.2	6.5	3.1	2.4	2.1	180
Inhibition of differentiation of Friend erythroleukemia cells ED_{50} (ng/ml)	1.0	0.2	2.0	0.4	n.d.[a]	150
Inhibition of specific binding of [^{3}H]PDBu ED_{50} (ng/ml)	3.0	n.d.	5.0	8.0	4.0	52
Tumor-promoting activity in Week 30 (%)	100	90	100	80	93	53

[a] n.d., Not determined.

tumor promoters. Because indole alkaloids are as potent as TPA in promoting tumors, we studied their binding to the phorbol ester receptor on the cell surface. Results showed that the indole alkaloids, dihydroteleocidin B, teleocidin, and lyngbyatoxin A, strongly inhibited the specific binding of [^{3}H]phorbol dibutyrate ([^{3}H]PDBu) by cloned rat embryo fibroblasts (CREF) (Umezawa et al., 1981).

The presence of one bromine residue in the phenol group changes the weak tumor-promoting activity of debromoaplysiatoxin to the strong activity of aplysiatoxin. Moreover, by comparison of the effects of these two polyacetates we could classify various biological effects induced by tumor promoters into effects that are more and less relevant to tumor promotion.

II. STRUCTURES

Teleocidin was first isolated from mycelia of *Streptomyces mediocidicus* (Takashima and Sakai, 1960). This compound was separated from a methanol extract of mycelia by column chromatographies on LH-20 and silica gel. The resulting preparation gave a single spot on thin-layer chromatography. However, this preparation has since been shown to be a mixture of teleocidin A and teleocidin B by HPLC (Fujiki and Sugimura, 1982). Teleocidin A, which has a molecular weight of 437, has two isomers, and teleocidin B, with a molecular weight of 451, has four isomers, C-14 and C-17 diastereomers (Fig. 1). Dihydroteleocidin B should be obtained by catalytic hydrogenation of one of the isomers of teleocidin B (Takashima et al., 1962).

Lyngbyatoxin A was isolated as a possible causative agent of swimmer's itch from the blue-green alga *Lyngbya majuscula* (Cardellina et al., 1979; Moore, 1981a). As Fig. 1 shows, we found that one isomer of teleocidin A corresponds to lyngbya-

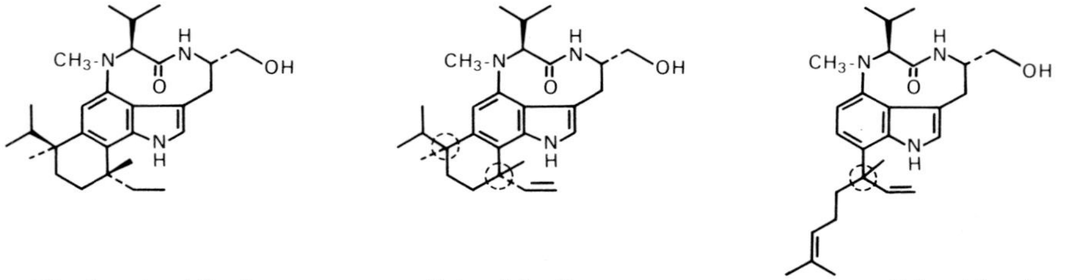

Dihydroteleocidin B   Teleocidin B   Teleocidin A
                                                   Lyngbyatoxin A

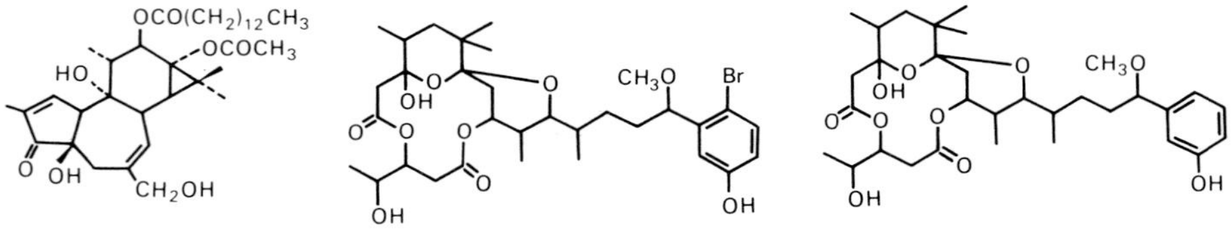

TPA   Aplysiatoxin   Debromoaplysiatoxin

Fig. 1.   Structures of various tumor promoters.   The carbon atoms shown in dashed circles have two variable positions,
positions R and S.   One isomer of teleocidin A corresponds to
lyngbyatoxin A.

toxin A, and that teleocidin A is a mixture of lyngbyatoxin A
and its C-14 epimer.   It was surprising to find that the same
compound was present in *Streptomyces* and a blue-green alga.

Aplysiatoxin and debromoaplysiatoxin were isolated from
another variety of *L. majuscula* (Mynderse *et al.*, 1977; Moore,
1982).   These compounds were found to be the causative agents of
swimmer's itch outbreak on windward Oahu, Hawaii in 1980
(Serdula *et al.*, 1982).   The two polyacetates were first found
in the digestive tract of the sea hare, *Stylocheilus longicauda*
(Kato and Scheuer, 1974).   Debromoaplysiatoxin differs from
aplysiatoxin in not having a bromine residue on the phenol
group.

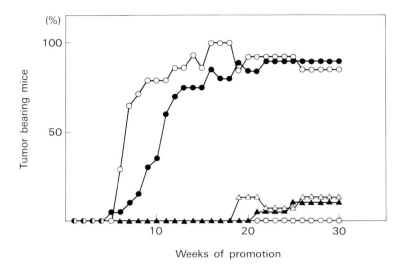

Fig. 2.   Effects of dihydroteleocidin B and TPA in tumor
formation.   Values are numbers of surviving mice bearing at
least one skin tumor as percentages of the number of survivors.
DMBA + dihydroteleocidin B (●), DMBA + TPA (O), dihydroteleocidin B (▲), TPA (Δ), and DMBA (◯).

III.   TWO-STEP CARCINOGENESIS EXPERIMENT

Carcinogenesis was initiated in the skin of the back of

8-week-old female CD-1 mice with 100 µg of DMBA.   From 1 week

later, 2.5 µg of dihydroteleocidin B were applied twice a week

until Week 30.   For comparison, 2.5 µg of TPA were given as a

positive control.   Figure 2 shows the time course of tumor for-

mation.   The tumor incidence in the group treated with DMBA

plus dihydroteleocidin B was 90%, and that in the group treated

with DMBA plus TPA was 100%.   Thus dihydroteleocidin B, which

is structurally unrelated to TPA, had the same tumor-promoting

activity as the latter (Fujiki et al., 1981b; Sugimura et al.,

1982).   Histological examination showed that dihydroteleocidin

B had the same effect as TPA in inducing squamous cell carcino-

mas.

Two-step carcinogenesis experiments were also carried out
by the same procedure with two other indole alkaloids (teleocidin and lyngbyatoxin A) and two polyacetates (aplysiatoxin
and debromoaplysiatoxin). Teleocidin, lyngbyatoxin A, and
aplysiatoxin showed tumor-promoting activity as potent as TPA
and dihydroteleocidin B (Fujiki *et al.*, 1981c, 1982a,b; Fujiki
and Sugimura, 1982). However, debromoaplysiatoxin, which has
no bromine residue, was a weaker tumor promoter than TPA. The
tumor incidences in Week 30 in the groups treated with these
compounds are shown in Table I.

IV. *IN VIVO* AND *IN VITRO* EFFECTS OF NEW TUMOR PROMOTERS

Tumor promoters exert many biological effects *in vivo* and
in vitro in cultured cells. Some of them are membrane-
associated effects. The results on new promoters are given in
Table I. It is important to notice the difference between the
potencies of the strong promoter aplysiatoxin and the weak promoter debromoaplysiatoxin on various biological parameters.
This difference led us to consider that there are two categories of biological effects of tumor promoters, one category
being more relevant and the other less relevant to tumor promotion. Various effects induced by aplysiatoxin and debromoaplysiatoxin are shown in the last two columns in Table I.
These effects could be classified into two types: category A,
those induced by both aplysiatoxin and debromoaplysiatoxin at
the same concentrations, and category B, those induced only by
strong promoters such as aplysiatoxin. For induction of the
effects in category B, a 100 times higher concentration of the
weak promoter, debromoaplysiatoxin, than of the strong promoters
was required. The effects of category B include more important
phenotypic changes associated with tumor-promoting activity than
those of category A (Table II).

TABLE II.   Classification of Various Effects of Tumor Promoters

---

Category A

1. Irritation of mouse ear
2. Induction of ODC
3. Release of arachidonic acid and formation of prosta-
    glandins
4. Release of choline
5. Induction of dark keratinocytes
6. Induction of cell-binding phenotype (CBP)
7. Inhibition of EGF binding
8. Inhibition of specific binding of $[^3\text{H}]$PDPr, $[^3\text{H}]$PDBu,
    and $[^3\text{H}]$TPA

Category B

1. Adhesion and induction of differentiation of HL-60 cells
2. Aggregation of NL-3 cells
3. Inhibition of differentiation of Friend erythroleukemia
    cells
4. Increase of membrane lipid fluidity
5. Increase of ^{32}P incorporation into phospholipids
6. Enhancement of 32,000-dalton protein
7. Induction of EB virus (EA and VCA)

A.   Category A of Biological Effects of Tumor Promoters

1. Irritation Test on Mouse Ear

     Compounds dissolved in acetone were applied to the inside
of the ear. This test was originally used by Hecker for purification of TPA from croton oil. The ID_{50}^{24} value is the amount
that causes reddening of the ears of 50% of the mice 24 h after
application of the compound (Hecker, 1963). As Table I shows,
TPA, dihydroteleocidin B, teleocidin, lyngbyatoxin A, aplysiatoxin, and debromoaplysiatoxin were all very potent irritants,
and their ID_{50}^{24} values were 0.005-0.017 nmol per ear (Fujiki *et
al.*, 1979, 1981b; Fujiki and Sugimura, 1982).

2. *Induction of ODC Activity*

ODC activity was determined 4 h after application of test compounds to the skin of the back of 8-week-old female CD-1 mice (Fujiki *et al.*, 1979). Test compounds dissolved in 0.2 ml acetone were applied to the skin after removing the hair with a depilatory agent. The assay procedure used was essentially that of O'Brien *et al.* (1975). After treatments with 5.0 µg of these six compounds, the amounts of $^{14}CO_2$ released in the test were similar, being 1.45-2.15 nmol CO_2/mg protein (Fujiki *et al.*, 1979, 1981b; Fujiki and Sugimura, 1982).

3. *Release of Arachidonic Acid and Formation of Prostaglandins*

The addition of TPA to C3H 10T1/2 cell cultures led to rapid release of [^{3}H]arachidonic acid into the medium, due to increased phospholipid degradation. Like TPA, dihydroteleocidin B, teleocidin, lyngbyatoxin A, aplysiatoxin, and debromoaplysia-toxin induced release of [^{3}H]arachidonic acid from C3H 10T1/2 cells, CREF cells, and HeLa cells (Sakamoto *et al.*, 1981; Umezawa *et al.*, 1981; Horowitz *et al.*, 1983). In all cases, the release of arachidonic acid was associated with increased synthesis of prostaglandins. It was especially remarkable that aplysiatoxin and debromoaplysiatoxin induced release of [^{3}H]arachidonic acid from C3H 10T1/2 cells. The ED_{50}, which is the dose producing 50% of the maximal effect, was 5.9 nM with aplysiatoxin and 5.5 nM with debromoaplysiatoxin (Horowitz *et al.*, 1983).

4. *Release of Choline*

The assay procedure used was that of Mufson *et al.* (1981). These workers reported that in contrast to TPA, the first-stage promoter A23187 did not release [^{3}H]choline from prelabeled cells. However, release of [^{3}H]choline was observed with both strong promoters, including aplysiatoxin, and a weak promoter, debromoaplysiatoxin. The ED_{50} value of aplysiatoxin was 4 nM, and that of debromoaplysiatoxin was 3.5 nM in CREF cells (Horo-witz *et al.*, 1983).

5. *Induction of Dark Keratinocytes*

A good correlation between tumor-promoting activity and increase in the number of dark keratinocytes in the epidermis was reported by Klein-Szanto *et al.* (1980). We determined the increase in number of dark keratinocytes 48 h after application of test compounds. Application of TPA induced 37.1 dark kera-tinocytes per 1000 basal cells, teleocidin induced 40.9, lyng-byatoxin A induced 44.8, and debromoaplysiatoxin induced 36.7. After application of acetone alone, 10.2 dark keratinocytes were found (Arai *et al.*, 1981).

6. *Induction of the Cell-Binding Phenotype (CBP)*

Phorbol esters induce morphological changes and aggregation of human lymphocytes. This phenomenon had been interpreted as an expression of the "cell-binding phenotype" (Patarroyo *et al.*, 1982). All the potent promoters as well as the very weak pro-moter PDBu induced cell-to-cell binding, which was measured as the percentage of cells aggregated with concentrations of over 7.5 ng/ml of test compounds. Therefore, induction of CBP may be a common effect of tumor promoters (Eliasson *et al.*, 1983).

7. *Inhibition of EGF Binding*

Epidermal growth factor (EGF) prelabeled with radioactive iodine binds to the specific EGF receptor on the cell membrane. TPA inhibits the binding of $[^{125}I]$EGF to the receptor. This in-hibition results from a secondary change produced by binding of TPA to the membrane receptor, and thus EGF does not compete with TPA for the receptor. Teleocidin inhibited the binding of $[^{125}I]$EGF and was as effective as TPA (Umezawa *et al.*, 1981). The ED$_{50}$ value of aplysiatoxin was 5.1 nM, and that of debromoaplysiatoxin was 55 nM in CREF cells (Horowitz *et al.*, 1983). Thus there was only a 5- to 10-fold difference in the

ED_{50} values of the two polyacetates, aplysiatoxin and debromoaplysiatoxin.

8. *Inhibition of Specific Binding of* $[^3H]PDPr$, $[^3H]PDBu$, *and*
    $[^3H]TPA$

Specific binding of $[^3H]$phorbol-12,13-dipropionate
($[^3H]$PDPr) to a particulate fraction of mouse skin was inhibited
by several tumor promoters. The inhibition coefficient (K_i) of
TPA was 1.7×10^{-9} M, and that of teleocidin was 3.1×10^{-9} M
(Schmidt *et al.*, 1981, 1982). Similar inhibition of binding of
$[^3H]$PDBu to rat embryo fibroblast monolayers in cultures was
also observed, 50% inhibition being achieved with 3.8 ng/ml of
TPA and 2.5 ng/ml of teleocidin (Umezawa *et al.*, 1981). It was
of great interest to see whether aplysiatoxin and debromoaplysiatoxin had similar effects in these cells. Results showed
that aplysiatoxin and teleocidin were equally effective in in-
hibiting $[^3H]$PDBu binding, but debromoaplysiatoxin had 5-10
times less inhibitory effects: The ED_{50} value of aplysiatoxin
was 14 nM and that of debromoaplysiatoxin was 94 nM (Table I)
(Horowitz *et al.*, 1983).

Two research groups independently developed a method for
direct measurement of specific binding of $[^3H]$TPA to a mouse
particulate fraction (Ashendel and Boutwell, 1981; Hergenhahn
and Hecker, 1981). Aplysiatoxin and debromoaplysiatoxin were
tested for ability to inhibit the specific binding of $[^3H]$TPA
by this method. Aplysiatoxin inhibited specific binding as effectively as debromoaplysiatoxin: The ED_{50} value of aplysiatoxin was 6.6 nM, and that of debromoaplysiatoxin was 8.0 nM
(T. Tahira, M. Suganuma, H. Fujiki, and T. Sugimura, unpublished). Therefore, the results of binding tests were not
correlated with the tumor-promoting potencies *in vivo*. For
example, compounds such as mezerein, 12-*O*-retinoylphorbol
13-acetate, and milliamine C strongly inhibited the binding
but had little, if any, promoting action (Schmidt *et al.*, 1982).

B.   Category B of Biological Effects of Tumor Promoters

1. *Adhesion and Induction of Differentiation of HL-60 Cells*

HL-60 Cells consist of 80% promyelocytes and about 20%
myeloblasts and myelocytes. Treatment with tumor promoters induced macrophage-like cells with disappearance of azurophilic
granules (Huberman and Callaham, 1979; Rovera *et al.*, 1979).
Cell adhesion was tested by measurement of the number of cells
that were not firmly attached to the surface of the flask
(Fujiki *et al.*, 1979, 1981b; Nakayasu *et al.*, 1981). All six
compounds induced differentiation of HL-60 cells, characterized
by increased phagocytosis, increased release of lysozyme, and
morphological change to macrophage-like cells. However, to
achieve the same extents of cell adhesion and differentiation
of HL-60 cells, about 100 times higher concentration of debromoaplysiatoxin than of the other five compounds was required
(Fujiki and Sugimura, 1982). The potencies of the six compounds in inducing phagocytosis are summarized in Table I.

2. *Aggregation of NL-3 Cells*

Human lymphoblastoid cells transformed by Epstein-Barr
virus aggregated rapidly in the presence of tumor promoter
(Hoshino *et al.*, 1980). The degree of cell aggregation was
estimated by counting the numbers of single cells in the dishes
after cultivation for 6 h. The abilities of all six promoters
to aggregate cells corresponded well with their effects on
HL-60 cells. Namely, a 100-times higher concentration of
debromoaplysiatoxin than of the other five compounds was required to achieve the same effect.

3. *Inhibition of Differentiation of Friend Erythroleukemia*
    Cells

Dimethyl sulfoxide (DMSO) induces differentiation of
Friend erythroleukemia cells into cells with ability to synthesize hemoglobin. This induction was inhibited by tumor pro-

moters. The concentrations of promoters required for 50% reduction of benzidine-reactive cells are shown in Table I
(Fujiki *et al.*, 1979, 1981b). The ED_{50} values of potent tumor
promoters were 0.2-2.0 ng/ml, whereas that of debromoaplysiatoxin was 150 ng/ml.

4. *Increase of Membrane Lipid Fluidity*

Fluorescence polarization of 1,6-diphenyl-1,3,5-hexatriene
was used to examine the dynamics of membrane lipid in Friend
erythroleukemia cells displaying sensitivity or resistance to
TPA (Fisher *et al.*, 1981). The TPA-resistant clones showed
higher fluorescence anisotropy values, indicating decreased
lipid fluidity. When tested at 100 ng/ml, TPA, teleocidin,
and aplysiatoxin were active in decreasing the fluorescence polarization of the membrane of C3H 10T1/2 cells, whereas debromoaplysiatoxin was inactive at up to 1000 ng/ml (P. L. Tran,
A. D. Horowitz, H. Fujiki, D. Schachter, T. Sugimura,
M. Castagna, and I. B. Weinstein, unpublished).

5. *Increase of ^{32}P Incorporation into Phospholipids*

The incorporation of radioactive inorganic phosphate ^{32}P
into phospholipids in HeLa cells was increased by several tumor
promoters (Nishino *et al.*, 1983). TPA, Dihydroteleocidin B,
teleocidin, lyngbyatoxin A, and aplysiatoxin induced alteration
in phospholipid metabolism. Debromoaplysiatoxin was efficient
only at about 100 times higher concentration than the other
compounds.

6. *Increased Synthesis of 32,000-Dalton Protein*

In BALB/c 3T3 cells the synthesis of a polypeptide with a
molecular weight of 32,000 and an isoelectric point of 6.4 increases about twofold in 2 h after addition of TPA (Hiwasa *et
al.*, 1982). The synthesis of this protein was increased to the
same extent when the cells were treated with 20 ng/ml of dihydroteleocidin B, teleocidin, lyngbyatoxin A, and aplysiatoxin.

Debromoaplysiatoxin stimulated synthesis of this protein only when added at higher concentrations (>200 ng/ml) (T. Hiwasa, H. Fujiki, T. Sugimura, and S. Sakiyama, unpublished).

7. *Induction of EB Virus*

Early antigen (EA) and/or viral capsid antigen (VCA) of EBV is induced by TPA and teleocidin in cell lines C-6 and P3HR-1, which carry the EBV genome (zur Hausen *et al.*, 1978; Hoshino *et al.*, 1981; Yamamoto *et al.*, 1981). Teleocidin enhanced both EA and VCA synthesis in P3HR-1 cells additively with *n*-butyrate but not with TPA (Yamamoto *et al.*, 1981). In combination with 3 mM *n*-butyrate, maximal induction of EA synthesis was achieved at concentrations of 5 to 10 ng/ml of the five potent promoters, but at 250 ng/ml of the weak promoter debromoaplysiatoxin (Eliasson *et al.*, 1983).

V. DISCUSSION

TPA and phorbol esters had been used as a unique class of potent tumor promoters and investigated extensively in studies on tumor promotion. A three-step screening test was used to find new tumor promoters other than TPA and phorbol esters. In this test, dihydroteleocidin B, which is a hydrogenated derivative of teleocidin B and a very strong skin irritant, was found to be as effective as TPA in inducing redness of mouse ear, ODC activity in mouse skin, and cell adhesion of HL-60 cells. The potent tumor-promoting activity of dihydroteleocidin B was then shown in a two-step *in vivo* carcinogenicity experiment. The parent compound of dihydroteleocidin B, teleocidin B, was isolated from mycelia of *Streptomyces*.

On purification, teleocidin was found to be a mixture of teleocidin A and teleocidin B. From its structural similarity to teleocidins, lyngbyatoxin A, which was isolated from blue-

green algae, was also supposed to be a new tumor promoter, and
results showed that it did have tumor-promoting activity in
mouse skin as high as dihydroteleocidin B and teleocidin.

In the late 1970s, lyngbyatoxin A was isolated from *L. majuscula* collected at Kahala Beach, Oahu and found to be a possible causative agent of swimmer's itch in Hawaii. In August
1980, over 400 people suffered from seaweed rash at Kailua beach
in Hawaii. Two compounds, aplysiatoxin and debromoaplysiatoxin,
were isolated from *L. majuscula* from this beach (Moore, 1981a).
Swimmer's itch was also reported in Okinawa (Hashimoto *et al.*,
1976). We found that the blue-green alga that grows in
Okinawa contains the same two compounds as the blue-green alga
in Hawaii. The finding that aplysiatoxin is a strong tumor
promoter and debromoaplysiatoxin is a weak promoter increased
our interest in the structure-function relationship of tumor
promoters. The derivatives of polyacetate bromoaplysiatoxin
and oscillatoxin A were found in a mixture of *Oscillatoria
nigroviridis* and *Schizothrix calcicola* from Enewetak (Mynderse
and Moore, 1978). We found that these two polyacetate derivatives induced less ODC activity in mouse skin than aplysiatoxin
and debromoaplysiatoxin, and that dibromoaplysiatoxin did not
induce ODC activity. Aplysiatoxin and debromoaplysiatoxin and
several other derivatives of polyacetates should be representatives of a new class of tumor promoters differing from phorbol
ester and indole alkaloid.

By comparison of the effects of aplysiatoxin, a strong
promoter, and debromoaplysiatoxin, a weak promoter, the biological effects of tumor promoters could be classified into two
categories: effects that are less (A) and more (B) relevant
to tumor promotion. Several other effects, such as production
of superoxide anion radicals (O_2^-) (Troll *et al.*, 1982), inhibition of melanogenesis in B-16 cells and of creatine kinase
isoenzyme transition (Fisher *et al.*, 1982), colony formation

of EBV-infected cord blood lymphocytes (Hoshino *et al.*, 1981), inhibition of pseudoemperipolesis (Hiai and Nishizuka, 1981; Kaneshima *et al.*, 1983), inhibition of metabolic cooperation assay (Jone *et al.*, 1982; K. Scott, personal communication), and rapid alteration of cytoskeletal organization (Rifkin *et al.*, 1979; Nakamura and Schliwa, 1982; H. Esumi, J. J.-C. Lin, J. R. Feramisco, H. Fujiki, and T. Sugimura, unpublished) were observed with teleocidin and TPA at similar concentrations. Malignant transformation of cultured mouse cells (A31-1-1) induced by 3-methylcholanthrene was enhanced by both dihydroteleocidin B and TPA. The effective concentration of TPA for these effects was at least 100 times more than that of dihydroteleocidin B (Hirakawa *et al.*, 1982). However, the effects described in this paragraph have not yet been classified into two categories, because aplysiatoxin and debromoaplysiatoxin have not been tested by these procedures.

Varshavsky (1981) reported that TPA enhances the amplification of dihydrofolate reductase gene in cultured mouse cells by methotrexate. This result indicated that TPA has an effect on DNA or chromatin. In addition to the fact that the advanced stage of promotion in mouse skin is not reversible, these studies strongly suggested that tumor promoters have not only epigenetic but also genetic effects in the cells. Hayashi in our laboratory found that tumor promoters of three classes, TPA, teleocidin, and aplysiatoxin, enhanced the appearance of Chinese hamster lung cells that were resistant to $CdCl_2$. Overproduction of metallothionein I mRNA and amplification of the metallothionein I gene in these cadmium-resistant cells was shown by northern and southern blot experiments (Hayashi *et al.*, 1982).

The blue-green alga *Lyngbya majuscula* sometimes grows epiphytically on edible algae, such as *Acanthophora spicifera* which is eaten in Indonesia and the Philippines (Moore, 1981b). The

problem as to whether these new tumor promoters, indole alkaloids and polyacetates, are relevant to human carcinogenesis
has not yet been investigated. There is a case report of a
resident in Hawaii who suffered from escharotic stomatitis
after eating the blue-green alga accidentally, because *L.
majuscula* grossly resembles the edible seaweed *Enteromorphe
prolifera* (called "limu ele ele" in Hawaii) (Sims and Zandeee
von Rilland, 1981).

2,3,7,8-Tetrachlorodibenzo-*p*-dioxin (TCDD) was shown to
be a potent tumor promoter in two-stage carcinogenesis in rat
liver (Pitot *et al.*, 1980). Furthermore, TCDD was found to
have strong tumor-promoting activity in the skin of HRS/J
hairless mice (Poland *et al.*, 1982). It is interesting that
TCDD appears to act by a different mechanism from TPA, teleocidin, and aplysiatoxin. It is certainly worthwhile to consider the risk of environmental tumor promoters to human
beings, because this approach is important for preventing human
cancer. We think that various other classes of tumor promoters
must be present in our environment and believe that further
screening for tumor promoters in human carcinogenesis is necessary.

VI.   CONCLUSION

To screen for new tumor promoters in our environment, we
developed a convenient short-term method consisting of three
tests: irritation of mouse ear, induction of ODC in skin of
the back of mice, and adhesion of HL-60 cells. Finally we carried out *in vivo* experiments with a two-step protocol. We
found two new classes of tumor promoters, indole alkaloids and
polyacetates, which are structurally unrelated to TPA. The indole alkaloids included dihydroteleocidin B, teleocidin, and
lyngbyatoxin A; the polyacetates included aplysiatoxin and de-

bromoaplysiatoxin. Dihydroteleocidin B, teleocidin, lyngbyatoxin A, and aplysiatoxin showed strong tumor-promoting activity, like TPA, on mouse skin. Debromoaplysiatoxin was only a
weak tumor promoter. We found that these compounds inhibited
the specific binding of $[^3H]$TPA to mouse particulate fraction.

By comparison of the effects of a strong promoter, aplysiatoxin, and a weak promoter, debromoaplysiatoxin, we could classify various biological effects induced by tumor promoters into
effects less relevant (category A) and those more relevant
(category B) to tumor promotion.

ACKNOWLEDGMENTS

This work was supported in part by Grants-in-Aid for Cancer
Research from the Ministry of Education, Science and Culture and
the Ministry of Health and Welfare of Japan, and the Princess
Takamatsu Cancer Research Fund. Work on the isolations of lyngbyatoxin A, aplysiatoxin, and debromoaplysiatoxin used in this
study was supported by Grant CA 12623-09 to Dr. R. E. Moore at
the University of Hawaii from the National Cancer Institute,
Health and Human Services, United States. We thank Dr. I. B.
Weinstein for valuable collaboration.

REFERENCES

Arai, M., Hibino, T., Fujiki, H., Sugimura, T., and Ito, N.
    (1981). *Proc. Annu. Meet. Jpn. Cancer Assoc. 40th,* p. 49.
Ashendel, C. L., and Boutwell, R. K. (1981). *Biochem. Biophys.
    Res. Commun. 99,* 543-549.
Berenblum, I. (1941). *Cancer Res. 1,* 807-814.
Boutwell, R. K. (1964). *Prog. Exp. Tumor Res. 4,* 207-250.
Cardellina, J. H., II, Marner, F. J., and Moore, R. E. (1979).
    Science (Washington, D.C.) 204, 193-195.
Eliasson, L., Kallin, B., Patarroyo, M., Klein, G., Fujiki, H.,
    and Sugimura, T. (1983). *Int. J. Cancer 31,* 7-11.
Fisher, P. B., Cogan, U., Horowitz, A. D., Schachter, D., and
    Weinstein, I. B. (1981). *Biochem. Biophys. Res. Commun.
    100,* 370-376.

Fisher, P. B., Miranda, A. F., Mufson, A., Weinstein, L. S.,
    Fujiki, H., Sugimura, T., Weinstein, I. B. (1982).
    Cancer Res. 42, 2829-2835.

Fujiki, H., and Sugimura, T. (1982). *In* "P&S Biomedical
    Sciences Symposia Genes and Proteins in Oncogenesis"
    (I. B. Weinstein, H. Vogel, eds.), in press.

Fujiki, H., Hori, M., Nakayasu, M., Terada, M., and Sugimura,
    T. (1979). *Biochem. Biophys. Res. Commun. 90,* 976-983.

Fujiki, H., Sugimura, T., and Moore, R. E. (1981a). *EHP
    Environ. Health Perspect. 50,* in press.

Fujiki, H., Mori, M., Nakayasu, M., Terada, M., Sugimura, T.,
    and Moore, R. E. (1981b). *Proc. Natl. Acad. Sci. USA
    78,* 3872-3876.

Fujiki, H., Mori, M., and Sugimura, T. (1981c). *Proc. Annu.
    Meet. Jpn. Cancer Assoc. 40th,* p. 50.

Fujiki, H., Suganuma, M., Nakayasu, M., Hoshino, H., Moore,
    R. E., and Sugimura, T. (1982a). *Gann 73,* 495-497.

Fujiki, H., Suganuma, M., Matsukura, N., Sugimura, T., and
    Takayama, S. (1982b). *Carcinogenesis (N.Y.) 3,* 895-898.

Hashimoto, Y., Kamiya, H., Yamazato, K., and Nozawa, K. (1976).
    In "Animal, Plant, and Microbial Toxins" (A. Ohsaka, K.
    Hayashi, and Y. Sawai, eds.), Vol. 1, pp. 333-338.
    Plenum, New York.

Hayashi, K., Fujiki, H., and Sugimura, T. (1982). *Proc. Annu.
    Meet. Jpn. Cancer Assoc. 41th,* p. 188.

Hecker, E. (1963). *Z. Krebsforsch. 65,* 325-333.

Hecker, E. (1967). *Naturwissenschaften 54,* 282-284.

Hecker, E. (1978). *Naturwissenschaften 65,* 640-648.

Hergenhahn, M., and Hecker, E. (1981). *Carcinogenesis (N.Y.)
    2,* 1277-1280.

Hiai, H., and Nishizuka, Y. (1981). *J. Natl. Cancer Inst.
    (U.S.) 67,* 1333-1340.

Hirakawa, T., Kakunaga, T., Fujiki, H., and Sugimura, T.
    (1982). *Science (Washington, D.C.) 216,* 527-529.

Hiwasa, T., Fujimura, S., and Sakiyama, S. (1982). *Proc. Natl.
    Acad. Sci. USA 79,* 1800-1804.

Horowitz, A. D., Fujiki, H., Weinstein, I. B., Jeffrey, A. M.,
    Okin, E., Moore, R. E., and Sugimura, T. (1983). *Cancer
    Res. 43,* 1529-1535.

Hoshino, H., Miwa, M., Fujiki, H., and Sugimura, T. (1980).
    Biochem. Biophys. Res. Commun. 95, 842-848.

Hoshino, H., Miwa, M., Fujiki, H., Sugimura, T., Yamamoto, H.,
    Katsuki, T., and Hinuma, Y. (1981). *Cancer Lett. (Shannon,
    Irel.) 13,* 275-280.

Huberman, E., and Callaham, M. F. (1979). *Proc. Natl. Acad.
    Sci. USA 76,* 1293-1297.

Jone, C. M., Trosko, J. E., Chang, C.-C., Fujiki, H., and
    Sugimura, T. (1982). *Gann 73,* 874-878.

Kaneshima, H., Hiai, H., Fujiki, H., Oguro, Y. B., Iijima, S., Sugimura, T., and Nishizuka, Y. (1983). *Leukemia Res.*, in press.

Kato, Y., and Scheuer, P. J. (1974). *J. Am. Chem. Soc.* 96, 2245-2246.

Klein-Szanto, A. J. P., Major, S. K., and Slaga, T. J. (1980). *Carcinogenesis (N.Y.)* 1, 399-406.

Moore, R. E. (1981a). *In* "The Water Environment: Algal Toxins and Health" (W. W. Carmichael, ed.), pp. 15-23. Plenum, New York.

Moore, R. E. (1981b). *In* "Marine Natural Products" (P. J. Scheuer, ed.), Vol. 4, pp. 1-52. Academic Press, New York.

Moore, R. E. (1982). *Pure Appl. Chem.* 54, 1919-1934.

Mottram, J. C. (1944). *J. Pathol. Bacteriol.* 56, 181-187.

Mufson, R. A., Okin, E., and Weinstein, I. B. (1981). *Carcinogenesis (N.Y.)* 2, 1095-1102.

Mynderse, J. S., and Moore, R. E. (1978). *J. Org. Chem.* 43, 2301-2303.

Mynderse, J. S., Moore, R. E., Kashiwagi, M., and Norton, T. R. (1977). *Science (Washington, D.C.)* 196, 538-540.

Nakamura, T., and Schliwa, M. (1982). *Proc. Int. Cancer Congr. 13th*, p. 381.

Nakayasu, M., Fujiki, H., Mori, M., Sugimura, T., and Moore, R. E. (1981). *Cancer Lett. (Shannon, Irel.)* 12, 271-277.

Nishino, H., Fujiki, H., Terada, M., and Sato, S. (1983). *Carcinogenesis (N.Y.)* 4, 107-110.

O'Brien, T. G., Simsiman, R. C., and Boutwell, R. K. (1975). *Cancer Res.* 35, 1662-1670.

Patarroyo, M., Yogeeswaren, G., Biberfeld, P., Klein, E., and Klein, G. (1982). *Int. J. Cancer 30*, 707-717.

Pitot, H. C., Goldsworthy, T., Campbell, H. A., and Poland, A. (1980). *Cancer Res.* 40, 3616-3620.

Poland, A., Palen, D., and Glover, E. (1982). *Nature (London) 300*, 271-273.

Rifkin, D. B., Crowe, R. M., and Pollack, R. (1979). *Cell 18*, 361-368.

Rovera, G., Santoli, D., and Damsky, C. (1979). *Proc. Natl. Acad. Sci. USA 76*, 2779-2783.

Sakamoto, H., Terada, M., Fujiki, H., Mori, M., Nakayasu, M., Sugimura, T., and Weinstein, I. B. (1981). *Biochem. Biophys. Res. Commun. 102*, 100-107.

Schmidt, R., Fujiki, H., Hecker, E., and Sugimura, T. (1981). *J. Cancer Res. Clin. Oncol.* 99, CH37 (Abstr.).

Schmidt, R., Adolf, W., Marston, A., Roeser, H., Sorg, B., Fujiki, H., Sugimura, T., Moore, R. E., and Hecker, E. (1982). *Carcinogenesis (N.Y.)* 4, 77-81.

Serdula, M., Bartolini, G., Moore, R. E., Gooch, J., Wiebenga, N. (1982). *Hawaii Med. J. 41*, 200-201.

Sims, J. K., and Zandee von Rilland, R. D. (1981). *Hawaii Med. J. 40,* 243-248.

Sugimura, T. (1982a). *Cancer (Philadelphia) 49,* 1970-1984.

Sugimura, T. (1982b). *Gann 73,* 499-507.

Sugimura, T., Fujiki, H., Mori, M., Nakayasu, M., Terada, M., Umezawa, K., and Moore, R. E. (1982). *In* "Carcinogenesis--A Comprehensive Survey, Cocarcinogenesis and Biological Effects of Tumor Promoters" (E. Hecker, N. Fusenig, F. Marks, and H. W. Thielmann, eds.), Vol. 7, pp. 69-73. Raven, New York.

Takashima, M., and Sakai, H. (1960). *Bull. Agric. Chem. Soc. Jpn. 24,* 652-655.

Takashima, M., Sakai, H., and Arima, K. (1962). *Agric. Biol. Chem. 26,* 660-668.

Troll, W., Witz, G., Goldstein, B., Stone, D., and Sugimura, T. (1982). *In* "Carcinogenesis--A Comprehensive Survey, Cocarcinogenesis and Biological Effects of Tumor Promoters" (E. Hecker, N. Fusening, F. Marks, and H. W. Thielmann, eds.), Vol. 7, pp. 593-597. Raven, New York.

Umezawa, K., Weinstein, I. B., Horowitz, A., Fujiki, H., Matsushima, T., and Sugimura, T. (1981). *Nature (London) 290,* 411-413.

Van Duuren, B. L. (1969). *Prog. Exp. Tumor Res. 11,* 31-68.

Varshavsky, A. (1981). *Cell 25,* 561-572.

Yamamoto, H., Katsuki, T., Hinuma, Y., Hoshino, H., Miwa, M., Fujiki, H., and Sugimura, T. (1981). *Int. J. Cancer 28,* 125-129.

zur Hausen, H., O'Neill, F. J., Freese, U. K., and Hecker, E. (1978). *Nature (London) 272,* 373-375.

14

PROMOTION OF HUMAN PREMALIGNANT EPITHELIAL CELLS

Eileen A. Friedman

Department of Gastrointestinal Cancer Research
Memorial Sloan-Kettering Cancer Center
New York, New York

I.   INTRODUCTION

There is increasing evidence that many human neoplasms arise through a series of progressive cellular changes. These sequential premalignant changes have been clearly demonstrated during human colon carcinoma evolution. Malignant colonic cells first appear within benign tumors or adenomas in all, or

at least in the vast majority of cases. This implies an
adenoma-to-carcinoma progression. The three histological
classes of colonic adenomas can themselves be ranked by their
malignant potential. In a study of over 2000 adenomas, Muto
et al. (1975) measured the incidence of the invasive carcinoma
within adenomas and found marked differences. The malignancy
rate was 5% for tubular adenomas, 40% for villous adenomas,
and 22% for the intermediate or mixed-type villotubular adenomas. The incidence of carcinoma in situ without invasion
across the muscular layer of the gut showed a similar distribution in the three types of adenomas.

These data are consistent with a cascade of cellular
changes beginning with the alteration, possibly by mutation,
of a normal colonic epithelial stem cell into a tubular adenomatous stem cell and then into a villotubular and finally a
villous cell. Carcinoma in situ would then arise within a
focus of villous cells, and the malignant cells would in turn
move through the basement membrane and muscular layer and form
a frank carcinoma. Supporting this simple progression model
is a clinical study in which adenomas were removed from a study
group of 18,000 patients. This led to a seven- to eightfold
decrease in the incidence of colon cancer over a 25-year
period (Gilbertson, 1974). Also, individuals with a hereditary
predisposition to develop numerous tubular adenomas invariably
develop colon cancer if the colon is not removed (Lipkin et al.,
1980). In addition, villous adenomas are usually much larger
than tubular adenomas (Muto et al., 1975), implying that they
arose during longer periods of aberrant growth. The existence
of the villotubular adenoma, which has histological properties
of both villous and tubular adenomas and an intermediate rate
of transition to malignancy, also supports the hypothesis that
adenomas progress through stages toward frank carcinoma.

Because of the slow evolution of colon carcinoma, 5-30 years in some documented cases (Muto *et al.*, 1975), colonic adenomas of macroscopic size are readily available. They can be removed during endoscopic examination without the necessity for general surgery. Adenomas are berry-like nodules or flat plaques composed of groups of very elongated crypts extending from the intestinal wall into the lumen of the colon. The epithelial cells of the colon are arranged as a single layer of columnar cells lining the sides of tubular indentations into the gut wall, called the crypts of Lieberkühn. Replicating epithelial cells are only found in the lower 2/3 of normal crypts, but in adenomas they are found all along the crypt column and even at the luminal surface of the gut (Lipkin *et al.*, 1980). The crypts elongate abnormally because of an increase in the fraction of proliferating cells and a concomitant decrease in production of mature nonreplicating cells that slough off. Adenomatous epithelial cells appear to be arrested at immature states of differentiation. They exhibit, in addition to an enhanced proliferative capacity, an altered nuclear morphology and, in general, decreased differentiation into mucus-secreting goblet cells. A stem cell at the base of the crypt must be altered, possibly mutated, as all adenomatous epithelial cells in a crypt appear similar in morphology.

A new approach to the study of human colonic premalignant cells was our development of methods for their *in vitro* culture (Friedman *et al.*, 1981). We have cultured over 90 adenomas with approximately equal frequency of success (85-90%) from each histological class. The washed, minced tissue was digested in hyaluronidase, neuraminidase, and collagenase with vigorous shaking to dislodge many of the intercryptal lymphocytes, which were then removed by differential centrifugation. The tissue was plated as partially digested colonic crypts, not single cells as these did not proliferate. The explants gave

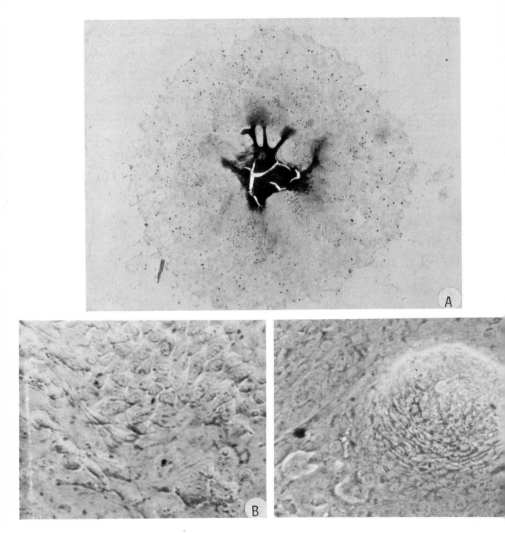

Fig. 1.   (A) Morphology of primary cultures used in this study. Colony of premalignant epithelial cells from a benign tumor after labeling for 64 h in 5 μCi [³H]thymidine/ml and 10^{-7} M DOC, followed by methanol fixation, autoradiography, and staining with hematoxylin and rhodamine B. The monolayer is intact with close-packed cells. Nuclei labeled with [³H]thymidine are found throughout the monolayer (×80). (B) Phase contrast micrograph of living colonic adenomatous cells in a section of another colony, washed extensively and then incubated in phosphate-buffered saline without calcium to show individual cell outlines (×256). (C) Phase contrast micrograph of part of an epithelial culture showing a dome (×251).

rise to islands of epithelial cells (Fig. 1A). Fibroblasts, in the very great majority of cases, did not grow out. They are a minority population in the colonic mucosae, where they line the colonic crypts. The epithelial islands consisted of hundreds to a few thousand very close-packed cells. Epithelial colonies from early-stage (tubular) adenomas were morphologically indistinguishable from those cultured from late-stage (villous) adenomas. Colon carcinoma cells were established in primary culture in identical fashion from tumors received from the surgical pathology department at Memorial Hospital and formed patches of several hundred cells before they were used.

II. CULTURED CELLS IDENTIFIED AS EPITHELIAL BY MORPHOLOGICAL AND FUNCTIONAL CRITERIA

The cells composing the epithelial monolayers exhibited in general a closely packed polygonal morphology nearest the explant (Figs. 1B and 3B) and a more flattened, elongated appearance at the colony periphery. The monolayer was one cell thick and did not form over a fibroblast layer, as shown by sectioning four monolayers. Irradiated fibroblasts were pushed aside by the continuous front of epithelial cells in cocultivation experiments. Colonic epithelial colonies formed whorls like keratinocytes (Sun et al., 1979). Tight packing of the cells gives the colonies a compact, dense circular shape (Fig. 1A) very different from diffuse fibroblast cultures with cells in parallel assay.

The cells elaborated typical epithelial structures such as brush borders and junctional complexes, and exhibited polarity of structures and subcellular organelles as seen in vivo. The cells were coupled by tight junctions, gap junctions, and des-

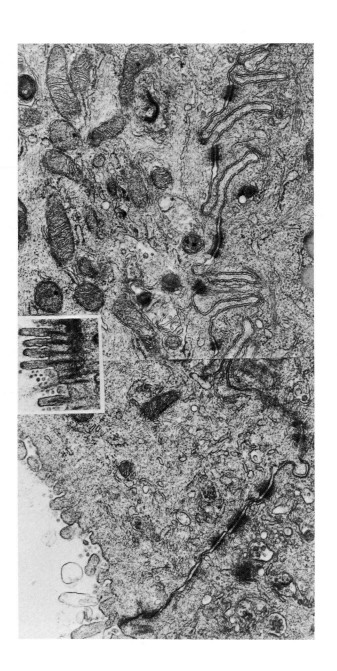

Fig. 2. Electron micrograph illustrating characteristic epithelial structures in cultured cells. At the extreme lower left corner a junctional complex begins at the medium face with a tight junction, followed by a gap junction, then a desmosome. Numerous membrane interdigitations alternating with desmosomes connect the two cells shown. Numerous mitochondria can also be seen (×14,110). A brush border was elaborated from the plasma membrane next to the medium (inset, ×14,370).

mosomes, in that order, starting at the apical or medium face
(Fig. 2). The lateral edges of adjoining cells were further
connected by extensive membrane interdigitations, interspersed
with desmosomes. The epithelial cells of the intestine are
subject to great mechanical stress, because they line a lumen
that undergoes large volume changes. Cells are also strengthened internally by numerous keratin filaments. The cultured
colonic epithelial cells contained numerous fibrils in their
cytoplasm as seen by transmission electron microscopy. These
fibrils are probably keratin bundles in that the cells stained
positively with rhodamine B, a keratin stain. This dense intracellular meshwork probably aided the cell in maintaining
its characteristic *in vivo* shape and organization. Monolayers
from four adenomas were sectioned. The cells were either
columnar or cuboidal, with a brush border at the apical end
and the nucleus basal, as is seen *in vivo*.

One of the major functions of colonic epithelial cells is
ion and water absorption. The brush border seen on the cultured
cells (Fig. 2, inset) predicts this function, which was shown
directly by the formation of domes in culture (Fig. 1C).
Groups of neighboring monolayer cells form domes or hemicysts
when they transport water and salts from the medium through
their basal surfaces to the impenetrable plastic petri dish.
Areas of the monolayer are lifted from the dish surface because
of the pressure of the trapped fluid that cannot leak out between the cells that are tightly coupled by junctional complexes. The position of the domes seen in the colonic epithelial cultures varied from day to day. Domes collapsed when
the monolayer was fixed in methanol. These observations indicate that domes were caused by trapped liquid and were not areas
where cells piled up. Dome formation is characteristic of
transporting epithelium and has been seen in primary cultures of
mammary epithelial cells (Pickett *et al.*, 1975) and mammary epi-

thelial and kidney epithelial cell lines (Leighton *et al.*, 1970; Dulbecco *et al.*, 1979).

III.   EPITHELIAL MONOLAYERS CONTAIN DIVIDING CELLS

Viable intact epithelial monolayers surrounding a small explant have been maintained routinely for 7 to 8 weeks. During this time colonies grow to contain several thousand cells by migration of cells from the explant followed by division of the migrating cells. The presence of replicating cells has been demonstrated by labeling with [^{3}H]thymidine. Parallel cultures were established from the same adenoma, cultured for 3 weeks, and then incubated with 5 μCi/ml of [^{3}H]thymidine for 72 h. The percentage of labeled cells gradually reached a plateau of 20% after 48 h. The labeled cells were seen throughout the monolayer, not just at the periphery or near the explant (Fig. 1A). This experiment was repeated with six different adenomas with similar results and with labeling indices of 38, 26, 21, 29, 36, and 23%, respectively.

IV.   VARIATION IN PROPERTIES OF CULTURED PREMALIGNANT CELLS
WITH HISTOLOGICAL CLASS

The purpose of initiating these studies was to determine whether the cultured cells derived from these three types of adenomas would reflect different stages of premalignancy by exhibiting different properties. A corollary to the adenoma-to-carcinoma progression model states that the cells derived from villous adenomas will have a phenotype closer to the malignant than will the tubular adenomatous epithelial cells. This was found to be the case. Epidermal growth factor (EGF) stimulated

TABLE I. Phenotypic Markers of Cultured Premalignant and Malignant Cells

Premalignant stage	Response of human colonic epithelial cells to:			Fetal-specific antibody (reactivity)
	EGF	DOC	TPA	
Early (tubular adenoma)	Increased DNA replication	Increased DNA replication	Increased DNA replication	18%
Mixed (villotubular adenoma)	No effect on DNA replication or morphology	No effect on morphology	a. Multilayering b. Plasminogen activator (PA) release c. Disruption of gap junctions	43%
Late (villous adenoma)	No effect on DNA replication or morphology	No effect on DNA replication or morphology	a. Multilayering b. PA Release c. Disruption of gap junctions	70%
Malignant-- primary culture (carcinoma)	Not tested; expect no response under our growth conditions	Not tested; expect no response	a. Multilayering b. PA Release c. Gap junctions already disrupted	71%

the proliferation *in vitro* of epithelial cells cultured from
tubular adenomas but not those cultured from villous adenomas
(summarized in Table I) under the same growth conditions
(media supplemented with 15% fetal calf serum).   Epidermal
growth factor has a very strong structural homology to uro-
gastrone, a tropic hormone in the intestine (Elder *et al.*,
1972).   These data imply that villous cells have lost normal
response to a hormone that controls cellular proliferation in
the gut.   Loss of growth control is characteristic of neoplasms.   In a second study (Higgins *et al.*, 1982), the reactivity of several cultured adenomas and carcinomas to an antibody raised against human fetal tissue was measured.   Reactive
cells were found more frequently in cultures derived from villous adenomas and carcinomas, less frequently in those from
villotubular adenomas, and least often in cultures from tubular adenomas (Table I).   Many tumors synthesize proteins whose
expression is otherwise limited to the time of fetal development.   Again, of all the adenomas, the premalignant villous
cells displayed characteristics closest to the carcinoma.

V.   DIFFERENTIAL RESPONSE OF PREMALIGNANT CELLS TO PROMOTING
     AGENTS

The adenoma cell classes are not the only premalignant
cell types that have been described in the human colon.   Lipkin
and collaborators (1980) have found proliferative abnormalities
in the colonic crypts of patients with one of three hereditary
predispositions to develop colonic carcinoma: familial polyposis, Gardner's syndrome, and hereditary colon cancer syndrome
without intestinal polyposis.   In these disorders colonic epithelial cells lining the crypts continue to divide even when
they reach the gut lumen, as do adenomas, even though the

crypts do not always elongate to form an adenoma. The adenoma cell types therefore appear to be at later stages in the progression than these cells. In analogy to the two-stage mouse skin carcinogenesis model (Van Duuren, 1969; Boutwell, 1974; Berenblum, 1975), the adenoma cells should already be initiated, as initiation is the first step in carcinogenesis. They have sustained a heritable alteration in their DNA. Initiated cells, again in analogy to the mouse skin model, are expected to respond to promoting agents. Thus we tested the effects of two tumor promoters, deoxycholic acid (DOC) and 12-O-tetradecanoyl-phorbol 13-acetate (TPA), on adenoma cell classes and found differential effects.

Deoxycholic acid, a secondary bile acid found in the colon, has been implicated in the etiology of colon cancer by several investigators. Increasing the concentration of bile acids in the intestines of laboratory animals pretreated with a carcinogen by biliary diversion (Chomchai et al., 1974), administration of the bile-sequestering agent cholestryamine (Nigro et al., 1973), direct intracolonic bile acid installation (Narisawa et al., 1974; Deschner and Raicht, 1979), direct feeding of bile acids (Cohen et al., 1980), or a high-fat diet (Reddy et al., 1976, 1977) in all cases caused an increase in the number of colonic tumors. An increase in bile acid concentration, by any of these methods, was not by itself tumorigenic. Therefore, bile acids have been postulated to act as promoting agents *in vivo*. Bile acids, cholesterol derivatives that function in fat, cholesterol, and fat-soluble vitamin absorption, may also play this role in humans (Miettinen, 1972). Epidemiological studies have suggested a link between high-fat diets, and therefore high bile acid concentrations, and an increased incidence of human colon cancer (Armstrong and Doll, 1975). TPA has been known for many years to induce tumors when applied locally to the skin of mice pretreated with a subthreshold level of a

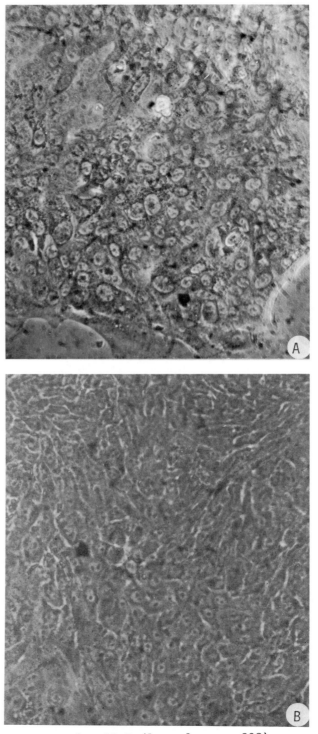

Fig. 3A,B (legend on p. 338)

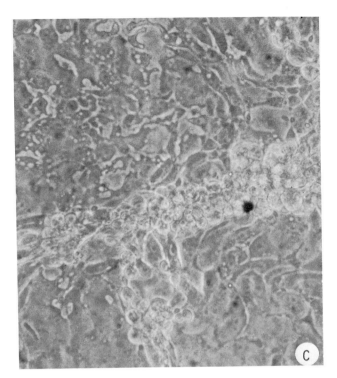

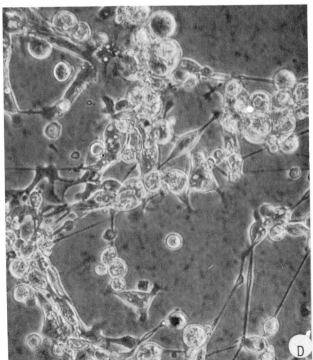

Fig. 3C,D (legend on p. 338)

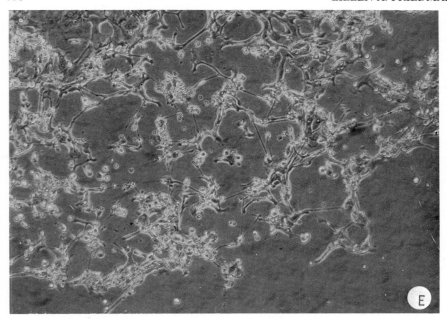

Fig. 3E

Fig. 3. Morphological alterations in parallel cultures
of premalignant epithelial cells exposed to TPA. (A) Control
culture of epithelial cells cultured from a villous or late-
stage adenoma 24 h in the presence of the diluent, 0.1% DMSO.
(B) Parallel culture incubated 24 h in 100 ng/ml of the inactive TPA analog 4αPDD. (C) Parallel culture incubated 16 h in
100 ng TPA/ml showing ridge or rill of cells. (D) Parallel
culture of epithelial cells incubated for 24 h in 100 ng of
TPA/ml. (E) Lower magnification of (D) (×80) showing networks
of colony-like aggregates throughout the culture. (A-D) Phase
micrographs of living cells (×265).

carcinogen. It has now been found that TPA induces gastroin-

testinal tumors when applied intragastrically in carcinogen-

pretreated mice (Goerttler et al., 1979). These data imply

that TPA can act as a promoting agent on gastrointestinal epi-

thelial cells as well as on epidermal tissue.

A. Differential Effects on Morphology

Premalignant epithelial cells at an early, an intermediate, or a late adenomatous stage in their development toward colon carcinoma were tested for their response to the phorbol ester tumor promoter TPA, and to DOC, a bile acid known to increase the incidence of colonic tumors (Friedman, 1981). Epithelial cell cultures were grown in the presence of (1) TPA, (2) its analog, 4-α-phorbol 12,13-didecanoate (4αPDD; inactive in promotion), (3) 0.1% dimethylsulfoxide (DMSO), the diluent, or (4) DOC. There was no observable alteration in morphology of early-stage premalignant epithelial cells following TPA treatment. When TPA was added to cultures of intermediate-stage villotubular (i.e., containing villous element) or late-stage 100% villous premalignant cells, however, marked morphological changes were seen, although culture conditions were identical for each cell type. After 6 h the cells began to elongate, then multilayer into long rills. By 24 h the majority of the colony had formed dense cellular clusters (Fig. 3D). Cell-to-substratum adhesion was decreased, and cell-to-cell adhesion was also altered. Networks of these cellular aggregates were seen throughout the entire colony (Fig. 3E). These changes were distinct from those seen when cells were exposed to a cytotoxic agent, such as a high (10^{-9} M) concentration of cholera toxin. Dying cells balloon, do not form clusters, and rapidly slough off the dish. Cell clustering and multilayering were not seen when parallel cultures were treated with either the nonpromoting analog 4αPDD or the diluent, 0.1% DMSO (Fig. 3A and B). In some experiments, TPA-treated cells remained as clusters attached to other cells on the dish for as long as 2 weeks. In others, patches of cells remained adherent.

Adenocarcinoma cells in primary culture responded to TPA in the same manner as did late-stage premalignant cells. Cell

clustering was marked within 24 h. To examine the generality
of this response, five colon adenocarcinomas (primary tumors,
not metastases) were placed in primary culture and treated
with TPA or 4αPDD. In three cases cell clustering was induced
by TPA, analogous to the response of premalignant cells. Cell
rilling and clustering, especially at colony peripheries, were
constitutive in the other two cases but enhanced by TPA (Table
II). Therefore, morphological changes inducible by TPA were a
property of primary transformants as well as classes of advanced
premalignant cells. In contrast, three human colon carcinoma
cell lines, SW1116, SW1417, and HT29, exhibited no clustering
or rilling when grown in the presence of TPA (Table II). One
of these lines, SW1116, induced tumor formation in a Swiss
nu/nu nude mouse in this laboratory during the period when the
experiments in Table II were performed. Line HT29 has been reported to be tumorigenic. Apparently these established lines,
although retaining malignancy, lost the clustering response to
TPA after adaptation to cell culture conditions.

In contrast to TPA, DOC induced no apparent morphological
changes in early-, intermediate-, or late-stage premalignant
cells or in malignant cells. For example, when parallel cultures, derived from one villous or late-stage adenoma, were
treated with either 10^{-7} M DOC or 100 ng TPA/ml, the TPA-
treated culture underwent cellular aggregation whereas the
DOC-treated culture remained morphologically unchanged.

To demonstrate the generality of this differential morphological response of premalignant cells to TPA and to DOC,
cultures from a large number of patients were assayed in a
double-blind study. The pathology diagnosis of each adenoma
was not decoded until completion of the experiment. Epithelial
colonies from 16 tubular (early) adenomas, 4 villotubular (intermediate) adenomas, and 6 villous (late) adenomas were ex-

TABLE II. Differential Effects of TPA and DOC on the Morphology of Malignant and Premalignant Epithelial Cells[a]

Epithelial pathology	Agent	Number of cultures	Clustering	Secreted protease
Tubular adenomatous (early-stage premalignant)	TPA	14	−	−
	4αPDD	14	−	−
	TPA	2	+	+
	4αPDD	2	−	−
	DOC	5	−	NT
Villotubular (inter-mediate-stage pre-malignant)	TPA	4	+	+[b]
	4αPDD	4	−	−
	DOC	2	−	NT[c]
Villous (late-stage premalignant)	TPA	6	+	+
	4αPDD	6	−	−
	DOC	5	−	−
Adenocarcinoma primaries (malignant)	TPA	5	+	+
	DOC	1	−	NT
Established carcinoma cell lines (malignant	TPA	3	−	+
	4αPDD	3	−	−

[a]Primary cultures of adenoma-derived premalignant epithelial cells and adenocarcinomas were grown for 2 to 3 weeks. The individual adenoma colonies contained several hundred to a few thousand cells in monolayer culture, and each plate contained on the average 5–10 colonies. Many more colonies were obtained from the adenocarcinomas. The carcinoma cell lines were grown to subconfluence (1–6 × 10^6 cells) in T75 flasks before assay. Both TPA and 4αPDD were added to 100 ng/ml, whereas DOC was added at 10^{-7} M. Secreted protease was assayed by the cleavage of a fluorescent tripeptide substrate.

[b]Protease was detected in culture medium from TPA-treated cultures at an average of fourfold the activity in medium controls.

[c]NT, not tested.

posed to TPA, 4αPDD, or DMSO diluent. Cells from 5 tubular, 2 villotubular, 5 villous adenomas, and 1 primary colon carcinoma were treated with DOC. DOC caused no morphological changes in any of the cultures, confirming the earlier observations (Table II). Of the 16 tubular (early-stage) epithelial

cultures, 14 (88%) exhibited no morphological changes (Table
II) in response to TPA. However, all of the epithelial colonies cultured from villotubular or villous adenomas responded
to TPA by marked cell clustering. Clustering did not occur in
parallel cultures treated with 4αPDD or DMSO. Reduction of the
TPA concentration from 100 to 50 ng/ml caused no obvious difference in cell response, whereas clustering was reduced at
10 ng/ml and minimal at 1 ng/ml. Pretreatment with the inactive analog 4αPDD did not noticeably alter response to TPA.
Cultures of villotubular cells from 2 different adenomas were
treated with 4αPDD for 2 days without any morphological changes.
The analog was removed and replaced with TPA. Cell clustering
followed within 24 h.

B. Stimulation of DNA Replication

        The mechanism by which promoting agents exert their ef-
fect in tumorigenesis is unknown, but the phorbol ester tumor
promoters have diverse effects on cultured cells (Weinstein *et
al.*, 1979), including a stimulation of DNA replication, a
property also exhibited by bile acids. Addition of the primary
bile acid, cholic acid, to the diet of laboratory rats caused
an enhanced rate of cellular proliferation in the colon
(Cohen *et al.*, 1980). Similarly, bile acid deprivation by bile
fistula markedly depressed colonic cell proliferation (Deschner
and Raicht, 1979). Therefore, the effects of both TPA and DOC
on the proliferation of different classes of premalignant cells
were assayed.

        Primary cultures from four different early-stage or tubu-
lar adenomas were tested with 10^{-8} to 10^{-7} M DOC (A, B, C, D)
or 100 ng TPA/ml (A, C, E, F). Primary cultures from four different late-stage or villous adenomas (A, B, C, D) were tested
with 10^{-7} M DOC. Late-stage (villous) cells clustered after

TABLE III. DOC and TPA Enhancement of the Proliferative Fraction in Colonies of Early-Stage Premalignant Epithelial Cells[a]

Pathology of premalignant cells	Stage in premalignancy	[3H]Thymidine-labeled nuclei (%)[b]		DOC Concentration (M)	Increase (%)
		Control	+DOC		
Tubular A	Early	30.8 ± 4.2	57.9 ± 6.3	10^{-7}	88
Tubular B	Early	22.2 ± 5.7	42.9 ± 4.7	10^{-7}	93
Tubular C	Early	22.6 ± 1.7	35.1 ± 4.7	10^{-8}	55
Tubular D	Early	22.5 ± 1.7	40.3 ± 1.4	10^{-8}	79
Tubular D	Early	22.5 ± 1.7	56.5 ± 1.3	5×10^{-8}	150
Villous A	Late	24.7 ± 3.8	18.1 ± 2.5	10^{-7}	0
Villous B	Late	32.3 ± 3.4	31.6 ± 1.7	10^{-7}	0
Villous C	Late	19.0 ± 0.1	21.5 ± 0.9	10^{-7}	0
Villous D	Late	30.4 ± 4.3	23.9 ± 4.0	10^{-7}	0
		Control	+4αPDD	+TPA	
Tubular A	Early	30.8 ± 4.2	31.3 ± 0.2	42.3 ± 3.0	37
Tubular E	Early	13.4 ± 0.8	9.8 ± 0.8	26.3 ± 0.3	96
Tubular C	Early	NT	22.6 ± 1.7	30.3 ± 2.9	34
Tubular F	Early	28.9 ± 0.7	NT	62.8 ± 4.2	117

[a] Colonies of premalignant epithelial cells were allowed to grow to several hundred cells by culture for 1 to 3 weeks. Then, 100 ng/ml of TPA or 4αPDD, 10^{-8}–10^{-7} M DOC, or 0.1% DMSO (the diluent) were added to parallel cultures. [3H]Thymidine at 5 µCi/ml was then added (DOC cultures), or was added 3 h later (TPA cultures) for 52 to 70 h of labeling. The cells were methanol fixed, processed for autoradiography, and then stained with hematoxylin. An average of 700 cells from an average of five separate adenoma colonies were counted for each value.
[b] Mean ± SD. [c] NT, Not tested.

TPA treatment, as described in the preceding section, and were
unsuitable for autoradiography. DOC was added to cultures from
tubular adenomas A and B and villous adenomas A and B at the
time of plating and with every medium change (Table III). DOC
was added to the remaining two villous cultures (C and D) at
the time of labeling. TPA was added 3 h prior to addition of
[^{3}H]thymidine in each case. The proliferative fraction of colonies from each tumor was measured by incubation with [^{3}H]thymi-
dine for 52 to 70 h, a period long enough to label all dividing
cells. In each of the four early-stage adenomas tested, the
growth fraction was enhanced (34-117%) by TPA (Table III). At
10^{-7} M DOC also caused a large increase (88 and 93%) in the percentage of replicating cells in epithelial colonies derived
from early-stage benign tumors, the tubular adenomas (Table
III). A lower concentration of DOC (10^{-8} M) caused a lower but
still significant enlargement (55 and 79%) of the proliferative
fraction in cultures from two other early-stage premalignant
adenomas (tubular adenomas C and D). In one experiment,
5×10^{-8} M DOC also caused a substantial (150%) increase in the
labeling index (tubular adenoma D). In contrast, 10^{-7} M DOC
had no discernible effect on the number of DNA-synthesizing
cells in colonies derived from four villous adenomas whether it
was added at the time of plating or after the cells had been
cultured for several days. At 10^{-7} M DOC was apparently not
toxic to the villous cells, as the labeling index is untreated
and treated cultures was indistinguishable (Table III).

Although both TPA and DOC caused an increase in the fraction of dividing cells in cultures from early-stage premalignant or benign tumors, DOC was more stimulatory. In the two
tumors in which parallel cultures were assayed with both agents
(A and C), TPA enhanced replication by an average of 36%, whereas DOC at 10^{-7} and 10^{-8} M stimulated 88 and 55%, respectively.
The effect of 50 ng of EGF/ml on culture A was 48.8 ± 3.5%

stimulation. In this one case, 10^{-7} M DOC was more effective in increasing proliferation (88%) than either TPA (37%) or EGF (58%). DOC affected replication in only the early-stage cells and had no measurable effect on the proliferation or morphology of late-stage cells. TPA stimulated replication in early-stage cells while not affecting morphology. Its effect on replication of late-stage cells could not be measured by autoradiography, because TPA induced cell clustering.

C. Protease Secretion

The cell clustering described in this study was very similar to that seen when Rous sarcoma virus-transformed chicken embryo fibroblasts were treated with TPA (Goldfarb and Quigley, 1978). The morphological alterations seen in the virally transformed cells (Quigley, 1979) were caused by enhanced levels of plasminogen activator secretion. Therefore, the media from TPA-treated premalignant and malignant epithelial cells in primary culture and appropriate controls were tested for proteolytic activity (see Section IV,C,1). Secretion of a protease(s) occurred in each case concomitantly with cell clustering (Table II). Protease levels in these cultures were three- to fivefold greater than levels found in fresh medium and were designated as + in Table II. The premalignant epithelial cells that did not cluster in response to TPA (from 14 of 16 tubular adenomas) also did not secrete detectable levels of protease (Table II). In contrast to these results from cells in primary culture, three established lines of colon carcinoma cells secreted enhanced levels of protease but did not form clusters in response to TPA. Secreted protease could be detected in media without concentration. In contrast, 10^7 Rous sarcoma virus-transformed chicken embryo fibroblasts did not secrete enough protease to be seen without concentration of medium (data not shown).

TABLE IV.   Protease Secretion in Response to TPA by Premalignant Epithelial Cells and Malignant Cells[a]

Epithelial pathology	Promoting agent	Secreted protease $(mU/10^3$ cells)
A. Controls for effect of serum		
Late premalignant villous adenoma F	TPA, No serum	480
Colon carcinoma cell line SW1116	TPA, No serum	1.63
	TPA, 1.5% Serum	1.06
	TPA, 15% Serum	1.30
B. Premalignant and nonclustering[b]		
Tubular adenoma A	TPA	<60[c]
Tubular adenoma A	4αPDD	<60[c]
C. Premalignant and clustering[d]		
Villous adenoma C	TPA	936
Villous adenoma C	4αPDD	<34[c]
Villous adenoma C	0.1% DMSO	<39[c]
Villous adenoma A	TPA	590
Villous adenoma D	TPA	1326
Villous adenoma E	TPA	1020
Tubular adenoma M	TPA	520
Tubular adenoma N	TPA	740
Villotubular adenoma B	TPA	1720
Villotubular adenoma C	TPA	380
D. Primary transformants		
Adenocarcinoma B	TPA	1.91
Adenocarcinoma B	0.1% DMSO	0.26
Adenocarcinoma C	TPA	14.9
Adenocarcinoma C	4αPDD	0.78
Adenocarcinoma C	0.1% DMSO	0.75
E. Established lines		
Human carcinoma cell line HT29	TPA	0.38
	0.1% DMSO	0.07
Human carcinoma cell line SW1417	TPA	2.22
	0.1% DMSO	0.49

(Table IV Continued)

Epithelial pathology	Promoting agent	Secreted protease (mU/10^3 cells)
Human carcinoma cell line SW1116	TPA	1.30
	4αPDD	0.92
	0.1% DMSO	0.50

[a]The number of cells in primary adenocarcinoma (nearly confluent 60-mm dishes) and cell line cultures (T75 flasks) was determined by trypsinization using a three-times crystallized 0.05% solution of trypsin (Worthington Biochemical Corp.) to achieve a single-cell suspension before counting in a Coulter counter. The adenoma cultures contained fewer cells, so the cell number was calculated as follows. Representative sections of each colony were photographed, and the number of cells was counted. The area of each colony was measured using an eyepiece with a micrometer on a phase-inverted microscope (Leitz). Appropriate calculations then gave an estimation of the number of adenoma cells per dish. Two assays, one with villous adenoma F and one with colon carcinoma cell line SW1116, were performed in the absence of serum. The difference in levels of protease secretion was still observed.

[b]Cells do not cluster in response to TPA.

[c]A representative calculation: a culture containing 3×10^3 cells and secreting less than 10 mU/0.1 ml of medium (1 ml total) was calculated to secrete less than 35 mU of protease per 10^3 cells.

[d]Cells cluster in response to TPA.

1. Quantitation of Protease Production

A direct fluorimetric assay was used in these studies instead of the more standard indirect assay for plasminogen activator, which relies on plasmin generation followed by the degradation of iodinated fibrin. The fluorimetric assay (Zimmerman et al., 1978) measures the cleavage of a single peptide bond, that following the synthetic tripeptide, glutaryl-glycyl-arginyl, to release a fluorescent compound. The proteolytic activity secreted from adenoma cells had a similar dose-response curve in the fluorimetric assay to human urokinase, a known plasminogen activator. All adenoma and carcinoma protease activity is expressed relative to standard Ploug units of urokinase activity (Tables IV and V).

The heat-inactivated fetal calf serum used in growth medium, and thus present in the assay, did not obviously potentiate or inhibit the protease secreted from adenoma or carcinoma cells. Appropriate controls with fresh medium were included in each experiment, and the adenoma-carcinoma protease values were corrected for this background activity. Cultures of TPA-treated SW1116 carcinoma cells were incubated in medium with no serum, 1.5% serum, or 15% serum. After subtraction of medium control values, there was no significant difference in the protease values obtained: 1.63, 1.06, and 1.30 $mU/10^3$ cells (Table IV, A). Serum does contain plasmin inhibitors, but the assay does not depend on plasmin generation. Therefore, the protease induced by TPA from adenomas and carcinomas (Table IV, B-E) was secreted into growth medium. Culture conditions were unchanged to optimize survival of the fastidious epithelial cells during TPA treatment.

The amount of protease produced from nine cultures of premalignant cells averaged 904 $mU/10^3$ cells (Table IV), with a range of 380 to 1720 $mU/10^3$ cells. The cultures assayed were derived from five villous adenomas, two villotubular adenomas, and the only two TPA-sensitive tubular adenomas detected. It was quite surprising to find that two colonic adenocarcinomas, under identical conditions of primary culture as the premalignant cells, secreted much less protease, 14.9 and 1.9 $mU/10^3$ cells (Table IV), respectively, in response to TPA. These colon tumors were at the primary site and did not arise from metastasis. Three established human colon carcinoma cell lines, SW1116, SW1417, and HT29, secreted about as much protease in response to TPA as the lower of the two adenocarcinomas in primary culture (0.38, 2.22, and 1.30 $mU/10^3$ cells, respectively).

This difference was still seen when protease was secreted into serum-free medium (Table IV, A). A TPA-treated late-stage premalignant culture secreted 480 $mU/10^3$ cells, whereas TPA-induced carcinoma cells secreted 1.63 $mU/10^3$ cells. The 480-mU value falls in the range seen in cultures treated with TPA in growth medium (Table IV, C, 380-1720 mU). Therefore, premalignant epithelial cells can be induced by a promoting agent, TPA, to secrete many times as much protease as fully transformed cells.

The cell lines and the primary carcinomas secreted low but measurable levels of protease constitutively (Table IV). This level was enhanced by TPA in all five cases assayed. Because of the relatively low number of cultured adenoma cells, it was not possible to determine whether any constitutive protease secretion occurred at the level detected from the carcinomas. Cells from villous adenoma C secreted <34 and <39 $mU/10^3$ cells in response to the nonpromoting TPA analog 4αPDD and the diluent 0.1% DMSO, respectively (for calculations, see footnotes to Table IV). A representative culture of tubular adenoma cells, unresponsive to TPA, secreted <60 $mU/10^3$ cells. These values indicate the lower levels of detection in each experiment and cannot be compared to the low but measureable values of protease secreted from much larger numbers of carcinoma cells. Protease secretion does not continue from premalignant cells at the high levels measured 2 days after TPA addition (Table IV). Even if additional aliquots of TPA were added, protease levels decreased and became undetectable after 4 to 6 days of treatment (experiments with four different adenomas).

TABLE V.   Effect of Protease Inhibitors[a]

Inhibitor[b]	Concentration	Adenoma protease (mU)	Human urokinase (mU)
None		104	112
Leupeptin	200 μM	0	0[d]
	100 μM	28[c]	NT
	80 μM	31[c]	NT
	20 μM	42[c], 27[e]	NT
	10 μM	52[c]	NT
NPGB	2 μM	0	0
	0.3 μM	0[c]	NT
	0.1 μM	31[c]	NT
Benzamidine	1 mM	0	0
	0.5 mM	52[c]	NT
	0.16 mM	59[c]	NT
ε-ACA	1.7 mM	96	96
Trasylol	15 U/ml	92	105
SBTI	1.7 μg/ml	100	108
TLCK	0.3 mM	96	108

[a]Dilutions of urokinase (112 mU each) or aliquots of medium from villous adenoma treated with TPA for 48 h (104 mU each) were added to reaction mixtures containing glt-gly-arg-AMC and one of the inhibitors listed. The values shown under adenoma protease were corrected for low background levels of proteolytic activity in the serum. The table summarizes experiments with three villous adenomas differentiated by footnotes c and e or none.

[b]Abbreviations: ε-ACA, ε-aminocaproic acid; SBTI, soybean trypsin inhibitor; TLCK, N-α-tosyl-L-lysylchloromethane.

[c]Protease secreted into medium without serum.

[d]NT, Not tested.

[e]Added in vivo; assayed in vitro 2 days later; different adenoma from that in footnote c.

2. Properties of the Adenoma Protease

The data shown so far only demonstrate that the adenomas reactive to TPA secrete a protease that cleaves after arginine, as does the plasminogen activator urokinase. To further define this activity, inhibitors of plasmin, plasminogen activator, or trypsin were assayed on medium from three TPA-treated late-stage

adenomas. The effect of these inhibitors was tested in parallel experiments on urokinase, a known plasminogen activator
(Table V).

Leupeptin (an arginine-containing peptide aldehyde),
NPGB (an active-site titrant of certain serine enzymes), and
benzamidine (an arginine analog) completely inhibited both the
adenoma protease and urokinase. A lysine analog, ε-aminocaproic
acid, and trasylol, both inhibitors of plasmin, had little inhibitory effect on either urokinase or the adenoma protease.
Soybean trypsin inhibitor, a general inhibitor of trypsin-like
proteases, and the lysine analog, N-α-tosyl-L-lysylchlorometh-
ane, did not inhibit (<4%) the adenoma protease or urokinase
(Table V).

In a second series of inhibitor studies, protease was secreted into medium containing 1.4 μg bovine serum albumin/ml
instead of serum. Parallel cultures from a villous adenoma
were washed in serum-free media and then incubated for 24 h
in this medium with either 100 ng TPA/ml or 100 ng 4 PDD/ml.
Cell clustering occurred only in the presence of TPA. The secreted protease was inhibited by three plasminogen-activator
inhibitors: 10-100 μM leupeptin, 0.1 and 0.3 μM NPGB, and
0.16 and 0.5 mM benzamidine (Table V). Thus, the major proteolytic activity assayed had an inhibitor profile characteristic
of a plasminogen activator, not plasmin or trypsin.

Cell clustering was inhibited *in vitro* by a plasminogen-
activator inhibitor. Epithelial cultures from three different
villotubular adenomas were treated for 24 h with 50 ng TPA/ml
and 1 mM benzamidine. Cells in parallel cultures remained
viable in 1 mM benzamidine as shown by their ability to exclude
trypan blue dye. There was no cell clustering and no detectable
level of protease released (<10 mU/0.1 ml medium). The cells
were washed several times and then incubated with 50 ng TPA/ml
alone. Cell clustering was apparent within 24 h, together with

protease release. The concordance of the two events suggests
strongly that cell clustering was the result of plasminogen activator release.

The adenoma protease secreted into medium containing serum
(and thus plasminogen) was still stimulated by added plasminogen. Addition of 15 U of purified human plasminogen to aliquots
of media from three different TPA-treated villous adenoma cultures stimulated proteolytic activity 7-21%. The similarity of
inhibitor profiles and dose-response curve to the known plasminogen activator, urokinase, plus the stimulation of adenoma
protease by plasminogen, strongly suggest that the major proteolytic activity secreted into TPA-treated adenoma culture medium is a plasminogen activator.

D.   Intercellular Communication Assay

We have shown that in response to 50 to 100 ng/ml TPA,
late-stage premalignant cells cultured from histologically distinct benign villous tumors with high malignant potential form
multilayers and then cell clusters, and at the same time secrete a plasminogen activator. These pronounced alterations
in cellular morphology suggested that membrane structures were
altered by TPA. Many studies have shown TPA to have pleotropic
effects at cell surfaces (Weinstein et al., 1979). However,
investigators have begun to focus on membrane structures that
may play a role in cell communication. Gap junctions are
thought to have this function by allowing the passage of low
molecular weight molecules between cells (Revel and Karnovsky,
1967; Loewenstein, 1979). A current hypothesis suggests that
gap junctions may provide the channels necessary for transmission of diffusible signals governing growth control. Cellular
communication has been shown to be modulated by the tumor promoter, TPA. TPA has been shown to inhibit electrical coupling

reversibly in a human cell line (Enomoto *et al.*, 1981) and to inhibit metabolic cooperation between cultured cells, a complex process that includes the physical exchange of molecules (Yotti *et al.*, 1979). Aberrant communication between cells is correlated with emergence of the neoplastic phenotype. A broad range of cells in adult tissues exhibit extensive communication, as shown by fluorescent dye transfer, electrical coupling, or transfer of radiolabeled molecules (Loewenstein, 1979).

In sharp contrast, many different types of neoplastic cells in explanted tissue or in primary culture exhibit an altered communication pattern, with decreased cellular coupling. We decided that use of primary cultures of adenomas and adenocarcinomas might yield relevant information about the degree of cellular communication associated with premalignant and malignant stages and its possible modulation by tumor promoters. We did not believe that our studies would merely repeat the earlier studies that were all performed with cell lines, which may not accurately reflect the properties of the tissues from which they were derived. For example, primary cultures of adenocarcinomas exhibited cell clustering in response to TPA, whereas established carcinoma cell lines did not (Table II), although both cultures secreted a plasminogen activator. This may imply alterations in the cell membranes of the cell lines, and it certainly implies that significant changes in the carcinoma cells have taken place when they became established in culture.

1. Premalignant Cells

Cellular communication was assayed by the injection into a single cell in randomly selected areas of the cultures of a fluorescent tracer molecule, fluorescein (MW322), which is small enough to pass through gap junctions (Friedman and Steinberg,

TABLE VI.   Extent of Intercellular Communication in Malignant
            and Premalignant Cell Cultures[a]

Tumor pathology	Number of injection sites with mean number of dye-coupled cells numbering:		Presence of areas with many dye-coupled cell
	3	39-69[b]	
Early-stage premalignant			
Tumor 392[c]	6	6	+
Tumor 504	4	8	+
Tumor 504 + TPA	0	2	+
Tumor 402	15	2	+
Tumor 402 + TPA	3	1	+
Late-stage premalignant			
Tumor 378	0	10	+
Tumor 428	0	2	+
Tumor 428 + TPA	7	0	−
Tumor 432	3	3	+
Tumor 432 + 4αPDD	1	6	+
Tumor 432 + TPA	8	0	−
Tumor 506 + 4αPDD	1	3	+
Tumor 506 + TPA	3	0	−
Malignant			
Adenocarcinoma 406	3	1[d]	±
Adenocarcinoma 484	3	1[d]	±
Carcinoma cell line			
SW1116	8	0	−
SW1116 + TPA	12	0	−

[a] *Individual cells were injected with fluorescein (METHODS) and the injection site photographed using UV optics. The identical area was also photographed by phase contrast microscopy. The two sets of photographs were compared and the number of fluorescing cells counted.*
[b] *Mean number of dye-coupled cells per injection site in early-stage premalignant cultures was 39. Mean number of dye-coupled cells in late-stage premalignant cultures per injection site was 69.*
[c] *When no additive is indicated the cultures were incubated in the TPA diluent, 0.1% DMSO, in culture medium.*
[d] *Patchwork pattern of fluorescence with dye skipping adjacent cells as seen in Fig. 4p.*

1982). Cultured premalignant cells were known to contain gap junctions by electron microscopy (Friedman *et al.*, 1981). Dye spread was followed by visualization of the injected cell and its neighbors by fluorescence microscopy. Epithelial cells were cultured from four villous adenomas and then exposed in parallel cultures either to TPA (50 ng/ml for 24 h) or to 0.1% DMSO (the diluent). In each case (Table VI), the TPA-treated cells first elongated, then rounded up, disrupting the mono- layer, and then clustered into small groups (Fig. 4i and m). The cells appeared to retain some physical connection, often by long cytoplasmic bridges. Were the morphological changes caused by TPA treatment sufficient to prevent some of these late premalignant cells from communicating with neighboring cells? Parallel cultures, treated with DMSO or TPA, consisted of petri dishes with one to about four epithelial cell patches (colonies). Injected cells in each of the DMSO-treated cul- tures (tumors 378, 428, 432) and the two TPA analog (4αPDD)- treated cultures (tumors 432 and 506) displayed one of three patterns: (1) The dye remained in the injected cell, which was completely uncoupled from other cells, (2) dye spread was limited to two to five adjacent cells (partial coupling), or (3) the dye spread to most of the neighboring cells until it was too dilute to be seen, and so the cells were considered highly coupled. The uncoupled and partially coupled injection sites are summed in the first column of Table VI, whereas the highly coupled areas are listed in the second. These highly coupled regions varied from 25 to 200 cells in size with a mean of 69 and a median of 48. (Fig. 4g, h, k, and l show representative regions.) The presence of these highly dye- coupled regions in DMSO- and 4αPDD-treated cultures was drama- tic because it showed that many, if not most, late-stage pre- malignant epithelial cells within a colony were communicating.

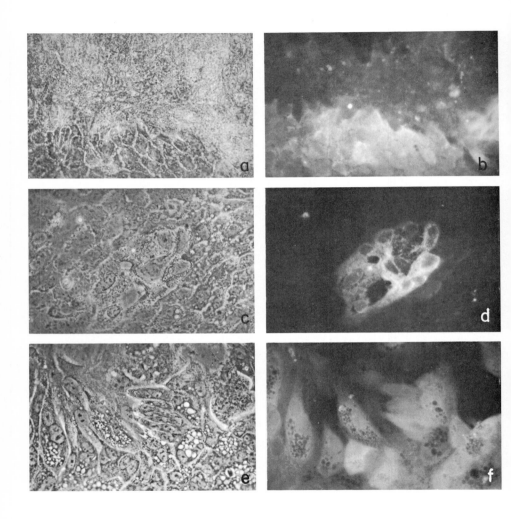

Fig. 4. Pattern of fluorescein dye spread in a series of
premalignant and malignant cell cultures. (a) Phase contrast
photomicrograph of early-stage premalignant cell culture from
tumor 504. (b) Fluorescence photomicrograph of some field as
(a) showing distribution of dye throughout the monolayer. Dye
injected at lower center has diffused through the entire field
but is less intense in the upper half of the field. Some

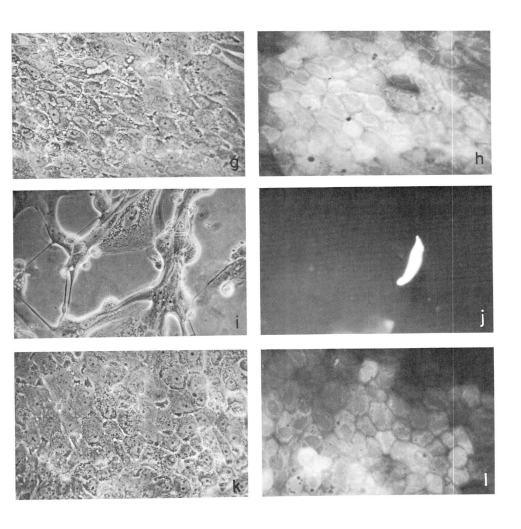

(Fig. 4 Continued) apparently uncoupled cells are visible in
the upper half of the field. Some apparently uncoupled cells
are visible in the upper left and upper center. (c) and (d)
Phase contrast and fluorescence photomicrographs of identical
field from tumor 504 showing a smaller group of coupled cells.
(e) Phase contrast photomicrograph and (f) fluorescence photomicrograph of parallel culture from tumor 504, treated in 24 h

(continued)

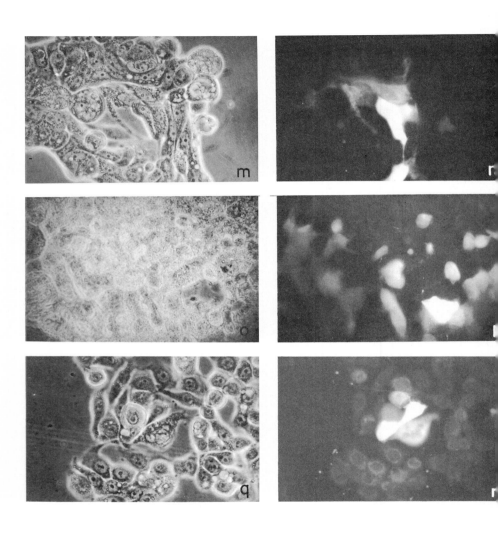

(Fig. 4 Continued) with 50 ng/ml TPA. No changes in fluorescein distribution or cell morphology were seen in TPA-treated parallel cultures. (g) Phase contrast photomicrograph of late-stage premalignant cell culture from tumor 432. (h) Fluorescence photomicrograph of same field as (g) showing extensive dye spread. (i) Phase contrast photograph of parallel culture from tumor 432, treated for 24 h with 50 ng/ml TPA and showing

When cells adhering to the petri dish were injected with fluorescein in the TPA-treated parallel cultures from tumors 428, 432, and 506, only partially coupled or uncoupled cells were seen. TPA completely abolished the highly coupled areas in each of the late-stage tumor cultures tested (zeros in Table VI; compare Fig. 4g and h with i and j, k and l with m and n). Therefore, TPA significantly decreased the extent of junctional communication in late-stage premalignant epithelial cell cultures.

Epithelial cells from three tubular (early-stage premalignant) adenomas were cultured and exposed in parallel cultures to either 50 ng/ml TPA or 0.1% DMSO for 24 h. There were no morphological changes. Dye injection experiments showed that DMSO-treated cultures from three tumors (392, 504, and 402) contained uncoupled, partially coupled, and highly coupled areas (Table VI). The number of cells in the highly coupled regions varied from 9 to 120 with a mean of 39 and a median of 18 (Fig. 4a-d). TPA-treated parallel cultures from tumors 504 and 402 also contained highly coupled regions (Fig. 4e and f). The presence of even one highly coupled area was considered

(Fig. 4 Continued) disruption of monolayer and multilayering of cells. (j) Fluorescence photomicrograph of identical field to (i) showing a completely uncoupled cell, which is a common finding in such cultures. (k) and (l) Phase contrast and matching fluorescence photomicrograph from late-stage premalignant cultures from tumor 428. (m) and (n) Phase contrast and matching fluorescence photograph from parallel tumor 428 cultures treated for 24 h with 50 ng/ml TPA. (o) Phase contrast photomicrograph of human colon adenocarcinoma 484 in primary culture. (p) Fluorescence photomicrograph of identical field to (o) showing patchwork fluorescence. (q) Phase contrast photomicrograph of colon carcinoma cell line SW1116. (r) Fluorescence photomicrograph of identical field to (q) showing two coupled cells, possibly undergoing division, with some dye spread to three surrounding cells (all photographs at 150× magnification).

significant because (a) it was easily distinguished from the
less coupled areas as it included so many more cells (mean of
39 versus mean of 3), and (b) TPA had eliminated this highly
coupled class in late-stage premalignant cell cultures. We
conclude that TPA decreased intercellular communication, probably by altering cellular morphology in late-stage premalignant cultures. In contrast, TPA had no observable effect on
the morphology of early-stage premalignant cell cultures and
did not eliminate extensive areas of intercellular dye coupling.

2. *Malignant Cells*

    Two adenocarcinomas in primary culture displayed a general-
ly uncoupled phenotype (Table VI). Each adenocarcinoma had an
area in which several cells (17-18 per field) were coupled.
However, dye spread was irregular, skipping many cells and
yielding a patchwork pattern of fluorescence (Fig. 4o and p),
in contrast to the almost uniform spread of dye through almost
every adjacent cell in highly coupled areas (e.g., Fig. 4b and
h) in untreated premalignant epithelial cultures. The reason
for this odd pattern of dye spread is unknown; however, the
adenocarcinoma in primary cultures does not always form the
flat monolayer seen in established cell lines from colon carcinomas. Some adenocarcinoma cells form elongated extensions
that may pass between and under nearby cells and end at other
cells not immediately adjacent. These long processes may be
responsible for the unusual patchwork pattern of fluorescence
seen in some areas of these cultures. TPA-treated adenocarcinoma primary cultures underwent morphological changes similar to
the late-stage premalignant cultures, as some cell clustering
was observed. No injection studies were performed as many
cells had been uncoupled before addition of TPA.

    The effects of TPA on the morphology and intercellular
communication of carcinoma cells was further studied using a

tumorigenic cell line, SW1116, established from a human colon
adenocarcinoma. The cell clustering seen in late-stage premalignant epithelial cell cultures, and to a lesser extent in
adenocarcinoma primary cultures, after TPA treatment, was not
seen in SW1116 cultures (Table II). Parallel cultures treated
with TPA and with DMSO were morphologically indistinguishable.
They were also indistinguishable in dye injection studies
(Table VI). Both types of cells were either completely uncoupled or coupled to at most four cells (Fig. 4q and r). No
areas of highly coupled cells were seen in TPA- or DMSO-treated
cultures (Table VI).

VI. DISCUSSION

The effects of two agents, TPA and DOC, that act as tumor
promoters in the gastrointestinal tract of experimental animals
were compared using primary cultures of human premalignant
colonic epithelial cells at different stages in tumor progression. DOC affected only the early-stage premalignant cells.
Of the three mitogenic compounds tested on early-stage cells
(DOC, TPA, and EGF), DOC had the greatest stimulatory effect
on DNA replication. Its major role in tumor progression *in
vivo* may be to enlarge significantly the early-stage premalignant cell population.

TPA Stimulated the growth of these cells to a lesser degree. Possibly the action of TPA on early-stage premalignant
cultures represents the reversible part of promotion, as the
major effect is hyperplasia. In contrast, TPA's action in
late-stage cells appears irreversible. When TPA was applied
to cells from late-stage (100% villous) and intermediate-stage
(with variable fraction of villous histology) benign tumors,
it induced cell clustering, multilayering, and concomitant

MODEL FOR
COLON CARCINOMA DEVELOPMENT

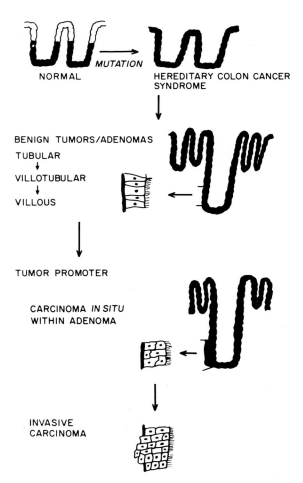

Fig. 5. Model for development of human colon carcinoma through several premalignant stages. The epithelial layer of the colonic crypt is indicated diagrammatically. The stem cell is near the base of the crypt. Cells divide and differentiate as they migrate up the crypt. Mature cells are shed at the lumenal surface. The filled-in areas indicate those cells capable of cell division. In the normal colonic crypt cell, division is limited to the lower 2/3, whereas dividing cells are found all along the length of the crypt and even at the lumenal surface in patients with hereditary colon cancer

release of a protease with many properties similar to a plasminogen activator. In the colon, epithelial cells are arranged in a single layer. Premalignant cells sometimes are pseudostratified and show morphological distortion *in vivo*. However, carcinoma *in situ*--that is, without rupture of the basement membrane and invasion of the muscular layer--can appear in the colon as a multilayering of cytologically aberrant cells (Muto *et al.*, 1975; Mughal and Filipe, 1978) within a benign tumor or adenoma (Fig. 5). Possibly the TPA-induced protease degrades membrane proteins, including those in tight junctions and gap junctions, leading to morphological alterations and inhibition of cellular communication.

Loss of junctional communication may actually play a role in the transition of premalignant cells to malignancy by allowing a cell with a malignant genotype to be freed of the growth control exerted by neighboring premalignant cells to which it is coupled in a benign tumor. Neighboring cells can inhibit the tumorigenicity of malignant cells, possibly because the cells are coupled. For example, normal embryonic cells in the mouse blastocyst completely inhibit the malignancy of added tumor cells, although these tumor cells contribute information to the developing animal (Mintz and Ilmensee, 1975). Moreover,

(Fig. 5 Continued) syndromes such as familial polyposis. In adenomas the length of the crypt is greatly increased as the immature, dividing cells are not shed from the lumenal face consistently. The elongated crypts are folded upon themselves to form an adenoma, or benign tumor, which projects into the lumen of the gut. Colonic epithelial cells are columnar and single-layered in normal tissue. In the adenoma the cells are distorted in shape but remain attached to the basal lamina in a single layer. Carcinoma *in situ* is a focal multilayering of epithelial cells within the adenoma that may be caused by the action of an endogenous tumor promoter initiating release of plasminogen activator. These cells would become invasive when they penetrated the basal lamina.

much of embryonic tissue is highly coupled (Loewenstein, 1979).
TPA, which enhances tumor formation in the gastrointestinal
tract (Goerttler *et al.*, 1979) and in the skin (Van Duuren,
1969; (Boutwell, 1974; Berenblum, 1975), disrupts communication
between late-stage premalignant cells from benign tumors.
Therefore, some of the capacity of TPA to act as a tumor promoter *in vivo* may be attributed to its activity on cells at this
specific stage in tumor development.

Perhaps the adenoma-to-carcinoma transition occurs *in vivo*
by a release of a protease such as a plasminogen activator from
the premalignant late-stage epithelial cells in response to an
endogenous promoting agent. There is reason to believe that
endogenous promoting agents exist and, furthermore, that phorbol
esters are their analogs. Mouse epidermal cells, the target
organ for the classic promoter studies, have specific binding
sites for phorbol ester tumor promoters (Delclos *et al.*, 1980).
A naturally occurring tumor promoter, teleocidin B (Fujiki *et
al.*, 1979), is structurally unrelated to TPA but inhibits its
binding (Horowitz *et al.*, 1981). These data suggest that compounds may exist in the body that may have other physiological
functions but can act as tumor promoters if they bind to the
proper receptors.

There has been much speculation about the possible interaction between TPA and the hormone EGF. Both compounds stimulate the proliferation of many different cell types. Phorbol
12,13-dibutyrate, a promoting agent less lipophilic and hence
more specific in membrane binding than its analog TPA, did not
block the binding of EGF and presumably has another receptor
(Driedger and Blumberg, 1980). In the study presented here,
the premalignant epithelial cells that responded to TPA by secreting protease and clustering were predominantly (83%) restricted to the villous and villotubular classes (Table II).
These cells were not stimulated to divide by EGF (added to

growth medium) (Table I). Proliferative response to EGF under our culture conditions was limited to the early-stage premalignant (tubular-derived) cells. These data suggest that a premalignant epithelial cell loses responsiveness to EGF as it gains the ability to respond to TPA by multilayering.

The relationship between malignancy and plasminogen activator release has remained unclear. Many normal cells (Astrup, 1978) such as macrophages and trophoblasts secrete this protease. It has also been known for years that some human tumors secrete a fibrinolytic activity (Cliffton and Grossi, 1955). However, similar levels of plasminogen activator were released from primary cultures of normal and malignant human mammary cells (Yang et al., 1980). In another study (Wilson and Dowdle, 1978), no consistent relationship between plasminogen activator secretion rate and malignant status was found for many types of epithelial tissues cultured in vitro. In contrast, the plasminogen activator content was found to be two- to fourfold higher in lung tumors than in normal tissue resected with the tumor (Markus et al., 1980), although there was a wide variation between individual tumors. Similar results were found in an extensive study of colon tumors, benign colonic tumors, and normal colonic tissue (Corasanti et al., 1980). Premalignant fibroblasts, Syrian hamster embryo fibroblasts that spontaneously transformed during long-term passage in culture, acquired fibrinolytic activity before becoming capable of either growth in agar or tumor formation in vivo (Barrett and Ts'o, 1978; Barrett, 1980).

In our studies it was observed that premalignant cells secreted much more protease in response to TPA than either colonic adenocarcinomas under similar conditions of primary culture or three human colon carcinoma cell lines as exposed to TPA (Table IV). TPA induced morphological changes in malignant cells in primary culture but not in tumorigenic-established

colon carcinoma cell lines. Perhaps the capacity to undergo
cell clustering due to protease secretion is needed for, or is
concomitant with, the transition to malignancy but is not required once malignant status is reached.

REFERENCES

Armstrong, B., and Doll, R. (1975). *Int. J. Cancer 15,* 617-
    631.
Astrup, T. (1978). *In* "Progress in Chemical Fibrinolysis and
    Thrombolysis" (J. F. Davidson, R. M. Rowan, M. M. Samama,
    and P. C. Desnoyers, eds.), Vol. 3, pp. 1-57. Raven, New
    York.
Barrett, J. C. (1980). *Cancer Res. 40,* 91-94.
Barrett, J. C., and Ts'o, P. O. P. (1978). *Proc. Natl. Acad.
    Sci. USA 75,* 3761-3765.
Berenblum, I. (1975). *In* "Cancer" (F. F. Becker, ed.), Vol. 1,
    pp. 323-344. Plenum, New York.
Boutwell, R. K. (1974). *CRC Crit. Rev. Toxicol. 2,* 419-443.
Chomchai, C. C., Bhadrachari, N., and Nigro, N. D. (1974).
    Dis. Colon Rectum 17, 310-312.
Cliffton, E. E., and Grossi, C. E. (1955). *Cancer (Philadel-
    phia) 8,* 1146-1154.
Cohen, B. I., Raicht, R. F., Deschner, E. E., Takahashi, M.,
    Sarwal, A. N., and Fazzini, E. (1980). *J. Natl. Cancer
    Inst. (U.S.) 64,* 573-578.
Corasanti, J. G., Celik, C., Camiolo, S. M., Mittelman, A.,
    Evers, J. L., Barbasch, A., Hobika, G. H., and Markus, G.
    (1980). *J. Natl. Cancer Inst. (U.S.) 65,* 345-351.
Delclos, K. B., Nagle, D. S., and Blumberg, P. M. (1980).
    Cell 19, 1025-1032.
Deschner, E. E., and Raicht, R. F. (1979). *Digestion 19,*
    322-327.
Driedger, P. E., and Blumberg, P. M. (1980). *Proc. Natl. Acad.
    Sci. USA 77,* 567-571.
Dulbecco, R., Bologna, M., and Unger, M. (1979). *Proc. Natl.
    Acad. Sci. USA 76,* 1256-1260.
Elder, J. B., Williams, G., Lacey, E., and Gregory, H. (1972).
    Nature (London) 271, 466-467.
Enomoto, T., Sasaki, Y., Shiba, Y., Kanno, Y., and Yamasaki,
    H. (1981). *Proc. Natl. Acad. Sci. USA 78,* 5628-5632.
Friedman, E. A. (1981). *Cancer Res. 41,* 4588-4599.
Friedman, E. A., and Steinberg, M. L. (1982). *Cancer Res. 42,*

Friedman, E. A., Higgins, P. J., Lipkin, M., Shinya, H., and Gelb, A. M. (1981). *In Vitro 17*, 632-644.

Fujiki, H., Mori, M., Nakayasu, M., Terada, M., and Sugimura, T. (1979). *Biochem. Biophys. Res. Commun.* 90. 976-983.

Gilbertson, V. (1974). *Cancer (Philadelphia) 34*, 936-939.

Goerttler, K., Loehrke, H., Schweizer, J., and Hesse, B. (1979). *Cancer Res. 39*, 1293-1297.

Goldfarb, F. H., and Quigley, J. P. (1978). *Cancer Res. 38*, 4599-4607.

Higgins, P. J., Friedman, E., Lipkin, M., Hentz, R., Attiyeh, F., and Stonehill, E. H. (1982). *Oncology 40*, 26-30.

Horowitz, A. D., Greenebaum, E., and Weinstein, I. B. (1981). *Proc. Natl. Acad. Sci. USA 78*, 2315-2319.

Leighton, J. L., Estes, W., Mansukhani, S., and Brado, Z. (1970). *Cancer (Philadelphia) 26*, 1022-1028.

Lipkin, M., Sherlock, P., and De Cosse, J. J. (1980). *Curr. Probl. Cancer 4*, 147-272.

Loewenstein, W. R. (1979). *Biochim. Biophys. Acta 560*, 1-65.

Markus, G., Takita, H., Camiolo, S. M., Corasanti, J. G., Evers, J. L., and Hobika, G. H. (1980). *Cancer Res. 40*, 841-848.

Miettinen, T. A. (1972). *In* "The Bile Acids: Chemistry, Physiology and Metabolism" (P. P. Nair and Kirtchevsky, eds.), Vol. 2, pp. 191-247. Plenum, New York.

Mintz, B., and Illmensee, K. (1975). *Proc. Natl. Acad. Sci. USA 72*, 3585-3589.

Mughal, S., and Filipe, M. (1978). *J. Natl. Cancer Inst. (U.S.) 60*, 753-767.

Muto, T., Bussey, H. J. R., and Morson, B. C. (1975). *Cancer (Philadelphia) 36*, 2251-2270.

Narisawa, T., Magadia, N. E., Weisburger, J. H., and Wynder, E. L. (1974). *J. Natl. Cancer Inst. (U.S.) 53*, 1093-1097.

Nigro, N. D., Bhadrachari, N., and Chomchai, C. C. (1973). *Dis. Colon Rectum 16*, 438-443.

Pickett, P. B., Pitelka, D. R., Hamamoto, S. T., and Misfeldt, D. S. (1975). *J. Cell Biol. 66*, 316-332.

Quigley, J. P. (1979). *Cell 17*, 131-141.

Reddy, B. S., Narisawa, T., Vukusich, D., Weisburger, J. H., and Wynder, E. L. (1976). *Proc. Soc. Exp. Biol. Med. 151*, 232-239.

Reddy, B. S., Watanabe, K., Weisburger, J. H., and Wynder, E. L. (1977). *Cancer Res. 37*, 3238-3242.

Revel, J. P., and Karnovsky, M. J. (1967). *J. Cell Biol. 33*, 7-12.

Sun, T.-T., Shih, C., and Green, H. (1979). *Proc. Natl. Acad. Sci. USA 76*, 2813-2817.

Van Duuren, B. L. (1969). *Prog. Exp. Tumor Res. 11*, 31-68.

Weinstein, I. B., Lee, L.-S., Fisher, P. B., Mufson, A., and Yamaski, H. (1979). *J. Supramol. Struct. 12,* 195-208.

Wilson, E. L., and Dowdle, E. (1978). *Int. J. Cancer 22,* 390-399.

Yang, N.-S., Kirkland, W., Jorgensen, T., and Furmanski, P. (1980). *J. Cell Biol. 84,* 120-130.

Yotti, L. P., Chang, C. C., and Trosko, J. E. (1979). *Science (Washington, D.C.) 206,* 1089-1091.

Zimmerman, M., Quigley, J. P., Ashe, B., Dorn, C., Goldfarb, R., and Troll, W. (1978). *Proc. Natl. Acad. Sci. USA 75,* 750-753.

IV. Cellular Lesions Caused by Chemical Carcinogens

15

MECHANISMS OF NEOPLASTIC TRANSFORMATION OF HUMAN CELLS

*Takeo Kakunaga, Janet D. Crow,
Hiroshi Hamada, and Tadashi Hirakawa*

Cell Genetics Section
Laboratory of Molecular Carcinogenesis
National Cancer Institute
Bethesda, Maryland

John Leavitt

Linus Pauling Institute of Sciences and Medicine
Palo Alto, California

I. CHARACTERISTICS OF HUMAN CELL TRANSFORMATION

A. Advantages of the Use of Human Cells

There are many advantages in using human cells for studying neoplastic transformation as compared to using the cells of
other species. It eliminates the species barrier, which is a
serious obstacle in extrapolating the results obtained with the
nonhuman system to human carcinogenesis. In addition, human
cells show one of the most stable karyotypes in culture and undergo a relatively low frequency of nonspecific changes in biological and biochemical properties during cultivation. This
feature is very helpful in identifying the molecular changes
specific to transformed cells. It is well known that rodent
cells such as mouse and hamster cells, especially after being
transformed, produce progeny cells with diverse properties including tumorigenicity at high frequencies in culture. In contrast, human cells are relatively stable in culture even after
being transformed (J. Fogh *et al.,* personal communication; see
also our data in this chapter).

Functional chromosomal mapping is well established with
human chromosomes compared to other mammalian chromosomes.
Another important feature in the use of human cells is the
availability of cells derived from cancer-prone genetic disease
patients. These cells obtained from a patient serve as the mutant cells, which provide precious materials for studying the
genetic factors and molecular process involved in the induction
of cell transformation. The use of human cells also enables us
to investigate the environmental and genetic factors *in vitro*
in conjunction with epidemiological studies. Because of these
advantages, the development of a transformation system using
human cells will facilitate our understanding of the mechanisms
of cell transformation as well as establishing the optimum method to assess human risk against environmental carcinogens.

TABLE I. Classification and Characteristics of the Transformation Systems Using Human and Rodent Cells

Transformation system	Species	Assay indicators[a]	Quanti- tation	Assay period
I. Full transformation				
Diploid cell to tumorigenic cell	Hamster	Tumorigenicity (focus and AI)	–	2–5 months
	Human	Tumorigenicity (focus and AI)	–	3–12 months
II. Partial transformation				
1. Diploid cell to partially transformed cell	Hamster	Clonal morpholo- gy	+	7–10 days
	Human	AI	+	2–6 weeks
2. Partially transformed cell (nonpermanent line) to tumorigenic cell	Hamster	Tumorigenicity and AI	+	1–6 months
	Human	Not yet developed		
3. Partially transformed cell (permanent line) to tumorigenic cell	Mouse	Focus formation	+	3–6 weeks
	Hamster	AI	+	3–5 weeks
	Human	Tumorigenicity	–	1–3 months

[a]AI, *Anchorage independence.*

B.   Classification of Transformation Systems

The multistep nature of neoplastic transformation of mammalian cells has been documented by several lines of evidence (Rous and Beard, 1935; Foulds, 1954, 1969, 1975; Vogt and Dulbecco, 1963; Kakunaga and Kamahora, 1968, 1969; Enders, 1969; Barrett and Ts'o, 1978). The cells morphologically transformed by virus or chemicals undergo qualitatively different changes in one or more of their characteristics to become tumorigenic. Depending on which stages in this multistep development are chosen as assay end points, the systems for neoplastic transformation of mammalian cells are divided into three classes (Kanunaga, 1979). As summarized in Table I, this classification is also applicable to the transformation systems using human cells that have been reported by many laboratories (Igel *et al.*, 1975; Benedict *et al.*, 1975; Rhim *et al.*, 1975; Freedman and Shin, 1975; Shimada *et al.*, 1976; Kakunaga, 1977, 1978; DeMar and Jackson, 1977; Freeman *et al.*, 1977; Milo and DiPaolo, 1978; Namba *et al.*, 1978; Borek, 1979; Sutherland *et al.*, 1980; Silinskas *et al.*, 1981; Zimmerman and Little, 1981; Parsa *et al.*, 1981).

In the first class, full transformation, which covers the entire process of the neoplastic conversion from normal diploid cells to neoplastic cells, has been demonstrated by several groups using the fibroblasts from an adult skin or foreskin and the pancreatic epithelial cells. As far as the fully transformed phenotype (i.e., tumorigenicity upon transplantation into immunoincompetent animals) is used as the end point of the assay, no quantitative system has been developed, as will be discussed later.

Another class is based on partial transformation, which covers a part of the neoplastic transformation process. The systems of partial transformation are divided further into two classes, depending on the types of cells used as the target cells. One system is the conversion of normal diploid cells into partially transformed cells. The partially transformed cells usually show anchorage-independent growth or morphological alteration but not tumorigenicity. This is analogous to the morphological transformation of hamster embryonic cells by a carcinogen, and the quantitation of phenotypic change is possible. The other system is the conversion of partially transformed cells into tumorigenic cells. In this case, the partially transformed cells have already acquired immortality and aneuploidy, but they are morphologically normal and their growth is anchorage dependent. This system is similar to the transformation system using 10T1/2 or BALB/3T3 cell lines.

With the hamster and mouse cells, there is plenty of evidence indicating that neoplastic transformation of diploid cells by chemical carcinogens is a multistep process. The diploid rodent cells treated with chemical carcinogens acquire distinguishable transformed phenotypes one by one. For example, they usually show morphological alteration first, then aneuploidy, anchorage-independent cell growth, escape from senescence, tumorigenicity, and finally metastatic potentials. Because of the multistep nature of neoplastic transformation, the frequency of transformation is extremely low and the time required is very long before the full transformation is observed. Thus, it is feasible that every quantitative assay system for transformation using rodent cells adopts one step in conversion as an assay end point. For example, alteration of growth pattern due to loss of contact inhibition of cell growth and movement is used as an end point of the quantitative assay of the transformation of the primary culture of hamster embryonic cells or 10T1/2 and BALB/3T3 cell lines. Transformation of human cells seems to be a multistep process similar to that of the rodent cells.

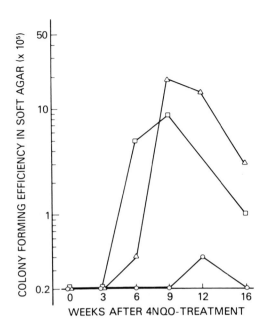

Fig. 1. Anchorage-independent cell growth of human skin fibroblasts treated with 4-nitroquinoline 1-oxide (4NQO). The KD cells were treated with 0 (O), 0.1 (□), and 0.3 μg/ml (△) 4NQO and then subcultured. At weekly intervals, the cells were tested for the ability to form colonies in soft agar. (From Kakunaga *et al.*, 1979.)

C. Differential Multistep Progress of the Transformation between Human and Rodent Cells

When an early passage of human diploid fibroblasts, KD cells, were treated with 4-nitroquinoline 1-oxide (4NQO) and then continuously subcultivated for 2 to 3 weeks, they showed a slight but significant increase in the anchorage-independent cell growth (Fig. 1). It is possible to estimate the induced frequency of anchorage-independent conversion on the basis of the number of cells that survived or were treated. During further subcultivation, however, the 4NQO-treated KD cells lost their increased ability to grow in soft agar. The

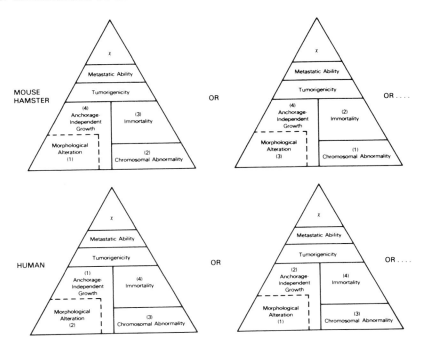

Fig. 2. Pyramid model for the multistep progress of neoplastic transformation of cultured mouse, hamster, and human
cells. Vertical height of pyramid represents the degree of
malignancy of cells. Bottom line of the pyramid corresponds
to the state of normal diploid cells. The cells increase
their malignancy by acquiring each phenotype one by one. Acquisition of phenotypes of the lower level is prerequisite to
acquisition of the phenotypes at upper level. Numbers in parentheses indicate the sequential order of the acquisition.
The sequential order within the species may vary, but two each
of examples shown are representatives that fit most cases.

anchorage-independent cells (i.e., the cells recovered from the
colonies in soft agar) showed senescence and failed to produce
nonregressive tumors upon injection into *nude* mice. Thus,
these anchorage-independent cells (partially transformed cells)
seem to need one or more of the other phenotypic conversions to
become fully tumorigenic (fully transformed) cells.

   Early induction of anchorage-independent cell growth of
human diploid cells after chemical treatment also has been

reported by several other groups (Freedman and Shin, 1975; DeMar and Jackson, 1977; Freeman *et al.*, 1977; Milo and DiPaolo, 1978; Sutherland *et al.*, 1980; Silinskas *et al.*, 1981; Zimmerman and Little, 1981). This phenomenon is in contrast with the observations made on the transformation of rodent cells (Kakunaga and Kamahora, 1968, 1969; Barrett and Ts'o, 1978). One of the most striking differences in transformation between human cells and rodent cells is the sequential order of the acquisition of different phenotypes as summarized in Fig. 2. Hamster fibroblasts show morphological alteration in a short time after the carcinogen treatment, and later they acquire both anchorage-independent cell growth and tumorigenicity almost simultaneously. Thus, the anchorage-independent cell growth of hamster fibroblasts has been closely correlated with their tumorigenicity (Kakunaga and Kamahora, 1968).

In contrast, human cells appear to acquire anchorage-independent cell growth relatively quickly, but they acquire all of the other phenotypic changes later. Another peculiar feature of the human cell transformation is the extremely low frequency of the acquisition of immortality compared to the rodent cells. All the tumorigenic rodent cells have become immortal cell lines. From human tumors, the successful rate of establishing immortal cell lines has been gradually increasing, being currently 20-50%, whereas no cell line has been established from non-neoplastic human tissues. It is expected that the technical improvement of culturing human tumor cells will elevate further the success rate of obtaining immortal cell lines from human tumor tissues. As far as we know, all the culturable human cells capable of forming progressively growing tumors upon injection into *nude* mice have shown immortality. These observations strongly suggest that the acquisition of unlimited cell proliferation is a prerequisite for full

transformation of human cells. Thus, the immortalization process is likely to be the rate-limiting step in the transformation of human diploid cells (Kakunaga, 1979).

II.   MACROMOLECULAR CHANGES IN THE CHEMICALLY TRANSFORMED
      HUMAN CELL LINE

A.   Comparison of Proteins Synthesized between Normal and
     Transformed Human Cells

The cellular mechanisms as described in the preceding section are still speculative in some aspects and would require
further study to prove them. However, such a multistep model
for the transformation process should reflect on the study of
the molecular mechanisms of transformation. It will be more
practical to explore the molecular changes underlying each step
of the conversion rather than to explore the almighty molecule
that causes all phenotypic changes associated with neoplastic
transformation. Among the various advantages of using human
cells for studying transformation, the relatively low frequency
of spontaneous changes in properties during cultivation and the
availability of mutant cells from cancer-prone genetic disease
patients are of extreme importance for studying the molecular
mechanisms of transformation.

Maher et al. (1982) reported that skin fibroblasts from
xeroderma pigmentosum patients showed a much higher sensitivity to the induction of anchorage independency by some carcinogens as compared to the normal skin fibroblasts, in a manner similar to the induction of HGPRT⁻ mutation. This result
suggests that the induction of anchorage-independent growth
of human cells by carcinogens is a mutational process.
There are many other pieces of indirect evidence suggesting
the involvement of the mutational process in the carcinogen-

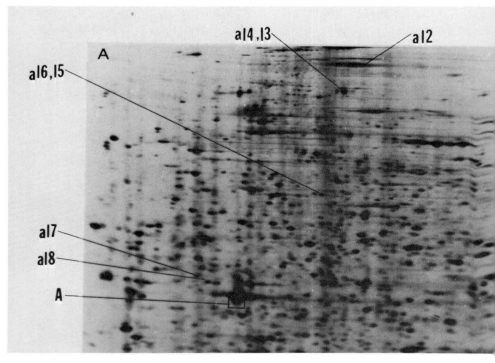

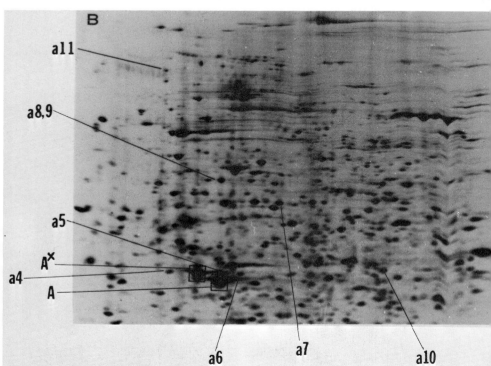

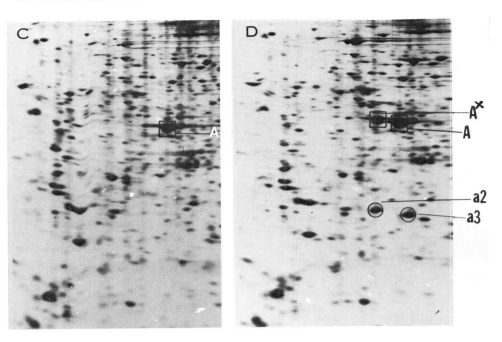

Fig. 3. Autoradiographs of two-dimensional gels containing [^{35}S]methionine-labeled, Triton-soluble polypeptides. Cells were incubated with the isotope for 4 h. The first dimension was isoelectric focusing between pH range from 4 (right) to 7 (left). (A) and (C) Polypeptides of KD cells; (B) and (D) polypeptides of HuT-14 cells. (A) and (B) 9% Acrylamide gels; (C) and (D) 12.5% acrylamide gels. A, β- and γ-actin; A^x and a2 through a78, polypeptides present in only one of the two cell types. (From Leavitt and Kakunaga, 1980.)

induced cell transformation. However, this indirect evidence, usually an observation of the parallelism between mutational events and neoplastic transformation, does not provide precise information on the type of mutation, much less on what kinds and portions of genes were mutated and how the mutation led the cells to express the transformed state.

In order to obtain molecular evidence for the mechanisms of neoplastic transformation, we have compared the proteins synthesized in normal and transformed human cells. This study

is based on the widely accepted conception that the changes in
the proteins synthesized in the transformed cells reflect the
alteration of gene structure or expression, mutational or regulatory, that is associated with neoplastic transformation.
Clonal transformed human fibroblast lines were obtained by a
single treatment of human diploid fibroblasts with 4NQO
(Kakunaga, 1978). They exhibited stable neoplastic properties
and provided us with a pair of normal and transformed cells of
which biochemical alteration may be closely related to the expression of transformed phenotypes. [^{35}S]Methionine-labeled
proteins were extracted with Triton-X buffer from the human fibroblasts transformed by 4NQO and compared with those from parental normal counterparts using two-dimensional gel electrophoresis developed by O'Farrell (1975) and Garrels (1979).
About 2% of the proteins of nearly 1000 polypeptide electrophoretic species were lost or newly gained in the transformed
cells (Fig. 3).

One new polypeptide designated A^x in Fig. 3 (pI 5.2, molecular weight 42,000), migrating very close to β- and γ-actin,
was found in one of the transformed cell lines (HuT-14). This
new polypeptide was also found in the Triton-insoluble fraction
and identified as a variant form of actin by immunoprecipitation with anti-actin antibody and its tryptic peptide finger-
print pattern (Leavitt and Kakunaga, 1980).

B. A Point Mutation Responsible for a Protein Change

The significant phenotypic characteristics of transformed
malignant cells are alterations of cell shape, motility, movement, mobility of cell surface component including receptors,
phagocytosis, or endocytosis, and responses of these functions
to contact inhibition. Actin is a major component of the cytoskeleton that is responsible for these cellular functions.

Thus, it is a feasible hypothesis that the alteration of the actin molecule induced by carcinogens results in the changes of these cellular functions--that is, the expression of trans- formation. Disorganization of the actin cable network in asso- ciation with the expression of transformed state has been re- ported with many transformed cells (Pollack et $al.$, 1975; Pollack, 1980). Thus, we have investigated the molecular mechanisms of the alteration of the actin form (designated A^x-actin) and its role in the expression of transformed pheno- types. Several possibilities could explain why A^x-actin is expressed in HuT-14 cells and not in other human cells: (1) al- tered posttranslational processing or modification, (2) altered processing of actin mRNA, (3) derepression of a silent actin gene, and (4) mutation in actin genes.

The first possibility, alteration of posttranslational processing or modification, was examined by analyzing in $vitro$ translation products in the presence of poly(A)$^+$RNA extracted from HuT-14 cells (Hamada et $al.$, 1981). Two-dimensional gel electrophoresis analysis showed that A^x-actin and its precursor unacetylated form as well as β- and γ-actin and their precursors were abundant in $vitro$ translation products. A^x-Actin was not found among the translation products in the presence of poly(A)- $^+$RNA from any other human cells. These results indicated that A^x-actin is encoded from the altered mRNA species in HuT-14 cells and excluded the possibility that A^x-actin is derived from the alteration of posttranslational processing or modifi- cation.

In order to assess the complementarity of the human actin genes expressed in HuT-14 cells to pcDd actin, which was used as a specific probe for actin mRNA or genes, poly(A)$^+$RNA was isolated from HuT-14 cells and hybridized to pcDd insert DNA. The RNA that hybridized was isolated and then assayed for its ability to direct the synthesis of actin in the reticulocyte lysate translation system. Two-dimensional gel electrophoresis of the translation products showed that HuT-14 mRNA that hybridized to pcDd was capable of directing synthesis of A^x- and β-actin but not γ-actin (Hamada *et al.*, 1981). Thus, pcDd actin sequence is similar to the human β-actin gene sequence in that it hybridizes to β-actin mRNA, and dissimilar to the human γ-actin sequence to the degree that it fails to hybridize to γ-actin mRNA. These results indicate that A^x-actin gene is similar to β-actin gene.

The sizes of A^x- and β-actin mRNA were compared by two different methods. First, HuT-14 poly(A)$^+$RNA was fractionated on a sucrose gradient under undenaturing conditions, and then each fraction was tested for its ability to direct the synthesis of actin polypeptides in the reticulocyte lysate translation system. Two-dimensional gel electrophoresis of *in vitro* translates showed that A^x-actin as well as β- and γ-actin mRNAs are slightly larger than 18S ribosomal RNA (Hamada *et al.*, 1981). Second, total RNAs from HuT-14 cells that synthesize A^x-actin or from HuT-11 cells that do not synthesize A^x-actin were fractionated on an agarose gel, transferred to diazobenzyl-oxymethyl paper, and hybridized to nick-translated pcDd insert DNA, which hybridizes with A^x- and β-actin mRNA. Only one band was observed in gels containing either HuT-14 or HuT-11 RNA. Thus, the sizes of A^x- and β-actin mRNA seem to be similar. The complete amino acid sequences of A^x- and β-actin that were isolated from HuT-14 cells were determined in collaboration with Drs. Vandekerckhove and Weber (Fig. 4). A^x-Actin differed from β-actin by only a single amino acid substitution; that is, glycine at the 244 position in β-actin was replaced by aspartic acid in A^x-actin (Vandekerckhove *et al.*, 1980). This substitution corresponds to a GC → AT transition point mutation in the coding sequence of β-actin gene. It is an interesting observation that such a single amino acid substitution contributes to

Fig. 4. Amino acid sequence of human cytoplasmic β- and A^X-actin isolated from HuT-14 cells determined by Vandekerckhove et al. (1980). The only amino acid difference between β-actin (glycine) and A^X-actin (aspartic acid) at position 244 is enclosed in the box.

2   10   20   30
Bl-Asp-Asp-Asp-Ile-Ala-Ala-Leu-Val-Val-Asp-Asn-Gly-Ser-Gly-Met-Cys-Lys-Ala-Gly-Phe-Ala-Gly-Asp-Asp-Ala-Pro-Arg-Ala-Val-

                                        40   50   60
Phe-Pro-Ser-Ile-Val-Gly-Arg-Pro-Arg-His-Gln-Gly-Val-Met-Val-Gly-Met-Gly-Gln-Lys-Asp-Ser-Tyr-Val-Gly-Asp-Glu-Ala-Gln-Ser-

            70 3Me   80   90
Lys-Arg-Gly-Ile-Leu-Thr-Leu-Lys-Tyr-Pro-Ile-Glu-His-Gly-Ile-Val-Thr-Asn-Trp-Asp-Asp-Met-Glu-Lys-Ile-Trp-His-His-Thr-Phe-

            100   110   120
Tyr-Asn-Glu-Leu-Arg-Val-Ala-Pro-Glu-Glu-His-Pro-Val-Leu-Leu-Thr-Glu-Ala-Pro-Leu-Asn-Pro-Lys-Ala-Asn-Arg-Glu-Lys-Met-Thr-

            130   140   150
Gln-Ile-Met-Phe-Glu-Thr-Phe-Asn-Thr-Pro-Ala-Met-Tyr-Val-Ala-Ile-Gln-Ala-Val-Leu-Ser-Leu-Tyr-Ala-Ser-Gly-Arg-Thr-Thr-Gly-

            160   170   180
Ile- Val-Met-Asp-Ser-Gly-Asp-Gly-Val-Thr-His-Thr-Val-Pro-Ile-Tyr-Glu-Gly-Tyr-Ala-Leu-Pro-His-Ala-Ile-Leu-Arg-Leu-Asp-Leu-

            190   200   210
Ala-Gly-Arg-Asp-Leu-Thr-Asp-Tyr-Leu-Met-Lys-Ile-Leu-Thr-Glu-Arg-Gly-Tyr-Ser-Phe-Thr-Thr-Thr-Ala-Glu-Arg-Glu-Ile-Val-Arg-

            220   230   234a
Asp-Ile-Lys-Glu-Lys-Leu-Cys-Tyr-Val-Ala-Leu-Asp-Phe-Glu-Gln-Glu-Met-Ala-Thr-Ala-Ala-Ser-Ser-Ser-Leu-Glu-Lys-Ser-Tyr-

240   250 [Gly]   260
Glu-Leu-Pro-Asp-Gln-Val-Ile-Thr-Ile-Gly-Asn-Glu-Arg-Phe-Arg-Cys-Pro-Glu-Ala-Leu-Phe-Gln-Pro-Ser-Phe-Leu-Gly-Met-Glu-

            270   280   290
Ser-Cys-Gly-Ile-His-Glu-Thr-Thr-Phe-Asn-Ser-Ile-Met-Lys-Cys-Asp-Val-Asp-Ile-Arg-Lys-Asp-Leu-Tyr-Ala-Asn-Thr-Val-Leu-Ser-

            300   310   320
Gly-Gly-Thr-Thr-Met-Tyr-Pro-Gly-Ile-Ala-Asp-Arg-Met-Gln-Lys-Glu-Ile-Thr-Ala-Leu-Ala-Pro-Ser-Thr-Met-Lys-Ile-Lys-Ile-Ile --

            330   340   350
Ala-Pro-Pro-Glu-Arg-Lys-Tyr-Ser-Val-Trp-Ile-Gly-Gly-Ser-Ile-Leu-Ala-Ser-Leu-Ser-Thr-Phe-Gln-Met-Trp-Ile-Ser-Lys-Gln-

            360   370   374
Glu-Tyr-Asp-Glu-Ser-Gly-Pro-Ser-Ile-Val-His-Arg-Lys-Cys-Phe

the significantly lower electrophoretic rate of actin molecules in the SDS dimension of the two-dimensional gel.

All the results described here indicate that A^x-actin is a product of a β-actin gene with a point mutation in HuT-14 cells. Hereinafter, A^x-actin is designated mutated β-actin or $β^x$-actin.

III.   ROLE OF THE MUTATION IN β-ACTIN GENE IN THE NEOPLASTIC TRANSFORMATION

A.   Correlation of the Alteration of β-Actin with the Increase in Cell Malignancy

One of the approaches we have taken to study the relationship between a point mutation and the expression of transformed phenotypes in HuT-14 cells is the isolation of cell variants of HuT-14 cells with increased malignancy and the characterization of the expression of β-actin in these variant cells.   First, we attempted to obtain the cell variants without treatment with mutagens and carcinogens.   However, we found that HuT-14 cells are very stable in their tumorigenic potentials and did not spontaneously produce progeny with increased malignancy at a frequency higher than 10^{-8} during cell generation.   Even the cells (HuT-14-T) recovered from tumors that were produced in *nude* mice by subcutaneous injection of 2×10^6 HuT-14 cells showed change in neither their tumorigenicity nor anchorage-independent cell growth (Table II).

So, HuT-14 cells were exposed to UV light, and many subclones were isolated.   Actually, the isolation of variant cells had two aims: (1) to obtain cells with different malignancies and (2) to isolate cells with no hypoxanthine-guanine phosphoribosyl transferase (HGPRT) activity and ouabain resistance (Oua^r). Thus, the first series of subclones was obtained in the presence of 6-thioguanine (6TG).   Many 6TG-resistant ($6TG^r$) subclones

TABLE II. Transformed Phenotypes of HuT-14 Subclones

Cells	Cloning efficiency in soft agar (%)	Tumorigenicity[a] (TD_{50})
Normal diploid fibroblasts (KD)	<0.0001	>1×10^7
HuT-14	1.1	3×10^5
HuT-14-11[b]	0.9	3×10^5
HuT-14-12[b]	0.9	NT[c]
HuT-14-13[b]	1.0	NT
HuT-14-T[d]	0.8	3×10^5
HuT-14-3[e]	3.5	8×10^5
HuT-14-3-1[e]	3.8	3×10^4
HuT-14-3-1 T[f]	8.5	<1×10^4

[a]Cell doses required for formation of tumors in 50% of nude mice injected subcutaneously.
[b]Subclones isolated from HuT-14 cell populations.
[c]NT, Not tested.
[d]Cells derived from the tumor that was produced by the subcutaneous injection of 2×10^6 HuT-14 cells in nude mice.
[e]Subclones isolated from UV-irradiated HuT-14 cell populations.
[f]Cells derived from the tumor that was produced by the subcutaneous injection of 2×10^6 HuT-14-3-1 cells in nude mice.

were selected and tested for their ability to grow in soft agar. One $6TG^r$ subclone, HuT-14-3, showed a significantly increased anchorage-independent cell growth compared to HuT-14 cells. Then HuT-14-3 cells were exposed again to UV irradiation, and Oua^r subclones were selected in the presence of ouabain in the culture medium. The $6TG^r$-Oua^r subclone, HuT-14-3-1, maintained a significantly increased anchorage-independent cell growth and showed a slightly increased tumorigenicity in nude mice compared to HuT-14-3 cells (Table II). The cells were recovered from the tumor produced by inoculating 2×10^6 HuT-14-3-1 cells, and designated HuT-14-3-1 T cells,

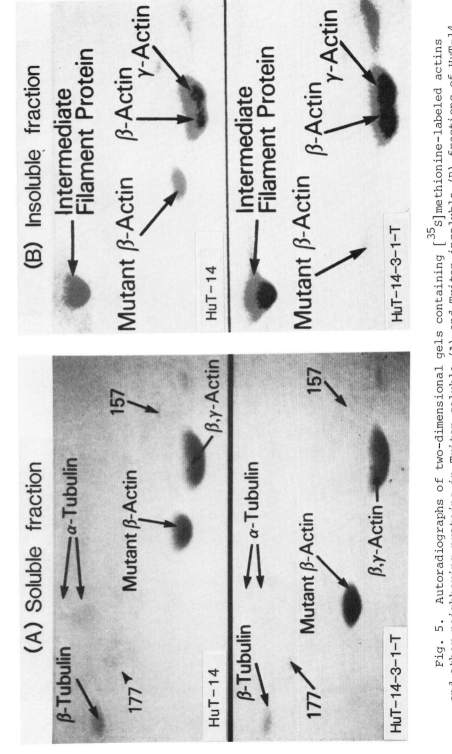

Fig. 5. Autoradiographs of two-dimensional gels containing [^{35}S]methionine-labeled actins and other neighboring proteins in Triton-soluble (A) and Triton-insoluble (B) fractions of HuT-14 and HuT-14-3-1 T cells. (From Leavitt et al., 1982a.)

after determining that their karyotypic patterns were similar
to HuT-14-3-1 cells. The HuT-14-3-1 T cells showed a further
increase in both tumorigenicity and anchorage-independent cell
growth (Table II). Because other 6TG^r subclones obtained from
HuT-14 cells did not show any change in their transformed phenotypes, it is likely that the acquisition of 6TG^r (or loss of
HGPRT) had no relationship with the increased malignancy of
HuT-14-3, HuT-14-3-1, and HuT-14-3-1 T cells.

Examination of [^{35}S]methionine-labeled polypeptides in
the variant cells using two-dimensional gel electrophoresis
showed that the mutant β-actin in HuT-14-3-1 T cells was
slightly more acidic than that of β-tubulin subunit (Fig. 5).
The mutant β-actin in HuT-14-3-1 T cells was shifted one additional unit negative charge compared to the mutant β-actin in
HuT-14 cells. The electrophoretic mobility of the new mutant
β-actin in the SDS dimension was reduced like the original mutant β-actin of HuT-14 cells. This new species protein was
identified as a variant form of actin by tryptic peptide finger-
print pattern and tentatively designated new mutant β-actin or
β^{xx}-actin. Two-dimensional gel electrophoresis of actin polypeptides of other subclones such as HuT-14-3, HuT-14-3-2, and
HuT-14-3-3 revealed that the additional change in isoelectric
point for the mutant β-actin occurred during the first step of
isolation of HuT-14-3 line from HuT-14 cells with UV irradiation. The new mutant β-actin was produced by *in vitro* translation of poly(A)$^+$RNA extracted from either HuT-14-3-1 or
HuT-14-3-1 T cells, indicating that the new change in mutant
β-actin is ascribed to the alteration at the level of mRNA
and/or DNA.

The amounts of newly synthesized mutant β-actins (β^x and
β^{xx}) and normal β- and γ-actins were compared with KD, HuT-14,
HuT-14-3-1, and HuT-14-3-1 T cells with each fraction (i.e.,
Triton-soluble fraction, Triton-insoluble fraction, and *in vitro*

TABLE III.   The Stepwise Changes in the Cytoplasmic Actins and
             Transformed Phenotypes in the Variants of HuT-14
             Cells

Changes	KD	HuT-14	HuT-14-3-1	HuT-14-3-1 T
			Cells	
Plating efficiency in soft agar (%)	<0.0001	1.1	3.8	8.5
Tumorigenicity[a] (TD_{50} in *nude* mice)	$>10^7$	3×10^5	3×10^4	$<10^4$
Relative ratio of actin[b] in cellular soluble fraction				
β^x or β^{xx}	0	1.2	NT[c]	1.7
β	1.0	1.0	NT	1.0
γ	1.2	1.2	NT	1.2
$\beta^x + \beta^{xx}/\beta + \gamma$	0	0.53	--	0.7
In insoluble fraction cytoskeleton)				
β^x or β^{xx}	0	0.6	NT	0.04
β	1.0	1.0	NT	1.0
γ	1.2	1.2	NT	1.2
$\beta^x + \beta^{xx}/\beta + \gamma$	0	0.27	--	0.02
In *in vitro* translation				
β^x or β^{xx}	0	0.8	0.7	1.7
β	1.0	1.0	1.0	1.0
γ	1.0	2.0	1.1	2.0
$\beta^x + \beta^{xx}/\beta + \gamma$	0	0.26	0.36	0.57

[a]*See footnotes to Table II.*
[b]*Relative density ratio of the actin species to the β-actin (1.0) on the autoradiograph of two-dimensional gels containing [^{35}S]methionine-labeled proteins. β^x, Mutant β-actin; β^{xx}, new mutant β-actin.*
[c]*NT, Not tested.*

translation products), respectively.   They were measured by
quantitating the density of each actin species on the autoradiographs of two-dimensional gels containing [^{35}S]methionine-

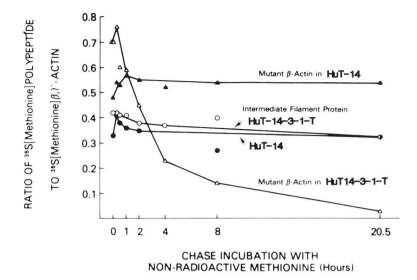

Fig. 6. Ratio of [^{35}S]methionine labeling of mutant β-actins to [^{35}S]methionine labeling of normal β- plus γ-actin in HuT-14 (▲) and HuT-14-3-1 T (△) cells after a 15-min pulse-labeling incubation. The ratio was determined by micro-densitometry scanning of autoradiographs of two-dimensional gels containing total cellular proteins isolated from each cell line for each time. Intermediate filament protein in HuT-14 (●) and Hut-14-3-1 T cells (○).

labeled (4 h) polypeptides. Values were corrected to relative ratio to the density of normal β-actin (1.0). As summarized in Table III, the ratio of mutant β-actin to normal β- plus γ-actin was increased in soluble fraction of HuT-14-3-1 T, and in the *in vitro* translation products synthesized in the presence of poly(A)$^{+}$RNA of HuT-14-3-1 and HuT-14-3-1 T com-pared to those in HuT-14 cells. In contrast, the ratio of mutant β-actin to normal β- plus γ-actin of the cytoskeletal fraction was lower than that of soluble fraction and of *in vitro* translation products, and was markedly reduced in HuT-14-3-1 T cells. There was no change in the ratio of nor-mal β-actin to γ-actin between soluble and cytoskeletal frac-tions in normal and variant cells.

When the cells were labeled with $[^{35}S]$methionine for a short time, either 8 or 15 min, the density of the new mutant β-actin in HuT-14-3-1 T cells was greatly enhanced, indicating both the increased rate of synthesis and the short life of the new mutant β-actin. The amounts of the two mutant β-actins measured by densitometry performed on Coomassie Blue-stained two-dimensional gels showed that the quantity of mutant β-actin relative to normal β- and γ-actin was reduced by 95% in HuT-14-3-1 T cells compared to that in HuT-14 cells (Leavitt *et al.*, 1982a). To know the half-life of actin polypeptides, the cells pulse-labeled with $[^{35}S]$methionine for 8 min were incubated in the absence of label but in the presence of excess nonradioactive methionine. The density of label in the new β-actin in HuT-14-3-1 T cells decreased rapidly, with a half-life of approximately 2 h, whereas the mutant β-actin of HuT-14 cells was almost as stable as the normal β-actin and γ-actin (Fig. 6).

These results indicate that mutant β-actin is defective in incorporation into cytoskeleton, and that the stepwise increase in malignancy of HuT-14 variant cells was associated with the increased synthesis and incremental deficiency of mutant β-actin.

B. Defects of β-Actin and Expression of the Transformed Phenotypes

The mutant β-actin was detected only in the HuT-14 and its subclones, and was found in neither other transformed human cell lines nor the cells freshly cultured from human embryo or various adult tissues. The uniqueness of the mutant β-actin among the transformed cells may arouse the hasty argument that the mutation in β-actin found in HuT-14 cells has nothing to do with expression of the transformed phenotypes. However, the cytoskeletal dysfunction similar to that caused by a point mutation in β-actin gene may also be induced by mutations in one of the actin-associated proteins or other unknown proteins controlling cytoskeletal structures and functions (Fig. 8). Alteration of modification, such as phosphorylation, of the regulatory proteins may result in similar phenotypic changes.

In general, similar phenotypic changes can be derived from the different alteration of genes or gene products. For example, the synthesis of one cellular component is affected by the mutation in any one of the genes coding for enzymes participating in its synthesis. Alteration of enzymatic activity of each enzyme can result from the mutation of the different mutable sites in one gene. Furthermore, alteration of enzyme molecules can result from different mutations of the same mutable site. In addition, the neoplastic cell transformation consists of multistep and complex processes as described. Transformed phenotypes are qualitatively and quantitatively diverse depending on the types of cells and tissues, stage of progression, and even the individual transformed cell. Thus, it is rather unwise to focus only on the identification of changes that are common and specific to all the transformed or tumor cells until we have more information on the molecules responsible for the expression of each transformed phenotype. Our approach is to investigate thoroughly the nature of the molecular changes associated with neoplastic transformation of human fibroblasts, regardless of whether the changes are common to many transformed cells. A universal picture of the mechanisms of neoplastic transformation will be evolved from particulars.

Alterations in cellular morphology, motility, and membrane fluidity are the most universal and remarkable characteristics of the neoplastic cells *in vitro* as well as *in vivo*. Cytoplasmic β- and γ-actins are the major components of the cytoskeleton, which has key roles in maintaining and controlling

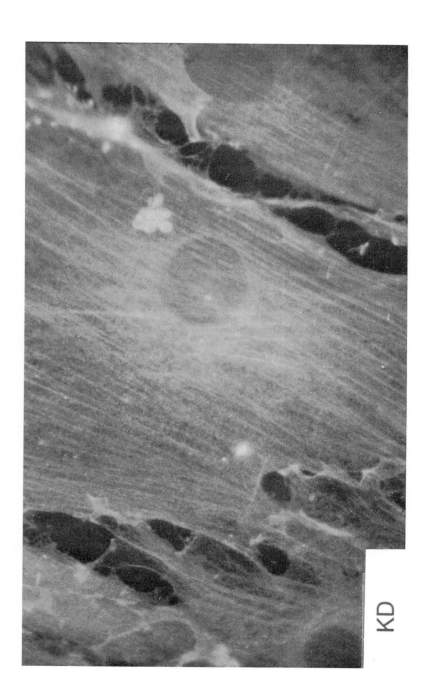

KD

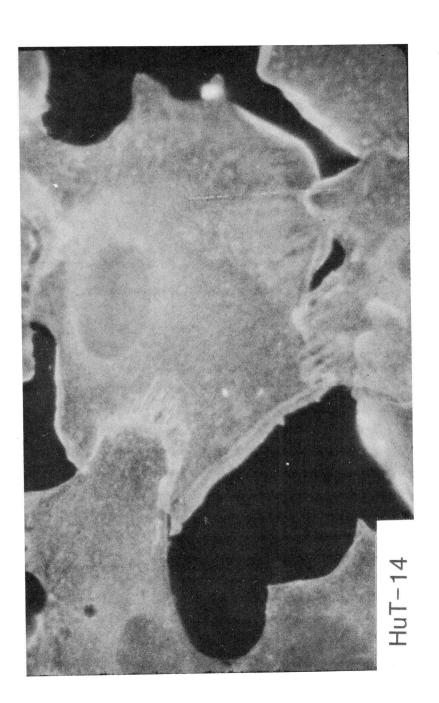

HuT−14

Fig. 7. Indirect immunofluorescence microscopy of KD (A) and HuT-14 (B) cells reacted with monoclonal anti-actin IgM provided by Lin.

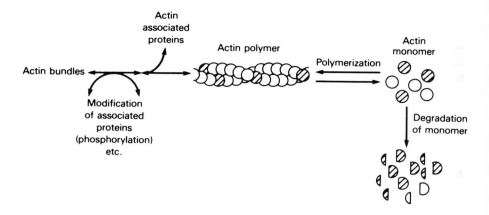

Fig. 8.   Schematic representation of the actin microfilament dysfunction caused by mutations in β-actin (O). Mutant
actins (◍) are deficient in polymerization and/or unstable.
The actin polymer containing mutant actins may also be abnormal
in stability, binding with actin-associated proteins, and sensitivity to the modification that regulates cytoskeletal functions.

the cell shape, motility, contractility, and membrane fluidity.
The results described previously indicate that a mutation in
β-actin may be responsible for the expression of the transformed phenotypes of HuT-14 and its subclones. Indirect immunofluorescence staining with monoclonal anti-actin antibody
showed the disorganization and disappearance in HuT-14 cells
of actin stress fibers, which are distinctly visible in untransformed KD cells (Fig. 7). This disorganization of actin
stress fibers was more marked in HuT-14-3-1 and HuT-14-3-1 T
cells than in HuT-14 cells.

       The changes in the distribution and organization of actin
microfilament proteins have been reported with many transformed
cells (Pollack *et al.*, 1975; Edelman and Yahara, 1976; Wang
and Goldberg, 1976; Boschek *et al.*, 1981). The results shown
in Table II indicate the deficiency of the mutant β-actins in
the ability to be incorporated into cytoskeletal structures as

well as in stability. Furthermore, the mutant β-actin has shown deficiency in the polymerization *in vitro* from G form (G-actin) to F form (F-actin) (S. Taniguchi and T. Takunaga, unpublished).

Figure 8 shows a hypothetical scheme of the pathways by which the mutant β-actins cause disruption of microfilament functions. Mutant β-actins are unstable and/or deficient in polymerization, resulting in less incorporation into actin polymer. The presence of mutated β-actin molecules in actin polymer, even though a minor component, compared to normal actin molecules, may make the polymer unstable or modulate the interaction of polymer with actin-associated proteins such as tropomyosin, vinculin, and α-actinin. Incorporated mutant actin may disturb the mechanisms that regulate the cytoskeletal functions through phosphorylation or other types of modification of regulatory cytoskeletal proteins. The resulting dysfunction of cytoskeleton may lead the cells to express the transformed phenotypes. Similar phenotypic changes may also be induced by mutations or alteration of modification, such as phosphorylation of actin-associated proteins or other molecules regulating cytoskeletal functions. Alteration of tropomyosin has been observed in various transformed cells (F. Matsumura, personal communication). Elevation of tyrosinephosphorylation of vinculin has been reported in the Rous sarcoma virus-transformed cells (Sefton *et al.*, 1981). Mimicry of morphological transformation by tumor-promoting agents is preceded by changes in the distribution and organization of actin microfilament protein (T. Kakanuga, unpublished). Many other observations on the cytoskeletal changes associated with cell transformation are consistent with the hypothesis as shown in Fig. 8.

ACKNOWLEDGMENTS

We thank Drs. R. Firtel and J. J. Lin for providing us with pcDd actin ITL-1 and monoclonal anti-actin IgM, respectively. Thanks are also owed to Ms. M. Petrino, Ms. C. Augl, and Ms. G. Bushar, and Mr. A. Leavitt for their excellent technical assistance, and Ms. L. Nischan for typing the manuscript.

REFERENCES

Barrett, J. C., and Ts'o, P. O. P. (1978). *Proc. Natl. Acad. Sci. USA 75,* 3761-3765.

Benedict, W. F., Jones, P. A., Laug, W. E., Igel, H. J., and Freeman, A. E. (1975). *Nature (London) 256,* 322-324.

Borek, C. (1979). *Nature (London) 283,* 776-778.

Boschek, C. B., Jockusch, B. M., Friis, R. R., Back, R., Grundmann, E., and Bauer, H. (1981). *Cell 24,* 175-184.

DeMar, R., and Jackson, J. L. (1977). *J. Environ. Pathol. Toxicol. 1,* 55-77.

Edelman, G. M., and Yahara, I. (1976). *Proc. Natl. Acad. Sci. USA 73,* 2047-2051.

Enders, J. F. (1969). *Proc. R. Soc. London Ser. B 171,* 431-433.

Foulds, L. (1954). *Cancer Res. 14,* 327-339.

Foulds, L. (1969). "Neoplastic Development," Vol. 1. Academic Press, New York and London.

Foulds, L. (1975). "Neoplastic Development," Vol. 2. Academic Press, New York and London.

Freedman, V. H., and Shin, S. (1975). *J. Natl. Cancer Inst. (U.S.) 58,* 1873-1875.

Freeman, A. E., Lake, R. S., Igel, H. J., Gernard, L., Pezzutti, M. R., Malone, J. M., Mark, C., and Benedict, W. F. (1977). *Proc. Natl. Acad. Sci. USA 74,* 2451-2455.

Garrels, J. I. (1979). *J. Biol. Chem. 254,* 7961-7977.

Hamada, H., Leavitt, J., and Kakunaga, T. (1981). *Proc. Natl. Acad. Sci. USA 78,* 3634-3638.

Igel, H. J., Freeman, A. E., Spiewak, J. E., and Kleinfeld, K. L. (1975). *In Vitro 11,* 117-129.

Kakunaga, T. (1977). *In* "Origin of Human Cancer" (H. H. Hiatt, J. D. Watson, and J. A. Winsten, eds.), pp. 1537-1548. Cold Spring Harbor Lab., Cold Spring Harbor, New York.

Kakunaga, T. (1978). *Proc. Natl. Acad. Sci. USA 75,* 1334-1338.

Kakunaga, T. (1979). *Adv. Mod. Environ. Toxicol. 1,* 355-382.

Kakunaga, T., and Kamahora, J. (1968). *Biken J. 11,* 313-332.

Kakunaga, T., and Kamahora, J. (1969). *Saibo Kagaku Shimpojiumu (Symp. Cell.)Chem. 20,* 135-148.

Kakunaga, T., Crow, J. D., and Augl, C. (1979). *In* "Radiation Research" (S. Okada, M. Imamura, Y. Terashima, and H. Yamaguchi, eds.), pp. 589-595. Jpn. Assoc. Radiat. Res., Tokyo.

Leavitt, J., and Kakunaga, T. (1980). *J. Biol. Chem. 255,* 1650-1661.

Leavitt, J., Bushar, G., Kakunaga, T., Hamada, H., Hirakawa, T. Goldman, D., and Merril, C. (1982a). *Cell 28,* 259-268.

Leavitt, J., Goldman, D., Merril, C., and Kakunaga, T. (1982b). *Carcinogenesis (N.Y.) 3,* 61-70.

Maher, V. M., Rowan, L. A., Silinskas, K. C., Kateley, S. A., and MaCormick, J. J. (1982). *Proc. Natl. Acad. Sci. USA 79,* 2613-2617.

Milo, G. E., and DiPaolo, J. A. (1978). *Nature (London) 275,* 130-132.

Namba, M., Nishitani, K., and Kimoto, T. (1978). *Jpn. J. Exp. Med. 48,* 303-311.

O'Farrell, P. H. (1975). *J. Biol. Chem. 250,* 4007-4021.

Parsa, I., Marsh, W. H., and Sutton, A. L. (1981). *Cancer (Philadelphia) 47,* 1543-1551.

Pollack, R. (1980). *In* "Cancer: Achievements, Challenges and Prospects for the 1980s" (J. H. Burchenal and H. F. Oettgen, eds.), Vol. 1, pp. 501-515. Grune & Stratton, New York.

Pollack, R., Osborn, M., and Weber, K. (1975). *Proc. Natl. Acad. Sci. USA 72,* 994-998.

Rhim, J. S., Park, D. K., Arnstein, P., Huebner, R. J., Weisburger, E. K., and Nelson-Rees, W. A. (1975). *Nature (London) 256,* 751-753.

Rous, P., and Beard, J. W. (1935). *J. Exp. Med. 62,* 523-548.

Sefton, B. M., Hunter, T., Ball, E. H., and Singer, S. J. (1981). *Cell 24,* 165-174.

Shimada, H., Shibata, H., and Yoshikawa, M. (1976). *Nature (London) 264,* 547-548.

Silinskas, K. C., Kateley, S. A., Tower, J. E., Maher, V. M., and McCormick, J. J. (1981). *Cancer Res. 41,* 1620-1627.

Sutherland, B. M., Ciminov, J. S., Delihas, N., Shih, A. G., and Oliver, R. P. (1980). *Cancer Res. 40,* 1934-1939.

Vandekerckhove, J., Leavitt, J., Kakunaga, T., and Weber, K. (1980). *Cell 22,* 893-899.

Vogt, M., and Dulbecco, R. (1963). *Proc. Natl. Acad. Sci. USA 49,* 171-179.

Wang, E., and Goldberg, A. R. (1976). *Proc. Natl. Acad. Sci. USA 73,* 447-451.

Zimmerman, R. J., and Little, J. B. (1981). *Carcinogenesis (N.Y.) 2,* 1303-1310.

16

ROLE OF DNA LESIONS AND DNA REPAIR IN MUTAGENESIS AND TRANSFORMATION OF HUMAN CELLS

J. Justin McCormick and Veronica M. Maher

Carcinogenesis Laboratory
Departments of Microbiology and of Biochemistry
Michigan State University
East Lansing, Michigan

I.   INTRODUCTION[1]

A.   Role of DNA Repair and of Replication in Mutagenesis and Transformation

To examine the mechanisms by which physical and chemical carcinogens cause cancer, we have developed quantitative assays for measuring the frequency of mutations (Maher and McCormick, 1976; Maher *et al.*, 1976a,b, 1977, 1979) and of neoplastic transformation (McCormick *et al.*, 1980, 1981; Silinskas *et al.*, 1981) induced in diploid human fibroblasts in culture by these agents.

---

[1]*Abbreviations: diol epoxide of benzo[a]pyrene, (±)-7β,8α-dihydroxy-9α,10α-epoxy-7,8,9,10-tetrahydrobenzo[a]pyrene; Asynch., asynchronously growing population; G_1, period in the cell cycle between mitosis and DNA synthesis phase; G_0, resting, noncycling state (in this work, cells entered this state because of density inhibition of replication); N-AcO-AABP, N-acetoxy-4-acetylaminobiphenyl; N-AcO-AAF, N-acetoxy-2-acetyl-aminofluorene; N-AcO-AAP, N-acetoxy-2-acetylaminophenanthrene; N-AcO-AAS, N-acetoxy-4-acetylaminostilbene; S phase, semiconservative DNA synthesis phase of the cell cycle; UV, ultraviolet radiation (254 nm); XP, xeroderma pigmentosum.*

To examine the role of DNA lesions and DNA repair in the mutagenesis and transformation process, we have carried out comparative studies with DNA repair-proficient cells from normal
persons and DNA repair-deficient cells from xeroderma pigmentosum (XP) patients (Maher *et al.*, 1976a,b, 1977, 1979, 1982;
Konze-Thomas *et al.*, 1979, 1982; Heflich *et al.*, 1980; Yang
et al., 1980, 1982; Simon *et al.*, 1981). We have compared
these cells for their ability to remove the potentially cytotoxic, mutagenic, and transforming lesions during various
lengths of time in the noncycling state (held confluent)
(Konze-Thomas *et al.*, 1979; Maher *et al.*, 1979, 1981; Heflich
et al., 1980; Yang *et al.*, 1980). In addition, we have made
use of synchronized populations of these human cells to examine
the role of semiconservative DNA replication in these processes
(Konze-Thomas *et al.*, 1982; Maher *et al.*, 1982; Yang *et al.*,
1982).

B. Relationship between Mutation Induction and Neoplastic
    Transformation

The working hypothesis for these comparative studies is
that chemical carcinogens and radiation cause cancer by acting
as mutagens, and that the initial event leading ultimately to
the neoplastic transformation of normal cells into tumor-forming
cells results from damage to DNA, which is converted into a
somatic cell mutation. It is instructive to recall that not
long ago this idea was not commonly accepted, even though
Brookes and Lawley (1964) had shown that the carcinogenicity
of a series of polycyclic aromatic hydrocarbons correlated with
their binding to DNA, rather than to RNA or proteins. Early
demonstrations that there was a good correlation between carcinogenicity and mutagenicity of reactive derivatives of chemical carcinogens (Maher *et al.*, 1968, 1970) were followed by

those of a number of workers (see McCann *et al.*, 1975), which
revived interest in the discarded theory of Boveri (1929) that
somatic cell mutations were responsible for the induction of
cancer. The development of assays for quantitating the induction of mutations and transformation of mammalian cells in culture, including human cells, made it possible to examine these
questions more closely and determine the basic cellular mechanisms involved.

Indirect support for the involvement of mutations in neoplastic transformation came from the finding (Cleaver, 1968)
that cells derived from XP patients, who are genetically predisposed to sunlight-induced skin cancer (Robbins *et al.*,
1974), were deficient in the rate of excision of UV-induced
DNA lesions. We demonstrated that these XP cells were abnormally sensitive to the cytotoxic and mutagenic effects of UV
(Maher and McCormick, 1976; Maher *et al.*, 1979) and also those
of broad-spectrum sunlight (Patton *et al.*, 1983). In addition, we compared NF and XP cells for their rate of excision
of DNA lesions (adducts) formed by a series of chemical carcinogens and compared them for their response to the mutagenic
and/or cytotoxic effects of these agents. Cytotoxicity was
defined as the inability of a cell to form a colony (i.e.,
reproductive death); mutagenicity was defined as an increase
in 8-azaguanine- or 6-thioguanine-resistant cells in the population (resulting from the loss of active hypoxanthine(guanine)-
phosphoribosyltransferase). The results indicated that mutations by these particular agents are not introduced during excision repair but result from semiconservative DNA synthesis
on a template containing unexcised lesions, that is, by mis-
replication or failure to replicate a portion of the DNA.
However, the genetic marker used for these mutagenesis studies
served only as a model for the kinds of mutational events by
which carcinogens are considered to affect cellular processes
or structures involved in neoplastic transformation.

Once we had developed a quantitative assay for the formation of diploid human fibroblasts (McCormick *et al.*, 1980, 1981;
Silinskas *et al.*, 1981), we took a more direct approach to determining whether DNA is the principal target for transformation. We compared the frequency of UV-induced neoplastic transformation of normal diploid human fibroblasts with that of XP
cells to see if the latter were significantly more sensitive.
If DNA is the target, the cells that cannot repair UV-induced
DNA damage or can excise it only very slowly should be at a
much higher risk of being transformed. By analogy with the results of our UV-induced mutagenesis studies, if the two populations initially receive the same level of DNA damage, the cells
with the more rapid rate of excision should exhibit the lower
frequency of transformation. The results showed that XP cells
are significantly more susceptible than normal cells to UV-
induced transformation to anchorage independence (Maher *et al.*,
1982). They also showed that excision repair taking place
before DNA replication occurs can eliminate the lesions responsible for this transformation. The cells derived from
these anchorage-independent colonies produced fibrosarcomas
upon injection into appropriate host animals. Further
studies to determine the number and nature of the steps involved in the multistepped process of neoplastic transformation are now possible and are in progress.

II.   RELATIONSHIP BETWEEN RATE OF EXCISION REPAIR OF UV LIGHT-
      INDUCED DNA LESIONS AND SENSITIVITY OF CELLS TO CYTOTOXIC
      AND MUTAGENIC EFFECTS OF UV

Our earliest studies with human fibroblasts showed that
the sensitivity of the cells to the potentially lethal or mutagenic effect of UV (254 nm) paralleled their excision repair

capability. Cells with the normal rate of excision were much
more resistant to the potentially lethal and mutagenic effect
of UV than were repair-deficient XP strains. After exposure
to low doses (1 J/m^2), XP12BE cells with little or no excision
repair capacity (Petinga et al., 1977) exhibited ∿5% survival;
XP7BE cells that excise very slowly, exhibited a survival of
∿18%; XP2BE cells, which excise damage more rapidly, had a
survival of ∿25%; and normally repairing cells exhibited 100%
survival. The corresponding frequency of thioguanine-resistant
cells in the population after this dose of UV was 315×10^{-6}
for strain XP12BE, 300×10^{-6} for XP7BE, and background level
($\sim15 \times 10^{-6}$) for the normal cells. An 8- to 10-fold higher
dose of radiation was required to cause comparable cytotoxicity and mutagenicity in the normal cells (Maher et al.,
1979, 1982). This is the result expected if the excision-
minus XP12BE cells exhibit essentially the maximum potential
cytotoxicity and mutagenicity of a given dose of UV, whereas
XP2BE or XP7BE cells can reduce their load of DNA damage to a
level 20-40% of that initially received, and the normal cells,
with rapid excision repair, can reduce their load to an insig-
nificant number of photolesions.

Because an essential difference between these strains is
their respective rates of excision repair of UV-induced damage,
the data are consistent with the hypothesis that there is a
finite amount of time for excision repair between the initial
radiation and the onset of the critical events responsible for
cell killing and/or mutation induction in these cells. We
suggested that the loss of ability to form a clone and the
frequency of mutations induced in these cells reflected the
number of unexcised lesions remaining in DNA at the time of
some "critical cellular event" that translated the DNA lesions
into their biological manifestations, and that this critical
event could be semiconservative DNA synthesis on a damaged
template (Maher et al., 1977, 1979).

III.   HOLDING CELLS IN NONCYCLIC STATE AFTER DAMAGE AND
       DECREASE IN POTENTIALLY CYTOTOXIC AND MUTAGENIC EFFECTS
       OF CARCINOGENS

A.   Evidence of Biological Recovery from Effects of UV Radiation

If the mutagenic event occurs during semiconservative DNA synthesis on a template containing unexcised lesions rather than by excision repair processes, extending the period between the introduction of the lesions in DNA and the onset of DNA replication in cells that have repair capacity should decrease the frequency of mutant cells induced. Similarly, if cell killing reflects replication on a DNA template that contains lesions, then extending the time available for excision repair before allowing cells to begin to replicate their DNA should result in increased survival. We tested this hypothesis by growing cells to confluence to cause density inhibition of cell replication. The cells were then irradiated or treated with a DNA-damaging agent and were allowed various lengths of time in this non-cycling state (G_0) to remove potentially cytotoxic or mutagenic DNA lesions before being released and assayed for the frequency of mutant cells (resistance to 6-thioguanine) and for percentage survival. Autoradiography studies demonstrated that under our conditions <0.5% of these confluent cells incorporated tritiated thymidine during an 8-h labeling period (Maher *et al.*, 1979). However, such noncycling cells are capable of excision repair (Konze-Thomas *et al.*, 1979; Heflich *et al.*, 1980; Yang *et al.*, 1980).

Confluent cultures of repair-proficient cells and repair-deficient XP12BE cells were UV irradiated with doses large enough to cause significant cell killing and mutation induction in exponentially growing populations, and held in the nonreplicating state for 7 days. They were then trypsinized, plated at lower densities, and assayed for survival and induction of

mutations. The normal cells showed no cell killing and no
mutation induction. In contrast, the XP12BE cells exhibited
essentially the same degree of cell killing and mutation induction as in cycling cells (Maher et al., 1979).

To determine how much time was required for normal cells
to remove all the potentially cytotoxic and/or mutagenic
lesions, we irradiated a series of confluent cultures with
9 J/m^2 UV and assayed one immediately and the others after 4,
8, 16, and 24 h. We found a gradual decrease in the lethal
and mutagenic effect of the radiation. The survival of the
cells released immediately was ∿20%; the frequency of mutants
was ∿60 × 10^{-6}. Cells held 8 h showed a survival of ∿45% and
∿30 mutants per 10^6 cells. Cells assayed after 16 h showed
100% survival, and the frequency of mutants reached the background level of the unirradiated population (i.e., ∿15 × 10^6).
Note that the frequency of mutant cells observed even in the
cells released immediately was significantly lower than that
expected for normal cells irradiated in exponential growth.
Cells released from the noncycling state under our experimental
conditions are synchronized and do not begin DNA synthesis
(S phase) for ∿24 h (Konze-Thomas et al., 1982). Therefore, a
reasonable explanation for this lower frequency is that mutations are "fixed" during semiconservative DNA replication, and
this extended G_1 phase gives the cells time for excision repair
processes to remove the majority of the potentially mutagenic
lesions from the DNA (Maher et al., 1979).

B. Correlation between Rate of Excision of Lesions and Rate
    of Recovery from Potentially Cytotoxic and Mutagenic Effect
    of Chemical Carcinogens

One may measure the rate of excision of UV-induced pyrimidine dimers in human cells with reasonable accuracy at doses
greater than 10 J/m^2, but not the rate of removal of the low

number of photoproducts induced by the doses of UV used in these experiments. To get around this difficulty, we made use of a series of labeled chemical carcinogens of high specific radioactivity which we had found caused lesions in DNA (covalently bound adducts) that the XP12BE cells were unable to excise (e.g., aromatic amide and polycyclic aromatic hydrocarbon derivatives). Using the same procedures as described for UV-irradiated cultures, Heflich *et al.* (1980) and Maher *et al.* (1981) showed that the rate of recovery of normally repairing cells treated in confluence with the cytotoxic effect of *N*-AcO-AABP, *N*-AcO-AAF, *N*-AcO-AAPh, or *N*-AcO-AAS was directly related to the rate of removal of the bound carcinogen residues from DNA (Fig. 1). (Note that the removal took days as opposed to a few hours.) In the population of XP12BE cells there was little or no removal of the bound material from cellular DNA and no evidence of recovery from the potentially lethal effects of the initial exposure, even after a period of 6 days in confluence.

Yang *et al.* (1980) used this same approach to investigate the kinetics of removal of DNA adducts formed by radioactive diol epoxide of BP and the rate of recovery from its potentially cytotoxic and mutagenic effects. Large populations of density-inhibited cells were treated in G_0, and a fraction of them were harvested immediately and assayed for DNA adducts, survival, and mutation induction. The rest were assayed after 2, 4, or 8 days in confluence. The results (Fig. 2) showed that the potentially cytotoxic and mutagenic lesions were removed with about the same kinetics as were the total number of DNA adducts. Residues were removed by the confluent normal cells over a period of 4 days, but then excision repair slowed considerably. Similarly, the survival of the cell increased during that same period, and the mutation frequency decreased almost to background. There was no loss of adducts from the

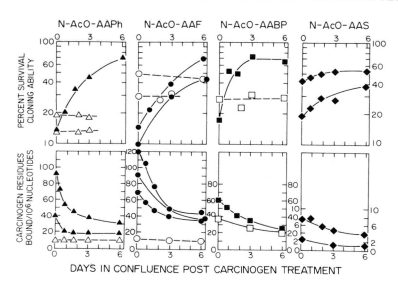

Fig. 1. Comparison of the rates of recovery from the potentially lethal effects of four aromatic amine derivatives with the rate of removal of radioactive labeled residues from the DNA of normal (▲,●,■,◆) of XP12BE cells (△,○,□). Cells were treated at confluence as described and then assayed after the designated period of time in the G_0 state. (Some data taken from Heflich et al., 1980.)

excision-deficient XP12BE cells and no change in survival or mutation frequency. This strongly suggests that the excision repair capability of the normal cells is responsible for reducing the potentially cytotoxic and potentially mutagenic effects of exposure to these chemical carcinogens, just as with UV-irradiated cells. (HPLC Characterization of the DNA adducts indicated that the major adduct was the N^2-guanyl derivative and that the kinetics of decrease of tritium label in the specific HPLC peak corresponded to the kinetics of recovery from the mutations and the cytotoxicity.)

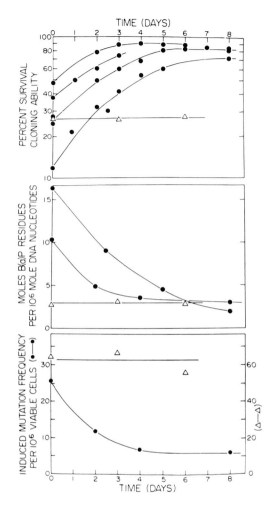

Fig. 2. Kinetics of removal of covalently bound adducts (middle) and recovery of normal (●) or XP12BE cells (Δ) from the potentially cytotoxic (top) or mutagenic (bottom) effects of anti-BPDE. The cells were treated in the G_0 state, released on the designated days, and assayed for survival of colony-forming ability, for the number of residues bound to DNA, and-- after a suitable expression period--for the frequency of induced mutations to TG resistance. (Taken from Yang et al., 1980, with permission.)

IV.   SHORTENING OF INTERVAL BETWEEN EXPOSURE OF CELLS TO DNA-
      DAMAGING AGENTS AND ONSET OF DNA SYNTHESIS (S PHASE):
      INCREASE IN MUTAGENIC EFFECT

A.   Evidence That Mutations Are "Fixed" by DNA Replication

     The results of these "plateau phase recovery" experiments
suggested that the cellular event responsible for killing and
mutation induction was semiconservative DNA replication on a
damaged template. They predicted that if the time available
for excision before S phase was shortened by synchronizing
cells and irradiating them or treating them with chemical carcinogens just prior to the onset of DNA synthesis, this should
significantly increase the frequency of mutations induced and
the cell killing observed in excision-proficient cells, but not
in XP12BE cells. We tested these predictions using UV (Konze-
Thomas et al., 1982) and the diol epoxide of benzo[a]pyrene
(Yang et al., 1982) as the DNA-damaging agents in cells synchronized by density inhibition. Cultures of normal and XP12BE
cells were released from confluence, allowed to attach at lower
densities and elongate, irradiated in early G_1 ($\sim$18 h prior to
the onset of S) or just prior to S phase, and assayed for the
frequency of mutations and survival. The slope of the dose response for mutations induced in the normal cells irradiated or
treated with diol epoxide of BP just prior to S was about 10-
fold steeper than that of cells irradiated 18 h earlier (Figs.
3 and 4). The frequencies induced in cells treated in confluence and then released so as to have at least a 24 h interval
prior to the onset of S phase were still lower. These are shown
in Figs. 3 and 4 for comparative purposes. As expected, the
frequency of mutations induced in the XP cells was the same
whether they were irradiated just before S, 18 h prior to S,
or 24 h before DNA synthesis began. These results support the

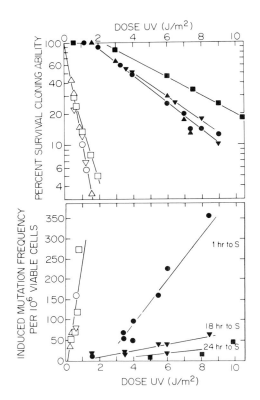

Fig. 3. Cytotoxicity and mutagenicity of UV in normal (closed symbols) or XPl2BE cells (open symbols) irradiated under conditions designed to allow various lengths of time for excision repair to take place prior to the onset of S phase. Cells irradiated in confluence (G$_0$) and then released and plated at lower densities (■,□ ; 24 h to S phase); cells released from G$_0$ and irradiated 6 h later (▼,▽; 18 h to S phase); cells released and irradiated 24 h later (●,○; 1 h to S phase); cells replated from asynchronously growing cultures and irradiated 16 h later (▲,△). (Taken from Konze-Thomas *et al.*, 1982, with permission.)

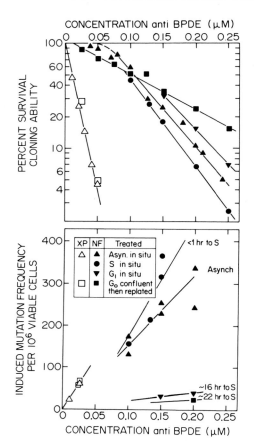

Fig. 4. Cytotoxicity (top) and frequency of mutations to TG resistance (bottom) induced by low doses of the diol epoxide of BP in normal (▲ , ● , ▼ , ■) and XP12BE cells (△ , □) treated under conditions designed to allow various lengths of time between treatment and the onset of S phase. Time to S phase: ● , <1 h; ▼ , ~16 h; ■ , □ , ~22 h; ▲ , △ , asynchronous. (Taken from Yang et al., 1982, with permission.)

idea that mutations are "fixed" by DNA replication, and the frequency is determined by the number of unexcised lesions remaining during DNA replication.

Note that the normal cells treated with the diol epoxide of benzo[a]pyrene just prior to onset of DNA synthesis exhibited a mutation induction dose-response curve that approximates that extrapolated for the XP12BE cells at these higher concentrations (Fig. 4). This is not the case with UV as the agent (Fig. 3). These results were expected because our data indicate that UV-induced DNA lesions are excised much more rapidly than the diol epoxide adducts can be removed. Therefore, even if DNA synthesis does not begin immediately, is abnormally extended, or is halted by the lesions themselves, the diol epoxide residues remain at a relatively higher frequency for a much longer time than do UV-induced lesions.

B. Evidence that Cell Death Is Not Determined Principally by Number of Unexcised DNA Lesions Remaining during Replication

Although the mutagenic effect of these agents in excision repair-proficent human cells was inversely correlated with the amount of time available for repair before S phase, the cell survival results did not show this. We observed no significant difference in the survival of the normal cells UV irradiated (Fig. 3) or treated with the diol epoxide of benzo[a]pyrene (Fig. 4) at various times prior to the onset of S phase. The XP12BE cells, of course, were not expected to exhibit any real difference, but the repair-proficient cells were. A more detailed investigation of the survival of synchronized normal cells UV-irradiated *in situ* with low doses (>6% survival) at various times prior to S phase failed to yield any significant differences between the various sets. Each set of normal cells was 10-fold more resistant than sets of XP12BE cells, but no striking cell cycle dependence was found (Konze-Thomas *et al.*, 1982). We therefore suggest that after DNA is damaged by these agents, the time available for repair of potentially lethal lesions is determined by the cell's need for critical cellular proteins and their respective mRNAs. If the DNA template for transcription of these mRNAs is still blocked by lesions at the time the cell has need of them, reproductive death (i.e., inability to form a colony) is the result. This would explain why holding cells in a resting state following exposure to DNA-damaging agents before releasing them into the cycling state results in a higher survival than does immediate release. If cells held in a confluence have a lower metabolic state than cells in exponential growth, fewer critical proteins would be needed before the cell has time to remove the blocking DNA damage. We suggest that reproductive death from exposure to UV radiation or these chemical agents results indirectly from faulty or blocked transcription from DNA-containing photoproducts or adducts, because of the resulting lack of required protein synthesis (Konze-Thomas *et al.*, 1982; Yang *et al.*, 1982). This conclusion is consistent with the fact that the XP12BE cells, which do not remove such lesions from their DNA, show no dose-modifying effect on being held in the resting state.

V. EVIDENCE THAT NEOPLASTIC TRANSFORMATION OF HUMAN CELLS INVOLVES A MUTAGENIC EVENT

A. Common Characteristics between Induction of Anchorage Independence in Diploid Human Cells and Induction of Thioguanine Resistance

As indicated in Section I, the underlying purpose of our research is to determine the number and nature of the steps involved in the transformation of cells in culture in order to understand the mechanisms of human carcinogenesis. Although results obtained with cells in culture cannot fully represent the *in vivo* process of carcinogenesis, such an approach permits a more direct experimental manipulation and quantitation of the individual steps involved and can yield information on the nature of these steps. A further advantage of using cell culture systems is that they allow experimental studies with human cells, which would otherwise be impossible for obvious ethical reasons. In fact, dissection of the steps involved in the neoplastic transformation of human cells in culture may represent the only experimental approach to obtaining such information.

Because in the past workers who were developing transformation assays have assumed either explicitly or implicitly that the transformation event(s) was not the result of mutations, most transformation assays were not designed to yield information on transformation frequencies and mutation frequencies simultaneously using the same treated cell populations. Furthermore, the protocols used, as well as the type of cell line (aneuploid), often precluded recognition of whether mutation(s) were involved in transformation. Even when early-passage diploid cells derived from Syrian hamster embryos are used (Berwald and Sachs, 1965; DiPaolo *et al.,* 1972; Barrett and Ts'o, 1978; Barrett *et al.,* 1980), the earliest end point—morphological transformation—develops at such a high frequency (0.1-1%) as to rule out genetic mutations as the cause. The cells in these morphologically transformed colonies are not tumorigenic *per se* (Barrett *et al.,* 1980). Cells able to cause tumors arise randomly in progeny of the carcinogen-treated cultures only after 35 to 70 population doublings posttreatment. By that time control cells from nontreated cultures have senesced, and the surviving treated cell population has become aneuploid. This delay makes it difficult to associate the ultimate tumorigenicity with the original carcinogen treatment.

For many years, workers had tried without success to induce the transformation of human fibroblasts with carcinogens.
Finally in 1977, Kakunaga demonstrated that human fibroblasts
treated with a carcinogen could give rise to cells that formed
foci (small areas, apparently clonal in origin, where cells
grow in a three-dimensional array) on the top of confluent monolayers. The progeny of these cells proved to be tumorigenic
when injected subcutaneously into athymic mice. Work by
Milo and DiPaolo (1978), Borek (1980), Sutherland et al.
(1980, 1981), and ourselves (McCormick et al., 1980, 1981;
Silinskas et al., 1981; Maher et al., 1982) has extended this
research.

Because of our extensive experience with mutation assays
for diploid human fibroblasts before we began developing a
transformation assay, and because of our conviction that the
transformation process was likely to involve one or more mutagenic events, we deliberately designed a human cell transformation assay modeled after our human cell mutagenesis assays
(McCormick et al., 1980). For example, we expected the process
of transformation of human fibroblasts to have in common with
the process of mutagenesis (1) an expression period, that is,
a period of time between carcinogen damage of cells and their
ability to express the new (i.e., transformed) phenotype,
(2) a linear increase in the frequency of transformants with
increase in carcinogen dose, (3) a concentration dependence
for the carcinogenic agent that resembled that required for induction of mutations, so that strong mutagens would usually be
strong transforming agents, (4) a low but measurable frequency
of transformed cells in non-carcinogen-treated cell populations,
just as one finds low but measurable frequency of mutant cells
in such populations, (5) a higher frequency of transformation
per dose in DNA repair-deficient cells than in normal cells,

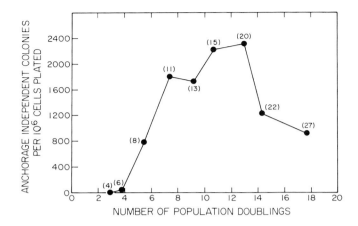

Fig. 5. Kinetics of expression of anchorage independence. Cells were treated with 21.5 µg/ml of propane sultone for 14 h after the cells had entered S phase. The surviving population (∿28%) as well as the control population were trypsinized, diluted 1:2, replated, and kept in exponential growth by continuous subculturing as required. On each of the days indicated in parentheses, 2–5 × 10^6 cells were trypsinized, pooled, and counted to determine the number of population doublings that had occurred. Then, for each determination, 10^6 cells were assayed for anchorage-independent growth (5 × 10^4 cells/ dish), and the rest were replated for continued propagation and subsequent assay. (Taken from Silinskas et al., 1981, with permission.)

as we had shown for the induction of mutants in XP cells, and (6) a cell cycle dependence similar to that which occurs for mutation induction, so that populations of cells treated just before S phase would show a higher frequency of transformation than cell populations treated with the same dose of the agent far from S phase. Our results described next confirmed each of these predictions.

Our assay, unlike that of Kakunaga (1977) is based on the induction of ability of the cells to grow in an anchorage-independent manner following carcinogen treatment. Human fibroblasts are treated with reactive derivatives of chemical carcinogens or radiation (UV or ionizing) using doses that

lower the survival, as judged by cloning, to between 80 and
10% of the control population. The surviving cells (10^6 or
more) are kept in exponential growth for 8 to 10 population
doublings to allow full expression of the anchorage-
independent phenotype (Fig. 5) and are then plated as single
cells into medium containing 0.33% agar. Colonies of
anchorage-independent cells develop to a size that can be
counted (∿0.2 mm diameter) after about 3 to 4 weeks. These
anchorage-independent cells have been repeatedly tested for
tumorigenicity by isolating colonies, propagating them into
large populations, and injecting 10^7 cells sc into immunologically depressed athymic mice. Tumors of ∿1 cm diameter
develop at the site of injection in less than 2 weeks. These
regress after several weeks. No tumors have developed in
the animals when they were injected with nontransformed
control populations ($>2 \times 10^7$/injection). Pathology examination identified representative tumors as fibrosarcomas.
Cells from several of the tumors have been returned to
culture. They all have a diploid human karyotype.

B. Ability of DNA Excision Repair to Decrease Potentially
    Transforming Lesions induced by UV Radiation

    Further evidence that loss of anchorage dependence with
its subsequent tumorigenicity is induced as a genetic event
in human diploid cells derives from a study in our laboratory
(Maher et al., 1982) comparing the frequency of induction in
normal human cells and in cells derived from two excision
repair-deficient xeroderma pigmentosum patients, XP7BE
(complementation group D) and XP12BE from group A. Note
that these XP cells are not malignant; the biopsies from
which they are derived are always obtained from non-sunlight-

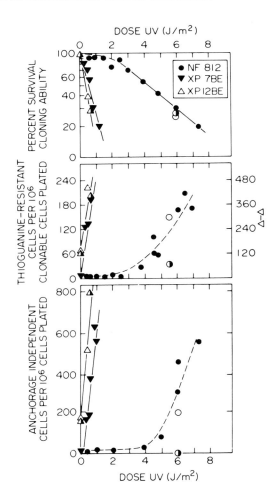

Fig. 6. Cytotoxicity, mutagenicity, and transforming ability of UV radiation in normal (O, ●, ◑) and XP cells (XP12BE, △ , ▲; XP7BE, ▼). The frequency of TG-resistant cells was assayed after 6 doublings, that of anchorage-independent cells after 9 to 11 doublings. The former were corrected for cloning efficiency on plastic. Solid symbols, populations irradiated in exponential growth; open symbols, cells synchronized by release from confluence and irradiated shortly before onset of S phase; half-solid symbols, cells irradiated 18-20 h prior to S phase. See text for details.

exposed areas of the skin. This is confirmed by the fact
that injection of >2 × 10^7 into athymic mice did not produce
tumors (Maher et al., 1982). The results are shown in
Fig. 6.

The survival data (Fig. 6, top) show that the XP cells
are significantly more sensitive than NF cells to the lethal
effect of UV; for example, a dose of 0.5 or 1.1 J/m^2
decreased their survival to 20%, whereas 7.5 J/m^2 were
required to cause the same decrease in NF cells. The mutagenicity data (Fig. 6, middle) show that the XP cells are
significantly more sensitive than normal cells to the mutagenic action of UV. The mutant frequencies were corrected
for the cloning efficiency of the cells, because we showed
that, under the selection conditions, their cloning efficiency is similar to that of cells plated at cloning density
in the absence of selection (Maher et al., 1977).

The transformation frequency data (Fig. 6, bottom) indicate
that the XP cells are also significantly more sensitive than
normal cells to UV-induced loss of anchorage dependence. These
particular data were obtained by assaying the progeny of the irradiated cells after an expression period of about 9 population
doublings. However, in the majority of cases, the frequency of
anchorage-independent cells was assayed twice (i.e., after 9
and 11 doublings) and yielded approximately the same frequencies both times. (Note that these data are the observed frequencies of agar colonies counted directly without a correction
factor.) The data indicate that to achieve a particular degree of cell killing, mutagenesis, and transformation, NF cells
have to be exposed to 8- to 10-fold higher doses of UV radiation than XP cells. As discussed previously, this is the result expected if induction of anchorage independence as well
as thioguanine resistance results ultimately from DNA damage
remaining unexcised in the cell at some critical time after

irradiation and if, because of the difference in their respective rates of excision repair, the average number of lesions
remaining at this critical time is approximately equal in the
three populations.

C.   Dependence of Frequency of Anchorage-Independent Cells on
     Duration of Period between UV Irradiation and Onset of DNA
     Synthesis

As discussed previously (Fig. 3), if synchronous populations of NF cells are irradiated shortly before the onset of
S phase, the frequency of thioguanine-resistant cells induced
is about eightfold higher than in the same cells treated 18 h
prior to S. No such difference is observed when the target
cells were virtually incapable of excision repair.

To determine if a similar cell cycle effect occurred for
induction of transformation, we irradiated NF and XP12BE
cells in early and late G_1 and assayed their progeny for
frequency of anchorage-independent cells. The results are
included in Fig. 6 as open and half-solid symbols. The transformation frequencies of the repair-proficient normal cells
showed a strong cell cycle dependence, that is, cells irradiated
with 6 J/m^2 ∿3 h prior to onset of S phase yielded 200 anchorage-independent cells per 10^6 cells plated; those irradiated in
early G_1 gave 0 colonies per dish ($<1 \times 10^{-6}$), the control cells
in this experiment also gave no colonies from $<1 \times 10^{-6}$ cells.
In contrast, the frequency of anchorage-independent cells in the
XP12BE population irradiated in early G_1 did not decrease; in
fact it was somewhat higher. In the corresponding mutation experiment, the frequencies were equal. In the mutagenesis experiments with normal cells from which the data in Fig. 6B
were taken, the frequency of mutant cells did not decrease completely to the background level. However, in this mutagenesis

experiment, the cells irradiated in G_1 had somewhat less time
for excision repair before onset of S than was available in the
transformation experiments. The fact that allowing substantial
time for excision before DNA synthesis eliminated the potentially mutagenic and transforming effect of UV radiation in
normal cells but not in XP12BE cells suggests that DNA synthesis
on a template still containing unexcised lesions is the cellular
event responsible for "fixing" the mutations and transformation.

An experiment reported by Kakunaga (1974) is consistent
with this interpretation. He showed that when confluent cultures of a mouse cell line were exposed to 4-nitroquinoline 1-
oxide and then allowed to carry out excision repair but not to
replicate, the potential for foci formation was gradually eliminated. However, when the cells were allowed to undergo a single
population doubling after treatment before attaining confluence,
additional time in confluence did not decrease the transformation frequency.

In addition to the information that can be gained by anal-
izing the 8- to 10-fold differences between XP and NF cells in
Fig. 6, it is useful to compare the frequencies of anchorage-
independent cells with those of thioguanine-resistant cells.
The similarity of the dose responses for the two phenotypes is
obvious and supports the idea that acquisition of anchorage independence (transformation) in human cells occurs as the result
of a single mutational event. The frequencies of mutations and
transformation differ by a factor of $\sim$2.5. In our earliest experiments, using propane sultone, the difference was $\sim$22-fold
(Silinskas et al., 1981). However, a ratio of 2.5 is much
closer to the ratios we now observe with a number of agents.
Part of the reason for the higher value reported in the early
experiments can be attributed to the use of a different lot of
serum and a different type of agar (J. J. McCormick, unpublished)
Small technical differences in the way the cells were handled

may also have contributed to the difference. A third consideration is that in those early experiments, the agar colonies per dish were so numerous that only a representative fraction of them was counted, and the calculated numbers may have been systematically overestimated. In the subsequent experiments with propane sultone, in which fewer cells per dish were assayed and every macroscopic colony was counted, the frequency was one-fourth of the early value (see Fig. 5).

If we assume that anchorage independence results from a mutation, we might speculate about the size of the DNA target involved. The observed number of thioguanine-resistant colonies (selected on plastic at a density equivalent to 10^4 cells per 60-mm dish) had been corrected for the cells' intrinsic cloning efficiency (i.e., 30-50%). The number of anchorage-independent cells (selected at a density of 10^5 cells per 3 ml of soft agar), however, was determined directly from the observed number of agar colonies without correction. There is no simple way to determine the "intrinsic cloning efficiency" under these conditions in which 10^5 cells are plated per dish. If the cloning efficiency in agar were less than 100%, the frequencies would have to be increased accordingly. Nevertheless, the relationship between the frequencies observed for thioguanine resistance as well as anchorage independence in the three strains that differ in DNA repair capacity support the hypothesis that mutations are involved in transformation.

VI.   CONCLUSION

In summary, these studies indicate that although the transformation of diploid human fibroblasts into tumor-forming cells is a multistepped process, an initial step is a mutagenic event. The data indicate that excision repair in these fibroblasts is essentially an error-free process and that the ability to excise potentially cytotoxic, mutagenic, or transforming lesions induced in DNA by UV radiation or by several classes of chemical carcinogens determines their ultimate biological consequences.

Other classes of carcinogens that form "bulky" lesions in DNA can be expected to give similar results, whereas the results with carcinogens that methylate DNA and with ionizing radiation may be different, because the damage produced by these latter agents is repaired by pathways at least partially different from those studied here. Such studies are in progress. The data presented here suggest that there is a certain limited amount of time available between the initial exposure and the onset of the cellular events responsible for mutation induction, for cell transformation, and for cell killing, and that the critical event for the mutation and transformation to anchorage independence is DNA replication on a template containing unexcised lesions (photoproducts, adducts). Cells deficient in excision repair, such as those derived from cancer-prone xeroderma pigmentosum patients, proved abnormally sensitive to the cytotoxic, mutagenic, and transforming effects of carcinogens. The accompanying cytotoxicity studies indicated that although a population's survival is determined by the extent of excision repair of potentially lethal damage from DNA before some critical cellular event, no single cell cycle-related event such as DNA synthesis on a damaged template is responsible for cell death.

ACKNOWLEDGMENTS

We wish to express our indebtedness to our colleagues, A. E. Aust, J. C. Ball, N. R. Drinkwater, R. H. Heflich, B. Konze-Thomas, J. W. Levinson, J. D. Patton, K. C. Silinskas, and L. L. Yang for their invaluable contributions to the research summarized here. The excellent technical assistance of M. Antczak, R. Corner, D. J. Dorney, R. M. Hazard, S. A. Kateley, T. E. Kinney, L. D. Milam, M. M. Moon, T. G. O'Callaghan, D. Richmond, L. A. Rowan, J. E. Tower, and T. VanNoord is gratefully acknowledged. The labeled anti-BPDE was provided by the Cancer Research Program of the National Cancer Institute and the labeled aromatic amines by Dr. John Scribner of the Pacific Northwest Research Foundation. The research summarized in this report was supported in part by Contract ES-78-4659 from the Department of Energy and by Grants CA 21247, CA 21253, CA 21289, and ES 07076 from the Department of Health and Human Services, NIH. Additional financial assistance was provided by the Michigan Osteopathic College Foundation.

REFERENCES

Barrett, J. C., and Ts'o, P. O. P. (1978). *Proc. Natl. Acad. Sci. USA 75*, 3761-3765.

Barrett, J. C., Crawford, B. D., and Ts'o, P. O. P. (1980). *In* "Mammalian Cell Transformation by Chemical Carcinogens" (N. Mishra, V. Dunkel, and M. Mehlman, eds.), pp. 467-501. Princeton Senate Press, Princeton, New Jersey.

Berwald, Y., and Sachs, L. (1965). *J. Nat. Cancer Inst. (U.S.) 35*, 641-661.

Borek, C. (1980). *Nature (London) 283*, 776-778.

Boveri, T. (1929). "The Origin of Malignant Tumors," 2nd ed. Williams and Wilkins Co., Baltimore.

Brookes, P., and Lawley, P. D. (1964). *Nature (London) 202*, 781-784.

Cleaver, J. E. (1968). *Nature (London) 218*, 652-656.

DiPaolo, J. A., Nelson, R. L., and Donovan, P. J. (1972). *Nature (London) 235*, 270-280.

Heflich, R. H., Hazard, R. M., Lommel, L., Scribner, J. D., Maher, V. M., and McCormick, J. J. (1980). *Chem. Biol. Interact. 29*, 43-56.

Kakunaga, T. (1974). *Int. J. Cancer 14*, 736-742.

Kakunaga, T. (1977). *In* "Origins of Human Cancer" (H. H. Hiatt, J. D. Watson, and J. A. Winsten, eds.) Vol. C, pp. 1537-1548. Cold Spring Harbor Lab., Cold Spring Harbor, New York.

Konze-Thomas, B., Levinson, J. W., Maher, V. M., and McCormick, J. J. (1979). *Biophys. J. 28*, 315-326.

Konze-Thomas, B., Hazard, R. M., Maher, V. M., and McCormick, J. J. (1982). *Mutat. Res. 94*, 421-434.

Maher, V. M., and McCormick, J. J. (1976). *In* "Biology of Radiation Carcinogenesis" (J. M. Yuhas, R. W. Tennant, and J. D. Regan, eds.), pp. 129-145. Raven Press, New York.

Maher, V. M., Miller, E. C., Miller, J. A., and Szybalski, W. (1968). *Mol. Pharmacol.* 4, 411-426.

Maher, V. M., Miller, J. A., Miller, E. C., and Summers, W. C. (1970). *Cancer Res.* 30, 1473-1480.

Maher, V. M., Curren, R. D., Ouellette, L. M., and McCormick, J. J. (1976a). *In* "*In Vitro* Metabolic Activation in Mutagenesis Testing" (F. J. deSerres, J. R. Fouts, J. R. Bend, and R. M. Philpot, eds.), pp. 313-336. Elsevier-North Holland, Amsterdam.

Maher, V. M., Ouellette, L. M., Curren, R. D., and McCormick, J. J. (1976b). *Nature (London) 261,* 593-595.

Maher, V. M., McCormick, J. J., Grover, P. L., and Sims, P. (1977). *Mutat. Res. 43,* 117-138.

Maher, V. M., Dorney, D. J., Mendrala, A. L., Konze-Thomas, B., and McCormick, J. J. (1979). *Mutat. Res. 62,* 311-323.

Maher, V. M., Heflich, R. H., and McCormick, J. J. (1981). *In* "Carcinogenic and Mutagenic N-Substituted Aryl Compounds" (E. K. Weisberger and S. S. Thorgeisson, eds.), pp. 217-222. Nat. Cancer Inst., Washington, D.C.

Maher, V. M., Rowan, L. A., Silinskas, K. C., Kateley, S. A., and McCormick, J. J. (1982). *Proc. Natl. Acad. Sci. USA 79,* 2613-2617.

McCann, J., Choi, E., Yamasaki, E., and Ames, B. N. (1975). *Proc. Natl. Acad. Sci. USA 72,* 5135-5139.

McCormick, J. J., Silinskas, K. C., and Maher, V. M. (1980). *In* "Carcinogenesis, Fundamental Mechanisms and Environmental Effects" (B. Pullman, P. O. P. Ts'o, and H. Gelboin, eds.), pp. 491-498. Reidel, Dordrecht.

McCormick, J. J., Silinskas, K. C., Kateley, S. A., Tower, J. E., and Maher, V. M. (1981). *Proc. Am. Assoc. Cancer Res. 21,* 122.

Milo, G. E., Jr., and DiPaolo, J. A. (1978). *Nature (London) 275,* 130-132.

Patton, J. D., Rowan, L. A., Mendrala, A. L., Maher, V. M., and McCormick, J. J. (Submitted 1983). *Photochem. Photobiol.*

Petinga, R. A., Andrews, A. D., Tarone, R. E., and Robbins, J. H. (1977). *Biochim. Biophys. Acta 479,* 400-410.

Robbins, J. H., Kraemer, K. H., Lutzner, M. A., Festoff, B. W., and Coon, H. G. (1974). *Ann. Intern. Med. 80,* 221-248.

Silinskas, K. C., Kateley, S. A., Tower, J. E., Maher, V. M., and McCormick, J. J. (1981). *Cancer Res. 41,* 1620-1627.

Simon, L., Hazard, R. M., Maher, V. M., and McCormick, J. J. (1981). *Carcinogenesis (N.Y.) 2,* 567-570.

Sutherland, B. M., Cemino, J. S., Delihas, N., Shih, A. G., and Oliver, R. P. (1980). *Cancer Res. 40,* 1934-1939.

Sutherland, B. M., Delihas, N. C., Oliver, R. P., and Suther-
    land, J. C. (1981). *Cancer Res. 41*, 2211-2214.
Yang, L. L., Maher, V. M., and McCormick, J. J. (1980). *Proc.
    Natl. Acad. Sci. USA 77*, 5933-5937.
Yang, L. L., Maher, V. M., and McCormick, J. J. (1982). *Mutat.
    Res. 94*, 435-447.

17

IN VITRO TRANSFORMATION OF HUMAN CELLS: MODULATION OF EARLY GENE EXPRESSION PRECEDING CARCINOGEN-INDUCED EVENTS

George E. Milo

Department of Physiological Chemistry and
Comprehensive Cancer Center
The Ohio State University
Columbus, Ohio

I. INTRODUCTION

Many investigators have reported on the transformation of human cells *in vitro* by different types of carcinogenic insults (Milo and DiPaolo, 1978; Kakunaga, 1978, Zimmerman and Little, 1981; Namba, 1982; Maher *et al.*, 1982). Many of these investigators have treated the cells when they were proliferating

in a logarithmic stage of growth (Silinskas et $al.$, 1981;
Sutherland et $al.$, 1981; Namba, 1982). However Zimmerman and
Little (1981), Borek (1980), Greiner et $al.$, (1981), and Milo
and DiPaolo (1978, 1980), using either an amino acid-deficient
growth medium or a small amount of fetal bovine serum-
supplemented growth medium, blocked the cells in a G_1 stage of
the cell cycle, released the cells from the block, and treated
the cells with a carcinogen as they exhibited S-phase entry.

Data from Milo and DiPaolo (1980) suggest to us that cells
released from G_1 block and treated in G_2 (4.5 h) or M (1.5 h)
were not transformed by the carcinogen. Moreover, there is a
period in early G_1 that the cells are refractory (will not
respond to the carcinogenic insult). The movement of cells
from G_1 block in the cell cycle following release from the
block into S phase was determined to be 10 h in length. The
intracellular localization of a cell cycle-regulatory protein,
calmodulin (Yasuhanu and Hidaka, 1982; Cheung, 1982), was followed by indirect immunofluorescence, over the time of release of the cells from the G_1 block into S. For a 2-h period
of time prior to release of the cells from the G_1 block and 4 h
into S, the cells were treated every hour for 1 h with methylazoxymethanol acetate (MAMA). This carcinogen treatment during a 16-h time span was followed in order to discern whether
a programmed release of the cells from G_1 block would alter the
extent of carcinogenic response to the treatment as measured by
the expression of anchorage-independent growth of carcinogen-
treated cells.

II. METHODS OF PROCEDURE

A. Cell Cultures

Neonatal human foreskin fibroblast cell populations (HNF) were seeded into 25-cm^2 flasks and produced confluent monolayers in 48 h (Riegner *et al.*, 1976). The cells were serially passaged and the incremental radiolabeling index determined as a measure of the growth phase (Cristofalo and Sharf, 1973). The cultures were maintained in complete growth medium composed of Eagle's minimum essential medium (MEM) supplemented with nonessential amino acids, sodium pyruvate, gentocin, glutamine, 25 mM Hepes at pH 7.2 (Milo and DiPaolo, 1980), and 10% fetal bovine serum. The routine serial passaging of the cells at 1:4 split ratios was done in the aforementioned complete growth medium (CM).

B. Preparation of Cells for G_1 Block

To arrest the cell population in the late G_1 phase of the cell cycle 10 h prior to S phase, the logarithmically growing cell population at 70% confluent density was transferred by seeding the cells into a modified Dulbecco's minimum essential medium (DM) deficient in arginine and glutamine for 24 h. Dialyzed fetal bovine serum (d-FBS) was prepared by dialysis against DM deficient in arginine and glutamine. DM Was supplemented with 10% d-FBS over the 24-h period in G_1. Sister cultures were prepared for each time point, and one culture was treated with [*methyl*-^{3}H]thymidine (60 Ci/mmol) at 1.0 μCi/ml. Samples were taken every hour from the time the cultures went into the block until midway into S period 38 h later. The other sister culture was treated with the carcinogen in the G_1 block, at time of release from the block, and midway into S period. All of the cultures were incubated in a 4% carbon dioxide-enriched air atmosphere at 37°C.

C.   Chemical Preparation

   The chemicals of interest--insulin (IN at 0.5 U/ml) methylazoxymethanol acetate (MAMA), 7β,8α-dihydroxy-9α,10α-epoxy-
7,8,9,10-tetrahydrobenzo[a]pyrene (BPDE I), N-methyl-N-nitro-
N-nitrosoguanidine (MNNG), and benzamide (BZ)--were solvated in
either ethanol or acetone (Milo et al., 1981) and used immediately. MAMA (3.6 µg/ml), MNNG (0.5 µg/ml), or BPDE I
(0.114 µM) were added to the cultures at the time the cells
were released from the block. In addition, MNNG (Milo and
DiPaolo, 1980) and BPDE I (Tejwani et al., 1982) were added
when the cells were in S.

   Finally, MAMA was added at each hour for 1 h of treatment
from 2 h prior to the release point until the cells were 4 h
into S.   Benzamide was added at 1 mM final concentration at
the G_1 cell block period after release from the block, removed
at S-phase entry, and then added again in a sister culture at
S-phase entry.

D.   Transformation Regimen

   Proliferating cell populations at a cell density of 5000
cells/cm^2 were transferred from CM to DM minus arginine and
glutamine and blocked in G_1 (Milo and DiPaolo, 1980; Zimmerman
and Little, 1981). The cells were released from the block by
removal of DM medium and readdition of CM (plus deficient amino
acids) with and without IN, and 10 h later the cells exhibited
S-phase entry. Treatment with the carcinogen was carried out
as described previously. The treated populations were serially
passaged (Milo and DiPaolo, 1978; Zimmerman and Little, 1980;
Silinskas et al., 1981) into CM containing 8x nonessential amino acids and 2x vitamins for 20 PDL, and at this time the
treated cells were seeded into a semisolid medium to measure
anchorage-independent growth (0.33% agar).

E. Anchorage-Independent Growth

The treated populations were serially passaged into 2 ml of soft agar (0.33%) containing Dulbecco's modified lo-Cal medium (Biolabs, Northbrook, Illinois) supplemented with 20% FBS (Milo *et al.*, 1981) over a 5-ml 2% agar base containing McCoy's 5A supplemented as described previously (Milo *et al.*, 1981) with 20% FBS.

The treated cultures were kept at a high humidity in a 4% carbon dioxide-enriched atmosphere at 37°C. After 21 days, colonies that contained ≥50 cells/colony were scored as positive.

F. Assay for Neoplasia

After counting the colonies in soft agar they were removed, pooled, dispersed into single-cell suspensions, and seeded into 25-cm^2 flasks containing 2 ml of CM supplemented with growth additive and 10% FBS. These transformed populations were evaluated for their neoplastic potential in *nude* mice (Donahoe *et al.*, 1982). The *nude* mice were irradiated with 450 rads (from a ^{137}Cs source) prior to the injection of the transformed cells. After 6 weeks, tumors were counted and excised for histopathological evaluation.

G. Calmodulin Localization

Cells seeded at ∿10,000 cells/cm^2 were fixed in 3% phosphate buffer formalin at pH 7.2 for 30 min. The slides were then postfixed in methanol at 20°C for 10 min, rinsed with PBS, and indubated 1 h at 37°C with the primary antibody toward calmodulin. This antibody was prepared against rat testis calmodulin protein in sheep. After rinsing the fixed cultures extensively with PBS, the secondary reagent, FITC-conjugated rabbit anti-

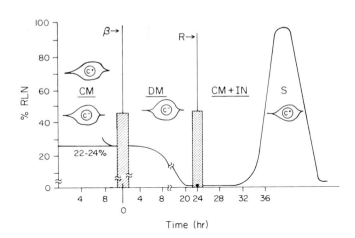

Fig. 1. Graphic representation of behavior of cells
leaving the block (R) G_1 traversing to S. β represents point
when proliferating cells in log growth are fed with DM minus
arginine, glutamine, and d-FBS. R is the point in time (h)
when the cells are released from the G_1 block and the incremental part of the cell population proceeds toward S phase of
the cell cycle. This population contains the maximum number
of cells that exhibit positively fluorescing antisera against
calmodulin localized in the nucleus at this time point. From
R to the time the population exhibits S-phase entry ([methyl-
³H]thymidine radiolabel nuclei), there is no further increase
in nuclei that fluoresce positive for the presence of calmodulin. S represents the point when the cell population enters
S phase of the cell cycle. The period R to S will be designated as S-phase entry time, and β to R will be designated as
G^1 transient period or late G_1 period.

sheep IgG, was incubated with the cells for 1 h at 37°C. Again
the slides were washed with PBS and examined under a Zeiss epi-
fluorescent microscope with 485-nm exciter filters and 520- to
560-nm barrier filters (Dedman et al., 1978; Markle et al.,
1981).

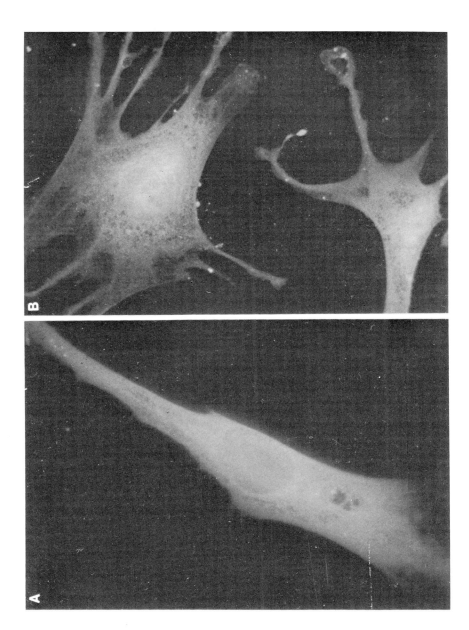

Fig. 2. (A) Photomicrograph of a fibroblast exhibiting fluorescence localized in the cytoplasm of the cell but not in the nuclear area (for the presence of calmodulin). The fluorescence is indicative of the localization of calmodulin in these cells when they are at point R (Figs. 1 and 3). (B) Localization of the fluorescence (calmodulin) in the nuclear area, and less intense fluorescence in the cytoplasmic area. These cells were evaluated 4 h after release from the block (DM, minus arginine and glutamine) (×35).

III.   RESULTS

Proliferating populations radiolabeled with $[methyl-^3H]$-
thymidine exhibited an incremental radiolabeling index from
22 to 24% (Fig. 1). When the CM medium over these populations
was replaced with DM (point β, Fig. 1), the radiolabeling index
(Cristofalo and Sharf, 1973) dropped to ≤0.1%. At point R
(Fig. 1), the DM medium was replaced with CM (Milo *et al.*,
1981), and IN was added to the CM. After 10 h the untreated
and treated cells exhibited S-phase entry (Milo and DiPaolo,
1980). Calmodulin, a cell-regulatory protein (Cheung, 1982)
associated with cell proliferation, localizes in the nucleus
before the cells enter S.   The protein can be located intra-
cellularly by indirect immunofluorescence, and following release of the cells from the block 2 h later fluorescence
staining properties for calmodulin were observed in the cytoplasm of the cells (Fig. 2A). Four hours later, the nuclei
fluoresced positive for the presence of the protein (Fig. 2B).
Six hours after release from the block the maximum number of
positive fluorescing calmodulin nuclei were observed. No
further increases in the number of positive fluorescing calmodulin nuclei (Table I) were found after the 6-h lapse of time.
We followed these events to S-phase entry, $(G_1^{10-11\ h})$. Concomitantly we examined the radiolabeling index over this same
time period. At G_1^{0-1} the radiolabeling index was ≤0.1%. At
G_1^{10-11} the incremental radiolabeling index increased from
≤0.1 to 3%, and at S^{13-14} the 1-hr Δ radiolabeling index was
28% for IN-treated cells.

Treatment of the sister cell populations with the carcinogens MNNG, BPDE I, and MAMA was initiated at G_1^{0-1} and S^{12-13}
following release of the cells from the block (Point R, Fig. 3).
Transformation was measured after 20 population doublings by
the ability of the treated cells to grow in soft agar (as

TABLE I.   The number of Calmodulin-Positive Fluorescing
           Nuclei Followed as a Function of Time of
           Release from the Block

% Calmodulin Fluorescing Nuclei[a]

$-IN^{c}$	$+IN^{c}$	Time in $G_1^{t-t_1}$ [b]
0	0	G_1^{0-1}
1	2	G_1^{3-4}
25	50	G_1^{6}
30	52	G_1^{8-9}
31	51	G_1^{9-10}
33	50	G_1^{10-11}

[a]*The number of calmodulin-positive fluorescing nuclei/
number of nonfluorescing nuclei × 100 expressed as a percentage.*
[b]*The notation G_1^{0-1} to G_1^{10-11} refers to the G_1 part
of the cell cycle, and $t-t_1$ was used to describe the beginning and end of the sampling time in hours following release from the block at point R (Fig. 1).*
[c]*-IN, Cultures released from the block receiving no
insulin treatment; +IN, sister cultures receiving insulin
treatment. These values are mean values for three readings.*

described herein). The number of colonies observed from G_1^{0-1}-
treated populations treated with MNNG, BPDE I, and MAMA was
zero (undetectable). At point G_1^{6-7}, when the optimum number
of calmodulin-positive nuclei were observed (Table I), the incidence of anchorage-independent growth of these carcinogen-
treated cells was 18 ± 3.0 for MAMA-treated cells, 0.0 for
MNNG-treated cells (undetected), and 0.0 for BPDE-I-treated
cells (undetected). When the populations were treated with the
carcinogen at S-phase entry (G_1 + S^{10-11}) with either BPDE I or
MNNG, the colony-forming incidence of these treated cells in
soft agar was 26 colonies/10^5 BPDE I-treated cells (Tejwani *et*

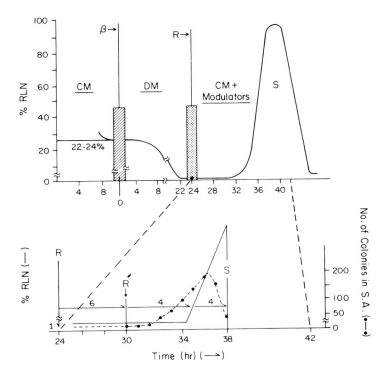

Fig. 3. The percentage of radiolabeled nuclei (% RLN) was plotted as a function of time following release from the cell cycle block at 24 h. The sections were divided into 6-h and 4-h periods. Six hours after release from the block at R' the maximum number of calmodulin-positive fluorescing nuclei was determined. The carcinogen treatment period was for 1 h in length from R' to S, 6-18 h after R (4 h into S). The number of colonies per 50,000 cells seeded into soft agar (S.A.) was plotted as a function of the length of treatment (1 h) at various time points, 30-38 h. These are mean values for three wells (see footnotes to Table II). The data presented here represent a combination of data from Table II and Fig. 1.

al., 1982) and 2.0 colonies/10^5 MNNG-treated cells (Milo *et al.*, 1981). When MAMA was used to treat populations at S-phase entry for 12 h we observed 700 colonies/10^5 cells (Kuhn *et al.*, 1982).

We therefore decided to titrate sister populations (Table II) with MAMA from G_1^{0-1} through to S^{13-14}. We treated the

TABLE II. Comparison of Treatment Time Following Release from G_1 Block (Hour R) into S Phase of the Cell Cycle with Number of Colonies that Exhibit Anchorage-Independent Growth

Number of colonies expressing anchorage-independent growth[a]		
$-IN^b$	$+IN^c$	Time $G_1{}^{t-t_1} + S^{t-t_1}{}^d$
0	0	$G_1{}^{0-1}$
0	0	$G_1{}^{3-4}$
1.4 ± 1.5	18 ± 3.0	$G_1{}^{6-7}$
1.4 ± 1.5	15 ± 2.3	$G_1{}^{7-8}$
1.4 ± 1.5	30 ± 17.0	$G_1{}^{8-9}$
20.3 ± 9.2	45 ± 3.1	$G_1{}^{9-10}$
12.3 ± 0.6	36 ± 2.5	$G_1 + S^{10-11}$
10.3 ± 3.5	150 ± 27.0	S^{11-12}
9.5 ± 3.0	271 ± 15.7	S^{12-13}
8.0 ± 0.0	65 ± 4.0	S^{13-14}

[a]*Treated cells (50,000) at 20 PDL were seeded into 2 ml of 0.33% agar overlayer over 5 ml of 2.0%. The growth medium in the agar overlayer was Dulbecco's lo-Cal medium (Milo et al., 1981) over McCoy's 5A in the 2.0% base; each contained supplements and FBS as described in Section II. Untreated cells seeded in the same manner yielded no colonies from 10^5 cells.*

[b]*The cells were released from the G_1 block, and no IN was added prior to administration of the carcinogen MAMA.*

[c]*The cells were released from the block and IN added prior to the administration of the carcinogen. The values reported here are mean values for three wells $\pm$ 1 standard deviation.*

[d]*The designation $G_1{}^{t-t_1} + S^{t-t_1}$ was used to describe the phase of the cell cycle such as G_1 or S, and the superscript $t-t_1$ is the beginning and end of the treatment time with carcinogen during that phase of the cell cycle. For example, $G_1{}^{0-1}$ is the time in G_1 when the cells were released from the block and were treated for 1 h. At this time the 1-h Δ radiolabeling index, using [methyl-^3H]thymidine (Milo and DiPaolo, 1980), was <0.01%. At the time of treatment, S^{13-14}, the incremental radiolabeling index was 22% for -IN carcinogen-treated cultures and 28% for +IN treated cultures.*

cells from the time of release, G_1^{0-1} for 1 h duration at each
hour up to S^{13-14}, that is, 13-14 h after release from G_1
(point R, Fig. 1 or Fig. 3). Over this time period we found
that -IN + MAMA-treated cells did not exhibit an increase in
colony formation in soft agar for G_1^{6-7}-treated populations
over the G_1^{0-1} period; that is, no colonies were found in soft
agar. Later, at S^{12-13} time period there was an increase in
colony formation to 9.5 ± 3.0 colonies per 50,000 seeded cells.
Insulin pretreatment of cells to be treated with MAMA at time
point S^{12-13} resulted in the formation of 271 ± 15.7 colonies
per 50,000 seeded cells (Table II). The 1-hr Δ radiolabeling
index at this time point was 28% (see footnotes to Table II).
At S^{13-14} treatment period there was a substantial decrease
from 271 ± 15.7 colonies to 65 ± 4.0 colonies. However, the
1-h incremental radiolabeling index increased to 75%. We did
not at this time carry the experiments beyond this point.

Previous experiments (Milo *et al.*, 1981), with treatments
in the later part of S with MAMA, MNNG, or BPDE I, prove that
the treated cells in this time period were less responsive to
the carcinogenic insult; that is, the treated cells did not
exhibit anchorage-independent growth. The relationship between
the release of the cells from the blocks and treatment regimen
with MAMA presented in Fig. 3 illustrates the profile of colony
formation versus treatment time (Table II) over a 14-h treatment period of time. Table II is a graphic representation of
the treatment regimen from point R through to midway into S.
Furthermore, data not presented here have revealed that the
carcinogenic response can be interfered with following the carcinogen treatment with BZ. Benzamide at 1 m*M*, added to the
cells at point R and removed at S (Fig. 3), reduced the number
of colonies formed to 67% of non-BZ-treated MAMA-treated cells.
When BZ was added at point $G_1 + S^{10-11}$ and removed at S^{14} (i.e.,
4 h later into S), it reduced the MAMA-induced colony-forming

frequency in soft agar from 10^3 colonies/10^5 seeded cells to
<2 colonies/10^5 cells (Kun and Milo, 1982). The 1-h Δ radio-
labeling index of BZ carcinogen-treated cells over the treatment time was not altered when compared to the sister MAMA-
treated cultures containing no BZ. There was no apparent cytotoxicity exhibited by the 1 mM BZ-treated cultures or change
in finite population doublings of these BZ-treated cells
(35 ± 5 population doublings). BZ-treated cell populations
would not grow in soft agar. Injection of the MAMA-transformed
cells into a *nude* mouse yielded a tumor that was excised from
the mouse and evaluated as an undifferentiated mesenchymal tumor. The frequency of tumor formation was two tumors per
16 mice that receive the injection (Donahoe *et al.*, 1982).

IV. DISCUSSION

   The transformation of human foreskin fibroblasts by carcinogen insults appears to be an operational phenomenon that
is logistically reproducible. There are several reports in
the literature that randomly proliferating cell populations
can be transformed following carcinogen administration
(Kakunaga, 1978, Sutherland, 1981, Maher *et al.*, 1982; Namba,
1982). There are reports also by other investigators that
blocking human diploid cell populations in G_1 by specific amino acid deprivation (Milo and DiPaolo, 1978, 1980; Zimmerman
and Little, 1981; Greiner *et al.*, 1981) or by reducing the fetal bovine serum requirement (Borek, 1980) followed by the addition of modulators (compounds that modify intracellular biochemical events without damage to the DNA), enhances the carcinogenic response. The heightened response to the carcinogen
treatment of the cells following treatment with the modulators
such as IN during the late G_1 phase of the cell cycle and into

S permits us to probe the system with the carcinogen to identify the time of optimum response to the carcinogen. Maher *et
al.* (1982) have found, using 6-thioguanine mutagenic selection
procedures, that the slope changes immediately prior to S-phase
entry, and there appears to be a correlation between the number
of mutants observed at this time and the number of transformants (express anchorage-independent growth).

We (Tejwani *et al.*, 1982) completed carcinogen-DNA adduct
studies on cell populations that will either respond to the carcinogenic insult and will exhibit anchorage-independent growth
(responsive) or will not exhibit anchorage-independent growth
(refractory). We found, in responsive cells treated with
BPDE I in early S, the period of heightened responsiveness to
carcinogen insult, that the carcinogen-dG adduct formation compared to refractory treated populations was quite similar.
Furthermore, the persistence of adducts in the refractory or
responsive carcinogen-treated cells over a 24-h period did not
appear to be a logical mechanism to explain why we observe the
differences in formation of colonies in soft agar, for BP-DNA
binding did not change in either treated cell population over
this time period. Moreover, Zimmerman and Little (1981) suggest that specific amino acid deprivation may contribute to
heighten response to the carcinogen treatment. This may indeed
occur; however, responsive or refractory cells, both those
blocked in G_1 by amino acid deprivation and those released from
the block in G_1, show no statistical significant differences in
binding of the radiolabel carcinogen to the DNA.

Maher *et al.* (1982) have shown that there is a dose-
dependent mutagenic response to UV light (254 nm) when cells
were treated in late G_1 3 h prior to onset of S and these
treated cell populations were examined for their capability to
grow in soft agar. It is interesting to note that the cells we
have treated with MAMA at 10 h prior to onset of DNA synthesis

exhibit anchorage-independent growth, whereas MNNG and BPDE I
treated cells do not exhibit this characteristic. In all
three treatments with BPDE I, MNNG, and MAMA, the time of optimum responsiveness to the carcinogenic insult appears to be
2-3 h into S. This response appears to be wiped out by BZ
treatment, lowering the expression of anchorage-independent
growth from ~700 colonies/10^5 treated cells seeded in soft
agar to <2 colonies/10^5 cells. Furthermore, we (Kuhn *et al*.,
1982) have found that BZ ameliorates the poly(ADP)ribosylase-
phosphorylated modification of acidic nuclear proteins of responsive cells.

We suspect that a complex series of events occurs in a
programmed manner as a function of time from the time of adding
a modulator through to the expression of the early carcinogenic
events. If, for example, one of these events is modified by
the administration of BZ while DNA damage, persistence of adducts, and repair of damage is in process, the cell responds
to the insult as a reversible or irreversible toxic event. We
propose that modification of nuclear protein covering the carcinogenic site sets in motion events leading to the expression
of a carcinogenic response (precancerous state), followed by an
expression of anchorage-independent growth and neoplastic potential. This of course presupposes that the correct genetic
damage (carcinogen-DNA adduct) was formed, and "error-prone
repair" is functional in S followed by chromosomal transposi-
tion (Klein, 1981). In any event, calmodulin, a cell-regulatory
protein in this system, apparently is active in the nucleus, is
expressed early in late G_1 prior to the onset of scheduled DNA
synthesis, and prefaces any subsequent event leading to cellular proliferation and fixation of the genetic damage in expression of a carcinogenic event.

V.   SUMMARY

Human foreskin fibroblast populations blocked in G_1, released, and treated with methylazoxymethanol acetate (MAMA)
from the time of release (late G_1) for 1-h treatment intervals
until 4 h into S, exhibited a differential sensitivity to MAMA
treatment at the different treatment times. A heightened response to the carcinogen treatment was not detected until calmodulin, a cell-regulatory protein, was optimally present in
the nuclei of the late G_1-treated cells 6 h after release from
the G_1 block. Moreover, there was a distinct increase in the
number of transformed phenotypes (cells that will grow in soft
agar), observed when the cells were treated with MAMA at the
onset of scheduled DNA synthesis. The time at which these
treated cells were optimally responsive to a carcinogenic insult was 12-13 h after release from the block 2-3 h into S.
Interestingly, this was followed by a decrease in the expression of anchorage-independent growth when the cells were
treated 13-14 h after release from the block 4 h into S. Benzamide interfered in the process when added at the onset of S,
and the resultant carcinogen-treated population did not exhibit
a comparable increase in expression of anchorage-independent
growth. Cells treated with MAMA at the point of release from
the block G_1^{0-1} to G_1^{3-4} did not express anchorage-independent
growth.

It is proposed that the heightened presence of calmodulin
in the nuclei 4 h prior to the onset of scheduled DNA synthesis
is a cell-regulatory function that sets in motion a complex
series of events (program) in carcinogen-initiated human fibroblasts that leads to a subsequent carcinogenic response.

ACKNOWLEDGMENT

We would like to acknowledge the assistance of Mrs. Inge Noyes for her technical assistance. This work was supported in part by AFSOR F 49620-80 and NIH-NCI P-30-CA-16058-09.

REFERENCES

Borek, C. (1980). *Nature (London) 283,* 776-778.
Cheung,   . (1982). *Ann. N.Y. Acad. Sci. 207,* 19-27.
Cristofalo, V., and Sharf, B. (1973). *Exp. Cell Res. 76,* 419-427.
Dedman, F. R., Welsh, M. J., and Means, A. (1978). *J. Biol. Chem. 253,* 7515-7521.
Donahoe, J., Noyes, I., Milo, G. E., and Weisbrode, S. E. (1982). *In Vitro 18,* 429-434.
Greiner, J. W., Evans, C. H., and DiPaolo, J. A. (1981). *Carcinogenesis (N.Y.) 2,* 359-362.
Kakunaga, T. (1978). *Proc. Natl. Acad. Sci. USA 75,* 1334-1338.
Klein, G. (1981). *Nature (London) 294,* 313-318.
Kun, E., Minaga, T., Kristen, E., Jackowski, G., Peller, L., Marton, L., Oredsson, S. M., and Milo, G. E. (1982). "Steinbock-Lily Symposium." Madison, Wisconsin.
Maher, V. M., Rowan, L. A., Silinskas, C., Kateley, S., and McCormick, J. (1982). *Proc. Natl. Acad. Sci. USA 79,* 2613-2617.
Markle, N. J., Dedman, J. R., Means, A. R., Chafouleas, F. G., and Sater, B. H. (1981). *J. Cell Biol. 89,* 695-699.
Milo, G. E., and DiPaolo, J. A. (1978). *Nature (London) 275,* 130-132.
Milo, G. E., and DiPaolo, J. A. (1980). *Int. J. Cancer 275,* 805-812.
Milo, G. E., Oldham, J., Zimmerman, R., Hatch, R., and Weisbrode, S. (1981). *In Vitro 17,* 719-729.
Namba, M., Fukushima, F., and Kimoto, T. (1982). *In Vitro 18,* 469-475.
Riegner, D., McMichael, T., Berno, J., and Milo, G. E. (1976). *Tissue Cult. Assoc. Man. 2,* 273-276.
Silinskas, K. C., Kateley, S. A., Tower, J. E., Maher, V. M., and McCormick, J. J. (1981). *Cancer Res. 41,* 1620-1627.
Sutherland, B. M., Delihas, N. C., Oliver, R. P., and Sutherland, J. C. (1981). *Cancer Res. 41,* 2211-2214.
Tejwani, R., Jeffrey, A. M., and Milo, G. E. (1982). *Carcinogenesis 37,* 727-732.

Yasuhanu, S., and Hidaka, H. (1982). *Biochem. Biophys. Res. Commun.* *104*, 451–456.

Zimmerman, R. J., and Little, J. B. (1981). *Carcinogenesis (N.Y.)* *2*, 1303–1310.

18

EFFECT OF DIMETHYLNITROSAMINE (DMNA) ON TARGET CELLS IN HUMAN PANCREAS EXPLANT

Ismail Parsa and Albert L. Sutton

State University of New York
Downstate Medical Center
Brooklyn, New York

I.   INTRODUCTION

Human pancreatic carcinoma, a fatal disease with no known cause, has been the subject of intensive studies. Environmental chemicals, and in particular nitrosamines and nitroso compounds, are considered possible factors in the development of human pancreatic carcinoma. This is supported in part by the

actions of these compounds in experimental pancreatic carcinogenesis in rodents. Druckrey and co-workers (1968) induced
pancreatic carcinoma in the guinea pig by methylnitrosourea
and methylnitrosourethane. The carcinogenic effect of methylnitrosourea was further demonstrated in the inbred strain 13
of the guinea pig model of pancreas carcinogenesis by Reddy
and Rao (1975). The tumorigenic effects of β-oxidized nitrosamine on Syrian hamster pancreas have been described (Kruger
et al., 1974; Pour et al., 1974; Mohr et al., 1977; Scarpelli
and Rao, 1979).

The majority of pancreatic carcinomas in humans are
classified as duct cell carcinoma, and on the basis of morphological appearance, embryological development, and the pattern of acinar cell differentiation, they are considered to
originate from preexisting ductal or ductular cells (Cubilla
and Fitzgerald, 1975; Morgan and Wormsley, 1977; Webb, 1977).
The diversity in experimental models of pancreas carcinoma and
the interpretation of experimental results in these models with
respect to histogenesis of pancreatic cancer have generated
serious controversy as to the origin of pancreatic carcinoma.
The controversy about the cell of origin in rodent pancreatic
carcinoma has often extended to human pancreatic tumors. Ductal adenocarcinoma was induced in Syrian hamster by β-oxidized
derivatives of N,N-dipropylnitrosamine. Numerous morphological
(Kruger et al., 1974; Pour et al., 1974, 1975, 1976, 1977,
1978) and ultrastructural (Altoff et al., 1976; Levitt et al.,
1977, 1978; Takahashi et al., 1977) studies of this model suggest the preexisting ductal and ductular cells as progenitors
of ductal adenocarcinoma.

Acinar cell carcinoma in the rat has been induced by
4-hydroxyaminoquinolone 1-oxide (Hayashi and Hasegawa, 1971),
azaserine (Longnecker and Curphy, 1975), nafenopin (Reddy and
Rao, 1977), and implantation of 7,12-dimethylbenz[a]anthracene

in pancreas (Dissin et al., 1975). The degree of differentiation of acinar cell tumors in rat and guinea pig (Reddy and
Rao, 1975) is reported to vary extensively according to the
carcinogen. The histogenesis of these tumors, however, is invariably reported to have a similar pathway, that is, degeneration of acinar cells with the loss of apical cytoplasm, dilatation of acinar lumen, and formation of ductlike structures
(pseudoductules) lined by acinar cells that may or may not contain zymogen granules (Reddy and Rao, 1975; Longnecker and
Curphy, 1975; Shinozuka et al., 1976; Bockman et al., 1978;
Rao and Reddy, 1980).

A potent carcinogen in rodents (Magee and Barnes, 1956,
1962), DMNA, can be produced in mammalian stomach under favorable conditions and is shown to be present at a low concentration in the blood of normal human volunteers. It is converted
by metabolism to an alkylating agent (Magee et al., 1973) able
to form covalent adducts with nucleophilic sites of macromolecules such as DNA, RNA, and proteins, DNA-carcinogen adducts
are most likely to bring about heritable genetic changes in
target cells and generate preneoplastic cells as steps toward
the development of neoplasia and carcinoma. Furthermore,
DMNA is reported to form adducts with nuclear proteins (histone
and nonhistone), and often to a greater extent and with a
longer half-life than with nuclear DNA. The persistence of
alkylated bases in DNA, particularly O-alkylated bases, is
thought to lead to cell transformation with a frequency that is
inversely related to their rate of removal (Kleihues and
Margison, 1974; Goth and Rajewsky, 1974a,b).

The induction of carcinoma in organ-cultured adult human
pancreas explants by DMNA was reported by this laboratory
(Parsa et al., 1981). DMNA Induced both ductal hyperplasia and
atypia within 6 weeks and carcinoma in 10 weeks. In this model,
within the first week of DMNA treatment, alteration of acinar

structures, degeneration and necrosis of some acinar cells, loss of apical cytoplasm, dilatation of acinar lumens, and proliferation of cells devoid of zymogen granules within the acinar complex were observed.

Monoclonal antibody to acinar cell surface, developed in this laboratory (Parsa, 1981), permitted the identification of normal and neoplastic acinar cells including undifferentiated tumors ultrastructurally devoid of zymogen granules or measurable amylase activity. We reported the development of a monoclonal antibody to duct cell surface determinant, allowing identification of duct cell (main duct, smaller ducts, and ductules) and the establishment of duct cell surface markers in six of six human pancreatic adenocarcinomas and one undifferentiated human pancreatic carcinoma (Parsa et al., 1982).

The distribution of [methyl-^{14}C]DMNA in organ-cultured adult human pancreas explants has been reported (Parsa and Butt, 1982). Autoradiographic sections of explants 6 h after exposure to [methyl-^{14}C]DMNA revealed a random pattern of grain distribution over nuclei and cytoplasm of all cell types. Selective concentration of grains was observed after 36 h incubation of labeled explants in the absence of DMNA and was pronounced by 72 h. The grains representing nucleic acid-carcinogen adducts appeared to persist over cells devoid of zymogen granules. Toward the establishment of the identity of cells with persistent labeled adducts, presumably progenitor cells of cancer in this system, we have used a combination of labeled carcinogen, monoclonal antibodies to acinar and ductal cell surface markers, autoradiography, and fluorescent microscopy. This chapter describes the identification of target cells in this model.

II. MATERIALS AND METHODS

A. Human Pancreas

Human pancreas including tail and a portion of body was obtained from four cadaveric donors, ages 30-55 years, who had no pancreatic disease. The warm ischemia time ranged from 5 to 15 min. The pancreases were cooled on removal and kept at 0 to 5°C for as long as 2 h before being cultured.

B. Organ Culture

The main pancreatic duct of each pancreas was opened by a longitudinal incision and was dissected out from the rest of the pancreas along with 4 to 5 mm of surrounding parenchyma. Explants of 1 mm thickness were prepared by cuts perpendicular to the main pancreatic duct. Thus each explant included a portion of the main pancreatic duct and its surrounding parenchyma (ducts, ductules, acini, and occasional endocrine islets). Four to eight explants were placed on a 4 × 100-mm strip of Millipore filter (Millipore Corp., Catalog No. HAWP-304-FO). As many as two strips were floated on 10 ml of prewarmed (37°C) medium in a roller tube (Bellco, Vineland, New Jersey, Catalog No. 7733-10535). The medium was a chemically defined medium (Parsa *et al.*, 1970) modified by the addition of 10 mg/liter of ascorbic acid and 8 mg/liter of bovine pancreas crystalline insulin (Sigma Chemical Co.). The roller tubes were incubated at 37°C in an atmosphere of 100% CO_2 in air saturated with water vapor and rotated at 0.5 rpm. The medium was changed daily during the first 4 days and biweekly thereafter.

C. DMNA

At the initiation of culture, 20 μg/ml of [*methyl*-^{14}C]DMNA, specific activity 15 Ci/mM (Amersham Co., Arlington Heights,

Illinois), were added to each roller vessel. DMNA (K & K
Laboratories, Inc., New York, New York) was added to the medium
twice a week after the fourth day of culture.

D. Microscopic Preparation

Cultured explants were fixed in Bouin's fluid, embedded
in paraffin, and cut at 2 to 4 μm thickness. Sections were
stained with hematoxylin and eosin or processed for autoradiography and/or fluorescence microscopy.

E. Autoradiography

Explants cultured for 2 h in the presence of 20 μg/ml of
$[methyl-^{14}C]$DMNA were washed three times with the medium containing no DMNA and incubated further in medium without DMNA
for 0, 12, 24, 36, 48, 72, 96, and 144 h. At each time point,
four explants were processed for autoradiography. The procedure was previously described in detail (Fitzgerald et al.,
1968b; Parsa et al., 1969). Sections 2-4 mm thick were used
with Kodak NTB-2 liquid emulsion. After 2 weeks of exposure,
autoradiographs were developed with D19 and stained with methyl
green thionin (Roque et al., 1965). Cells with more than two
silver grains were counted as positive. The average number of
silver grains per cell and the average number of grains per
positive cell were calculated for each time point.

F. Monoclonal Antibodies

AC1 antibody to acinar cell surface marker (Parsa, 1981)
and HP-DU-1 antibody to duct cell surface determinant (Parsa
et al., 1982) were diluted 1:200 and 1:400, respectively, with
phosphate-buffered saline (PBS) before use.

G. Fluorescence Microscopy

Tissue sections were deparaffinized in xylene, gradually hydrated (ethanol: 100, 95, 60, 40, and 30%), and placed in PBS, pH 7.2 for 10 min. Sections were then incubated in mono-clonal antibody or PBS (as control) for 30 min at room tempera-ture followed by three washes with PBS, incubated in fluorescein-conjugated goat anti-mouse IgG for 30 min at room temperature, rinsed three times with PBS, coverslip-mounted with glycerol, and examined for fluorescence. Autoradiographic sections were prepared for fluorescence microscopy after exami-nation for localization of silver grains by incubation in PBS at 60°C for 30 min to dissolve the emulsion, and then incu-bated with antibody.

III. RESULTS

A. Cultured Explants

Cultured explants showed great variation in the degree of degeneration, necrosis, and morphological alterations with each pancreas. There were no significant changes during the first 24 h. Degeneration of some acinar cells became apparent by the end of the second day of culture while other acinar cells re-mained intact. Gradual loss of apical cytoplasm and dilatation of acinar lumens occurred during the first week. Loss of zy-mogen granules even in the preserved acinar cells was a promi-nent feature of DMNA-treated explants during the first week. Ductal and ductular cell degeneration was minimal. Prolifera-tion of the main duct epithelium forming papillary projections was present.

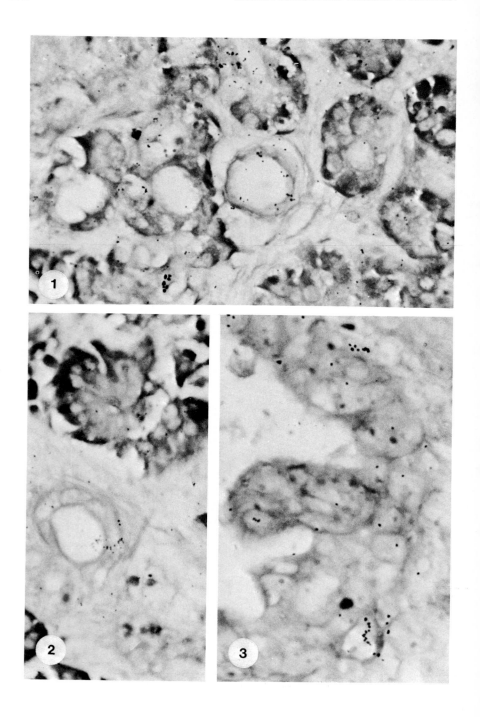

B. $^{14}CH_3$ Distribution

Autoradiographs from explants cultured for 2 h in the presence of [methyl-^{14}C]DMNA and those labeled for 2 h and further incubated for 6 h in the absence of DMNA showed a random pattern of distribution of silver grains over nuclei and cytoplasm of all cell types with an average of 7.6 grains/cell, although some cells (acinar and ductal) showed up to 30 grains. The average number of grains per cell declined rapidly to 5.9, 4.3, 3.7, 1.9, 0.2, and 0.2 after 12, 24, 36, 48, 72, and 96 h of incubation, respectively, in the absence of DMNA. In contrast, the average number of grains per positive cell (2 or more grains) showed a much slower decrease. As early as 36 h after incubation, a selective concentration of grains on some cells was apparent (9.3 grains/positive cell) (Fig. 1). The concentration of the grains on some cells persisted after 96 h of incubation (Figs. 2 and 3).

C. Fluorescence Microscopy

In more than 160 explants of various time points examined with fluorescence microscopy, AC1 specifically delineated acinar cells (Fig. 4). Degenerated acinar cells even after the loss of apical cytoplasm and zymogen granules showed positive surface fluorescence with AC1 (Fig. 5). HP-DU-1 antibody was specific for ductal epithelium and showed strong fluorescence

Fig. 1. Autoradiograph from explant labeled for 2 h with [14C]DMNA and then incubated for 36 h in control medium showing silver grains concentrated on ductal and centroacinar cells (×400).

Fig. 2. Autoradiograph from explant, 96 h after labeling; silver grains are noted on one of the ductular epithelial cells (×400).

Fig. 3. Portion of a large duct 96 h after labeling, with aggregates of silver grains on three of the epithelial lining cells (×800).

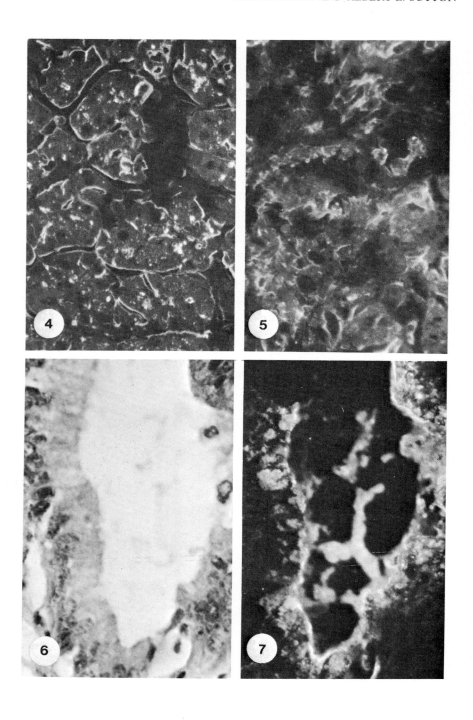

even with intraluminal ghost cells (Figs. 6 and 7). In all of
the 20 autoradiographs stained with HP-DU-1 after removal of
emulsion it was possible to distinguish between the ductular
cells and pseudoductular structures (Figs. 8 and 9).

IV. DISCUSSION

Like several other types of chemical carcinogens, DMNA
requires for its activation to an alkylating agent a metabolic
process involving enzymatic activity of target cells or other
cells in the target organ. The carcinogenicity of the activated compound, however, requires direct action on macromolecules of target cells. The ability of the pancreas to activate
carcinogens metabolically has been demonstrated in rat, hamster,
and guinea pig. Azaserine and N-(N-methyl-N-nitroso-carbamyl)-
L-ornithine have been reported to produce persistent DNA damage
in rat pancreas 1 h after administration (Lilja et al., 1977).
Similarly, the activation of nitrosamines in hamster was demonstrated by Scarpelli et al. (1980). DNA damage induced by
4-hydroxyaminoquinoline 1-oxide (Iqbal et al., 1976), N-methyl-
N-nitrosourethane (Iqbal and Epstein, 1978) in guinea pig pancreas, and metabolic activation of benzo[a]pyrene by the microsomal fraction of the guinea pig pancreas (Iqbal et al., 1977)
were described. The capability of human pancreatic duct to

Fig. 4. Fluorescent micrograph from explant labeled with
[14C]DMNA showing acinar cell surface fluorescence with AC1
antibody (×400).
Fig. 5. Fluorescent micrograph 96 h postlabeling, showing
surface fluorescence of degenerating acinar cells with AC1 (×400).
Fig. 6. Hematoxylin and eosin micrograph of portion of a
large duct (×800).
Fig. 7. Fluorescent micrograph of duct shown in Fig. 4,
demonstrating ductal cell surface fluorescence with HP-DU-1
antibody (×800).

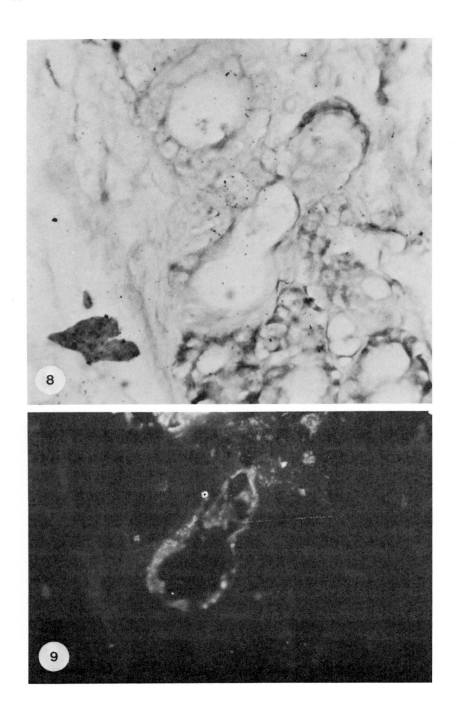

activate benzo[a]pyrene and 7,12-dimethylbenz[a]anthracene metabolically in culture was demonstrated by Harris and co-workers (1977). The present data further establish the ability of pancreatic epithelium to metabolize DMNA in organ culture.

An important consideration in analyzing the carcinogenic effects of chemical agents is that the modification of DNA is nonrandom. When tested with DMNA (Gronow, 1980), certain regions of DNA were disproportionately reactive with the carcinogen. It is significant that the accessibility of DNA sequences to carcinogens correlates with their accessibility to nuclease probes of chromatin structure. It follows that shielding of the DNA through association with histone and nonhistone proteins is likely to be a factor in the carcinogenic response. The role and the proportion of alkylated nuclear proteins in the present model is yet to be established.

The selective localization of $^{14}CH_3$ from labeled DMNA on ductular epithelium and its persistence after 6 days on the proliferating ductal lining suggest that the progenitor cells of carcinoma in this model are included in ductal epithelium and share antigenic determinants with ductal cells. A random pattern of distribution of $^{14}CH_3$ within 2 h of exposure to DMNA indicates that both ductal and acinar cells are capable of metabolizing DMNA. The accelerated degeneration and necrosis of acinar cells treated with DMNA appeared nonrandom, and indeed in spite of the loss of zymogen granules some acini were preserved better and longer than control explants (Parsa et al., 1981). This paradoxal effect may be attributed to the

Fig. 8. Autoradiograph from explant 72 h after labeling, showing silver grains on ductular cell lining. Pseudoductules are negative for silver grains (right lower corner) (×800).

Fig. 9. Fluorescent micrograph of ductules and pseudoductules, showing ductular cell surface fluorescence with HP-DU-1 antibody (×800).

toxicity of DMNA for some acinar cells and its trophic effect
on others, to be distinguished from acinar cell degeneration
and necrosis, which occurs upon change in environment (e.g.,
from *in vivo* to organ culture).

The cytotoxicity of chemical carcinogens, which may be
important for the development of neoplasia, often overshadows
their carcinogenic effect. It is considered that a chemical
carcinogen triggers a series of events in the cells of the
target organ that eventually, under "favorable" conditions,
lead to the appearance of malignancy. The sequence of events
begins with "initiation," that is, the induction of a new cell
type that can selectively proliferate and evolve from progenitor cells through preneoplastic and premalignant stages to
malignant tumor. Although the induction of a heritable lesion
is attributed to the effects of a chemical carcinogen on
nuclear DNA, the mitotic activity in embryonic, fetal, neonatal,
and regenerating organs is considered to be of importance in the
evolution of initiated cells to cancer. Thus the process of regeneration in a differentiated parenchymal organ such as pancreas may be an important factor in the development of pancreatic cancer (Konishi *et al.*, 1978).

It follows that the probability of the development of neoplasia in a regenerating parenchymal cell population is increased provided it contains the target cells and/or the
initiated cells. The process of regeneration per se, however,
is not sufficient to produce cancer. Such is the case with the
effect of ethionine on the acinar cell of rat pancreas
(Fitzgerald *et al.*, 1968a,b), wherein degeneration followed by
regeneration does not lead to an increased rate of acinar cell
carcinoma, even though ethionine is considered a potent hepatocarcinogen in the rat. Acinar changes in response to DMNA include loss of apical cytoplasm and zymogen granules, and dilatation of acinar lumens, resulting in the formation of "pseudo-

ductules," followed by partial regeneration. These changes may merely reflect the vulnerability of acinar cells to the toxic effects of carcinogens, unrelated to their carcinogenicity. Therefore, these changes are not sufficient to consider the acinar cell as the progenitor cell of cancer in this model. The presence of duct cell determinants on labeled cells in the present chapter and the demonstration of the same determinants on pancreatic carcinoma cells from seven patients (Parsa *et al.*, 1982; Parsa, 1982) strongly suggest that the progenitor cells of tumors induced by DMNA in this model are of ductal epithelium.

ACKNOWLEDGMENTS

In support of the acinar cell origin of pancreatic cell cancer, it has been postulated that during the carcinogenic process, the acinar cell is capable of dedifferentiating into a totipotential cell with the option to give rise to either ductal or acinar cell carcinoma of the pancreas. Although this postulate has its merits, there is no evidence thus far to support the acinar cell origin of ductal adenocarcinoma in humans. This work was supported in part by the NCI Grants 1RO1 CA3035401 and 2R26 CA 22682.

REFERENCES

Altoff, J., Pour, P., Malick, L., and Wilson, R. B. (1976). *Am. J. Pathol. 83,* 517-530.
Bockman, D. E., Black, O., Jr., Mills, L. R., and Webster, P. D. (1978). *Am. J. Pathol. 90,* 645-658.
Cubilla, A. L., and Fitzgerald, P. J. (1975). *Cancer Res. 35,* 2234-2248.
Dissin, J., Mills, L. R., Mainz, D. L., Black, O., Jr., and Webster, P. D., III (1975). *J. Natl. Cancer Inst. (U.S.) 55,* 857-864.
Druckrey, H., Ivankovic, S., Bucheler, J., Preussmann, R., and Thomas, C. (1968). *Z. Krebsforsch. 71,* 167-182.

Fitzgerald, P. J., Herman, L., Carol, B., Roque, A., Marsh,
    W. H., Rosenstock, L., Richardson, C., and Pearl, D.
    (1968a). *J. Am. Pathol. 52,* 983-1011.
Fitzgerald, P. J., Vinijchainkul, K., Carol, B., and Rosenstock,
    L. (1968b). *Am. J. Pathol. 52,* 1039-1065.
Goth, R., and Rajewsky, M. F. (1974a). *Z. Krebsforsch. Klin.
    Onkol. 82,* 37-64.
Goth, R., and Rajewsky, M. F. (1974b). *Proc. Natl. Acad. Sci.
    USA 71,* 639-643.
Gronow, M. (1980). *Chem. Biol. Interact. 29,* 1-30.
Harris, C. C., Autrup, H., Stoner, G., Yang, S. K., Lentz, J. C.
    Gelboin, H. V., Selkirk, J. K., Conner, R. J., Barrett,
    L. A., Jones, R. T., McDowell, E., and Trump, B. F. (1977).
    Cancer Res. 37, 3349-3355.
Hayashi, Y., and Hasegawa, T. (1971). *Gann 62,* 329-330.
Iqbal, Z. M., and Epstein, S. S. (1978). *Chem. Biol. Interact.
    20,* 77-87.
Iqbal, Z. M., Majdan, M., and Epstein, S. S. (1976). *Cancer
    Res. 36,* 1108-1113.
Iqbal, Z. M., Varnes, M. E., Yosyida, A., and Epstein, S. S.
    (1977). *Cancer Res. 37,* 1011-1015.
Kleihues, P., and Margison, G. P. (1974). *J. Natl. Cancer
    Inst. (U.S.) 53,* 1839-1841.
Konishi, Y., Denda, A., Inui, S., Takahashi, S., Ueda, N., and
    Namiki, M. (1978). *Cancer Lett. (Shannon, Irel.) 4,* 229-
    234.
Kruger, F. W., Pour, P., and Altoff, J. (1974). *Naturwissen-
    schaften 61,* 328.
Levitt, M. H., Harris, C. C., Squire, R., Springer, S., Wenk,
    M., Mollelo, C., Thomas, D., Kingsbury, E., and Newkirk,
    C. (1977). *Am. J. Pathol. 88,* 5-28.
Levitt, M., Harris, C. C., Squire, R., Wenk, M., Mollelo, C.,
    and Springer, S. (1978). *J. Natl. Cancer Inst. (U.S.)
    60,* 701-705.
Lilja, H. S., Hyde, S., Longnecker, D. S., and Yager, J. D.,
    Jr. (1977). *Cancer Res. 37,* 3925-3931.
Longnecker, D. S., and Curphy, T. J. (1975). *Cancer Res. 35,*
    2249-2258.
Magee, P. N., and Barnes, J. M. (1956). *Br. J. Cancer 10,*
    114-122.
Magee, P. N., and Barnes, J. M. (1962). *J. Pathol. Bacteriol.
    84,* 19-31.
Magee, P. N., Hawks, A. M., Stewart, W. B., and Swann, P. F.
    (1973). *In* "Pharmacology and the Future of Man,"
    (S. Karger, ed.) Vol. 2, pp. 140-149. Karger, Basel.
Mohr, U., Reznik, G., Emminger, E., and Lijinsky, W. (1977).
    J. Natl. Cancer Inst. (U.S.) 58, 429-432.
Morgan, R. G. H., and Wormsley, K. G. (1977). *Gut 18,*
    580-596.

Parsa, I. (1982). *Cancer Lett. (Shannon, Irel.)* 15, 115-121.

Parsa, I., and Butt, K. M. H. (1982). *Banbury Rep.* 12, 15-24.

Parsa, I., Marsh, W. H., and Fitzgerald, P. J. (1969). *Am. J. Pathol.* 57, 489-521.

Parsa, I., Marsh, W. H., and Fitzgerald, P. J. (1970). *Exp. Cell Res.* 59, 171-175.

Parsa, I., Marsh, W. H., Sutton, A. L., and Butt, K. M. H. (1981). *Am. J. Pathol.* 102, 403-411.

Parsa, I., Sutton, A. L., Chen, C. K., and Delbridge, C. (1982). *Cancer Lett. (Shannon, Irel.)* 17, 217-222.

Pour, P., Kruger, F. W., Altoff, J., Cardesa, A., and Mohr, U. (1974). *Am. J. Pathol.* 76, 349-358.

Pour, P., Kruger, F. W., Altoff, J., Cardesa, A., and Mohr, U. (1975). *Cancer Res.* 35, 2259-2268.

Pour, P., Altoff, J., Gingell, R., Kupper, R., Kruger, F. W., and Mohr, U. (1976). *Cancer Res.* 36, 2877-2884.

Pour, P., Altoff, J., Kruger, F. W., and Mohr, U. (1977). *J. Natl. Cancer Inst. (U.S.)* 58, 1449-1453.

Pour, P. M., Salmasi, S. Z., and Runge, R. G. (1978). *Cancer Lett. (Shannon, Irel.)* 4, 317-323.

Rao, M. S., and Reddy, J. K. (1980). *Carcinogenesis (N.Y.)* 1, 1027-1034.

Reddy, J. K., and Rao, M. S. (1975). *Cancer Res.* 35, 2269-2277.

Reddy, J. K., and Rao, M. S. (1977). *J. Natl. Cancer Inst. (U.S.)* 59, 1645-1647.

Roque, A. L., Jafarey, N. A., and Coulter, P. (1965). *Exp. Mol. Pathol.* 4, 266-274.

Scarpelli, D. G., and Rao, M. S. (1979). *Cancer Res.* 39, 452-458.

Scarpelli, D. G., Rao, M. S., Subbarao, V., Beversluis, M., Gurka, D. P., and Hollenberg, P. F. (1980). *Cancer Res.* 40, 67-74.

Shinozuka, H., Popp, J. A., and Konishi, Y. (1976). *Lab. Invest.* 34, 501-509.

Takahashi, M., Pour, P., Althoff, J., and Donnelly, T. (1977). *Cancer Res.* 37, 4602-4606.

Webb, J. N. (1977). *J. Clin. Pathol.* 30, 103-112.

19

CARCINOGEN-INDUCED CHANGES IN CULTURED HUMAN ENDOMETRIAL CELLS

*David G. Kaufman, Jill M. Siegfried, B. Hugh Dorman,
Karen G. Nelson, and Leslie A. Walton*

Departments of Pathology and of Obstetrics and Gynecology
and The Cancer Research Center
University of North Carolina School of Medicine
Chapel Hill, North Carolina

I.   INTRODUCTION

A thorough understanding of cancer as it occurs in human cells and tissues *in vivo* may require further knowledge about the specific features of each of the various human tissues and cell types that are targets for cancer development. Carcinogenesis studies in whole animals or in cell cultures have generally utilized inbred rodent strains selected for their proneness to cancer development or in derivative cell cultures that have been even further selected for their propensity for transformation in culture. Thus, it is necessary to determine whether malignant transformation in human cells or tissues differs either quantitatively or qualitatively from transformation in these selected rodents or rodent cell cultures.

As a step toward this goal it is necessary to develop suitable methods for studying human cells or tissues in culture and to explore the effects of chemical carcinogens on them. Because of existing clinical associations with members of the pathology and obstetrics and gynecology departments, we chose to undertake studies of this type with tissues from the female genital tract. We were aware of the presence of normal human endometrium in surgical specimens obtained for appropriate clinical indications. The potential availability of this tissue, coupled with the fact that the endometrium is a common site for malignancies in women, made this tissue attractive for carcinogenesis studies. This chapter traces our efforts to grow cell cultures of human endometrium and to determine the cells of origin for these cultures. The chapter also describes our observations of the effects of a chemical carcinogen and a promoting agent on these cells in culture.

II.   CULTURE OF TISSUE AND IDENTIFICATION OF CELL TYPES

A.   Establishment of Cell Cultures

Monolayer cell cultures were established from endometrial tissue obtained from over 200 hysterectomy specimens. All donors were patients offering informed consent. A careful review of their clinical histories offered no evidence of hormonal administration, pelvic inflammatory disease, or previous endometrial sampling consistent with hyperplasia or neoplasia (Kaufman et al., 1980). Immediately following abdominal or vaginal hysterectomy, the uterus was opened in the surgical suite using sterile techniques and examined for evidence of gross endometrial pathology. If no gross abnormality was evident, a portion of the endometrium was removed by scraping the surface with a large scalpel blade held perpendicularly to the surface. The specimen was placed in 10 ml of chilled culture medium containing high concentrations of antibiotics (1000 IU/ml penicillin and 1000 μg/ml streptomycin) and transported to the tissue culture laboratory.

Upon arrival at the laboratory, the tissue was minced and washed repetitively with Ca^{2+} and Mg^{2+}-free Hanks' balanced salt solution (CMF-HBSS) containing 25 mM Hepes buffer, pH 7.4. To obtain mixed cultures of epithelial and stromal cells, minced tissue was incubated in a solution containing 0.1% trypsin, 0.1% hyaluronidase, and 0.05% collagenase in CMF-HBSS. After incubation at 37°C for approximately 1 h, the tissue had dissociated into free cells and a few connective tissue strands. The liberated cells were plated onto 60-mm tissue culture dishes at a density of 5×10^4 cells/cm^2. To obtain enriched fractions of glands or stromal cells, the tissue fragments were incubated at 37°C in 0.25% collagenase in CMF-HBSS (5 ml per 0.5 cm^3 tissue). At 15-min intervals the tissue was pipetted up and down several times, and the progress of dissociation was monitored by phase contrast microscopy. This procedure yielded a suspension of glands relatively free of nonepithelial cells and single cells primarily of stromal cell origin. Glands were separated from stromal cells by repetitive washings with CMF-HBSS followed by gentle centrifugation at 500 rpm for 15 sec. These processes yielded a pellet of endometrial glands and single cells in suspension. Between 20 and 90% of isolated glands attached to the tissue culture dishes, and epithelial cells migrated and grew out from the glands. The stromal cell suspension was plated separately. Mixed cultures of stromal and epithelial cells were also obtained from explanted endometrial tissue. Endometrial tissue was minced and then placed directly onto culture dishes and partially covered with culture medium. Outgrowths began to emerge from the explants within 5 to 7 days, and confluence was reached after approximately 3 weeks. Scratching the plastic dishes with a scalpel blade facilitated the establishment of explant cultures.

The basic medium used for routine culturing was CMRL-1066 (Gibco) supplemented with 10% heat-inactivated fetal bovine serum (FBS, Gibco), glutamine (10 mM), Hepes (25 mM), penicillin (100 IU/ml), streptomycin (100 μg/ml), and insulin (4 μg/ml). The serum lots were analyzed, and only those that contained less than 1 pg/ml of estrogen and 1 ng/ml of progesterone were used in these studies. The medium CMRL-1066 was chosen initially for establishing cultures because it had provided the best preser-

vation of morphology in endometrial organ cultures (Kaufman
et al., 1980).

B. Morphology and Growth Properties of Endometrial Cell
    Cultures

Mature epithelial cells were best observed in cultures established from isolated glands. Glands attached and cells began to migrate from them 6-12 h after plating. The plating efficiency was enhanced by the use of fibronectin-coated plates
or irradiated 3T3 cells as a feeder layer. Epithelial colonies
contained cells that were polygonal and tighly packed or
"tadpole" shaped and grew in swirls (Fig. 1). Colonies ceased
to grow after 7 to 10 days, but the epithelial cells maintained
their normal appearance for 2 to 4 weeks, after which degenerative changes became evident. Seeding at high density helped
to extend the viability of epithelial colonies for periods of
as long as 2 months in culture. In addition, increasing the
serum concentrations to 20% increased the longevity of the colonies. Unfortunately, all efforts to subculture these normal
epithelial colonies by trypsinization and replating have proved
unsuccessful. We have documented several features of mature
epithelium in colonies in primary cultures (Varma *et al.,*
1982). The epithelial cells rested on a continuous basal lamina, and there were well-developed junctional complexes with
numerous desmosomes between cells. Following subculture, epithelial colonies could not be found; surviving cells lacked the
ultrastructural characteristics of epithelial cells. The lack
of survival of endometrial epithelial cells in continuous culture has also been described by others (Liszczak *et al.,* 1977;
Kirk *et al.,* 1978).

Cultures established from the single-cell suspension following collagenase dissociation initially gave rise to cells

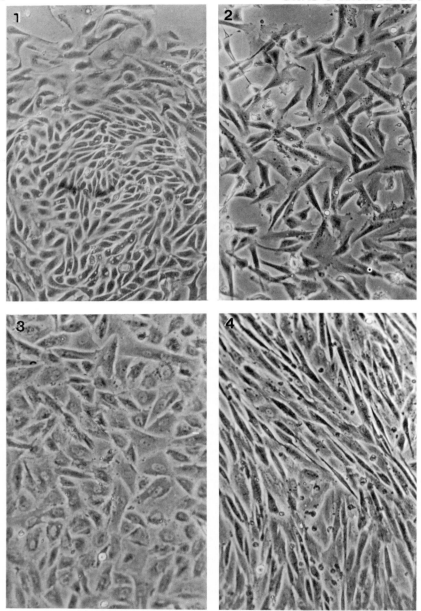

Figs. 1-4. Phase contrast photomicrographs (×400).
    Fig. 1. Colony of endometrial epithelial cells, primary culture.
    Fig. 2. Endometrial stromal cells, primary culture.
    Fig. 3. Endometrial stromal cells, passage 3 (CMRL-1066 medium.
    Fig. 4. Endometrial stromal cells, passage 7 (DMEM medium).

with a stellate or spindle-shaped appearance (Fig. 2). Cells
began to attach approximately 1 h after initial plating. As
with the glands, the plating efficiency was highly variable.
One to two weeks after an initial plating at 4.5×10^4 cells/cm^2,
these cells had grown to confluence and had crowded out any epithelial colonies present. These cells were easily subcultured.
Cells that initially displayed a stellate or polygonal morphology in primary culture became spread out and more polygonal in
shape after 1 or 2 passages (Fig. 3), and retained this morphology for at least 20 passages. Growth kinetic studies showed a
doubling time of 5 to 7 days. Cultures retrieved after prolonged storage in liquid nitrogen yielded cells with similar
morphological features and growth characteristics. Although
this cell type has an epithelioid appearance in monolayer culture plates, morphological studies showed characteristics of
the endometrial stromal cell. As evidenced by electron microscopy (Varma *et al.*, 1982), these polygonal cells also formed
a monolayer on a thin basal lamina, but the area of contact was
limited. The cells displayed random orientation, and no desmosomes were present.

The shape of stromal cells was also found to be dependent
on the medium used for culture. If medium other than CMRL-1066
was used, such as Ham's F12 or Dulbecco's modified Eagle's
medium (DMEM), the polygonal morphology gradually evolved into
a stellate appearance (Fig. 4). This process took about 6 weeks
and was reversible; if stellate cells were returned to CMRL-
1066, the cells returned to a polygonal shape. Agents such as
cholera toxin and 12-*O*-tetradecanoylphorbol 13-acetate (TPA)
caused stromal cells cultured in DMEM to assume a polygonal
morphology.

These findings demonstrate that stromal cell cultures are
capable of expressing a range of morphological patterns *in
vitro* that are similar to those observed *in vivo*. During the

proliferative phase of the menstrual cycle, endometrial stromal
cells undergo vigorous proliferation and change from small
spindle cells to larger stellate cells. During the secretory
phase of the cycle, the stromal cell cytoplasm increases in
volume and the cells develop a striking epithelioid appearance
in areas of predecidual change. It seems that CMRL-1066 potentiates this predecidual morphology.

Fibroblasts have also occasionally been found in our cultures. These cells emerged only when other cellular elements
of the endometrial specimens did not survive in culture.

C. Histochemical Characterization of Cell Cultures

The epithelial and stromal cell origins of the two cell
types derived from human endometrium have been confirmed by
comparing histochemical markers found in monolayer cultures to
markers found in frozen sections of endometrium. The methods
employed were standard histochemical techniques that demonstrate
the presence of enzymes by using coupling agents that form insoluble colored products at the site of enzyme activity. This
allows localization of activity with good resolution. The
enzyme-staining procedures of Bancroft (1975) were utilized.
Localization of γ-glutamyltranspeptidase was demonstrated by
the technique of Dorman *et al*. (1982). Tissue for frozen sections was obtained from endometrial specimens at the time that
tissue was obtained for culturing. Tissue was embedded in
Tissue-Tele II O.C.T. compound (Fisher Scientific), frozen in
liquid nitrogen, and stored at -20°C until sectioned and
stained. The results for stained sections were compared to
those with stained cells from primary culture and after passaging. Cells were grown on Lab-Tek chamber slides (Miles Laboratories), and fixation and staining were carried out within each
chamber. Fixation was carried out after enzyme assay in the
case of leucine aminopeptidase, which is destroyed by fixatives.

Whereas many enzyme activities were found in both glands and stroma of frozen sections, several enzymes were found to be specific for either glands or stroma. Glandular and surface epithelia were positive for alkaline phosphatase (ALP), β-glucuronidase (BG), and γ-glutamyltranspeptidase (GGT). The stroma was completely negative for ALP and GGT and contained a few scattered cells that showed some BG activity. Blood vessels also demonstrated ALP activity. However, ALP (Fig. 5) was found in greatest amount in endometrial specimens obtained in the proliferative phase, an observation previously reported by Flippe and Dawson (1968) and Dallenbach-Hellweg (1981). BG activity did not vary with the menstrual cycle. GGT activity was highest during the secretory phase and was found chiefly on the luminal surface of glands in the zona compacta and zona spongiosa. GGT activity disappeared within 24 h of culture; glandular epithelial cells that attached to the culture dish did not express the enzyme, whereas those that were floating remained positive. The ALP (Fig. 6) and BG activities were expressed by colonies of epithelial cells in primary culture. Stromal cells in culture were completely negative for GGT and ALP, and expressed a low level of BG in 10 to 20% of cells.

Stromal cells *in vivo* and *in vitro* were positive for many enzymes, but few markers clearly distinguished cells of stromal origin from cells of epithelial origin. In frozen sections, acid phosphatase (AP) was found in epithelial cells of glands and in the supporting stromal cells. AP activity was consistently higher in glands, but activity in stromal cells increased to nearly comparable levels during the secretory phase. High AP activity has been demonstrated in predecidual cells (Goldberg and Jones, 1956). AP activity was also high in stromal cultures; under high power, the lysosomal localization of the enzyme was apparent (Fig. 7). Leucine aminopeptidase (LAP) activity was found in sections of secretory-phase endometrium,

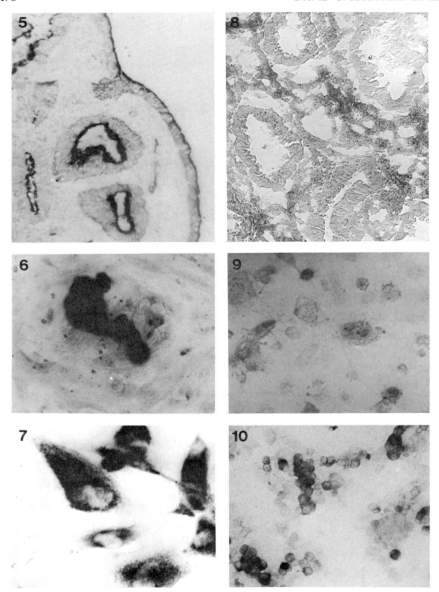

Fig. 5. Alkaline phosphatase staining of frozen section of endometrium showing positive reaction in glandular and surface epithelia; section is counterstained with methyl green (×100).

Fig. 6. Epithelial cells in primary culture stained positively for ALP, counterstained with methyl green; a fragment of gland (highly stained by methyl green) is also visible (×400).

especially in predecidual areas around blood vessels and under surface epithelium (Fig. 8); glands were generally negative for this enzyme. In culture, epithelial colonies were also generally negative for LAP, whereas stromal cultures demonstrated enzymic activity (Fig. 9). This enzyme is also a predecidual marker (Flippe and Dawson, 1968; Baron and Esterly, 1975). Fibronectin antibody conjugated with fluorescein also proved useful for distinguishing glands and stroma. Only stromal cells in frozen sections and stromal cells in culture were labeled by this fluorescent marker, whereas epithelial cells showed no reaction in sections or in culture.

These histochemical results confirm the earlier ultrastructural observations identifying the origin of cells previously classified as epithelial and stromal cells. These findings also reinforce our impression that epithelial cells do not survive subculture, because epithelial cell markers are found only in primary cultures. Furthermore, these observations support our opinion that stromal cells express predecidual characteristics under certain conditions of culture. We have utilized histochemical markers to identify single cells directly isolated from endometrial tissue after digestion of fresh tissue with trypsin at 4°C for 18 h, followed by separation by centrifugation through Percoll. Two bands, correspond-

Fig. 7. Cultured stromal cells stained for acid phosphatase showing activity localized in lysosomes, no counterstain (×1000).

Fig. 8. Leucine aminopeptidase staining of frozen section of endometrium (late secretory) showing positive areas in stroma; glands are negative. Counterstained with methyl green (×100).

Fig. 9. LAP Staining of cultured stromal cells, no counterstain (×400).

Fig. 10. Epithelial cell band isolated from Percoll gradient stained for ALP and GGT. Darker cells are positive for both enzymes (×100).

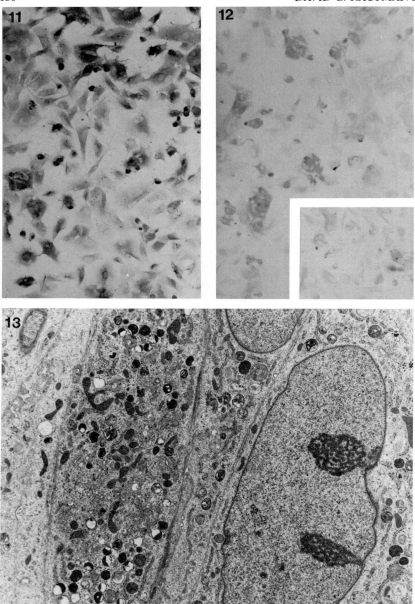

Fig. 11.   PAS Staining of stromal cell culture exposed to
0.1 μm DES for 1 week followed by 0.1 μm progesterone plus
0.01 μm DES for 1 week (×200).

Fig. 12.   Diastase digestion of cells treated as in Fig.
11, stained for PAS.   Inset: control culture exposed to DES
alone for 2 weeks, stained with PAS (×200).

ing to epithelial and stromal cells, formed after centrifugation through 35% Percoll for 20 min at 15,000 rpm. Figure 10
shows staining of the epithelial cell band; cells are highly
positive for ALP and GGT. Although complete purity was not
attained, 80-85% of cells in the stromal cell band were negative for these markers.

D. Response to Hormonal Cycling *in Vitro*

Production of glycogen and aggregation into predecidualized
areas are two features of the differentiation of stromal cells
in vivo that occur under the influence of progesterone during
the secretory phase of the menstrual cycle (Noyes, 1973). As
a further means of confirming the origin of stromal cells in
culture and to assess their physiological status, the biological responsiveness of cultured stromal cells to steroid hormones was studied. The steroid hormone concentrations in the
culture medium were varied to stimulate the changing steroid
hormone milieu during the menstrual cycle. Stromal cell cultures were treated with 0.1 μM progesterone plus 0.01 μM di-
ethylstilbestrol (DES) for 1 week after priming with 0.1 μM
DES alone for 1 week. At the end of this period the cultures
contained compact islands of crowded cells that were highly positive for PAS (Fig. 11). The cells in these areas were small
and oval with dense cytoplasm and appeared piled up into multiple layers. Continuous treatment with vitamin A (0.1 μM) or
hydrocortisone (0.1 μM) appeared to enhance this response.
The PAS staining was sensitive to diastase digestion (Fig. 12),
indicating that the stained product was glycogen. In all con-

Fig. 13. Transmission electron micrograph of stromal cell
aggregate found in hormonally cycled cultures. Multicellular
nature of aggregates is apparent (×16,000).

trol cultures examined, the cells were larger and stellate with
a relatively clear cytoplasm as compared to the hormonally
cycled cells. No aggregation or at most a minimum of loose
cellular aggregation was observed (Fig. 12, inset). Background
staining by PAS was observed, but this was not removed by prior
incubation with diastase.

The ultrastructural appearance of the cellular aggregates
in hormonally cycled cultures is shown in Fig. 13. The multiple
layers of cells in the aggregates are evident. Rough endoplasmic reticulum, Golgi apparati, and numerous lysosomes were
prominent in the cytoplasm of these cells. In some cases, large
gap junctions (nexi) and an occasional rudimentary cilium,
features of predecidual stromal cells, were observed (Dorman
et al., 1982). This response was usually observable only in
the first to third passage. These results provide further evidence of the stromal cell origin of the propagable monolayer
cultures derived from endometrium and indicate that the cells
retain some of their normal physiological properties *in vitro.*

E. Development of a Colony-Forming Assay

Quantitating growth of stromal cell cultures from single
cells provides a better measure of proliferative capacity of
stromal cells at the time of plating than evaluating the average growth of the population as a whole. Initial efforts to
perform a colony-forming assay with stromal cells cultured in
CMRL medium were disappointing. Stromal cells grew best in
CMRL medium when plated at high density, but scanty growth from
single cells was observed when cells were plated sparsely, even
when feeder layers of murine 3T3 cells, human myometrial smooth
muscle, or human fibroblasts were used. Coating tissue culture
plates with human fibronectin, type I collagen, or poly-*D*-
lysine failed to enhance clonal growth in CMRL. After fixation

TABLE I.   Media Conditions for Clonal Growth of Stromal Cells

Culture medium	Colony-forming efficiency (%)		
	Line 1	Line 2	Line 3
DMEM	7.0	10.7	15.8
IMEMZO	2.4	6.1	6.5
Waymouth MB752/1	3.9	10.2	16.2
BME	4.4	n.d.	19.0
RPMI	2.7	n.d.	n.d.
Ham's F12	3.6	8.1	13.7
199	n.d.[a]	n.d.	19.9
CMRL	0.3	0.0	0.3
DMEM + additives (see text)	n.d.	0.5	2.9

[a]n.d., Not done.

in 90% methanol–10% acetic acid and staining with Giemsa, only a few colonies consisting of degenerating cells were evident. In contrast, when other media were examined, colony-forming efficiencies (CFE) of up to 20% were obtained on plastic dishes without protein coatings or feeder layers (Table I). Considerable variability was found in the CFE of cells from different individuals. On the basis of these observations, DMEM was routinely used to assay clonal growth. Medium was supplemented with 4 µg/ml insulin and 20% fetal bovine serum (FBS). Under these conditions, cells doubled approximately every 3 days; plates were evaluated on Day 11 when colonies of 12 or more cells were scored (Fig. 14).

CMRL was the only medium tested that did not support clonal growth (Table I). There are several characteristics of CMRL-1066 medium that differ consistently from those of the other tested media: a high level of L-cysteine-HCl (260 mg/liter), a high level of ascorbic acid (50 mg/liter), the presence of glutathione (10 mg/liter), and the presence of cocarboxylase (1.0 mg/liter). When these ingredients were added to DMEM, a substantial reduction in CFE occurred (Table I), although it

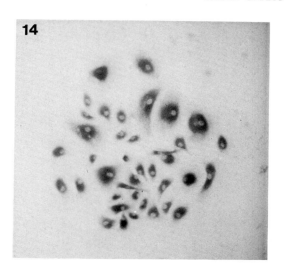

Fig. 14.   Light micrograph of stromal cell colony, Day 11,
stained for acid phosphatase and counterstained with methyl
green (×200).

was not as inhibitory as CMRL itself. This suggests that conditions that bring about a polygonal, predecidual morphology in
stromal cells also inhibit clonal growth, whereas conditions
that bring about a stellate morphology permit clonal growth.

The ability of stromal cell cultures to form colonies was
dependent on presence of FBS. Figure 15 illustrates results of
varying the percentage of FBS in culture medium; with less than
5% serum, no colonies were detected. Optimal colony formation
was observed with 20% FBS. This correlated with our previous
findings that 20% FBS gave optimal growth ratio of stromal
cells (Dorman *et al.*, 1982) and is an indication of the biological normalcy of these cultures. Because more rapid growth
was achieved with 20% FBS than with 10% FBS, the higher serum
level was routinely used in colony-forming assays.

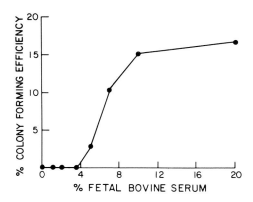

Fig. 15. Serum dependence of colony formation. Cells were seeded 500 per dish in DMEM medium with varying supplements of FBS. Colonies were stained on Day 11.

III. EFFECTS OF CARCINOGEN TREATMENT OF ENDOMETRIAL CELL CULTURES

A. Methods for Carcinogen Treatment

Because the most common human endometrial malignancy is adenocarcinoma, we studied effects of carcinogens on cultured epithelial cells. A direct-acting carcinogen, N-methyl-N'-nitro-N-nitrosoguanidine (MNNG), was chosen for these studies rather than agents requiring metabolism by the P-450 cytochrome system, because metabolic activity may vary between individuals (Dorman et al., 1981) and may be influenced by the duration and conditions of cell culture. Because of the difficulty in maintaining epithelial cells in culture, we utilized epithelial colonies in primary cultures and exposed the cultures to 0.5 or 0.1 µg/ml MNNG for 30 min during the first or second week after tissue obtainment. Cloning tubes were used to select epithelial colonies 1 to 2 weeks after MNNG exposure, and these colonies were transferred to dishes containing 3T3 cell feeder

layers. This procedure yielded epithelial cultures that survived for over a month after the first passage. Although
studies to date have yielded only isolated epithelial cell
colonies rather than a cell line, the goal of future studies
remains to obtain an epithelial cell line after carcinogen
treatment that can be used to monitor successive changes following further exposure to carcinogens or tumor-promoting
agents.

More extensive studies with MNNG have been conducted on
cultured endometrial stromal cells. Cultures containing approximately 95% endometrial stromal cells were treated with
MNNG while at subconfluent densities and actively growing.
Cells were treated for 30 min at 37°C in Hanks' balanced salt
solution (HBSS) to which MNNG (Aldrich Chemical Co., Milwaukee,
Wisconsin) dissolved in acetone was added to give final concentrations of MNNG of 0.5, 1.0, 2.0, and 4.0 µg/ml. The final
concentration of acetone was constant for all groups, and solvent controls received acetone (0.5% final concentration) in
HBSS. Medium controls received HBSS without additions. Both
solvent and medium controls were maintained in parallel to
carcinogen-treated cultures. Following carcinogen or control
treatment HBSS was removed and maintenance medium substituted.
Two protocols for carcinogen treatments were used. In one protocol, cultures were treated repetitively in the same plate.
In the other, carcinogen-treated cells were subcultured to
analyze growth characteristics prior to further treatment. In
the latter case, phenotypic alterations were analyzed following
each successive carcinogen treatment and subsequent passage.
Cultures were routinely examined by phase contrast microscopy
to monitor alterations in cellular morphology. Growth rate,
saturation density, and plating efficiency were analyzed with
methods described previously.

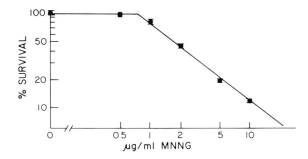

Fig. 16.   Toxicity of MNNG toward human endometrial stromal cells.   Cells were seeded 500 per dish 20 h before carcinogen exposure.   Cells were treated with MNNG in Hanks' buffer for 30 min, after which DMEM medium was replaced.

B.   Toxic Effects of Carcinogen Treatment

A single 30-min treatment of endometrial stromal cells with MNNG resulted in measurable cytotoxicity as analyzed by de-creased colony formation.   Figure 16 illustrates a dose-response curve for survival of stromal cells from one individual exposed to MNNG.   From this curve the concentration of MNNG estimated to cause a 50% reduction in survival of cultured cells was 1.8 μg/ml.   This level of cytotoxicity was constant in cultures from many individuals and supported findings from population studies in which the growth rate of cultures exposed to 1.0 μg/ml MNNG was reduced by 50%.   Decreases in cell survival and population growth were accompanied by the appearance of many vacuolated, multinucleated cells and floating cells.   Resistance to toxic effects of MNNG also developed in the cells surviving the initial exposure.   A second exposure to 1.0 μg/ml MNNG pro-duced no growth inhibition when assayed by plating efficiency, doubling time, or saturation density.   Phenotypic changes in cell cultures were best observed at MNNG concentrations that yielded 30-80% survival after initial exposure.

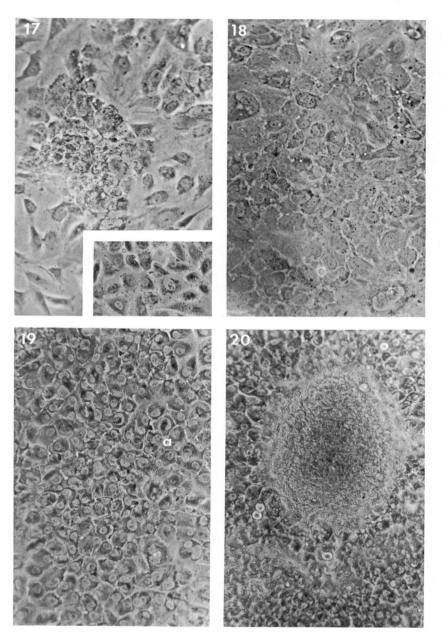

Fig. 17. Morphology alterations after MNNG exposure.
Small area of cellular crowding found 8 weeks after one carcinogen exposure (2 µg/ml) (×400). Inset: morphology of
acetone-treated cells (×200).

C. Carcinogen-Induced Changes in Morphology

Stromal cell cultures displayed progressive alterations of morphology with increasing numbers of carcinogen treatments. Solvent-treated control cells were uniform in size and evenly spaced (Fig. 17, inset). They had clearly delineated outlines and regular nuclear size and shape. Most nuclei contained several small, round nucleoli and the nuclear:cytoplasmic ratio was low. In contrast, 6 weeks after a single treatment with MNNG (2 μg/ml), there were areas with cellular crowding and with less distinct individual cell boundaries than normal (Fig. 17). These changes were observed even when the plates had low cell density. Following two exposures to MNNG (2 μg/ml) and four passages, the cell cultures had more atypical cellular morphology (Fig. 18). Crowded, small, irregular cells represented a larger fraction of the cell population.

After five exposures to MNNG, cellular crowding was more intense and involved a greater number of areas of larger size on the plates (Fig. 19). Nuclei appeared irregular in size and shape, and many had single prominent, centrally located nucleoli. The nuclear:cytoplasmic ratio also was increased. Even more abnormal morphological characteristics were observed after 10 treatments with MNNG. Figure 20 illustrates a densely crowded focus of cells. Within the focus, the cells were piled up and so intensely crowded that they obscured cellular bounda-

Fig. 18. Crowded areas became larger, and irregularity in cell shape developed 8 weeks after second MNNG treatment (×400).

Fig. 19. After five carcinogen exposures, the entire culture consisted of small, tightly packed cells with increased nuclear:cytoplasmic ratio (×400).

Fig. 20. After 11 treatments with MNNG, large foci of densely packed cells were visible (×400).

TABLE II.   Growth Properties of Stromal Cells Exposed to MNNG

Property	Acetone control	Number of exposures to MNNG (0.5 µg/ml)		
		2	4	12
Plating efficiency (%)	63	64	86	104
Doubling time (days)	7.1	6.5	5.0	3.8
Saturation density (cells/cm^2)	25,300	29,000	40,000	85,000

ries and cytological details.   Some of these foci were of sufficient size to be visible macroscopically.

D.   Alterations of Growth Parameters

Multiple treatments with MNNG resulted in enhanced growth potential in carcinogen-treated cultures as compared to control cultures.   Whereas the plating efficiency of untreated or solvent-treated endometrial cells averaged approximately 50%, cells displayed increased plating efficiencies following repetitive carcinogen treatments (Table II).   After multiple treatments with MNNG, cells also displayed increases in saturation density over that of solvent-treated controls.   In these studies, the saturation density was measured by monitoring cell counts 21-29 days after seeding cells as for growth curves.   The saturation density of control cells consistently averaged 2.5×10^4 cells/cm^2 and showed little variation over time.   In contrast, a two- to threefold increase in saturation density was observed in carcinogen-treated cultures after multiple exposures (Table II).

Elevated growth rates were also observed for cells treated repetitively with MNNG.   A progressive decrease in doubling time was observed after more than two exposures (Table II). The data in Table II represent the lowest MNNG concentration (0.5 μg/ml) at which changes were detected. Similar results were obtained at higher concentrations, but the number of successive exposures required before alterations were detected was lower than those shown (Dorman *et al.*, 1983). Cells treated with only one exposure to MNNG required up to a year of continuous culture before changes in morphology or growth properties were detected.

E. Other Phenotypic Changes

The capacity for anchorage-independent growth was also examined in carcinogen-treated cell populations sequentially after each carcinogen treatment. Untreated or solvent-treated human endometrial stromal cells remained as single cells or loose collections of several cells and were not able to proliferate in soft agar. In contrast, after four exposures to MNNG, cells developed the capacity to grow and form colonies from single cells in soft agar. The CFE of carcinogen-treated cells in soft agar ranged from 0.018 to 0.069%. From the fourth to sixth carcinogen treatment there was a progressive increase in the percentage of cells capable of anchorage-independent growth. The CFE in soft agar did not increase after the sixth MNNG treatment.

Higher levels of GGT were observed in cultures treated repetitively with MNNG than in control cultures. The proportion of treated cells with elevated GGT levels increased up to the sixth MNNG treatment, when most cells displayed elevated enzyme levels. The cells found to stain most intensely positive for GGT were observed in crowded, morphologically altered foci, where 100% of the atypical partially overlapping cells stained. Control populations displayed only faint background levels of GGT.

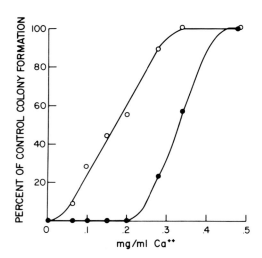

Fig. 21.   Calcium dependence of colony formation, control
(●) versus carcinogen-treated (O) cells.   Calcium-free DMEM
was prepared as described, and calcium levels were varied by
addition of CaCl$_2$.

The capacity for clonal growth in CMRL-1066 medium on
standard tissue culture dishes was analyzed for carcinogen-
treated and control cells.   Untreated or solvent-treated control cells did not form colonies in CMRL-1066 medium and degenerated rapidly following low-density plating.   Similarly,
cells treated one to five times with MNNG also were not capable
of clonal growth.   However, after six or more treatments with
1.0 μg/ml MNNG, cells capable of clonal growth were detected,
and they had a colony-forming efficiency of 10%.

Carcinogen-treated cells also showed a reduced dependence
on calcium for clonal growth (Fig. 21).   Calcium-free DMEM and
chelated FBS were prepared as described by Swierenga *et al.*,
(1978); the calcium content of the culture medium was 1-3 mg/
liter.   Calcium content was then varied by adding CaCl$_2$.   Control cells were highly dependent on calcium for growth; no
colonies were detected at 0.2 mg/ml calcium or less.   After

repeated MNNG treatment, however, cells were able to form colonies even at calcium levels as low as 0.06 mg/ml. The capacity for growth in medium with low calcium concentrations has been noted earlier in other transformed cells (Swierenga et al., 1978).

F. Tumorigenicity

Although many properties of these human stromal cells have been altered by treatment with MNNG, we have been unable to obtain tumors from these cells following their xenotransplantation into nude mice. To date, neither normal nor carcinogen-treated endometrial stromal cells have survived more than a few days in vivo after inoculation into nude mice (D. G. Kaufman and B. H. Dorman, unpublished). Because these cells are cleared so rapidly from our nude mice under the conditions we have employed, their inability to form tumors is not surprising. Further efforts are in progress to increase the duration of residence of injected cells in our mice and to reduce the capacity for rejection of xenotransplanted cells in mice of this colony. It should be noted that although a positive result would be confirming evidence of transformation, a negative result does not mean transformation has not been achieved. In fact, many human tumors (Shimosato et al., 1976) and cell lines derived from human tumors (Giovanella et al., 1974) are unable to grow in nude mice. Conversely, despite their numerous altered characteristics, the carcinogen-treated stromal cells may be only partially transformed.

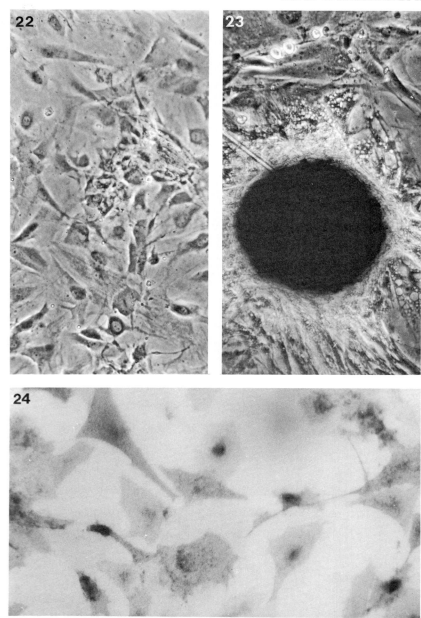

Fig. 22.   Primary stromal cell sarcoma culture showing overlapping of cells (×400).

Fig. 23.   Subcultured sarcoma cells showing dense region of packed cells rising above plane of monolayer (×400).

Fig. 24.   Stromal sarcoma in culture stained positively for ALP, no counterstain (×1000).

IV. COMPARISON OF CARCINOGEN-TREATED CELLS WITH STROMAL CELL
     TUMORS

A. Morphology and Growth Properties

We have begun to examine several properties of human endometrial stromal cell sarcomas as a standard for evaluating the
altered characteristics of endometrial stromal cells after
treatment with carcinogens. In effect, we are exploring whether
these sarcoma cells can be used as a positive control for carcinogenesis studies. Several properties of cell cultures
derived from stromal cell sarcomas have been compared with
those of stromal cell cultures treated with MNNG. Morphologically, the cultured sarcomas showed many features that were also
seen in MNNG-treated cultures. Cells varied in shape from stellate to polygonal, and formed crowded, overlapping areas (Fig.
22). At times this crowding resulted in the formation of macroscopic foci composed of multiple layers of cells raised above
the level of the surrounding monolayer (Fig. 23).

In general, stromal cell sarcoma cultures grew slowly,
with a doubling time of 6 days. The growth rate could be increased by adding fibroblast growth factor (FGF) to the medium.
These sarcoma cells were able to form colonies in CMRL-1066 or
DMEM medium if FGF (50 µg/ml) was present, indicating that these
media alone may not be optimal for the tumor. The growth rate
of sarcoma cells was also greatly influenced by the concentration of serum in the medium, in a manner analogous to the effect we had observed earlier in normal and carcinogen-treated
stromal cells. Sarcoma cultures also were able to form colonies
in reduced calcium medium as had been observed in carcinogen-
treated cultures.

B. Evaluation of Enzyme Markers

Enzymatic analysis of primary tumors and cell digests indicated that alkaline phosphatase and β-glucuronidase were
present in stromal cell sarcomas. These enzymes, as well as
γ-glutamyltranspeptidase, were also detected histochemically
(Fig. 24). All three of these enzymes have been detected histochemically in cultures treated extensively with MNNG. These
three enzymes normally are only demonstrable histochemically
in endometrial epithelium and not in stromal cells. The aberrant expression of these enzymes, which is observed in stromal
tumors and carcinogen-treated cells, may be useful as a marker
for transformation.

Another similarity that was found between cultured sarcoma cells and carcinogen-treated cells was an abnormal lactate
dehydrogenase (LDH) isoenzyme pattern. Results from a representative experiment are shown in Table III. Isoenzymes were
separated by electrophoresis on agarose gels (Corning Special
Purpose Electrophoresis Film) by standard techniques (Rosalki,
1974). Similar to normal endometrial tissue, normal cultured
stromal cells mainly express the heart form of LDH, as evidenced by the predominance of LDH1, 2, and 3 isoenzymes, and
have little of LDH5 isoenzyme (muscle form). The ratio of
LDH1:LDH5, a commonly used index of normalcy (Niklasson *et al.,*
1981), was 22.7. Carcinogen-treated cells displayed lower
levels of LDH1 than control cells; the pattern was shifted
toward the LDH5 isoenzyme, giving a ratio of LDH1 to LDH5 of
2.97. A stromal cell sarcoma culture and a Müllerian tumor of
mixed stromal and glandular origin both showed extreme changes
of their isoenzyme patterns. Both had pronounced shifts toward
the LDH5 isoenzyme, and their ratios of LDH1 to LDH5 were 0.02
and 0.36, respectively.

TABLE III. Lactate Dehydrogenase Isoenzymes

| Sample | % Isoenzyme | | | | | |
	LDH 1	LDH 2	LDH 3	LDH 4	LDH 5	Ratio 1:5
Acetone control	22.7	27.1	30.4	18.8	1.0	22.7
MNNG Treated	8.6	25.1	39.9	23.5	2.9	2.97
Stromal sarcoma	0.7	9.3	21.5	31.2	37.3	0.02
Müllerian tumor	4.6	15.8	35.6	31.3	12.7	0.36

Hormonal responsiveness, as evidenced by glycogen production following steroid hormone stimulation, was also demonstrable in both the sarcoma and in cell line treated repetitively with MNNG (Dorman et al., 1983). This finding,
coupled with the observations of biochemical markers, demonstrated that the carcinogen-altered cells are stromal in origin and have several properties in common with tumors of stromal cell origin.

V. EFFECTS OF TPA ON STROMAL CELLS

A. Responsiveness of Endometrial Stromal Cells to TPA

We have observed that multiple treatments with MNNG and
multiple population doublings are required before sufficiently
severe phenotypic alterations develop in stromal cell cultures
to suggest that the cells are transformed. Because of the slow
emergence of alterations in the carcinogen-treated cell populations, it was potentially interesting to study the effects of
tumor promoters on cells at different stages of progression
toward a transformed phenotype. Moolgavkar and Knudson (1981)
and Yuspa et al. (1980) have suggested that selective expansion
of premalignant cell populations by tumor promoters provides an
enlarged pool of altered cells and this increases the likelihood

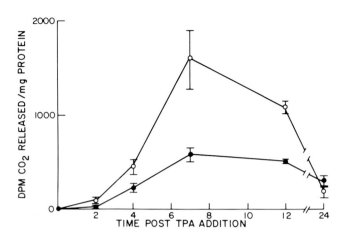

Fig. 25.   Induction of ODC by 0.1 µg/ml TPA in stromal cells.   Either TPA (O) or ethanol (●) was added without changing the medium; duplicate plates were harvested at times indicated.   The cytosol fraction was prepared by centrifuging the cellular homogenate at 100,000 g, and the ODC activity was quantitated by measuring the release of $^{14}CO_2$.

of tumor formation.   This hypothesis led us to explore whether differences in response to 12-*O*-tetradecanoylphorbol 13-acetate (TPA), a prototype tumor promoter, might be demonstrable between cells that had been exposed to MNNG and those that had only been exposed to acetone vehicle.

The responsiveness of normal human stromal cells to TPA *in vitro* was first tested by examining a well-documented effect of TPA, induction of ornithine decarboxylase (ODC) activity.   The assay was carried out as described by Yuspa *et al.* (1976). Ethanol was used as the vehicle for TPA.   Figure 25 illustrates the effect of 0.1 µg/ml TPA on ODC activity.   Although the extent of induction was not as high as has been reported in rodent skin, the time course was similar (Yuspa *et al.*, 1976).   This indicated that human stromal cells may respond to TPA in a manner similar to the response that occurs in tissues demonstrating tumor promotion. Furthermore, this induction suggests that TPA may be a relevant compound to test for other effects of tumor promoters in endometrial stromal cells.

B. Effects of TPA on Morphology

The ability of TPA to induce morphological changes in stromal cells with and without pretreatment with MNNG was examined. As has been reported in many other cell types, TPA induced a reversible morphological change in human stromal cells, but the extent of change was greater in initiated populations. Cells were pretreated with MNNG (1 µg/ml) or acetone at least 1 month prior to TPA exposure. At the time of TPA challenge, neither the MNNG-treated nor the acetone-treated cells exhibited changes in growth properties. The cultures consisted of polygonal cells as shown in Fig. 26. Within several hours of TPA addition (1 ng/ml), control stromal cells (not treated with MNNG) became more elongated and cellular membranes became more distinct than in controls treated with the ethanol vehicle used to solubilize TPA. The ethanol vehicle controls were polygonal in shape as in Fig. 3. These changes were much more pronounced in cultures that had previously been treated with MNNG (Fig. 27). Many more elaborate processes were visible in TPA-treated cultures, and many cells also detached from the dish. Cells not pretreated with MNNG reverted to normal morphology within 24 h even if TPA was not removed, whereas initiated cultures did not reverse until 48 to 72 h after application.

C. Effects of TPA on Colony-Forming Efficiency

Repetitive exposures to promoters over a long interval are necessary to increase skin tumor yields *in vivo* (Boutwell, 1964). This suggests that frequent or prolonged stimulation of

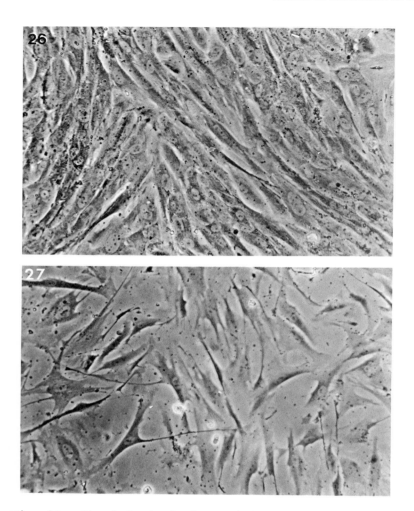

Fig. 26. Morphological change induced in acetone-treated stromal cells 4 h after addition of 1 ng/ml TPA (×400).

Fig. 27. Morphological change induced in MNNG-treated cells 4 h after addition of 1 ng/ml TPA (×400).

cellular processes by TPA may be required for promotion. For this reason we examined the effect of prolonged TPA exposure on the ability of stromal cells to form colonies from individual cells in "initiated" and noninitiated cultures. The CFE assay typically has been used as a measure of the relative viability

TABLE IV. Effect of 4 Months' Continuous TPA Exposure on
           Colony-Forming Ability

Number of carcinogen treatments	Colony-forming efficiency (%)		Ratio TPA:ETOH
	ETOH	TPA	
Acetone	8.0 ± 0.9	1.3 ± 0.2	0.163
1	15.9 ± 2.8	9.9 ± 1.0	0.623
6	9.2 ± 0.7	7.7 ± 1.7	0.837
10	11.8 ± 0.2	24.5 ± 0.2	2.07

and proliferative capacity of cultured cells. Data in Table IV
show observations from cultures of one individual pretreated
with either acetone or varying amounts of MNNG, and then grown
continuously in 0.01 μg/ml TPA for 4 months.

The percentage of acetone-treated cells that were capable
of forming colonies was profoundly decreased by TPA treatment
over this time. In carcinogen-treated populations, the response to long-term TPA was dependent on the extent of MNNG
treatment. Some inhibition was seen in cells exposed to only
1 or 6 MNNG treatments, although the extent of inhibition was
only 37.8 and 16.3%, respectively, as compared to 83.8% in acetone controls. Cells treated 10 times with MNNG showed an increased ability to form colonies after TPA exposure. Cells
treated once with MNNG had undergone little change in morphology and did not stain for the marker enzyme GGT, so they closely
resembled acetone controls. In contrast, the cells treated
6 times with MNNG had begun to express GGT activity, and cells
treated 10 times showed a 90% incidence of cells positive for
this enzyme. In addition, these extensively treated cultures
also displayed severe cellular crowding and occasional foci of
densely packed cells, indicating further deviation from normalcy than the other two groups. These findings indicate that
differences in response to TPA may be a function of the extent
to which cells have undergone preneoplastic changes.

Response of cell cultures to prolonged TPA may reflect a balance between stimulation of cell growth and induction of terminal differentiation. Yuspa and Morgan (1981) have demonstrated that TPA induces terminal differentiation in normal mouse epidermal cells, but not in initiated cells. A report by O'Brien *et al.* (1982) also supports this hypothesis. TPA prevented Syrian hamster embryo cells exposed to benzo[a]pyrene *in vitro*, but not normal cells, from undergoing senescence. If population dynamics such as these also occur *in vivo,* this could explain how repetitive long-term application of tumor promoters produces increased tumor yields. We have also noted that TPA can induce a predecidual-like morphology in stromal cells grown in DMEM, when under normal conditions the morphology would resemble proliferative phase. Thus, TPA may be able to induce differentiation of normal stromal cells. If initiated cells are resistant to terminal differentiation, or if TPA can selectively induce initiated cells to divide while inducing differentiation of normal cells, the net result could be an increase in colony forming of cells altered by carcinogen. This enhancement of growth of altered cells could also lead to an increased rate of phenotypic change in carcinogen-treated populations.

VI.   CONCLUSIONS

These studies show that cell cultures can be successfully established from normal human endometrial tissue. Epithelial cells with readily identifiable morphological and biochemical properties can be grown in primary culture. In agreement with the observations of several other investigators, however, these cells cannot be subcultured. We cannot presently explain the difficulty in subculturing these cells, nor can we explain how a single carcinogen treatment alters these cells so as to permit even the limited subculturability we have observed to date.

The endometrial stromal cell is the predominant cell type to emerge from cultured human endometrial tissue. These cells have been identified as endometrial stromal cells on the basis of their ultrastructural characteristics, their biochemical and histochemical properties, and their response to hormonal stimuli in culture. As experience with culture of human endometrial stromal cells has increased, it has been recognized that the morphological characteristics of the stromal cells are influenced by the choice of culture medium as well as by the hormonal content of the medium or the presence of exogenous agents such as TPA.

It is our current hypothesis that in most media, like DMEM, the stromal cells in culture assume a stellate shape and resemble stromal cells in endometrium during the proliferative phase of the menstrual cycle. In CMRL-1066 medium, these cells are more polygonal in shape and are larger. These cells seem to have assumed the state of differentiation of stromal cells as seen in the endometrium during the secretory phase of the menstrual cycle. Finally, when appropriately conditioned by ovarian hormones, these cells appear like the pseudodecidual stromal cells seen in late secretory phase.

Repetitive treatments of cultured human endometrial stromal cells with MNNG caused generally consistent and sequential changes in several biological properties of the stromal cells. These studies were conducted with endometrial stromal cells because they could be subcultured and survived in culture for many months. Concentrations of MNNG were chosen that produced limited toxic effects on these cells. Because of the inability initially to clone stromal cells in CMRL medium, the population treated with carcinogen and subsequently analyzed was not clonally derived. These observations therefore represent the

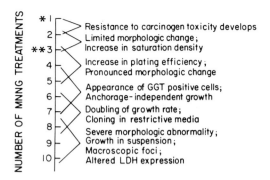

* Initiated: Abnormal morphology after 20 population doublings
** Initiated: TPA produces selective effects

Fig. 28. Progression of phenotypic changes in MNNG-treated human endometrial stromal cells in culture. *, Initiated: Abnormal morphology after 20 population doublings. **, Initiated: TPA produces selective effects.

detection and quantitation of altered characteristics within a mixed population. For this reason, we did not see consistent, precise transitions in phenotypic properties but rather more gradual emergence of altered phenotypic properties within the population over time as the number of treatments increased.

In Fig. 28 we show the general pattern of emergence of various phenotypic alterations in cultured stromal cells in relation to the number of carcinogen treatments. Among the earliest alterations we observed was that cells that survived the initial carcinogen treatment became resistant to the toxicity of further exposures to MNNG. Following this, differences in morphology and growth properties were observed. For purposes of discussion, these alterations can be broken down into early, intermediate, and advanced stages.

The early changes expressed by the third carcinogen treatment involved slight morphological deviation from normalcy and increased growth potential, as measured by plating efficiency and saturation density. After four or more carcinogen treatments, intermediate changes were expressed; cells acquired the capacity to grow in soft agar and demonstrated elevated levels of GGT activity. The cells also showed an increase in growth rate and acquired the capacity for clonal growth in CMRL-1066 medium and in medium with low concentrations of calcium. Concurrently, the cells developed altered morphological characteristics with pleomorphic appearance to cells and their nuclei. There was an increase in the ratio of nucleus to cytoplasm, and focal areas of cellular crowding were quite evident.

After eight or more treatments with MNNG, cells expressed more advanced alterations: severe morphological abnormalities with extreme cellular crowding and a marked increase in the nuclear:cytoplasmic ratio. Cytopathologists interpreted these cells to be malignant. Occasionally, macroscopic foci of highly crowded cells were visible on culture plates. These highly treated cells could also be grown in suspension in spinner flasks. These cells showed differences in histochemical staining patterns and LDH isoenzyme distributions from control cells, and they were able to grow at low density in restrictive media.

These properties were similar or identical to the properties observed in cultured human stromal cell sarcomas, suggesting that the phenotypic alterations induced in normal endometrial stromal cells by the repetitive MNNG treatments are similar to the alterations that have occurred in the stromal sarcoma cells. The sequential changes observed *in vitro* may therefore be related to malignant transformation as it occurs in these cells *in vivo*.

The successful growth of the carcinogen-treated cells in *nude* mice is an objective that has eluded us. As noted earlier, the lack of growth in *nude* mice does not constitute evidence that the cells are not malignantly transformed. Further efforts will be made to grow these cells as tumors in *nude* mice in order to provide important additional evidence for the malignant

nature of these cells and to relate our observations more effectively with those of other investigators. Our observation
that CMRL-1066 medium fosters the differentiation of cultured
endometrial stromal cells more than do other media may offer a
possible explanation for the previous lack of success in growing these cells in *nude* mice. The choice of CMRL-1066 medium
was made to achieve an acceptable state of differentiation in
the cultured stromal cells. This objective may be inimical to
the objective of obtaining growth in *nude* mice, as it may inhibit the establishment of transplanted cells in these animals.
Future studies will consider the effects of culture in media
that minimize the differentiation of these cells in culture
prior to their transplantation into *nude* mice.

The gradual, progressive nature of development toward a
transformed phenotype in cultured human endometrial stromal
cells makes this system attractive for studies *in vitro* that
stimulate the process of promotion as it occurs *in vivo*. Because stromal cells can be altered in varying degrees by different numbers of treatments with MNNG, the ability of promoting agents to bring about further transitions at each stage can
be tested. Also, the response of cells to promoters at different stages of progression can be compared. Initial studies
showed that human endometrial cells are responsive to treatments with TPA yielding biochemical and morphological responses.
Differences in responses were observed between control cells
and cells that had previously been treated with MNNG and thus
may be "initiated" cells.

Although dramatic responses to TPA treatment were observed
after a single exposure to TPA, perhaps the more intriguing alterations were observed following long-term culture in the
presence of TPA over a period of 4 to 6 months. TPA was shown
to cause the differentiation of stromal cells toward their
secretory stage-like appearance in culture, and TPA can gradual-

ly inhibit the further growth of these cells. In marked contrast, prolonged exposure to TPA seemed to enhance the growth of cells previously treated with MNNG. In other observations, TPA treatment of initiated cells led to the acquisition of phenotypic characteristics that would have developed with further MNNG treatment. These consequences of TPA treatments *in vitro* in endometrial stromal cells appear to be generally consistent with current hypotheses regarding tumor promotion *in vivo*, which suggests that promoters exert different and perhaps opposite effects on normal and initiated cells, fostering the growth of the initiated cells while fostering the differentiation of normal cells.

ACKNOWLEDGMENTS

    We thank Drs. Charles N. Carney and Vijay A. Varma for their assistance in the obtainment of human endometrial tissue. We also thank Jane L. Martin for assistance in preparation of illustrations and Carol A. Klevay for assistance in preparation of the manuscript. This research was supported by grant CA31733 and contract CP75956 from the National Cancer Institute. David G. Kaufman is supported by a Research Career Development Award (CA00431) from the National Cancer Institute. Jill M. Siegfried and Karen A. Nelson are the recipients of National Research Service Awards (CA09156 and ES07017, respectively). B. Hugh Dorman was supported by a predoctoral fellowship from the Chemical Industry Institute of Toxicology.

REFERENCES

Bancroft, J. D. (1975). *In* "Histochemical Techniques,"
        pp. 223-304. Butterworth, London.
Baron, D. A., and Esterly, J. R. (1975). *Am. J. Obstet. Gynecol. 123,* 790-796.
Boutwell, R. K. (1964). *Prog. Exp. Tumor Res. 4,* 207-250.
Dallenbach-Hellweg, G. (1981). *In* "Histopathology of the Endometrium" 3rd ed., pp. 38-41. Springer-Verlag, New York.

Dorman, B. H., Genta, V. M., Mass, M. J., and Kaufman, D. G.
    (1981). *Cancer Res. 41,* 2718-2722.
Dorman, B. H., Varma, V. A., Siegfried, J. M., Melin, S. A.,
    Adamec, T. A., Norton, C. R., Carney, C. N., and Kaufman,
    D. G. (1982a). *In Vitro 18,* 919-928.
Dorman, B. H., Siegfried, J. M., and Kaufman, D. G. (1983).
    Cancer Res. 43, 3348-3357.
Flippe, M. I., and Dawson, I. M. P. (1968). *J. Pathol.
    Bacteriol. 95,* 243-258.
Giovanella, B. C., Stehlin, J. S., and Williams, L. J. (1974).
    J. Natl. Cancer Inst. (U.S.) 52, 921-927.
Goldberg, B., and Jones, H. W. (1956). *Obstet. Gynecol. (N.Y.)*
    7, 542-546.
Kaufman, D. G., Adamec, T. A., Walton, L. A., Carney, C. N.,
    Melin, S. A., Genta, V. M., Mass, M. J., Dorman, B. H.,
    Rodgers, N. T., Photopulos, G. J., Powell, J., and
    Grisham, J. W. (1980). *Methods Cell Biol. 21B,* 1-27.
Kirk, D., King, R. J. B., Heyes, J., Peachey, L., Hirsch, P. J.,
    and Taylor, R. W. T. (1978). *In Vitro 14,* 651-662.
Liszczak, T. M., Richardson, G. S., MacLaughlin, D. T., and
    Kornblith, P. L. (1977). *In Vitro 13,* 344-356.
Moolgavkar, S. H., and Knudson, A. G. (1981). *J. Natl. Cancer
    Inst. (U.S.) 66,* 1037-1052.
Niklasson, O., Skude, G., Johansson, R., and Stormby, N. (1981).
    Acta Obstet. Gynecol. Scand. 60, 1-8.
Noyes, R. W. (1973). *In* "The Uterus" (A. T. Hertig, H. J.
    Norris, and M. R. Abell, eds.), pp. 110-135. Williams
    & Wilkins, Baltimore, Maryland.
O'Brien, T. G., Saladik, D., and Diamond, L. (1982). *Cancer
    Res. 42,* 1233-1239.
Rosalki, S. B. (1974). *Clin. Biochem. 7,* 29-40.
Shimosato, Y., Kameya, T., Nagai, K., Hirohashi, S., Tsutomu,
    K., Hayashi, H., and Nomura, T. (1976). *J. Natl. Cancer
    Inst. (U.S.) 56,* 1251-1255.
Swierenga, S. H. H., Whitfield, J. F., and Karasak, S. (1978).
    Proc. Natl. Acad. Sci. USA 75, 6069-6072.
Varma, V. A., Melin, S. A., Adamec, T. A., Dorman, B. H.,
    Siegfried, J. M., Walton, L. A., Carney, C. N., Norton,
    C. R., and Kaufman, D. G. (1982). *In Vitro 18,* 911-918.
Yuspa, S. H., and Morgan, D. L. (1981). *Nature (London) 293,*
    72-74.
Yuspa, S. H., Lichti, U., Ben, T., Patterson, E., Hennings, H.,
    Slaga, T., Colburn, N., and Kelsey, W. (1976). *Nature
    (London) 262,* 402-404.
Yuspa, S. H., Ben, T. B., Hennings, H., and Lichti, U. (1980).
    Biochem. Biophys. Res. Commun. 97, 700-708.

20

THE USE OF FIBROBLASTS FROM PATIENTS WITH HEREDITARY RETINOBLASTOMA FOR TRANSFORMATION STUDIES: RELEVANCE OF CELL CULTURE STUDIES TO HUMAN TUMORIGENICITY

William F. Benedict

Clayton Ocular Oncology Center
and the Division of Hematology/Oncology
Childrens Hospital of Los Angeles
and
Department of Pediatrics
University of Southern California School of Medicine
Los Angeles, California

A. Linn Murphree

Clayton Ocular Oncology Center
and the Division of Ophthalmology
Childrens Hospital of Los Angeles
and
Departments of Pediatrics and Ophthalmology
University of Southern California School of Medicine
Los Angeles, California

I. INTRODUCTION

The transformation of human cells to date has been extremely difficult. There may be less than a dozen documented cases of human transformation by either chemical or physical agents in which the morphologically transformed cells were aneuploid, had an unlimited life span in culture, and produced rapidly progressive, histologically malignant tumors in immunosuppressed animals. Because several chapters in this volume address the problems and successes in this area, they will not be emphasized in this chapter.

In this section we (1) describe one of our approaches to the transformation of human cells and the rationale for pursuing these studies, (2) discuss collaborative efforts designed to demonstrate the relevancy of human transformation studies, and (3) present our very preliminary studies on the transformation of human cells using fibroblasts from patients with retinoblastoma.

II. RATIONALE FOR USING FIBROBLASTS FROM RETINOBLASTOMA
PATIENTS FOR TRANSFORMATION STUDIES

Because previous studies suggested that reproducible transformation of human cells is particularly difficult, we decided to use fibroblasts from patients with a known genetic susceptibility to develop retinoblastoma as target cells for transformation studies in an effort to increase the frequency of detectable transformations. In 1971 Knudson proposed a "two-mutation" model for retinoblastoma. He suggested that in the hereditary form one mutation was prezygotic, and the second mutation was somatic. Our findings and those of others

support this concept (see Benedict *et al.*, 1983a). Thus
fibroblasts from patients with hereditary retinoblastoma have
a constitutional change predisposing to retinoblastoma. Such
cells may be particularly sensitive to transformation by
physical and chemical agents, because only one additional
genetic change might be necessary for transformation to occur.

We have been able to show in collaboration with others
that the initial genetic change predisposing to retinoblastoma
involves either a large deletion (Sparkes *et al.*, 1980) or a
small submicroscopic deletion and/or mutation within chromosomal region 13q14 (Sparkes *et al.*, 1983). The site of these
genetic changes have been shown to be tightly linked to the
locus for the polymorphic enzyme, esterase D (Sparkes *et al.*,
1980, 1983). Evidence from one of our patients with the 13-
deletion form of retinoblastoma suggests that the retinoblastoma gene acts as a recessive cancer gene at the cellular
level (Benedict *et al.*, 1983b). Clearly, retinoblastoma
appears to be particularly well suited for studying the genetic
mechanisms involved in the initiation and suppression of human
tumorigenesis.

Unfortunately, we do not have normal human retinoblasts
available in cell culture on which to carry out transformation
studies. However, it is known that patients with hereditary
retinoblastoma also have a high propensity to develop secondary
tumors. In a review of 706 survivors of bilateral retino-
blastomas and 18 unilaterally affected patients with a family
history of retinoblastoma, Abramson and colleagues have found
that approximately 50% of these individuals develop second
tumors within 20 years, and approximately 90% have second
tumors within 32 years after diagnosis of their primary tumor
(Abramson *et al.*, 1983). Thus the retinoblastoma gene appears
to be highly penetrant not only for retinoblastoma formation,
but also for producing a number of other human malignancies.

Consequently, we believe there is a rationale for using fibroblasts from patients with hereditary retinoblastoma as human target cells for transformation studies in an effort to increase the yield of bona fide human transformed cells that are aneuploid and produce progressively growing tumors in *nude* mice. If frequent transformation of these fibroblasts can be obtained, it also could be possible to investigate the molecular mechanisms involved in this transformation.

III.   CELL FUSION STUDIES BETWEEN FIBROSARCOMAS OR CHEMICALLY
       TRANSFORMED CELLS AND DIPLOID FIBROBLASTS

Stanbridge and colleagues have shown that when a human tumor cell of epithelial origin is fused with normal fibroblasts, the chromosomes from both parents are retained and tumorigenicity of the epithelial cells is suppressed (Stanbridge *et al.*, 1982). One of us (W. F. B.) has completed a similar study with E. J. Stanbridge and B. E. Weissman in order to determine whether suppression of tumorigenicity also occurred in hybrids in which the tumor cells used were of mesenchymal origin. The human fibrosarcoma cell line HT1080 was used for the study, and when these cells were fused with normal diploid fibroblasts the majority of chromosomes from both parents again were retained in the hybrids and tumorigenicity was suppressed.

Once it had been established that the tumorigenicity of a naturally occurring fibrosarcoma could be suppressed as just described, we decided it was important to determine if human fibroblasts transformed in culture could also be suppressed. Therefore, one of us (W. F. B.) has shown in a collaborative study with T. Kakunaga and colleagues that several hybrids

derived from the fusion of a diploid fibroblast with a
tumorigenic, chemically transformed human fibroblast line
retain most of the chromosomes from both parent cells, and are
not tumorigenic in *nude* mice. The parent chemically transformed cell used was obtained by Kakunaga (1978) and produced
fibrosarcomas in *nude* mice. Therefore, it appears that
studies done on human transformation in culture have relevancy
to actual human tumor formation, and we are encouraged to
pursue these studies further.

IV. PRELIMINARY OBSERVATIONS OF POTENTIAL TRANSFORMATION
     WITH FIBROBLASTS FROM A RETINOBLASTOMA PATIENT

Our studies utilizing fibroblasts from retinoblastoma
patients for transformation are in their early stages. However, a patient with bilateral retinoblastoma has been of
particular interest to us. She had one eye enucleated and
received a subsequent course of chemotherapy as well as radiation to the other eye. At the time the second eye was
removed, connective tissue attached to the outside of the eye
was taken for culture before the eye was opened and the tumor
exposed. This tissue was in the field that had received
maximum radiation. Several pieces of tissue were cultured
separately. In one culture dish the cells were noted to pile
up unlike the fibroblasts in the other dishes. This mass
culture also grew to a considerably higher saturation density
than the other cultures obtained from the same site, and it
produced numerous colonies in semisolid medium. The remaining
mass cultures of fibroblasts from the same patient did not
grow in semisolid medium. Therefore, the cells gained two
properties that have been associated with transformation,

namely morphological changes and growth in semisolid medium.
However, these cells have not been shown as yet to be aneuploid
or to produce progressively growing, histologically malignant
tumors in animals, which would be necessary to establish that
the cells are truly transformed to malignancy.

Nevertheless, the cells should prove interesting for
future studies, in that the transformed phenotype they show
may have resulted from their predisposition to malignancy and
their exposure to radiation *in vivo*. In the future we will
attempt to obtain fibroblasts from regions that have received
radiation to determine whether or not such transformation is a
common phenomenon. The unexpectedly high incidence of second
malignancies in patients with the hereditary form of retinoblastoma and the effect of radiation in reducing the latency
time to tumor appearance (Abramson *et al.*, 1983) suggests that
these cells could provide an ideal model in which to study
human transformation.

V.   CONCLUSIONS

It is our belief that we are entering a new era in the
history of human transformation studies utilizing human tissues
and culture systems. It should be possible to relate studies
done in organ and tissue culture to human cancer. Those
systems that show the most promise can then be utilized to
examine oncogenic progression and chemoprevention.

We also believe that the use of cells from patients with
a genetic predisposition to malignancy may provide a significant tool for probing the molecular biology of human cancer.
Because retinoblastoma is one of the best understood hereditary
human cancers, it is our goal to participate in the cloning

of the retinoblastoma gene and in the determination of its molecular function. We hope the transformation studies using fibroblasts from patients with hereditary retinoblastoma will help in this process.

ACKNOWLEDGMENTS

This work was supported in part by Grant EY-02715 from the National Eye Institute and was performed in conjunction with the Clayton Foundation for Research.

REFERENCES

Abramson, D. H., Ellsworth, R. M., Kitchin, F. D., and Tung, G. (1983). *Ophthalmology (Rochester, Minn.)*, in press.
Benedict, W. F., Banerjee, A., Mark, C., and Murphree, A. L. (1983a). *Cancer Genet. Cytogenet.* (New York), in press.
Benedict, W. F., Murphree, A. L., Banerjee, A., Spina, C. A., Sparkes, M. C., and Sparkes, R. S. (1983b). *Science (Washington, D.C.)* 219, 973-975.
Kakunaga, T. (1978). *Proc. Natl. Acad. Sci. USA* 75, 1334-1338.
Knudson, A. G., Jr. (1971). *Proc. Natl. Acad. Sci. USA* 68, 820-823.
Sparkes, R. S., Sparkes, M. C., Wilson, M. G., Towner, J. W., Benedict, W. F., Murphree, A. L., and Yunis, J. J. (1980). *Science (Washington, D.C.)* 208, 1042-1043.
Sparkes, R. S., Murphree, A. L., Lingua, R. W., Sparkes, M. C., Field, L. L., Funderburk, S. J., and Benedict, W. F. (1983). *Science (Washington, D.C.)* 219, 971-973.
Stanbridge, E. J., Der, C. J., Doersen, C., Nishimi, R. Y., Peehl, D. M., Weissman, B. E., and Wilkinson, J. E. (1982). *Science (Washington, D.C.)* 215, 252-259.

V. Cellular Lesions Caused by Physical Carcinogens

21

ONCOGENIC TRANSFORMATION OF NORMAL, XP, AND BLOOM SYNDROME CELLS BY X RAYS AND ULTRAVIOLET B IRRADIATION[1]

Carmia Borek
and Alan D. Andrews

Departments of Radiology, Pathology,
and Dermatology
Columbia University
College of Physicians and Surgeons
New York, New York

[1]*This investigation was supported by Grant No. CA 12536-11 to the Radiological Research Laboratory/Department of Radiology, and by Grant No. CA 13696 to the Cancer Center/Institute of Cancer Research, awarded by the National Institute, DHHS, and by Grant No. AM 26392-03, awarded by the National Institute of Arthritis, Metabolic, and Digestive Diseases.*

I. INTRODUCTION

In a letter written in 1657, William Harvey stated that
"Nature is nowhere accustomed more openly to display her secret
mysteries than in cases where she shows traces of her workings
apart from the beaten path ... (Garrod, 1928, p. 1055)."

Cancer, a manifestation of nature's "working apart from
the beaten path," is an old disease. It already afflicted
prehistoric animals (Moodie, 1918). Yet the awareness of
carcinogenic agents and the implication of environmental
factors in the causation of the disease are relatively recent.
This realization has emanated from epidemiological data
(Findlay, 1928; Brown, 1936; UNSCEAR, 1977, Doll and Peto,
1981), as well as from studies performed in animal systems
in vivo and *in vitro* (Upton, 1975; Heidelberger, 1975; Sugimura *et al.*, 1977; Urbach *et al.*, 1974; Nagao and Sugimura,
1978; Miller and Miller, 1978; Hecker *et al.*, 1981; Borek,
1982a,b).

Among the various suspected environmental carcinogens,
radiation has received much attention. Ionizing radiation is
present and is increasing in our environment, and in recent
years public attention has focused on the hazards of the low
dose range, doses used in medical diagnosis. Although it is a
weak carcinogen as compared to some chemicals, ionizing radiation is ubiquitous and measurable at low doses.

Nonionizing, ultraviolet (UV) radiation has been associated with skin cancer in humans (Urbach *et al.*, 1974).
Dose-response relationship and quantitative assessments of
UV-induced cancer in humans are often even more complicated
than those evaluated for other types of radiation. Besides
genetic factors and complex environmental cofactors, the risk
following exposure to sunlight varies with life-style, climate,

altitude, and pollution, where photochemical oxidants serve as additional modifiers (Borek and Mehlman, 1983).

Although epidemiological and animal studies have contributed much to our present knowledge on the oncogenic action of radiation, they are limited when trying to assess cancer risk at low doses and to elucidate underlying genetic and molecular mechanisms.

II. CELLULAR TRANSFORMATION *IN VITRO*

Cell culture systems of rodent and human origin offer valuable alternatives as tools to assess the carcinogenic action of various agents under conditions free from host-mediated effects and to evaluate a variety of cellular properties associated with a neoplastic state. These systems also afford us the opportunity to identify cocarcinogens, study cellular and molecular mechanisms, and define factors that may modulate oncogenic processes and prevent neoplastic development. A large volume of data has been accumulated from transformation studies in rodent cells. These studies serve as an important baseline and background for the investigation of the oncogenic potential of various agents in human cells.

A. Radiogenic Transformation of Rodent Cells

1. *Cell Cultures*

A limited number of rodent cell systems have been used in studies in radiation-induced transformation, and these have been reviewed in detail (Borek, 1981, 1982a, 1983). The earliest system used is the hamster embryo system (Borek and Sachs, 1966). These are primary or secondary cell strains,

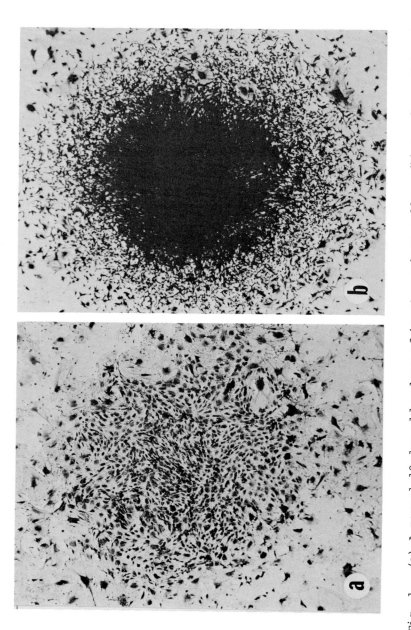

Fig. 1. (a) A normal 10-day-old colony of hamster embryo cells. (b) A colony of hamster embryo cells transformed *in vitro* by 0.1 rad 430-KeV neutrons. From Borek et al. (1978).

cultured from midterm embryos. The hamster cells, similar to human cells, are diploid and have a limited life span. Transformation assays consist of scoring colonies of transformed cells from among the survivors; thus toxicity and transformation are assessed in the same dishes (Borek and Hall, 1973). Upon neoplastic transformation these diploid hamster cells are endowed with an unlimited life span.

Another system often used is that of the mouse $C3H/10T\frac{1}{2}$ heteroploid cell line (Reznikoff et al., 1973a,b). Transformation is identified by the appearance of foci bearing a characteristic growth pattern differing from the underlying normal cells.

2. *Sequential Events in Transformation,*
   Initiation, and Expression

Cell culture systems of rodent cells, mostly of fibroblast-like cells, have enabled us to assess sequential events in the progression of radiogenic transformation from early events on initiation and fixation of the transformed state that require cell division shortly after exposure (Borek and Sachs, 1966, 1967, 1968) to later events associated with the expression of transformation and requiring additional cell divisions (Borek and Sachs, 1967). The transformed state in the fibroblast-like cells is expressed phenotypically by the appearance of morphologically distinct colonies or foci that differ from untransformed controls (Fig. 1).

Once transformed cells have been identified, they can be isolated and propagated, and a number of tests can be carried out to characterize the transformed state of the cells. Thus, other forms of expression of the neoplastic state have been characterized in radiation-transformed rodent cells, especially in the hamster embryo system, and have been discussed in detail elsewhere (Borek et al., 1977, 1978; Borek, 1979a, 1981,

1982a). These include changes in cell topography (Borek and Fenoglio, 1976), loss of intercellular ionic communication (Borek *et al.*, 1969), alterations in cellular ganglioside patterns (Borek *et al.*, 1977), an increased activity of membrane (Na^+, K^+)-ATPase (Borek and Guernsey, 1981), an increase in cellular proteolytic enzymes (Borek *et al.*, 1978), and ability to grow in semisolid agar and to give rise to tumors (Borek and Sachs, 1966; Borek and Hall, 1974; Borek *et al.*, 1978). The latter two properties are the most crucial in ascertaining the neoplastic nature of the cells. Growth in agar is suggestive of malignant potential but not indicative. Tumor formation is an unequivocal proof of the malignant nature of the transformed cells.

Whereas cellular radiogenic transformation is most likely associated with subtle genetic modifications, these are not reflected at early stages by marked chromosomal changes as ascertained by banding techniques. Transformed hamster cells at early passage, although exhibiting a variety of physiological and membrane-associated alterations, remain karyotypically diploid or near diploid (Borek *et al.*, 1977, 1978).

The involvement of DNA metabolism and the role of repair and replication in radiogenic transformation have been suggested by early experiments using liquid-holding recovery (Borek and Sachs, 1967), where exposure of nondividing cells to radiation and their maintenance in a replication state for a period as long as 72 h after irradiation resulted in a progressive decline in transformation rate following subsequent cloning. This decline was directly related to the period of maintenance in nondividing state, suggesting a recovery and reduced "misrepair" of damaged sites by preventing DNA replication. More direct evidence of the role of DNA metabolism in transformation is provided by our experiments, whereby 3-aminobenzamide, and inhibition of poly(ADPribose) synthesis,

TABLE I. Inhibition of X-Ray Induced Transformation in
C3H/10T$\frac{1}{2}$ Cells by Inhibitors of Poly(ADP)Ribosylation

Treatment	Transformed foci/surviving cells	Transformation frequency/surviving cells
Control	0/15930	0
3-Aminobenzamide[a]	0/15680	0
400 Rads	29/28720	1.0×10^{-3}
3-Aminobenzamide + 400 rads	1/27180	3.7×10^{-5}

[a]3-Aminobenzamide added at a concentration of 1 mM.

inhibits X-ray induced transformation in C3H/10T$\frac{1}{2}$ mouse cells
(Borek and Cleaver, 1983) (Table I). The unique involvement
of poly(ADP)ribosylation in regulating the ligation stage in
repair of alkylation damage and the slowing of this ligation
by 3-aminobenzamide (Creissen and Shall, 1982) implicates this
process in the induction of X-ray induced transformation.

3. A Baseline for Cancer Risk Estimates

From a pragmatic point of view, rodent cells *in vitro*
have provided important tools for assessing the oncogenic
potential of a variety of radiation over a wide range of doses
(for review see Borek, 1982a). The hamster diploid cell
system has been the most useful in the study of low-level
radiation. Thus, we have found that X rays can transform cells
at doses as low as 0.3 rad (Borek, 1982a) and that neutrons
are more than 10-fold more efficient in transforming cells as
compared to X rays at a comparable dose, though their high
oncogenic effect is matched by their higher toxicity (Borek
et al., 1978). We also found using the hamster cell system

that exposure of cells to protracted doses of X-irradiation at low doses but not at high doses may lead to a 70% enhancement of transformation as compared to the frequency following exposure to the same total given acutely (Borek and Hall, 1974; Borek, 1979b). The studies indicate that extrapolation from high to low dose may be neither conservative nor prudent when oncogenic transformation is the end point studied. Our findings that the oncogenic potential of X rays at low doses (3 rads) is twice as high as that of cobalt γ rays at that dose but that at higher doses of 150 rads their oncogenic action is equal (Borek *et al.*, 1983), is another case in point.

B. Transformation of Rodent Cells by Ultraviolet Radiation

    Similar to the utilization of rodent cells in studies on X-ray induced transformation, most *in vitro* studies of UV-induced transformation have utilized rodent cells as the quantitative test system using germicidal lamps as the source of UV light (Mondal and Heidelberger, 1976; Chan and Little, 1976; Kakunaga and Crow, 1980). Germicidal lamps emit light at a wavelength of 254 nm, a wavelength highly efficient at producing pyrimidine dimers in DNA. Pyrimidine dimers are considered the principal lethal lesion produced by 254-nm light (Selow and Setlow, 1972; Rothman and Setlow, 1979), although evidence is accumulating that other types of lesions are also important when UV light at longer wavelengths is used as the lethal treatment (Suzuki *et al.*, 1981). Pyrimidine dimers have been directly linked to neoplastic transformation in an *in vivo* study utilizing a species of fish in which specific photoreactivation of the dimers can be readily produced (Setlow and Hart, 1974). Doniger *et al.* (1981), studying *in vitro* transformation in Syrian hamster embryo

cells at different UV wavelengths (between 240 and 313 nm),
found a rough correlation between dimer production and transformation, suggesting that pyrimidine dimers were the important
lesions in UV-induced *in vitro* transformation as well. However, Suzuki *et al.* (1981), utilizing V 79 Chinese hamster
cells and C3H/10T$\frac{1}{2}$ mouse cells, found that broad-band UV light
>300 nm produces neoplastic transformation at rates appreciably
greater than expected if pyrimidine dimers are considered the
sole transforming lesion.

In general, whether using 254-nm or longer wavelengths of
UV, studies of UV-induced neoplastic transformation in rodent
cells have indicated a dose dependency (Borek, 1982a). Transformation of rodent cells by 254-nm UV light has been enhanced
by X rays (DiPaolo and Donovan, 1976) and by the promoter (TPA)
(Mondal and Heidelberger, 1976). Kakunaga and Crow (1980)
presented evidence for a wide variance in sensitivity to the
transforming effects of 254-nm UV light among clones of BALB/
3T3 mouse cells, even though the clones had similar sensitivities to the killing effects of this light. Ananthaswamy and
Kripke (1981) have transformed neonatal BALB/c mouse epidermal
cells with "long-wavelength" UV light (i.e., >290 nm) and
demonstrated the tumorigenicity of the transformants.

III. ONCOGENIC TRANSFORMATION OF HUMAN CELLS

Animal cell systems have yielded important information on
the oncogenic potential of environmental agents, including
radiation. Yet a logical goal has been to develop human cell
systems in which one can study in an analogous fashion, at a

cellular and molecular level, mechanisms and sequential events
in neoplastic development, and carry out quantitative assessments of cancer risk factors.

One is cognizant of the fact that there exists a wide
variation in seemingly nondiseased as well as in diseased
individuals, which could result in varied sensitivities to
particular agents. However, in cases where diseases are genetically transmitted and the genetic defects are defined, the
in vitro systems of human cells offer the opportunity to
investigate at a cellular level the susceptibility of the cells
to specific transforming agents. Of specific interest are
genetic syndromes with a high predisposition to cancer, such
as xeroderma pigmentosum (XP) and Bloom syndrome.

A.   Human Cell Transformation by X Irradiation

The induction of oncogenic transformation in human cells
by X rays was carried out using normal diploid human skin
fibroblasts (Borek, 1980a,b). These cells, defined as strain
KD (Kakunaga, 1978), were utilized at early passage to avoid
altered properties, such as changes in cell cycle kinetics,
which are inevitable in human cell strains, which possess a
limited life span.

Cells were synchronized and brought to quiescence (G_1) by
a 24-h incubation in medium supplemented with 1% fetal calf
serum and were released from G_1 by a medium change using complete medium fortified with 10% fetal calf serum and β-
estradiol or the protease inhibitor antipain (Borek, 1980).
Cells were irradiated at G_1-S, after which cells were split
equally into two flasks and propagated for several generations.
After 13 to 15 doublings, visible discrete foci were detected,
in which cells arranged themselves in multilayers that differed

from the flat background untransformed cells but were not as
dramatic in their haphazard arrangement as the X-ray transformed diploid hamster cells (Fig. 2a and b). The transformed
cells grew in low-calcium medium in contrast to the normal
cells, which died under those conditions (Fig. 2c). This
served as a useful selective factor to isolate transformants.
The transformed cells proliferated in medium containing 1%
serum agar (Fig. 2d). However, this property of growth in low
serum was not confined to the transformed human cells as in
the rodent systems (Borek et al., 1977; Borek, 1982a) but was
also a property of the normal KD cells.

The transformed KD cells grew in semisolid agar in
contrast to the normal cells, which could not, indicating that
the cells following irradiation had acquired a phenotype of
anchorage independence associated with a neoplastic state.
Some of these anchorage-independent cells formed tumors in
nude mice, indicating unequivocally that these transformants
were malignant (Borek, 1980a). The failure of some of the
clones derived from agar to grow in the animal illustrated
that anchorage independence is a step in neoplastic transformation and that the property of anchorage independence is
suggestive but not indicative of a malignant potential in vivo.

Similar to the X-ray transformed hamster cells, the
karyotype of the X-ray transformed human cells was near
diploid or diploid. Also, similar to the rodent system, DNA
replication within hours after initiation was required for
fixation of transformation. Cultures that were treated or
irradiated in a nondividing state, as well as those that were
allowed only four or five cell divisions before reaching confluency (and not subcultured further), did not exhibit
transformed foci.

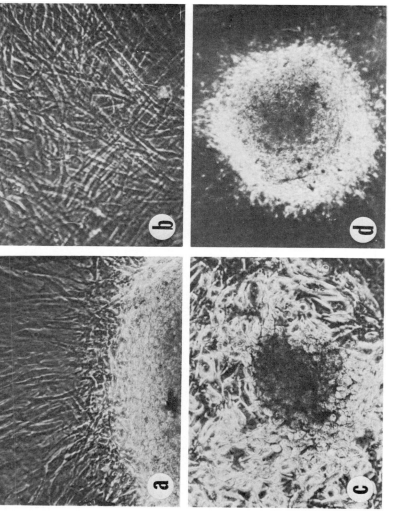

Fig. 2. (a) A focus of X-ray transformed human KD cells (phase x105). (b) A culture of irradiated transformed KD cells (phase x105). (c) The same cells as in (b) following a 24-h treatment in medium containing low calcium (phase x105). (d) Irradiated transformed KD cells growing as anchorage-independent cells in agar (x110). In part from Borek (1980a).

There are striking differences between the radiation-transformed hamster embryo cells and the X-ray transformed KD cells in the temporal sequences of neoplastic progression and in the transformation rate. Whereas anchorage independence in hamster cells is acquired several generations after the appearance of morphologically identifiable foci (Borek *et al.*, 1978; Barrett and T'so, 1978; Kakunaga, 1978), anchorage independence of human cells is observed at the time of the appearance of foci in culture and is acquired even earlier. Thus, whereas 13 to 15 cell doublings were required for the appearance of foci in culture, growth in agar could be observed within 6 to 10 doublings after exposure.

The rate of transformation in KD cells following exposure to 400 rads is approximately 10^{-6}. The frequency of transformation in hamster embryo cells exposed to 400 rads is close to 10^{-4}.

Although we know now that cell synchronization is not essential for radiogenic transformation of human cells, current experiments indicate that this procedure enhances the frequency of transformation and reduces the time period required for expression of transformation. Current experiments also indicate that susceptibility to transformation by X rays is reduced in the human cells with passage *in vitro*, similar to our early observations with hamster embryo cells (Borek and Sachs, 1967). It is still unclear whether cell senescence or progressive cellular differentiation is the cause of this phenomenon.

The mechanism of potentiation of radiogenic transformation in human cells by β-estradiol and antipain is unclear. Both have antiprotease activity (Borek, 1980a), and both can potentiate rodent cell transformation by X rays (Borek, 1982a).

If one speculates that oncogenic transformation may be
mediated in part via activation of cellular transforming genes
(Cooper, 1982), the biological activity of these genes may be
modified at different stages in the cycle and the life span of
the cells, as well as by modifying factors such as estradiol
or antipain.

Although anchorage independence did not always correlate
with malignancy *in vivo*, it seems a reproducible end point to
ascertain phenotypic changes induced by an oncogenic agent and
associated with a transformed state. Thus, experiments carried
out with UV radiation utilized this end point for quantitative
assessment of transformation (Andrews and Borek, 1982).

B.   Ultraviolet Transformation of Xeroderma Pigmentosum
     and Bloom Syndrome Cells

Sunlight exposure is clearly associated with development
of the most prevalent of all human cancer, namely skin cancer.
Evidence from epidemiological and animal studies indicates
that UV wavelengths in the "UVB" range (280-320 nm), which are
responsible for sunlight-induced erythema of human skin
(Parrish *et al.*, 1974), are probably also responsible for
sunlight-induced skin cancer (Urbach *et al.*, 1974; Setlow,
1974). To date, however, only certain rodent cell studies,
discussed previously, have examined *in vitro* transformation
utilizing UVB sources. Studies of *in vitro* neoplastic transformation of human cells have utilized only germicidal lamps,
which produce UV at 254 nm, a wavelength not present in natural
sunlight at the earth's surface. Nevertheless, these studies
have demonstrated that *in vitro* UV-induced transformation of
human cells is feasible (Sutherland *et al.*, 1980; Milo *et al.*,

1981; Maher *et al.*, 1982), and such systems promise to be of great value in further elucidating the details of UV-induced neoplastic transformation of human cells.

Our studies, however, were designed to examine transformation of human cells by UVB light (Andrews and Borek, 1982). We bagan with cells from patients with the rare genetic syndrome, xeroderma pigmentosum (XP), which are defective in DNA repair (Cleaver, 1968; Setlow *et al.*, 1968) and are particularly sensitive to the killing and mutagenic effects of UV light (Andrews *et al.*, 1978; Maher and McCormick, 1976). Patients with XP suffer from a markedly increased susceptibility to sunlight-induced skin cancer (Robbins *et al.*, 1974; Setlow, 1974; Cleaver *et al.*, 1981), and their cells are known to carry one of at least eight different genetic defects in the capacity to repair UV-induced damage to DNA (Kraemer *et al.*, 1975; Lehmann, 1975; Arase *et al.*, 1979; Keijzer *et al.*, 1979).

Fibroblast strains XP5BE, from a patient in XP group D (Robbins *et al.*, 1974), and CCD-25SK, a normal strain, were used. We also utilized line GM1492 from a patient with Bloom syndrome, another disorder in which patients are cancer prone (primarily internal malignancies) and in which the cells appear to have some as yet ill-defined alteration in DNA metabolism. The cells were partially synchronized by growth in medium containing 1% serum for 72 h. After a subsequent 6-h period of growth in complete medium with 20% serum, the cells were exposed, in buffer, to the first of a series of doses of UVB light from the Westinghouse FS20 sunlamps filtered through 1 mm of Pyrex glass. Daily doses of 8.4 to 33.6 J/m^2 were repeated at 24-h intervals for 4 to 8 days. Cells were incubated at 37°C in complete medium between each irradiation, and for a period of 2 weeks or more after the last irradiation. The cells were then plated in semisolid agarose (0.25%) and

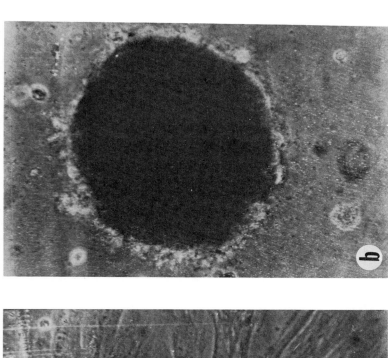

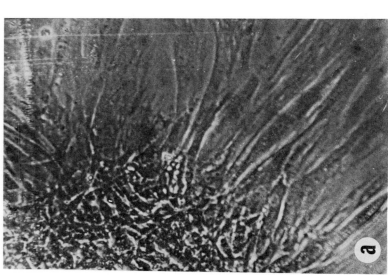

Fig. 3. (a) A focus of Bloom syndrome fibroblast transformed *in vitro* by UVB. (b) An anchorage-independent colony of UVB-transformed Bloom syndrome fibroblasts growing in agar. From Borek (1982a).

incubated for an additional period of 3 weeks before scoring. The frequency of oncogenic transformation was determined by the number of colonies that formed in agarose as a fraction of the total cells plated. Parallel cultures were screened for the appearance of multilayered transformed foci (Fig. 3); whereas irradiated normal cells showed no transformation at the low UVB doses used, both the XP and the Bloom syndrome strains yielded significant numbers of anchorage-independent colonies after irradiation, indicating their higher sensitivity to the oncogenic effects of UVB, as compared to normal.

1. XP Cells

Whereas no toxicity was observed in the normal cells exposed to the UV doses used (268.8 J/m^2), cell survival in the exposed XP cell was reduced to 50% of the unirradiated cells.

Oncogenic transformation as measured by anchorage ind independence was clearly related to total dose of exposure (Table II), whether delivered in four or eight protracted doses. The yield of colonies in agar increased with expression time in culture and was directly related to the number of cell doublings that took place between the exposure to UVB and subsequent culture in the semisolid medium (Table III). It is of interest to note that anchorage independence was observed

TABLE II. Oncogenic Transformation of XP Cells by UVB

Daily dose (J/m^2)	Total dose (J/m^2)	Anchorage-independent transformations/10^6 cells
0	0	0
16.8	67.2	37
8.4	67.2	35
33.6	268.8	79

TABLE III. Effect of Postirradiation Expression Time on the
            Yield of Transformation of XP Cells Exposed to UVB

Daily dose (J/m^2)	Total dose (J/m^2)	Population doublings	Transformants/10^6 cells
8.4	67.2	2	35
16.8	67.2	2	37
16.8	67.2	3	68
8.4	67.2	4	128

in the XP cells as well as in the Bloom syndrome cells (Table
IV) as early as two doublings after exposure.

2. *Bloom Syndrome Cells*

     Our results indicated that although no toxicity was
observed in the Bloom cells following exposure to the low UVB
doses employed, transformation was induced in these cells
(Table IV). However, transformation rate in these experiments
did not increase with dose within the small range of doses
used (Table IV), nor did we find the effect of expression time
that was so markedly obvious in the XP cells (Table II).

TABLE IV. Oncogenic Transformation of Bloom Syndrome Cells
           by UVB

Daily dose (J/m^2)	Total dose (J/m^2)	Population doublings	Anchorage-independent transformants/10^6 cells
0	0	—	1
8.4	33.6	4	63
16.8	67.2	2	61
16.8	67.2	4	57
33.6	134.4	2	50
33.6	134.4	4	57

A particular link between toxicity and induction of transformation is suggested and is currently under investigation over a wider range of doses.

IV. CONCLUSIONS

The field of oncogenic transformation by chemical and physical agents is young. Human fibroblasts *in vitro* have been transformed by a variety of chemical carcinogens (Kakunaga, 1978; Milo and DiPaolo, 1978; Silinskas *et al.*, 1981; Zimmerman and Little, 1981), by X rays (Borek, 1980a,b; Milo *et al.*, 1981), and by UV (Sutherland, 1980; Andrews and Borek, 1982; Maher *et al.*, 1982). Cells of patients with genetic syndromes in which enhanced cancer rates are observed and in which defects in DNA metabolism prevail appear to have a higher cellular sensitivity to transformation as compared to seemingly normal cells. This can be assessed by the response of XP cells to UVA (Maher *et al.*, 1982) and the response of XP and Bloom syndrome cells to UVB (Andrews and Borek, 1982).

When comparing the human cells to rodent cells, several differences can be recognized. A clear difference can be seen in the frequency of transformation as well as in its temporal progression. It appears that human diploid cells are far less sensitive to radiogenic transformation as compared to rodent diploid cells (Borek, 1980a). However one must be cognizant of the different experimental conditions that must be employed. Also, one cannot state these facts unequivocally until large volumes of data on transformation of seemingly normal human cells are accumulated. Humans vary genetically and are exposed to so many different life-styles (Harris, 1980; Dole and Peto, 1981), as compared to animals bred and maintained in cages.

Human cell transformation *in vitro* progresses in a somewhat different fashion than rodent cells. Hamster cells transformed by X rays show morphological changes within 2 weeks but acquire anchorage independence after progressive culture *in vitro* (Borek et al., 1978), whereas X-ray transformed human cells can grow in agar within 6 to 10 doublings after exposure, although morphological changes *in vitro* are observed after 13 to 15 doublings. Genetically defective XP and Bloom cells grow in agar within two doublings after exposure, although the yield of transformed colonies, as assessed by anchorage independence and growth in agar, increase with the number of doublings after UVB exposure.

Growth in agar is a useful indicator of the acquisition of a new phenotype associated with transformation, which under the same conditions employed is not expressed in normal cells derived from solid tissue. If one alters the conditions, normal cells of solid tissue can also express anchorage independence (Peehl and Stanbridge, 1981), indicating the importance of unified conditions in various experimental settings.

Although only a fraction of anchorage-independent colonies express malignant potential in the animal (Borek, 1980a), the acquisition of this phenotype following exposure to carcinogens under specific conditions is dose related (Silinskas et al., 1981; Andrews and Borek, 1982; Maher et al., 1982). Because of technical differences (purity and type of agar, media used, quality of serum) and scoring methods, one can expect differences in actual rates reported from various laboratories.

We are clearly ignorant of the mechanisms underlying the events in initiation — that is, to what extent oncogenes play a role (Cooper, 1982) and to what extent physiological competence of cells is involved (Borek, 1982b). We find that thyroid hormones play a crucial role as a permissive factor in making some hamster, mouse, and rat cells competent to be transformed by X rays, direct- and indirect-acting chemical carcinogens, and the Kirsten virus (Borek, 1983). This indicates that in rodent cells initiation can take place only under optimal physiological conditions, and it suggests that this may hold true also for human cells.

In addition, we find that in rodent cells cellular protective factors when added externally can inhibit transformation by radiation and chemicals and inhibit the enhancement of transformation by tumor promoters. These include a variety of retinoids, selenium (Borek, 1982b), as well as superoxide dismutase (Borek and Troll, 1983). Thus, these inherent cellular systems, which protect cells from the deleterious action of free radicals produced by a variety of carcinogens, probably play a role in the transformation process and serve as additional variables that determine the transformation frequency. These variables are related to the cellular level of these factors and may differ with cell type and species (Borek and Troll, 1983; Borek and Mehlman, 1983).

The malignant potential of human cells transformed *in vitro* is of great interest. Tumors produced by injection of transformed human cells into *nude* mice can regress and transformed human cells do not necessarily acquire immortality as do transformed rodent cells. The karyotype of the human transformed and malignant cells can be diploid or near diploid, although near diploid may be sufficient to produce instability. Human cells differ from rodent cells in their lower requirements for serum nutrients. Rodent cells transformed by X rays will grow in medium supplemented with 1% serum whereas normal cells will die (Borek *et al.*, 1977). In contrast, both normal and transformed human cells can grow in medium with 1% serum (Borek, 1980a,b).

It is too early to conclude how reproducible human cell transformation experimentation is and whether the system will be used for pragmatic risk evaluation and in mechanistic studies as efficiently as animal cell systems, but time will tell. Perhaps the development of human cell lines with indefinite life spans of both fibroblast and epithelial origin may be an important unifying step for future experimentations.

REFERENCES

Ananthaswamy, H. N., and Kripke, M. L. (1981). *Cancer Res. 41*, 2882-2890.

Andrews, A. D., and Borek, C. (1982). *Clin. Res. 30*, 574A.

Andrews, A. D., Barrett, S. F., and Robbins, J. H. (1978). *Proc. Natl. Acad. Sci. USA 75*, 1984-1988.

Arase, S., Kozuka, T., Tanaka, K., Ikenaga, M., and Takebe, H. (1979). *Mutat. Res. 59*, 143-146.

Barrett, J. C., and T'so, P. O. P. (1978). *Proc. Natl. Acad. Sci. USA 75*, 3297-3301.

Borek, C. (1979a). *Radiat. Res. 79*, 209-232.

Borek, C. (1979b). *Br. J. Radiol. 52*, 845-849.

Borek, C. (1980a). *Nature (London) 283*, 776-778.

Borek, C. (1980b). *In* "Carcinogenesis, Fundamental Mechanism and Environmental" (B. Pullman *et al.*, eds.), pp. 509. Reidel, Amsterdam.

Borek, C. (1981). *J. Supramol. Struct. Biochem. 16*, 311-336.

Borek, C. (1982a). *Adv. Cancer Res. 37*, 159-232.

Borek, C. (1982b). *In* "Molecular Interrelations of Nutrition and Cancer" (M. S. Arnott, J. Van Eys, and Y.-M. Wang, eds.), pp. 337-350. Raven, New York.

Borek, C. (1983. *Proc. Int. Cancer Congr. 13th*, in press.

Borek, C., and Cleaver, J. E. (1983). *Proc. Am. Assoc. Cancer Res. 74*, 56.

Borek, C., and Fenoglio, C. M. (1976). *Cancer Res. 36*, 1325-1334.

Borek, C., and Guernsey, D. C. (1981). *Stud. Biophys. 84*, 53-54.

Borek, C., and Hall, E. J. (1973). *Nature (London) 252*, 499-501.

Borek, C., and Mehlman, M. A. (1983). *Adv. Mod. Environ. Toxicol. 5*, 325-362.

Borek, C., and Sachs, L. (1966). *Nature (London) 210*, 276-278.

Borek, C., and Sachs, L. (1967). *Proc. Natl. Acad. Sci. USA* *57*, 1522-1527.

Borek, C., and Troll, W. (1983). *Proc. Natl. Acad. Sci. USA* *78*, 5708-5711.

Borek, C., Higashino, S., and Loewenstein, W. R. (1969). *J. Membr. Biol.* *1*, 274-293.

Borek, C., Pain, C., and Mason, H. (1977). *Nature (London)* *266*, 452-454.

Borek, C., Hall, E. J., and Rossi, H. H. (1978). *Cancer Res.* *38*, 2997-3605.

Borek, C., Zaider, M., and Hall, E. J. (1983). *Nature (London)* *301*, 156-158.

Brown, P. (1936). "American Martyrs to Science through Roentgen Ray." Thomas, Springfield, Illinois.

Chan, G. L., and Little, J. B. (1976). *Nature (London)* *264*, 442-444.

Cleaver, J. E. (1968). *Nature (London)* *218*, 652-656.

Cleaver, J. E., Zelle, B., Hashem, N., and German, J. (1981). *J. Invest. Dermatol.* *77*, 96-101.

Cooper, G. M. (1982). *Science (Washington, D. C.)* *217*, 801-806.

Creissen, D., and Shall, S. (1982). *Nature (London)* *296*, 271-272.

DiPaolo, J. A., and Donovan, P. J. (1976). *Int. J. Radiat. Biol.* *30*, 41-54.

Dole, R., and Peto, R. J. (1981). *J. Natl. Cancer Inst.* *66*, 1191-1308.

Doniger, J., Jacobson, E. D., Krell, K., and DiPaolo, J. A. (1981). *Proc. Natl. Acad. Sci. USA 78*, 2378-2382.

Findlay, G. M. (1928). *Lancet 2*, 1070-1073.

Garrod, A. (1928). *Lancet 1*, 1055.

Harris, C. C. (1980). *Ann. Intern. Med.* *92*, 809-825.

Hecker, E., Fusenig, J. E., Kunz, W., Marks, F., and Thielman, H. W. (1981). "Carcinogenesis." Raven, New York.

Heidelberger, C. (1975). *Annu. Rev. Biochem.* *44*, 79-121.

Kakunaga, T. (1978). *Proc. Natl. Acad. Sci. USA 75*, 1334-1338.

Kakunaga, T., and Crow, J. D. (1980). *Science (Washington D. C.)* *309*, 505-507.

Keijzer, W., Jaspers, A. G., Abrahams, P. J., Taylor, A. M., Arlett, C. F., Zelle, B., Takebe, H., Kinmont, P. D., and Bootsma, D. (1979). *Mutat. Res.* *62*, 183-190.

Kraemer, K. H., Deweerd-Kastelein, E. A., Robbins, J. H., Keijzer, H., Barrett, S. F., Petinga, R. A., and Bootsma, D. (1975). *Mutat. Res.* *33*, 327-340.

Lehmann, A. R., Kirk-Bell, S., Arlett, C. F., Paterson, M. C., Lohman, P. H. M., DeWeerd-Kastelein, E. A., and Bootsma, D. (1975). *Proc. Natl. Acad. Sci. USA 72*, 219-223.

Maher, V. M., and McCormick, J. J. (1976). *In* "Biology of Radiation Carcinogenesis" (J. M. Yuhas *et al.*, eds.), pp. 129-145. Raven, New York.

Maher, V. M., Rowan, L. A., Silinskas, K. C., Kateley, S. A., and McCormick, J. J. (1982). *Proc. Natl. Acad. Sci. USA* *79*, 2613-2617.

Miller, E. C., and Miller, J. A. (1979). *Int. Rev. Biochem.* , *123-165*.

Milo, G. E., and DiPaolo, J. A. (1978). *Nature (London) 275*, 130-132.

Milo, G. E., Weisbrode, S. A., Zimmerman, R., and McCloskey, J. A. (1981). *Chem. Biol. Interact. 36*, 45-59.

Mondal, S., and Heidelberger, C. (1976). *Nature (London) 260*, 710-711.

Moodie, R. L. (1918). *Surg. Clin. Chicago 2*, 319-331.

Nagao, M., and Sugimura, T. (1978). *Annu. Rev. Genet. 12*, 117-159.

Parrish, J. A., Ying, C. Y., and Pathack, M. A. (1974). *In* "Sunlight and Man" (T. Fitzpatrick *et al.*, eds.), pp. 131-141. Univ. of Tokyo Press, Tokyo.

Peehl, D. M., and Stanbridge, E. J. (1981). *Proc. Natl. Acad. Sci. USA 78*, 3053-3057.

Reznikoff, C. A., Brankow, D. W., and Heidelberger, C. (1973a). *Cancer Res. 33*, 3231-3238.

Reznikoff, C. A., Bertram, J. S., Brankow, D. W., and Heidelberger, C. (1973b). *Cancer Res. 33*, 3239-3249.

Robbins, J. H., Kraemer, K. H., Lutzner, M. A., Festoff, B. W., and Coon, H. G. (1974). *Ann. Intern. Med. 80*, 221-248.

Rothman, R. H., and Setlow, R. B. (1979). *Post. Chem. Photobiol. 29*, 57-61.

Setlow, R. B. (1974). *Proc. Natl. Acad. Sci. USA 72*, 3363-3366.

Setlow, R. B., and Hart, R. W. (1974). *Radiat. Res. 59*, 73-74.

Setlow, R. B., and Setlow, J. R. (1972). *Annu. Rev. Biophys. Bioeng. 1*, 293-346.

Silinskas, K. C., Kateley, S. A., Tower, J. E., Maher, V. M., and McCormick, J. J. (1981). *Cancer Res. 41*, 1620-1627.

Sugimura, T., Nagao, M., Kawachi, T., Honda, M., Yahasi, T., Seino, Y., Sato, S., and Matsukura, A. (1977). *In* "Origins of Human Cancer" (H. H. Hiatt, J. D. Watson, and J. Winsten, eds.), pp. 1561-1567. Cold Spring Harbor Lab., Cold Spring Harbor, New York.

Sutherland, B. M., Cimino, J. S., Delihas, N., Shih, A. G., and Oliver, R. P. (1980). *Cancer Res. 40*, 193401939.

Suzuki, F., Han, A., Lankas, G. R., Utsumi, H., and Elkind, M. M. (1981). *Cancer Res. 41*, 4916-4924.

United Nations Scientific Committee on the Effects of Atomic Radiation (UNSCEAR) (1977. "Report to the General Assembly on Sources and Effects of Ionizing Radiations." United Nations, New York.

Upton, A. C. (1975). *In* "Cancer-A Comprehensive Trestise" (F. F. Becker, ed.), Vol. 1, pp. 387–401, Plenum, New York.

Urbach, F., Epstein, J. H., and Forbes, P. D. (1974). *In* "Sunlight and Man" (T. Fitzpatrick, M. A. Pathak, L. C. Harber, M. Seiji, and A. Kukita, eds.), pp. 259–283. Univ. of Tokyo Press, Tokyo.

Zimmerman, R. J., and Little, J. B. (1981). *Carcinogenesis 2*, 1303–1310.

22

QUANTITATIVE STUDIES OF CYTOTOXICITY, MUTAGENESIS, AND ONCOGENIC TRANSFORMATION BY RADIOISOTOPES INCORPORATED INTO DNA

John B. Little, Peter K. LeMotte, and Howard L. Liber

Laboratory of Radiobiology
Harvard School of Public Health
Boston, Massachusetts

I. INTRODUCTION

The results reported in this chapter represent a part of our ongoing investigation of the role of specific cellular and molecular lesions in radiation-induced cytotoxicity, mutagenesis, and transformation. Of particular interest is the role of DNA damage in the initiation of transformation *in vitro*. In order to gain information on involvement of DNA damage as well as its molecular nature, we have studied the effects of two radioisotopes incorporated into cellular DNA and compared these with the effects of X rays. The radioisotopes are ^{125}I incorporated as ^{125}I-labeled dUrd and ^{3}H as [^{3}H]-thymidine ([^{3}H]-TdR). Upon disintegration, ^{3}H emits a

Copyright © 1983 by Academic Press, Inc.
All rights of reproduction in any form reserved.
ISBN 0-12-327660-8

low-energy β particle with a mean path length in tissue of
about 1 μm and a maximal path length of about 8 μm. In
contrast, ^{125}I emits a shower of low-energy, densely ionizing
Auger electrons with a very limited path length. The energy
deposition from ^{125}I is thus most intense in very small
regions of the DNA molecule within a few base pairs of the
radioactive disintegration (Martin and Haseltine, 1981). The
radiation from ^{3}H incorporated into DNA as [^{3}H]-TdR will be
restricted to the cell nucleus but relatively uniformly
distributed within it.

In this investigation, mutagenesis was studied in a human
diploid lymphoblast system (Thilly *et al.*, 1980), with 6-
thioguanine or ouabain resistance as the genetic end points.
These cells have the advantage of growing at high concentrations in suspension cultures, which greatly improves the
logistics of experiments and allows the accurate measurement
of induced mutations at lower frequencies than are feasible
with human diploid fibroblasts. Malignant transformation was
measured with the A31-11 BALB/3T3 transformation system
(Little, 1979). In both systems, the mutation and transformation frequencies induced by the incorporated radioisotopes
were compared with those induced by external X-ray exposure.

II. MATERIALS AND METHODS

The general methodology for measuring induced mutations
in human diploid lymphoblasts has been described in detail
elsewhere (Thilly *et al.*, 1980), as has the application of
this assay to the measurement of mutations induced by external
irradiation and incorporated radioisotopes (Liber *et al.*,
1983). Briefly, the cells are maintained in suspension
cultures at a density of approximately 400,000 cells/ml by

diluting them daily 1:2 with fresh medium. The cells were incubated with the appropriate radioisotope, rinsed, and returned to complete medium containing 10^{-5} thymidine and 10^{-6} M deoxycytidine. An aliquot of cells was removed for radioactive counting, and the determination of the actual amount of radioactivity was incorporated for each data point. A second aliquot was removed and seeded at 1 to 10 cells per well in microtiter dishes to determine cytotoxicity. The treated cells were then allowed the appropriate expression time for the locus being tested, before seeding in selective medium. The cells were seeded at a density of 40,000 cells per well in microtiter dishes; parallel dishes were seeded with 1 cell per well to measure plating efficiency.

The use of the A31-11 BALB/3T3 cell line for studies of radiation transformation has been described in detail elsewhere (Little, 1979), as well as its adaptation to the study of transformation induced by incorporated radioisotopes (LeMotte et al., 1983). DNA single-strand breaks were studied by the alkaline elution technique originally described by Kohn et al. (1974). Double-strand breaks were estimated by the neutral elution technique described by Bradley and Kohn (1979). The adaptation of these techniques to the investigation of DNA strand breaks induced by incorporated radioisotopes has been described in detail elsewhere (LeMotte and Little, 1983b).

Cytotoxicity was studied by standard colony formation techniques, following incorporation of radioactivity as described for the mutagenesis or transformation assay. For cells exposed to ^3H_2O, ^3H_2O was added to the culture medium and the cells allowed to continue growth at 37°C. At the end of the exposure period, the radioactivity was removed, the cells washed and overlaid with fresh medium containing no ^3H_2O. In other experiments, ^3H_2O was added to the culture medium, and the flasks cooled to 0°C. At the end of the exposure period the cells were removed from the cold, overlaid with nonradioactive medium, and returned to 37°C. These exposure conditions and techniques have been described in detail elsewhere (LeMotte and Little, 1983a).

III. RESULTS

The results for cytotoxicity and mutations induced in human diploid lymphoblasts by ^{125}I-labeled dUrd, [^{3}H]-TdR, and X rays are presented in Table I. As can be seen, ^{125}I-labeled dUrd was much more effective than [^{3}H]-TdR at killing cells and producing mutations. When the dose was expressed as total disintegrations per cell (dpc), the D_0 (inverse of the slope) of the survival curve for ^{125}I was 28 dpc and for ^{3}H was 385 dpc. The slopes of the mutation curves were approximately 75 x 10^{-8} 6-thioguanine resistant (6TG^r) mutants per cell per disintegration for ^{125}I and 2.3 x 10^{-8} 6TG^r mutants per cell

TABLE I. Induction of Cytotoxicity and 6TG^r Mutants in Human Diploid Lymphoblasts by Incorporated Radioisotopes[a]

Isotope	Survival D_0 (dpc)[b]	Mutations (per cell per disintegration x 10^{-8})[c]
^{3}H	385	2.3
^{125}I	28	75

[a]*Data from Liber et al. (1983).*

[b]*D_0 is inverse of slope of survival curve with dose expressed as total disintegrations per cell (dpc).*

[c]*Derived from initial slope of dose-response curve for induction of mutations.*

per disintegration for ^{3}H. The slope of the mutation curve for X rays was approximately 8 x 10^{-8} 6TG^r mutants/cell/rad. No ouabain-resistant mutants were induced by any of the three agents.

As ^{125}I was very efficient in producing both cytotoxicity and mutations, it was of interest to determine whether these two biological effects appeared to be produced by the same mechanism. One way of gaining information on this point is to compare the frequency of mutations induced by the different types of radiation at similar levels of survival. The dose-response curves for the induction of 6TG^r mutations by ^{125}I and X rays are plotted as a function of the surviving fraction in Fig. 1. As can be seen in Fig. 1, ^{125}I was much more effective than X rays in inducing mutations at very low doses (high survival levels). For example, a dose of 12 dpc of ^{125}I

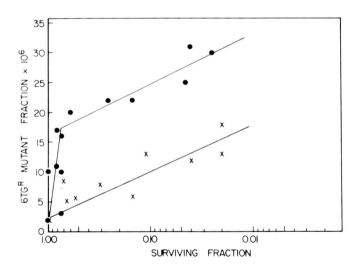

Fig. 1. Induction of 6-thioguanine resistant mutants in lymphoblasts by ^{125}I-labeled dUrd (●——●) and X rays (X——X) plotted as a function of the surviving fraction. Data from Liber *et al.* (1983).

yielded a mutation frequency of 15 x 10^{-6} and a survival level of 80 to 90%; the induction of a similar mutation frequency by X rays would require approximately 220 rads, which kills 98% of the lymphoblasts (Liber *et al.*, 1983). At ^{125}I doses that yielded significant cytotoxicity, however, the dose-response curve paralleled that of X irradiation, as can also be seen in Fig. 1. This result suggests that the mechanisms of mutagenesis and cytotoxicity were similar at higher dose levels. The available data for ^{3}H yielded an intermediate result.

Similar results were observed for malignant transformation of mouse 3T3 cells. The sensitivities of this cell line to transformation by ^{125}I-labeled dUrd and [^{3}H]TdR are shown in Fig. 2. As in the case of mutation (Table I), ^{125}I was much more efficient in inducing malignant transformation than was ^{3}H. These data are normalized for cell survival and compared to the results for X irradiation in Fig. 3. The results are qualitatively very similar to those observed for 6-thioguanine

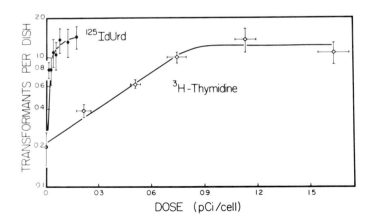

Fig. 2. Induction of oncogenic transformation in mouse A31-11 BALB/3T3 cells by [^{3}H]thymidine (O——O) or ^{125}I-labeled dUrd (●——●). Vertical and horizontal error bars represent standard error of the mean for data from five separate experiments. Reproduced from LeMotte *et al.* (1983).

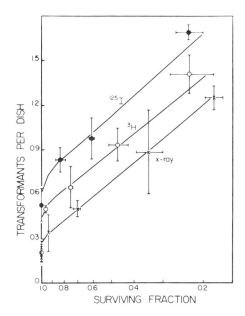

Fig. 3. Oncogenic transformation in 3T3 cells by [³H]TdR
(O——O), ¹²⁵I-labeled dUrd (●——●), and X rays (X——X) plotted
as a function of the surviving fraction as for induced mutations in Fig. 1. Mean and standard error of data from five
experiments. Reproduced from LeMotte *et al.* (1983).

resistant mutants in the human diploid lymphoblasts (Fig. 1).
A three- to four-fold increase in the yield of transformants
was seen with doses of ¹²⁵I that yielded no measurable cell
killing. The induction of comparable transformation frequencies by X irradiation required approximately 300 rads.

In order to gain information as to the nature of the
molecular damage associated with these incorporated radioisotopes, we have studied the induction of DNA strand breaks
by these agents in parallel experiments in human diploid
fibroblasts employing alkaline and neutral elution techniques.
In these experiments DNA damage occurred under frozen conditions; the results are summarized in Table II. As can be seen
in Table II, ¹²⁵I was particularly efficient in inducing DNA

TABLE II.   Induction of DNA Strand Breaks in Human Diploid
            Fibroblasts by Incorporated Radioisotopes[a]

Isotope	D_{37} (number of decays)[b]	Efficiency of production (breaks per disintegration)	Rad equivalent disintegration[c]
Single-strand breaks			
^{3}H	3,500	1.5	0.34
^{125}I	1,200	4.4	1.0
Double-strand breaks			
^{3}H	54,000	0.14	0.64
^{125}I	9,000	0.84	3.80

[a]*Data from LeMotte and Little (1983b).   Induction of DNA damage was under frozen conditions.*

[b]*Dose necessary to reduce DNA size to 37% of initial value.*

[c]*The rad dose of X rays necessary to produce a similar effect, based on efficiency of production of 4.4 SSB and 0.22 DSB/rad for γ or X rays (LeMotte and Little, 1983b).*

double-strand breaks (DSB) as compared with ^{3}H; the yield of double-strand breaks was sixfold higher, whereas the yield of single-strand breaks (SSB) was only threefold higher for ^{125}I as compared with ^{3}H.   Indeed, the efficiency of production of DSB for ^{125}I (0.84 per disintegration) indicates that on the average a single ^{125}I disintegration will produce approximately one double-strand break.   Yet, as can be seen in Table I, the mean lethal dose for ^{125}I was 28 dpc.   It is also interesting to note (Table II) that X rays produce double-strand breaks

quite efficiently (0.22 DSB/rad) but that the ratio of single-
to double-strand breaks (20) is much higher than for [125]I (~3).

An unexpected finding in these studies was that human
diploid cells appeared much more sensitive to the cytotoxic
effects of both ^{125}I and ^{3}H than did 3T3 cells. In order to
investigate this phenomenon in greater detail, the cytotoxic
effects of [3]H$_2$O were examined in several different human and
rodent cell lines. The results of some of these studies are
tabulated in Table III, which shows that the D_0 for the rodent
cells was consistently 5- to 10-fold higher than the D_0 for the
human cells. The rodent cells studied include an established

TABLE III. Survival of Human and Rodent Cells after Irradiation with [3]H$_2$O and X Rays[a]

Cells[b]	Temperature of irradiation (°C)	D_0 [3]H$_2$O (mCi/ml x hours exposed)	D_0 X rays (rads)
10T$\frac{1}{2}$	37	61.4	175
10T$\frac{1}{2}$	0	18.5	—·
AG1522	37	14.9	145
AG1522	0	10.5	—
RO4	37	70.3	—
C143	37	21.9	151

[a]Data from LeMotte and Little (1983a).

[b]10T$\frac{1}{2}$, established line of mouse embryo fibroblasts;
AG1522, human diploid fibroblasts; RO4, early-passage diploid
hamster embryo cells; C143, established human melanoma cell
line.

line of mouse embryo-derived fibroblasts ($10T\frac{1}{2}$), as well as
primary diploid Syrian hamster fibroblasts. The human cell
strains included a human diploid skin fibroblast and an
established human tumor cell line derived from a melanoma.
These results were obtained in cells incubated at 37°C with
^3H_2O for a period of 4 days. When the cells were incubated
with ^3H_2O, immediately cooled to 0°C for up to 3 days, and
subsequently returned to 37°C to simulate an "acute" irradiation, the difference between the rodent and human cells was
greatly diminished. These cells also showed similar sensitivity to acute X-ray exposure. These results suggest that the
difference in sensitivity shown in Table III between human and
rodent cells represents an effect of dose-rate; that is, human
cells are much more sensitive than rodent cells to low dose
rate radiation but show similar sensitivity to acute radiation
exposure.

IV. DISCUSSION

The results in Table I and Fig. 1 indicate that ^{125}I is
highly mutagenic when incorporated into DNA as ^{125}I-labeled
dUrd. On the assumption that the HGPRT gene contains about
1000 base pairs (about 10^{-6} of all of the DNA), these data
could imply that each ^{125}I disintegration within this gene
would lead to a mutation. The high efficiency of double-
strand break production by ^{125}I (Table II) suggests the
possibility that the double-strand break might be the mutagenic
lesion. However, it has generally been assumed that unrepaired
DNA double-str nd breaks are lethal lesions, as the integrity
of the DNA molecule is destroyed unless repair occurs. If
this is indeed true, repair must be occurring in these experiments as indicated by the cytotoxicity data in Table I. The

D_0 or mean lethal dose for cell killing by ^{125}I was 28 dpc. This means that, on the average, a cell must accumulate 28 disintegrations before it loses its reproductive capacity. On the basis of the hypothesis that unrepaired double-strand breaks are lethal lesions, this result would imply that many of them must be repaired and the integrity of the DNA thus restored.

It is important to note that the double-strand break produced by ^{125}I may be qualitatively different from that produced by X rays. Though relatively little is known about the precise structural nature of such breaks, X-ray induced double-strand breaks may represent staggered single-strand breaks; such breaks may involve only cleavage or damage to single bases. Repair and rejoining could therefore occur without disruption of the base sequence. In this case, X-ray induced mutation would likely be due to DNA lesions other than double-strand breaks. Martin and Haseltine (1981) have shown, however, that most of the DNA strand breaks that are induced following disintegration of ^{125}I occur within a few base pairs of the site of incorporation. This disintegration is associated with the release of on the average about 20 densely ionizing Auger electrons. It thus seems probable that the disintegration of the ^{125}I atom within the DNA could lead to destruction of several base pairs at the site of a DNA break. The integrity of the DNA could be restored by repair of such a break, but the base sequence would likely be altered as a result of the destruction or loss of one or more bases (unless repair occurred via recombination with homologous DNA). A frameshift mustation would be a likely result. Frameshift mutagens are known to be highly efficient at inducing 6-thioguanine resistant mutants, but they do not induce mutations to ouabain resistance.

We thus hypothesize that the extreme mutagenicity of ^{125}I at low doses results from misrepair of this latter class of DNA double-strand breaks (DSB). The intermediate result for ^{3}H would suggest that ^{3}H also produces some breaks of this type in which the base sequence is altered. These breaks would likely occur from transmutational effects: those resulting from the direct disintegration of the atom within the DNA chain. Other DSB would be similar to those induced by X rays and would result from interaction of the released β particles with DNA at sites distant from the site of incorporation. As in the case of X rays, some ^{3}H-induced mutations would result from lesions other than DSB produced distant from the site of disintegration.

Further evidence to support the hypothesis that there are two classes of DSB, one of which may be highly mutagenic, comes from an examination of the efficiency of induction of double-strand breaks by X rays and ^{125}I at equal levels of survival or mutation. In the experiments shown in Table II, the doses necessary to reduce survival to 20% were approximately 220 rads of X rays and 50 dpc for ^{125}I. The data on the yield of DNA strand breaks in Table II indicate that these doses would produce similar numbers of DSB (about 42 and 50, respectively). When one looks at the mutation figures in the human lymphoblasts, the results are quite different: The yield of mutations per DSB is about fivefold higher for ^{125}I. For example, a dose of 220 rads yields about 15 6TG^{r} mutations per 10^{6} cells. Again, this dose would produce about 50 DSB. In contrast, 15 x 10^{6} mutations are produced by approximately 12 dpc of ^{125}I, a dose that yields only 10 DSB. If the DSB is a mutagenic lesion in ^{125}I-treated cells, these results would suggest that the predominant type of DSB produced by ^{125}I is qualitatively different from DSB produced by X rays. Both types of DSB are equally cytotoxic, but the type produced by ^{125}I would in addition be mutagenic.

An examination of the data as plotted in Fig. 1 indicates that when the mutagenic effects of ^{125}I and X rays were compared at doses yielding similar levels of survival, ^{125}I was much more effective than X rays at low dose (high survival) levels. When the dose of ^{125}I was increased to the point where significant cytotoxicity occurred, the dose-response curve in Fig. 1 paralleled that for X rays. This latter result suggests that at higher doses the mechanisms of mutation production by ^{125}I and X rays are similar. The mechanisms for this effect are not clear. One might speculate that the error-prone repair process acting on the premutagenic lesions produced at low doses becomes saturated when significant cytotoxicity occurs, and cells with significant numbers of these lesions are killed. At higher doses, therefore, the mutations produced in cells surviving ^{125}I exposure result from radiation absorbed at sites distant from that of incorporation, with premutagenic lesions comparable to those induced by X rays.

It is particularly interesting to note that the results for malignant transformation plotted in Fig. 3 are very similar to those observed for mutagenesis. The transformation frequency in mouse 3T3 cells was enhanced three- to fourfold over background by doses of ^{125}I that produced no measurable cell killing. The induction of a similar level of transformation by X rays required 300 rads, a dose that killed over 50% of the cells. As ^{125}I irradiation is largely confined to the nucleus of the cell and cellular DNA, these findings also imply that DNA damage is indeed involved in the initiation of transformation by ionizing radiation.

Finally, we have shown that rodent cells are 5 to 10 times more resistant to the effects of these incorporated isotopes than are human cells. A large difference in sensitivity between cells from these two species was also seen after protracted irradiation from ^3H_2O at 37°C (Table III) but not when the cells were exposed to ^3H_2O under frozen conditions to simulate an "acute" radiation exposure. Both human and rodent cells showed generally similar sensitivities following acute exposures to X rays. We thus hypothesize that the differences we observe between rodent and human cells result from a difference in their capacity to tolerate protracted radiation exposure; specifically, rodent cells may possess a repair process that can efficiently deal with damage produced at low dose rates. This might be similar to the process that compensates for the relative inefficiency of excision repair in rodent as compared with human cells.

In sum, these results indicate that human cells experience much less enhancement in survival than rodent cells when intracellular irradiation is protracted over several days rather than given as an acute exposure. This apparent hypersensitivity of human cells to low dose rate irradiation is not evident upon comparison of survival curves obtained with acute exposure, which likely explains why previously it has largely gone unrecognized. These results suggest that rodent cells in some cases may not be an accurate model for radiation effects in human cells, and suggests that caution should be employed in such extrapolations.

REFERENCES

Bradley, M. O., and Kohn, K. W. (1979). *Nucleic Acids Res.* 7, 793-804.
Kohn, K. W., Friedman, C. A., Ewig, R. A. G., Iqbal, Z. M. (1974). *Biochemistry 13*, 4134-4139.
LeMotte, P. K., Adelstein, S. J., and Little, J. B. (1983). *Proc. Natl. Acad. Sci. USA 79*, 7763-7767.
LeMotte, P. K., and Little, J. B. (1983a). *Radiat. Res.*, in press.
LeMotte, P. K., and Little, J. B. (1983b). *Cancer Res.*, in press.
Liber, H. L., LeMotte, P. K., and Little, J. B. (1983). *Mutat. Res.*, in press.
Little, J. B. (1979). *Cancer Res.* 39, 1478-1484.
Martin, R. F., and Haseltine, W. A. (1981). *Science (Washington, D. C.) 213*, 896-898.
Thilly, W. G., DeLuca, W. G., Furth, E. E., Hoppe, H., IV, Kaden, D. A., Krolewski, J. J., Liber, H. L., Skopek, T. R., Slapikoff, S. A., Tizard, R. J., and Penman, B. W. (1980). *In* "Chemical Mutagens" (F. F. deSerres and A. Hollaender, eds.), Vol. 6, pp. 331-364. Plenum, New York.

23

EFFECTS OF ASBESTOS AND CARCINOGENIC METALS ON CULTURED HUMAN BRONCHIAL EPITHELIUM

John F. Lechner

Laboratory of Human Carcinogenesis
National Cancer Institute
Bethesda, Maryland

Aage Haugen

National Institute of Public Health
Oslo, Norway

Benjamin F. Trump

Department of Pathology
University of Maryland School of Medicine
Baltimore, Maryland

Takayoshi Tokiwa and Curtis C. Harris

Laboratory of Human Carcinogenesis
National Cancer Institute
Bethesda, Maryland

I. INTRODUCTION

    Carcinogenesis studies using normal human lung epithelial
tissues and cells have been hindered by both deficient methodological techniques and lack of knowledge of the cellular processes that control their growth and differentiation. Therefore, we have concentrated our initial efforts on developing
culture techniques and delineating the biology of normal adult
human bronchial epithelial and pleural mesothelial cells.

    Several methods of culturing these tissues and cells have
been devised. As a result, morphological normal bronchial
tissue can be maintained in culture for periods of time
exceeding 1 year (Trump *et al.*, 1980), tissue explanted onto
gelatin sponge will contain mitotic epithelial cells after
more than 3 months of incubation, fibroblast-free outgrowths
of epithelial cells can be obtained from explanted tissue
(Lechner *et al.*, 1981), and bronchial epithelial cells can be
grown clonally using either cultivation with mitotically
arrested feeder cells (Lechner *et al.*, 1981) or defined, serum-
free medium (Lechner *et al.*, 1982). These cultures have been
documented to consist of normal bronchial epithelial cells

using chromosomal, morphological, and antigenic marker criteria (Trump *et al.*, 1980; Stoner *et al.*, 1980b; Lechner *et al.*, 1981).

In addition, ciliated mucus-containing and squamous differentiated cells have been identified (Stoner *et al.*, 1980b; Lechner *et al.*, 1981, 1982). Subsequently, we have investigated the mechanisms that govern their multiplication and/or commitment to terminal squamous differentiation. We have found that the nutrient composition of culture medium and supplemental factors, especially serum and Ca^{2+} (Lechner *et al.*, 1982, 1983a), profoundly influence the percentage of squamous differentiated cells present within the culture.

In order to investigate mesothelial cell carcinogenesis, methods have been developed to culture cells obtained from pleural effusions of noncancerous donors. These cultures have also been characterized by morphological, antigenic marker (keratin), and chromosomal criteria. In addition, the cells have been found to be very sensitive to the cytotoxic effects of asbestos (Lechner *et al.*, 1983b).

Metallic ions (i.e., nickel, chromium, and arsenic) have been documented by human epidemiological studies as occupational causes of lung cancer (Doll *et al.*, 1980). In addition, asbestos is considered to be the major cause of mesothelioma (Kannerstein and Churg, 1980) and a cocarcinogenic factor in the etiology of bronchogenic carcinoma (Selikoff and Lee, 1978). In preliminary experiments, cells expressing altered terminal differentiation properties, as well as having changes in growth requirements, karyology, and population-doubling potential, have been isolated from bronchial epithelial and pleural mesothelial cell cultures after prolonged exposure to these agents.

II. MATERIALS AND METHODS

A. Tissue Obtainment and Culturing

Bronchial tissues were obtained from immediate and medical examiner autopsies (Trump *et al.*, 1974). The bronchi were cut into 2 x 3-cm^2 fragments and placed into culture in rocking chambers for 4 to 6 days to promote reversal of ischemia (Trump *et al.*, 1980). The tissues were then cut into 0.5-cm^2 pieces, explanted epithelium side up (four to five explants/60-mm dish), and incubated in explant growth medium (EGM) (Lechner *et al.*, 1981). After 8 to 11 days of incubation, the tissues were transferred to new culture dishes to initiate a second outgrowth of epithelial cells. After 2 to 4 days of incubation of the original outgrowth cultures in serum-free LHC-1 medium (Lechner *et al.*, 1982), the cells were dissociated using trypsin and inoculated into dishes coated with human fibronectin (10 µg/ml, collagen (Vitrogen®; 30 µg/ml, and crystallized bovine serum albumin (10 µg/ml) (Lechner *et al.*, 1982), or they were cryopreserved in liquid N$_2$ (Lechner *et al.*, 1980).

Mesothelial cells were obtained from pleural effusions obtained from donors without cancer. The fluid was centrifuged at 125 *g* for 5 min, and the pelleted cells were resuspended and inoculated into 100-mm culture dishes containing 10 ml of supplemented CMRL-1066 medium (Stoner *et al.*, 1980a) at a ratio of one dish/50 ml of pleural fluid. The cells were dissociated using trypsin when the cultures attained subconfluency. The cultures were further expanded and either cryopreserved or used according to experimental protocols.

B. Nutrient Media

Supplemented CMRL-1066 (Stoner *et al.*, 1980b): The glutamine concentration was adjusted to 0.3 m*M*, and the medium was supplemented with 1.0 µg/ml insulin (ISN), 1.0 x 10^{-4} m*M* hydrocortisone (HC), 1 m*M* putrescine, 1 m*M* pyruvate, 20 m*M* Hepes buffer, 50 µg/ml gentamicin, and 10% fetal calf (bovine) serum (FBS).

EGM medium (Lechner *et al.*, 1981): M199 with the Ca^{2+} concentration reduced to 0.6 m*M* and supplemented with 1.0 µg/ml ISN; 5 x 10^{-4} m*M* HC, 20 ng/ml epidermal growth factor (EGF), 20 m*M* Hepes buffer, 50 µg/ml gentamicin, trace elements (Lechner *et al.*, 1981), and 1.25% FBS.

LHC-1 medium (Lechner *et al.*, 1982): MCDB 151 (Peehl and Ham, 1980) with the Ca^{2+} concentration increased to 0.1 m*M* and supplemented with 5 µg/ml ISN, 5 ng/ml EGF, 10 µg/ml transferrin, 5 x 10^{-4} m*M* each of phosphoethanolamine and ethanolamine, 5 x 10^{-4} m*M* HC, 50 µg/ml gentamicin, and trace elements.

C. Morphological, Antigenic, and Karyotypic Characterization

Cell morphology was monitored by phase contrast microscopy. Cultures were also examined using transmission and scanning electron microscopy (TEM and SEM) (Trump *et al.*, 1980). The number of cross-linked envelopes were measured using a modification of the method of Sun and Green (1976).

Antigenic markers were detected using immunoperoxidase staining. Coverslip cultures were rinsed with two changes of Hepes-buffered saline (Lechner *et al.*, 1980) and fixed for 10 min with cold acetone (keratin) or 10% formalin (blood group antigens). Immunoperoxidase staining was then carried out as described (Stoner *et al.*, 1980b).

For chromosome studies, cells were exposed to colcemid
(0.05 µg/ml for 2 to 3 h, treated in 0.075 M KCl for 20 min,
and fixed in methanol:acetate acid (3:1). The cells were
then air dried onto glass slides. Scoring of 25 to 50
chromosome spreads permitted determination of the model
chromosome number. For banding analysis, slides were processed
to G-banding procedure according to a modification of the
method of Seabright (1971).

D. Clonal Growth and Cytotoxicity Assay

Mitogenicity and cytoxicity activities were assessed using
clonal growth dose-response assays. Coated dishes (60-mm-
diameter) were inoculated with 5000 bronchial epithelial
cells, 1000 pleural mesothelial cells, or 1000 bronchial
fibroblastic cells. Twenty-four hours after the cells were
inoculated, the medium was replaced with medium containing
increasing concentrations of growth factors, fibers, or metal
ions. Each dose was assayed in duplicate. The growth factors
and metal ions were retained for the duration of the incubation period; fiber-treated cultures were washed twice and re-
incubated in fiber-free media after 3 days of exposure. Ten
days postinoculation, the colonies were fixed in 10% formalin
and stained with 0.25% crystal violet. The number of colonies
per dish (colony-forming efficiency, CFE) and the clonal growth
rate (average number of population doublings per day, PD/D)
were then determined (Lechner and Kaighn, 1979). Student's
t test was used to evaluate the significance of differences
between experimental groups.

III. RESULTS

A. Epithelial Outgrowths from Bronchial Explant Cultures

Insulin (0.2 μg/ml), HC (5 x 10^{-4} mM), and serum (10%)
are growth stimulatory for primary explant outgrowth cultures
of human bronchial epithelial cells. However, fibroblastic
cells commonly contaminate these cultures, although to a lesser
extent when putrescine was incorporated into the medium
(Stoner et al., 1980b). It was found that reduction in the
serum level to 1.25% almost totally eliminated contamination
by fibroblastic cells. The populations of epithelial cells
multiplied at a slow rate when incubated in low (1.25%) serum-
supplemented medium, but marked growth stimulation was noted
by adding several factors: HC, ISN, EGF, and trace elements
(Lechner et al., 1981). This combination of factor-supple-
mented, low serum-containing medium proved to support rapid
growth of fibroblast-free populations of bronchial epithelial
cells.

Repeated transfer of explant tissue to a new dish was
found to be a good method to reinitiate primary cultures
(Lechner et al., 1981). To date, multiple sequential outgrowth
cultures (up to 20 times) from more than 100 donors (17 to 81
years old) have been initiated using this technique. Donor
age has not had any effect on the number of times the tissue
could be transferred. Using several criteria (i.e., keratin
and blood group immunostaining, and presence of ciliated cells),
no differences between the first and twentieth epithelial outgrowth of cells were noted.

B. Normal Bronchial Epithelial Replicative Cell Cultures

The epithelial cells continued to divide so long as the explant tissue remained contiguous with the monolayer portion of the culture. Removal of the explant tissue resulted in a rapid damping of mitotic activity and an increase in cell size. Four to five days later, the cells became squamous and eventually sloughed into the medium. Therefore, it was necessary to develop conditions that maintained mitotic activity in postexplant transferred cultures. Several media formulations (EGM, CMRL-1066, DMEM, L-15, M199, PFMR-4) were tested with limited success. Hoever, the bronchial epithelial cells continued to multiply when cocultured with Mitomycin C[®] mitotically inactivated Swiss mouse 3T3 feeder cells and incubated in EGM (Lechner *et al.*, 1981). These cocultured bronchial epithelial cells could be dissociated into single cells and replated at clonal density (5000 cells/60-mm dish). However, reattached cells failed to expand into colonies unless feeder cells were present. Colonies containing between 50 and 200 cells could be repeatedly subcultured with feeder cells as many as five more times before the cells failed to grow into colonies.

The cocultivation method was optimized for rapid clonal growth by adjusting the calcium concentration of the medium (Lechner *et al.*, 1981). However, ascertaining the response of the epithelial cells to exogenous agents (e.g., nutrients, growth factors, and carcinogens) was difficult, because the influence of the feeder cells could not be determined. Because continual propagation and mitotic inactivation of the 3T3 cells is time consuming and expensive, and viral contamination of the bronchial epithelial cells caused by the mouse feeder cells is a potential problem, we sought a method to grow these epithelial cells without feeder cells. We found that replicative cultures of adult human bronchial epithelial cells could be obtained using medium LHC-1 (Lechner *et al.*, 1982), a slight modification of the nutrient formula developed by Peehl and Ham (1980), to grow human newborn epidermal keratinocytes without feeder cells. In addition, an enhanced clonal growth rate was noted by coating the culture dish surface with a mixture of collagen, fibronectin, and bovine serum albumin (Lechner *et al.*., 1982) and incorporating 3,3',5-triiodo-*d*-thyronine and 35 µg/ml of aqueous pituitary extract protein (Lechner, 1983; Willey *et al.*, unpublished) into LHC-1 medium (LHC-4).

C. Control of Squamous Differentiation

The presence and concentrations of serum and Ca^{2+} profoundly influence both the rate of growth and/or the degree of squamous differentiation. It is generally accepted that most cell types require serum for growth unless the medium components are carefully adjusted to provide the cells with their correct balance of nutritional requirements, and often, specific factor and hormonal supplements are also necessary (Barnes and Sato, 1980). However, the serum dose response of the

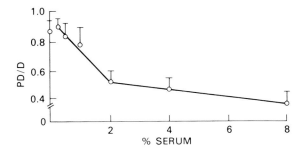

Fig. 1. Effect of serum supplementation on clonal growth rate of normal human bronchial epithelial cells incubated in LHC-1 medium ($[Ca^{2+}]$ 110 µ*M*). Five thousand cells were inoculated per dish. PD/D, population doublings/day; bars denote standard error of the mean.

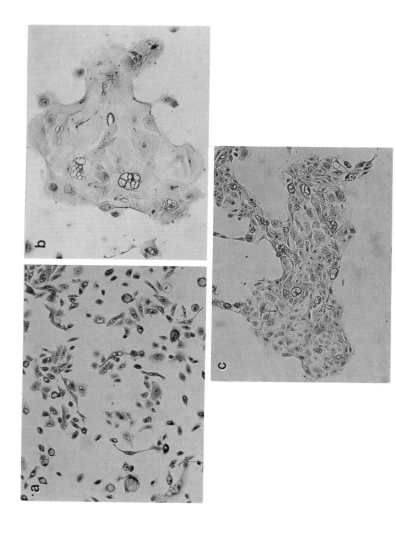

Fig. 2. Photomicrographs of normal human bronchial epithelial cells after 8 days of incubation in LHC-1 medium: (a) with standard Ca^{2+} concentration (110 μM) and without serum; (b) with standard Ca^{2+} concentration and 8% serum (x90); (c) with increased Ca^{2+} concentration (1000 μM) and without serum.

bronchial epithelial cells was markedly different from that noted for most cell types. As little as 2% serum supplementation significantly reduced the clonal growth rate (Fig. 1); inhibition increased in proportion to serum concentrations. Serum also changed cellular morphology and cell-cell arrangements within colonies (Fig. 2a,b). Cultures maintained 8-10 days in serum-free medium were composed primarily of small and migratory cells, and cell-cell junctions and tonofilaments were rarely noted. In contrast, large (squamous), closely adjacent, multilayering cells containing numerous desmosomes and extensive networks of keratin bundles were prevalent in cultures maintained in serum-supplemented media. The percentage of cross-linked envelopes also increased from less than 5% in serum-free medium to more than 80% in cultures incubated for 8 to 10 days in medium containing 8% serum (Lechner et al., 1983a).

The results of serum dose-response experiments with other cell lines showed that serum toxicity per se was not responsible for the appearance of squamous cells. Ten cultures, including normal human bronchial fibroblasts and human lung carcinoma cell lines A549, HuT 292, SW 900, CaLu 6, A427, SK-MES-1, A2182, A1188, and A1146, all showed typical serum dose responses when tested in LHC-1 medium. This difference in serum response—that is, growth inhibition of the normal bronchial epithelial cells and multiplication stimulation of human lung carcinoma cell lines—is being applied experimentally (see later) to select carcinogen-altered cells that are resistant to serum-induced squamous differentiation.

The Ca^{2+} concentration in medium is known to affect the extent of differentiation of epidermal keratinocytes (Hennings et al., 1980). A markedly different result was noted for normal human bronchial epithelial cells. Without serum supplementation, the clonal growth rate progressively increased

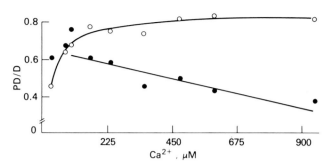

Fig. 3. Response of normal human bronchial epithelial
cells to various Ca^{2+} concentrations: (O), medium without
serum; (●), medium with serum. Data points represent mean of
18 randomly selected colonies; lines derived from variance-
weighted least squares regression.

as the Ca^{2+} concentration was increased from 30 to 100 μM Ca^{2+},
then remained constant up to 1000 μM Ca^{2+} (Fig. 3). The cells
within colonies became less migratory (Fig. 2c), and tonofilaments and desmosome junctions became more abundant as the
Ca^{2+} concentration was increased. In contrast, the percentage
of the cells acquiring cross-linked envelopes after 10 days of
incubation in 1000 μM Ca^{2+}, serum-free medium was not significantly greater than in cultures incubated in the standard
(110 μM) Ca^{2+} concentration. In the presence of a marginally
inhibitory amount of serum (1.25%; see Fig. 1), an interaction
between Ca^{2+} and serum was found; Ca^{2+} potentiated the
differentiation-inducing activity of serum. Further, whereas
less than 10% of the cells of cultures grown in 1.25% serum-
containing medium acquired envelopes, more than 70% were
envelope positive after 10 days of growth in medium containing
both 1000 μM Ca^{2+} and 1.25% serum.

D. Mesothelial Cell Cultures

Replicative cultures have been developed from more than 10 donors with nonmalignant diseases (Lechner *et al.*, 1983b). Cellular morphology and rate of growth are dependent on medium conditions. Cells incubated in serum-supplemented CMRL-1066 medium grow slowly (45–50 h generation time) and are morphologically epithelioid (Fig. 4). The same cells inoculated into PFMR-4 (Lechner *et al.*, 1980) medium supplemented with 3×10^{-4} m*M* HC, 5 ng/ml EGF, and 5% serum grow more rapidly (35 h generation time) and have a more fusiform shape. The cells grown in serum-supplemented CMRL-1066 mediums contain keratin tonofilament bundles. In addition, their surfaces are covered with abundant microvilli. The cultures undergo senescence after 15 to 20 population doublings; 20–30% of the senescent cells contain cross-linked envelopes.

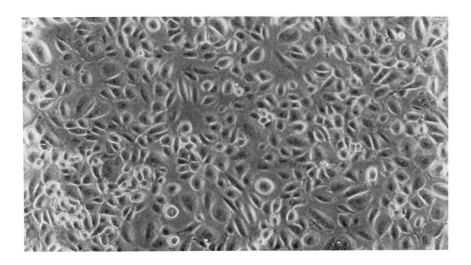

Fig. 4. Normal human pleural mesothelial cells incubated in serum-supplemented CMRL-1066 medium.

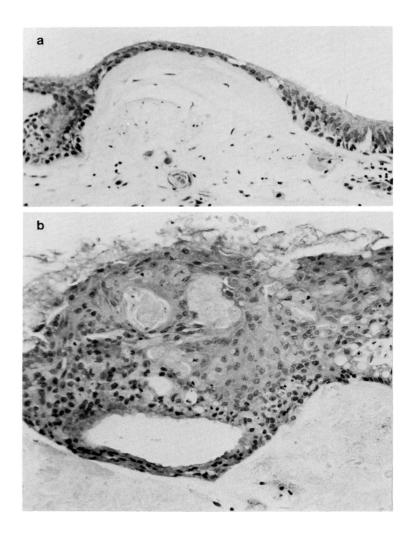

Fig. 5. Morphological appearance of human bronchial tissue after 12 weeks of incubation on Gelfoam supports: (a) control culture; (b) exposed to 10 µg/ml Ni^{2+}.

E. Cytotoxicity

The cytotoxic effects of asbestos and glass fibers and some metallic ions were determined for bronchial epithelial and fibroblastic as well as mesothelial cells (Haugen et al., 1982; Lechner et al., 1983b). The mesothelial cells were the most sensitive to fibers, whereas the bronchial fibroblasts were relatively resistant (amosite 50% cytotoxic dose: 0.3, 5, and 95 μg/ml, respectively). For all cell types, chrysotile was the most toxic fiber tested, and even glass fibers were quite deleterious for the mesothelial cells (50% cytotoxic dose for mesothelial cells: 0.3, 0.3, 1, and 5 μg/ml for chryso-tile, amosite, crocidolite, and glass fibers, respectively). Cell-type differential cytotoxic effects of Ni^{2+} or Cr^{6+} were not noted (50% cytotoxic dose: 15 and 1.5 μg/ml for Ni^{2+} and Cr^{6+}, respectively). However, a marked difference between bronchial epithelial and fibroblastic cell survival in the presence of As^{+5} was noted; the epithelial cells were 20 times more resistant (10 versus 200 μg/ml.

F. Carcinogenesis Studies with Metal Ions

Subsegmental bronchiolar tissue was cut with a scalpel into 0.2 x 0.2-cm^2 pieces, explanted onto Gelfoam® supports, and incubated in serum-supplemented CMRL-1066 medium. After 12 weeks of continuous exposure to Ni^{2+} (10 μg/ml, as $NiSO_4 \cdot 6H_2O$), histopathological differences were noted (Fig. 5a,b). The control cultures exhibited some squamous metaplasia, but the appearance of the glands was generally unremarkable and cellular atypia was not noted. Epithelium exposed to Ni^{2+} exhibited extensive cell growth, and amorphous glands as well as areas of cellular atypia with mitotic cells were common. Cultures exposed to Cr^{6+} (0.75 μg/ml, as Na_2CrO_4) also had

mitotic epithelial cells after 12 weeks of exposure. In
addition, lumen-like structures were frequent but atypia was
rare. Although the dose of As^{+5} used (50 µg/ml, as $Na_2HAsO_4 \cdot 7H_2O$) did not affect the growth of epithelial cells when cultured at clonal density, both stromal and epithelial cyto-
toxicity were noted in exposed tissue.

Replicative epithelial cell cultures were developed from
the exposed or control tissues by dissociating the explants
with trypsin and inoculating the cells into coated dishes.
These cultures became quiescent after four (1:3) subculturings.
After 4 additional weeks of incubation, colonies of mitotic
epithelial cells appeared only in the cultures developed from
the Ni^{2+}-exposed tissues. These latter cultures are being
expanded and will be assessed for tumorigenic properties.

Carcinogenesis experiments have also been conducted using
replicative cultures of bronchial epithelial cells. Cultures
were continuously exposed to a semitoxic dose of nickel (7.5–
10 µg Ni^{2+}/ml) for periods of time ranging from 21 to 40 days.
After 30 days of incubation, mitotic cells were exceedingly
rare, and, in general, the cultures consisted of large, flat,
quiescent cells. These cultures were then continually maintained in medium without Ni^{2+}. After 40 to 75 days, colonies
consisting of small mitotic cells appeared. Sufficient numbers
of experiments have not yet been undertaken to permit statistically significant rates (colonies per number of cells at
risk) to be established. However, for four experiments a rate
of one colony per 100,000 original cells at risk has been
obtained. No colonies appeared in control cultures or in
cultures exposed for 90 days to less than 5 µg Ni^{2+}/ml.

A partial characterization of several of the colonies
that arose in Ni^{2+}-treated cultures has been initiated. Some
of the isolates have been subcultured 10 times with a minimum

of 8 to 10 population doublings per passage. Thus, compared
to unexposed control cells, cultures isolated after prolonged
exposure to Ni^{2+} have exhibited an increase in their
population-doubling potential of at least 50 divisions. Escape
from serum-induced differentiation has also been ascertained
for some of these isolates; all have shown partial resistance
to serum. In addition, in contrast to normal cells one isolate
(81-D) has lost the requirement of EGF for clonal growth.

Karyotypic changes have also been noted. One phenotypically altered culture (81-D) was found to be diploid when
isolated, but the chromosome pattern changed with continued
subculturing. At the ninth passage the modal chromosome number
was in the hypotetraploid range. Marker chromosomes, including
dicentric chromosomes, were also observed. Culture 171-ND
also exhibited a diploid chromosome mode when isolated. However, these cells were determined to be eudiploid by banding
analysis. Twenty percent of the karyotypes were trisomic of
chromosomes Nos. 8 and 19, and a monosomic of chromosome No. 11.
By the fourth subculture, the chromosome modal number was
widely distributed, and five marker chromosomes were identified
(Fig. 6a).

G. Carcinogenesis Studies with Asbestos Fibers

Both long and short amosite asbestos fibers impaled
bronchial epithelial cells within a few minutes after exposure
(Haugen et al., 1982). During the initial phases of fiber
phagocytosis, a sleeve of cell membrane enveloped the fibers,
and by 2 h short amosite fibers (<12 μm) could be seen totally
within the cells. After 72 h, very long fibers completely
enveloped by the cell membrane protruded from the cells.
Numerous focal lesions including hyperplasia, epidermoid

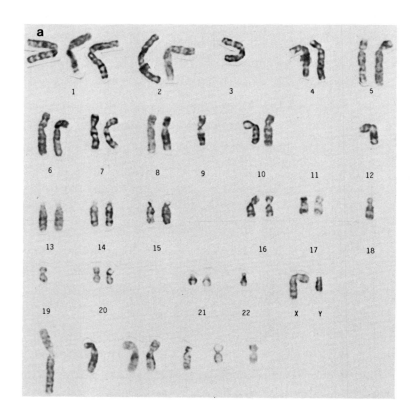

Fig. 6(a). Karyotypic changes resulting from exposure of bronchial epithelial cells to carcinogens: bronchial epithelial cells (isolate 171-ND) after exposure to Ni^{2+}.

metaplasia, and dysplasia were observed as early as 2 weeks after exposure to amosite asbestos. These lesions appeared as elevations of cells that varied considerably in size and shape and were either devoid of or sparsely populated with cilia. The surface features of the cells exhibited a high degree of variation; both stratified cuboidal epithelium and metaplastic areas were seen. The area surrounding these lesions was

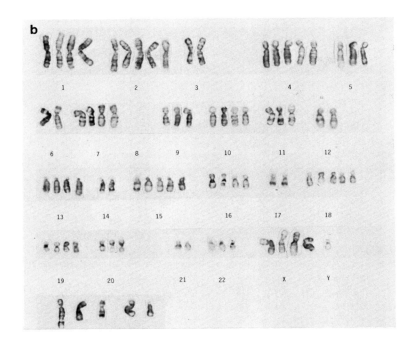

Fig. 6(b). Karyotypic changes resulting from exposure of pleural mesothelial cells to carcinogens: pleural mesothelial cells after exposure to amosite asbestos.

covered by closely packed cilia. Cytopathic alterations of the bronchial epithelium included irregular cell arrangements, cell polymorphism, variation in nuclear size, and nuclear hyperchromasia (Fig. 7). Cells involved in the lesions were examined for asbestos fibers utilizing X ray microanalysis in combination with TEM (Haugen et al., 1982), and both intracytoplasmic and intranuclear fibers were observed. These lesions became less discernible with continued incubation, and 12 weeks after asbestos treatment only a few small areas of abnormality were noted. The control tissues remained essentially normal for the duration of the experiment; areas of metaplasia were seen only rarely.

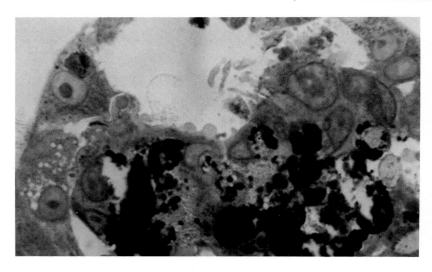

Fig. 7. Histotypic appearance of asbestos-induced focal lesion: variation in size of cells, cellular atypia, and loss of normal polarity were observed.

Replicative cultures of mesothelial cells have also been exposed to asbestos. After one exposure to amosite (2 µg/ml), changes in cellular phenotype were noted. After 2 weeks of incubation the experimental and control (glass fibers, 2 µg/ml) cultures were dissociated, subcultured, and reexposed to amosite or glass fibers. Ten days later, differences between the treated and control cultures were noticed. Colonies of phenotypically altered mitotic cells were present in the exposed cultures, whereas the control cultures underwent senescence. The amosite-treated cells have continued to pro-liferate (for six sequential 1:3 subcultures to date). Hyper-diploid and hypotetraploid metaphases have been noted in 80% of the karyotypes. In addition, the hypotetraploid cells have five marker chromosomes (Fig. 6b).

IV. DISCUSSION

Normal human bronchial epithelial cells in culture are capable of undergoing at least two distinctly different forms of terminal differentiation, most often squamous and to a much lesser extent ciliated (Lechner et al., 1981, 1983a). We found that the presence and concentration of certain medium components — notably serum and Ca^{2+} — profoundly influence whether growth or squamous differentiation occurs. A common characteristic of malignant (pseudo-) stratified epithelium is an aberration in the terminal differentiation program (Rheinwald and Beckett, 1980; Yuspa et al., 1981; Stanbridge et al., 1982). Accordingly, malignant cells escape the proliferative blocks that govern normal cell differentiation and multiplication. Serum contains both factors that induce epithelial differentiation and factors that stimulate cell growth. Transformed cells may have a reduced ability to recognize proliferation-blocking serum constituents but retained the capability to respond to the growth factors and thus to be stimulated to multiply more rapidly in serum-supplemented medium. This marked difference between normal and tumorigenic cells is being used in carcinogenesis experiments to isolate putative malignant cells.

Replicative cultures of normal bronchial epithelial cells can be maintained in an optimally formulated low-Ca^{2+} serum-free medium supplemented with selected growth factors and hormones in culture dishes coated with a mixture of collagen, fibronectin, and bovine serum albumin. The cells rapidly cease dividing when the medium is supplemented with serum and acquire properties commonly ascribed to squamous differentiation, such as multilayering (Sun and Green, 1976), increased cell size (Watt and Green, 1981), abundant tonofilaments and desmosomes (Hennings *et al.*, 1980), and cross-linked envelopes (Sun and Green, 1976). Cells incubated for 3 days in serum-supplemented media incorporate little [^{3}H]thymidine into DNA, whereas the synthesis of RNA is not markedly affected (Lechner *et al.*, 1983a). These observations argue against serum cytotoxicity and support the conclusion that normal bronchial epithelial cells incubated in serum differentiate because of factors in serum that induce this form of terminal differentiation. High concentrations of Ca^{2+} have been shown to trigger squamous differentiation of epidermal keratinocytes (Hennings *et al.*, 1980). In contrast, similar amounts of Ca^{2+} failed to induce normal human bronchial epithelial cells incubated in serum-free media at clonal density to differentiate. However, in the presence of serum, Ca^{2+} promotes squamous differentiation of bronchial epithelium in a dose-dependent fashion. Thus with regard to bronchial epithelial cells, factors in serum induce differentiation, and the activity of these factors can be potentiated by Ca^{2+}.

The metal ions Ni^{2+}, Cr^{6+}, and As^{5+} have been shown to be efficient transformation-inducing agents for animal cells in culture (Sunderman, 1978). We have found that Ni^{2+} will induce colonies of phenotypically altered human bronchial epithelial cells, some of which express characteristics noted in malignant cells, such as extended population-doubling potential, escape from induction to terminal squamous differentiation, reduced growth factor requirements for cell multiplication, and aneuploid karyotypes with marker chromosomes.

Human pleural mesothelial cells can be grown for more than 15 generations in cell culture. These cells exhibit the properties of mesothelial tissue including characteristic microvilli (Andrews and Porter, 1973), keratins (Wu *et al.*, 1983), and cross-linked envelopes at senescence (Wu *et al.*,

1983). Four types of fibers (amosite, crocidolite, chrysotile, and glass) were analyzed for their cytotoxic effects on pleural mesothelial, bronchial epithelial, and bronchial fibroblast cells. Chrysotile was found to be 10 times more toxic than either amosite or crocidolite and 100 times more toxic than glass fibers; these findings correspond to data previously obtained by other investigators using other cell systems (Harrington *et al.*, 1975). Asbestos or glass fibers were most toxic for the mesothelial cells, and bronchial epithelial cells were more sensitive than bronchial fibroblastic cells. A possible explanation for this difference in cytotoxicity could be that the cell surfaces of mesothelial and bronchial epithelial cells permit a more efficient uptake of fibers as compared to fibroblasts. Further, asbestos fibers produce profound effects in plasma membranes; the potency of these reactions for one cell type may not be equivalent for other cell types. For example, we noted a marked difference in the pinocytosis of fibers by macrophages and bronchial epithelial cells (Haugen *et al.*, 1982).

Asbestos fibers are considered to be the major factor in the etiology of mesothelioma (Kannerstein and Churg, 1980). We have noted differences between mesothelial and bronchial epithelial cells with respect to the response of these cell types to amosite fibers. Exposure of bronchial epithelial cells to a single dose of amosite stimulated the appearance of morphological lesions. However, these lesions became less noticeable with continued incubation (12 weeks), and we were unable to establish cultures of cells expressing altered phenotypic characteristics from trypsin-dissociated tissue. In contrast, phenotypically altered mesothelial cells with aneuploid karyotypes have been isolated 1 month after exposure.

REFERENCES

Andrews, P. M., and Porter, K. R. (1973). *Anat. Rec. 117,* 409-426.
Barnes, D., and Sato, G. (1980). *Anal. Biochem. 102,* 255-270.
Doll, R., Fishbein, L., Infante, P., Landrigan, P., Lloyd, J. W., Mason, T. J., Mastromattoo, E., Norseth, T., Pershagen, G., Saffiotti, U., and Saracci, R. (1981). *EHP Environ. Health Perspect. 40,* 11-20.
Harrington, J. S., Allison, A. C., and Badami, D. V. (1975). *Adv. Pharmacol. Chemother. 12,* 291-402.
Haugen, A., Schafer, P. W., Lechner, J. F., Stoner, G. D., Trump, B. F., and Harris, C. C. (1982). *Int. J. Cancer 30,* 265-272.
Hennings, H., Michaels, D., Cheng, C., Steinert, K., Holbrook, K., and Yuspa, S. H. (1980). *Cell 19,* 245-254.
Kannerstein, M., and Churg, J. (1980). *EHP Environ. Health Perspect. 34,* 31-36.
Lechner, J. F. (1983). *Fed. Proc. Fed. Am. Soc. Exp. Biol.,* in press.
Lechner, J. F., and Kaighn, M. E. (1979). *J. Cell. Physiol. 100,* 519-530.
Lechner, J. F., Babcock, M. S., Marnell, M., Narayan, K. S., and Kaighn, M. E. (1980). *In* "Normal Human Tissue and Cell Culture" (C. C. Harris, B. F. Trump, and G. D. Stoner, eds.), Academic Press, New York. *Methods Cell Biol. 21B,* 195-225.
Lechner, J. F., Haugen, A., Autrup, H., McClendon, I. A., Trump, B. F., and Harris, C. C. (1981). *Cancer Res. 41,* 2294-2304.
Lechner, J. F., Haugen, A., McClendon, I. A., and Pettis, E. W. (1982). *In Vitro 18,* 633-642.
Lechner, J. F., Haugen, A., McClendon, I. A., and Shamsuddin, A. M. (1983a). Differentiation, in press.
Lechner, J. F., Tokiwa, T., Curren, R. D., Yeager, H., Jr., and Harris, C. C. (1983b). *Proc. Am. Assoc. Cancer Res. 24,* 58.
Peehl, D. M., and Ham, R. G. (1980). *In Vitro 16,* 526-538.
Rheinwald, J. G., and Beckett, M. A. (1980). *Cell 22,* 629-632.
Seabright, M. (1971). *Lancet 30,* 971-972.
Selikoff, I. J., and Lee, D. H. K. (1978). *In* "Asbestos and Disease" (I. J. Selikoff and D. H. L. Lee, eds), pp. 307-336. Academic Press, New York.
Stanbridge, E. J., Der, C. J., Doersen, C.-J., Nishimi, R. Y., Peehl, P. M., Weissman, B. E., and Wilkinson, J. E. (1982). *Science (Washington D. C.) 215,* 252-259.
Stoner, G. D., Harris, C. C., Myers, G. A., Trump, B. F., and Connor, R. D. (1980a). *In Vitro 16,* 399-408.

Stoner, G. D., Katoh, Y., Foidart, J.-M., Myers, G. A., and
    Harris, C. C. (1980b). *In* "Normal Human Tissue and Cell
    Culture" (C. C. Harris, B. F. Trump, and G. D. Stoner, eds.),
    Academic Press, New York. *Methods Cell Biol. 22A*, 15-35.
Sun, T.-T., and Green, H. (1976). *Cell 9*, 511-521.
Sunderman, F. W., Jr. (1978). *Fed. Proc. Fed. Am. Soc. Exp.
    Biol. 37*, 40-46.
Trump, B. F., Valigorsky, J. M., Dees, J. H., Mergner, W. J.,
    and Kim, K. M. (1974). *Hum. Pathol. 4*, 89-109.
Trump, B. F., Resau, J., and Barrett, L. A. (1980). *In* "Normal
    Human Tissue and Cell Culture" (C. C. Harris, B. F. Trump,
    G. D. Stoner, eds.), Academic Press, New York. *Methods
    Cell Biol. 21A*, 1-14.
Watt, F. M., and Green, H. (1981). *J. Cell Biol. 90*, 738-742.
Wu, Y.-J., Parker, L. M., Binder, N. E., Beckett, M. A., Sinard,
    J. H., Griffiths, C. T., and Rheinwald, J. G. (1982). *Cell
    31*, 693-703.
Yuspa, S. H., Hawley-Nelson, P., Kochler, B., and Stanley, J.
    R. (1981). *Cancer Res. 40*, 4694-4703.

VI. Special Address

24

SOMATIC CELL GENETIC CHARACTERIZATION OF ONCOGENES

F. H. Ruddle

Departments of Biology and Human Genetics
Yale University
New Haven, Connecticut

P. E. Barker and D. Pravtcheva

Department of Biology
Yale University
New Haven, Connecticut

J. Ryan

Department of Human Genetics
Yale University
New Haven, Connecticut

I.   INTRODUCTION: SOMATIC CELL GENETICS

Mendelian genetic studies have contributed in a significant way to our understanding and control of the neoplastic
process.   It is now clear that somatic cell genetic approaches
will also contribute.   In this chapter we summarize briefly
some of the features of somatic cell genetics and show its
relevance to current studies on neoplasia.   Mendelian genetics
has certain disadvantages when applied to long-lived organisms
such as the mammals, and particularly humans.   The generation
time is long and the progeny size is small; moreover, for
humans one cannot direct mating.   The result is that with the
Mendelian approach the pace of investigation is slow and
costly.   Moreover, in many instances the mutations of interest
are lethal or produce early death, thus restricting their easy
study.

Many of these obstacles are overcome by the somatic cell
genetic approach.   By this methodology, whole chromosomes,
segments of individual chromosomes, even discrete genes are
transferred from the species, individual organism, or tissue
of interest into a foreign surrogate somatic cell—usually of
different species origin.   In this way, it is possible to infer
the linkage relationships of genes, to determine their functional properties, and to effect their physical isolation.
For cancer studies the somatic cell method is particularly
useful, because it permits a direct genetic analysis of neo-
plastically transformed cells, something that is impossible by
the sexual or Mendelian approach.

II. GENE MAPPING

The isolation, actually the cloning, of individual donor chromosomes into recipient, surrogate cells provides a simple way of mapping genes to individual chromosomes (Ruddle and Creagan, 1975). All that is required is that the donor genes be distinguished from their recipient homologs. This can be easily accomplished if the donor and recipient cells come from phylogenetically diverse species, such as mouse and human—a favorite duo. In this combination, the donor and recipient chromosomes can be easily identified, and the presence of specific donor genes can be identified by tests performed on the gene product or on the gene itself. The order of genes along the length of the chromosome can be established by the cloning of overlapping subchromosomal segments into surrogate cells. Using this general approach, approximately 500 genes have been mapped in humans since 1969; the great majority have been mapped to subregions of chromosomes (Berg et al., 1981).

Gene mapping by DNA hybridization techniques is particularly relevant to our discussion here. The current method of choice involves using differences in restriction enzyme patterns to distinguish donor from recipient homologous gene sequences. In most instances, the DNA probe is nonspecifically cross-hybridizing and therefore is not discriminating. The first genes mapped using restriction pattern differences in conjunction with cell hybrid panels were those that code for the immunoglobulins (Swan et al., 1979). Cloned Ig probes were hybridized to restricted hybrid cell DNA, and by this means the donor restriction pattern for a particular Ig class could be correlated with a particular donor chromosome. Subsequently the Ig loci were localized to a chromosome subregion either by correlation with a subchromosomal segment or by

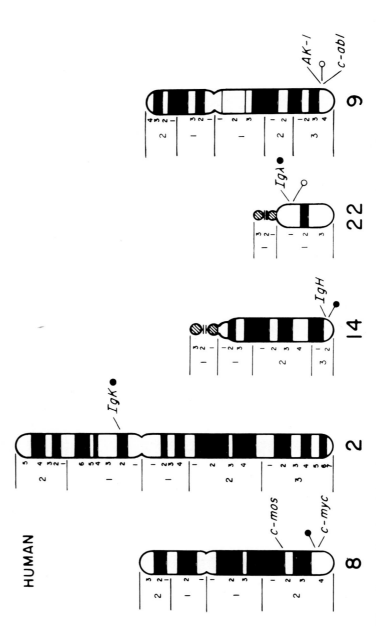

Fig. 1. Relationships between genes and chromosome translocation breakpoints. The gene marker and chromosomal breakpoint are presented on the same line if they are known to be close and if their distal-proximal relationships are unknown (i.e., *IgK* in humans for Burkitt chromosome translocation). In instances where the assignment of a locus to the region of a breakpoint has not been reported, the breakpoint symbol has been omitted (i.e., murine *Igλ*). See citations

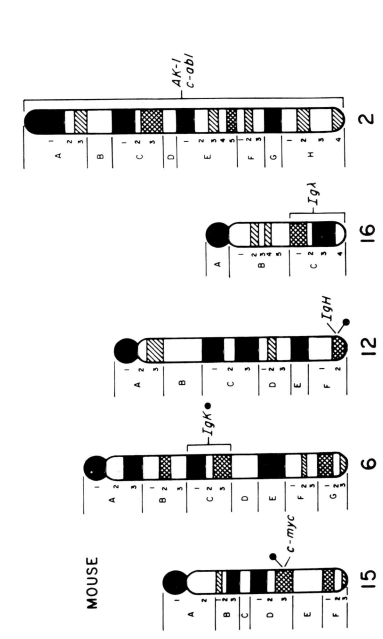

(Fig. 1 continued) in text. *Human:* ●, Burkitt translocations; *IgK* ●,
○ CML translocations; signifies that locus and breakpoint are in the same band but that distal/proximal relationships
are unknown. *Mouse:* ● plasmacytoma tx breakpoints.

in situ hybridization. *In situ* hybridization can be used
effectively in combination with somatic cell genetic mapping
procedures. If a gene has been mapped to a chromosome by the
somatic cell genetic technique, then one can employ *in situ*
hybridization to confirm the first result and also to fix a
subchromosomal location. This can be done easily with multi-
copy genes located within a single locus and, in certain
instances, can be extended as well to single-copy genes
(Ruddle, 1981). The chromosomal locations of human and mouse
Ig loci are given in Fig. 1.

The use of restriction pattern differences to identify
genes can also be extended to alleles in the context of
Mendelian genetics. It has been postulated and verified at
least in a preliminary way that nucleotide substitutions occur
frequently within a species, so that restriction pattern differences will be common (Botstein *et al.*, 1980). These are
recognized as restriction site polymorphisms (RSP). Such RSP
can be used as genetic markers for establishing the linkage
relationships between genes. RSP markers can be readily
assigned to chromosomal sites using somatic cell genetics
and/or *in situ* hybridization techniques (Wyman and White, 1980).

III.   THE CELLULAR ONCOGENES

The somatic cell genetic approach has been particularly
successful in establishing the map positions of the cellular
oncogenes. These genes were first identified by their sequence
homology with viral oncogenes isolated from oncogenic retroviruses (Weiss *et al.*, 1982). Thus, the viral oncogenes or
their cloned cellular oncogene counterparts serve as convenient
probes for establishing the map positions of these genes using
the somatic cell approaches already discussed. The chromosomal

TABLE I. Chromosome Locations of the Cellular Oncogenes[a]

c-onc	Mouse	Human	References
c-ras[N]		1p13-cen	J. Ryan, P. E. Barker, M. Rabin, and F. H. Ruddle (unpublished)
c-fos	15 or 19	2	P. E. Barker, I. M. Verma, and F. H. Ruddle (unpublished)
c-fms		5	M. Roussel, C. J. Sherr, P. E. Barker, and F. H. Ruddle (unpublished)
c-myb		6	Dalla-Favera *et al.* (1982a)
c-Ki-ras-1		6	O'Brien *et al.* (1983)
c-myc	15 (D2-3)	8q24	Dalla-Favera *et al.* (1982c), Crews *et al.* (1982), Neel *et al.* (1982)
c-mos	4	8q22	Neel *et al.* (1982), Prakash *et al.* (1982)
c-abl	2	9q34	Goff *et al.* (1981, 1982), Heisterkamp *et al.* (1982)
c-Ha-ras-1[b]	7	11	J. Ryan, P. E. Barker, and F. H. Ruddle (unpublished); Martinville *et al.* (1983), O'Brien *et al.* (1983), and McBride *et al.* (1982)
c-Ki-ras-2		12	J. Ryan, P. E. Barker, and F. H. Ruddle (unpublished, Sakaguchi *et al.* (1982)
c-fes[c]		15	Heisterkamp *et al.* (1982), Dalla-Favera *et al.* (1982a)
c-src		20	Sakaguchi *et al.* (1982)
c-sis[d]		22q11-qter	Dalla-Favera *et al.* (1982b)
c-Ha-ras-2		Xq26-cen	O'Brien *et al.* (1983)

[a]*Other c-onc genes reported for which no map position is known include, c-ski (Li et al., 1982), c-erb (Roussel et al., 1979), c-rel (Cohen et al., 1981, c-amv (Bergman et al., 1981), c-yes (Shibuya et al., 1982), and c-ros (Shibuya et al., 1982).*

[b]*Homology to c-bas (Santos et al., 1982).*

[c]*Homology to c-fps (Shibuya et al., 1982).*

[d]*Homology to oncogene of PI-FeSV (Besmer et al., 1983).*

locations of human and mouse cellular oncogenes are given in
Table I. It should also be pointed out that some of the cellular oncogenes have already been shown to be associated with
restriction site polymorphisms (see Table I). Their polymorphic character will be useful in establishing their linkage
relationship with other closely linked polymorphic sites and
in addition may serve to characterize the oncogenic potential
of individual alleles.

IV. GENE TRANSFER AND THE ISOLATION OF CELLULAR ONCOGENES

    Whereas cell hybridization can be used to introduce
chromosomes into surrogate recipient cells, the so-called gene
transfer methodologies have been used to transfer specific
genes. The range of options available have been discussed in
several reviews (Huttner and Ruddle, 1982; Scangos and Ruddle,
1981). Here, attention will be focused on the calcium
phosphate-DNA coprecipitation technique. In this system,
foreign DNA is extracted then coprecipitated with calcium
phosphate (CP). The CP-DNA precipitate is ingested by the
recipient cell, and, in a small proportion of cells, the
foreign gene of interest is stably expressed.
    The gene transfer approach has been effectively employed
in the characterization and isolation of cellular oncogenes
(Cooper, 1982). In this system, DNA is isolated from human
tumor cell populations, and then transfected into NIH/3T3
mouse fibroblasts using the CP-DNA procedure. Oncogenic
transformation is judged by the acquisition of neoplastic
phenotypes in the recipient cells, such as reduced cell-cell
adhesion, growth in agar, and tumorigenic growth potential in
nude mice. The system can be used to isolate individual

oncogenes by virtue of their linkage with repetitive sequences that are specific for the donor human species. Thus in practice, the donor DNA is serially passaged through mouse NIH/3T3 cells two to three times. At each transformation step, selection is exerted for the human oncogene of interest. Thus at the same time, serial transfer dilutes out nononcogenic gene sequences. Finally, the ultimate transformant DNA is used to construct a DNA libray, and the segments in the library are screened for one of the highly redundant human repeated sequences, such as the *Alu* repeats (Schmid and Jelinek, 1982). These serve as an identifying sequence for the oncogene, and provide a means of isolating the oncogene from the gene library. Subsequently, the cloned gene is verified as having oncogenic properties by another round of CP-DNA transformation in NIH/3T3 cells.

Once the oncogenes have been isolated by the procedures just outlined, it is possible to locate the position of the homologous cellular gene using somatic cell hybridization techniques. It is also possible on the basis of sequence homology to establish identity if any between the isolated human transforming gene and previously characterized *v-onc* genes. In the case of human transforming genes isolated from human bladder tumors, it could be shown that they possessed homology with Harvey *v-ras* sequences, and that their corresponding cellular oncogene mapped to human chromosome 11 (McBride *et al.*, 1982; Parada *et al.*, 1982; Santos *et al.*, 1982; Shimizu *et al.*, 1983; J. Ryan, P. E. Barker, and F. H. Ruddle, unpublished). In the case of human transforming gene sequences isolated from human lung and colon tumors, homology with Kirsten *v-ras* sequences was demonstrated (Shimizu *et al.*, 1983). The corresponding cellular oncogene *c-Ki-ras* mapped to chromosome 12 (J. Ryan, P. E. Barker, and F. H. Ruddle, unpublished). A human transforming gene has been isolated from

a human neuroblastoma (SK-N-SH), which maps to human chromosome
1 (Shimizu *et al.*, 1983; J. Ryan, P. E. Barker, and F. H.
Ruddle, unpublished). This sequence has also been shown to
possess homology with the *c-ras* family (Shimizu *et al.*, 1983).

V.   RELATIONSHIP BETWEEN CHROMOSOME TRANSLOCATIONS
     AND CELLULAR ONCOGENES

A.   Chronic Myeloid Leukemia (CML)

     It has long been recognized that certain chromosomal
rearrangements are associated with particular types of cancers.
One of the best examples is the Philadelphia chromosome and
chronic myeloid leukemia (CML) (Nowell and Hungerford, 1960).
Almost invariably, CML cells possess a reciprocal chromosomal
translocation between chromosomes 22 and 9.   The translocation
breakpoints occur in the long arm of chrmosome 22 (22q11), and
at the end of the long arm of chromosome 9 (9q34) (Rowley,
1982).   The result is an obviously shortened chromosome 22,
which has been designated the Ph^1 chromosome.   The nearly in-
variant association of CML with a specific chromosome rearrangement suggested an underlying genetic mechanism.   The
general validity of this notion and the details of the underlying genetic events are now becoming clear.

     Gene mapping studies played a crucial role in establishing
these relationships.   The first assignment of a cellular
oncogene was that of the murine *c-abl* gene to mouse chromosome
2 (Goff *et al.*, 1981, 1982).   Later, human mapping studies
indicated that the *c-abl* gene was located on human chromosome
9 (Heisterkamp *et al.*, 1982).   At this point, comparative
mapping data proved useful in predicting a subchromosomal
regional assignment of the gene.   It had been established that
the gene coding for adenylate kinase 1 (AK-1) mapped to mouse

chromosome 2 and to human chromosome 9 (Dalla-Favera *et al.*, 1982a). This suggested that *c-abl* and AK-1 might be closely linked in both species. It was already known that AK-1 mapped to the end of human chromosome 9 (9q34); therefore, it could be assumed that *c-abl* likewise mapped to this region. This has subsequently been verified by direct testing (de Klein *et al.*, 1982).

Meanwhile, chromosome mapping studies on human chromosome 22 provided additional useful information. First, it was shown that the *c-sis* gene mapped to the chromosome segment 22q11-qter (Dalla-Favera *et al.*, 1982b). Second, it was demonstrated that the human *Ig*λ locus mapped to the middle of the long arm of 22 in the vicinity of the chromosomal breakpoint involved in CML (22q11) (Taub *et al.*, 1982). The position of the relevant genes to the chromosome breakpoints is now becoming known. It appears that in three independent translocations, *c-abl* maps distal to the breakpoint on 9 and therefore is transferred to the Ph[1] chromosome (de Klein *et al.*, 1982). In contrast, AK-1 is proximal to the breakpoint and retains its position on chromosome 9 (de Klein *et al.*, 1982). These results indicate that a close relationship exists between the *c-abl* and the *Ig*λ loci in CML cells on the basis of cytogenetic studies. Whether an interesting interaction exists between *Ig*λ, *c-abl*, and/or *c-sis* on a molecular level remains to be demonstrated. However, we may presume this will be so, because such a relationship has been reported in the case of another chromosomal translocation associated with neoplastic disease, namely murine plasmacytoma.

B.   Murine Plasmacytoma

In murine plasmacytoma, there occurs a modification of
chromosome 15 at high frequency (Shepard *et al.*, 1974).   The
modification occurs as a reciprocal translocation with chromosome 6 or chromosome 12.   The translocation breakpoints are
relatively constant and occur at 15 (D2-3) and 6 (C) on the
one hand, and 15 (D3) and 12 (F2) on the other (Shepard *et al.*,
1978; Ohno *et al.*, 1979).   Mapping studies have shown that the
*Ig*κ and *Ig* heavy-chain loci map to chromosomes 6 and 12, respectively (Swan *et al.*, 1979; Crews *et al.*, 1982).   The *IgH*
locus maps at the translocation breakpoint site on chromosome 12
(Fig. 1) (Kirsch *et al.*, 1982).   The *c-myc* gene has been mapped
to murine chromosome 15 in the region of the translocation
breakpoint on 15 (D2-3) (Taub *et al.*, 1982).   These observations make a compelling case for an interaction between *c-myc*
and the *Ig* loci in the generation of the murine plasmacytomas.
As will be shown, such a relationship is borne out by studies
at the molecular level.   Unfortunately, the precise relationships between the relevant genes and the translocation breakpoints at the cytogenetic level have not yet been reported.
However, in a homologous case in humans involving the Burkitt
lymphomas, these relationships have been established at least
in a preliminary way (see later).
Molecular studies on murine plasmacytomas have shown that
the 12/15 chromosomal translocations involve regions of the *Ig*
locus of chromosome 12 and sequences that reside on chromosome
15.   The first report of this kind provided evidence for a
novel sequence covalently bonded to the *C*α gene at the switch
(S) region 5' to the unexpressed *C*α gene (Harris *et al.*, 1982).
This novel sequence, termed NIARD, was isolated and then mapped
to its normal genomic position using the technique of somatic
cell genetics as described previously.   The NIARD sequence

could be shown not to originate on murine chromosome 12 but on chromosome 15. A similar finding involving the *C*α S region has been reported (Crews *et al.*, 1982). In another comparable study, a more complex modification was observed. In this instance, the heavy-chain switch region for μ (chromosome 12) and the gene for κ constant region (chromosome 6) were joined to a chromosome 15 sequence (Van Ness *et al.*, 1982). Therefore, originally unlinked sequences from three chromosomes—namely 6, 12, and 15—have contributed to a novel structure. Complex chromosome rearrangements involving three chromosomes have been reported in humans in association with neoplastic disease (Rowley, 1982). These findings, together with others, indicate that the rearrangement may be variable and complex at the molecular as well as the chromosome level. Thus, three reports now indicate that the 12/15 chromosome translocations in mouse plasmacytomas involve exchanges within the *Ig* locus to sequences residing on chromosome 15. Just how these rearrangements occur and whether they are adaptive to the tumor cell remains as yet unresolved.

As described previously, the *c-myc* gene had been mapped to chromosome 15 by somatic cell genetic techniques. The *c-myc* gene became a natural candidate for the chromosome sequences that became linked to the *Ig* complex. This prediction has been shown correct. In studies at the mRNA and DNA levels, it was shown that in five mouse plasmacytoma lines the *C*α gene was joined in the switch region to *c-myc* sequences. It was also shown in all instances that the *c-myc* and *C*α genes were in the opposite transcriptional orientation (Shen-Ong *et al.*, 1982). In an independent study similar results were obtained (Crews *et al.*, 1982).

C. Burkitt Lymphoma

Burkitt lymphomas present a pattern of chromosomal translocations similar to those found in mouse plasmacytomas (Klein, 1981). In humans, the immunoglobulin loci, as in the mouse, map to three different chromosomes, namely 2, 14, and 22 (see Fig. 1). In the Burkitt lymphoma cells one character-istically observes translocations between chromosome 8 and chromosomes 2, 14, or 22. The 8/14 translocation is predomi-nant, and significantly, the breakpoint on 14 occurs in the region of the *Ig* locus (Taub *et al.*, 1982). Mapping studies have shown that two cellular oncogenes map to chromosome 8, namely *c-myc* (Dalla-Favera *et al.*, 1982; Neel *et al.*, 1982; Taub *et al.*, 1982) and *c-mos* (Prakash *et al.*, 1982). *c-myc* and *c-mos* have been mapped to the 8q24 and 8q22 subregions, respectively (Neel *et al.*, 1982; Taub *et al.*, 1982). Cyto-genetic analysis of the translocated chromosomes isolated in hybrid cells has shown that *c-myc* is distal to the breakpoint on chromosome 8, and therefore it is transferred close to the *IgH* locus, which itself is proximal to the chromosome 14 breakpoint (Dalla-Favera *et al.*, 1982c). The relationship of *c-mos* to the Burkitt translocation breakpoints remains to be worked out. If *c-mos* is at 8q22, it is above the breakpoint on chromosome 8, which is at band 8q24. Rearrangements of *c-mos* in Burkitt lymphomas, detected as novel restriction fragments, have been reported (Taub *et al.*, 1982). Evidence at the molecular level has shown that *c-myc* sequences have been joined to *Ig*μ sequences in the region of the μ switch region (Marcu *et al.*, 1983; Taub *et al.*, 1982). Thus, in many important respects, one sees a striking homology between the human and mouse B-lymphocytic tumors.

VI.   POSSIBILITIES

Approximately 20 cellular oncogenes have been identified. Of these, about 14 have been mapped to chromosomal sites (Table I).   The somatic cell genetic and *in situ* hybridization methods are ideally adapted to mapping the cellular oncogenes. It should be possible to establish the map positions of the full catalog of these genes in the near future.   As newly recognized cellular oncogenes are detected by the gene transfer and other procedures, their map positions can be rapidly established.

The map positions of the cellular oncogenes provide useful information on their structural and functional characterization.   Knowing the chromosomal locations of these genes permits one to infer relationships between particular cellular oncogenes and chromosomal rearrangements, such as reciprocal translocations, deletions, duplications, and other complex rearrangements.   An example is the 15/17 translocation frequently found in acute promyelocytic leukemia cells.   The existence of the *c-fes* gene on human chromosome 15 suggests that this gene may be situated at the chromosome 15 breakpoint.   This is a hypothesis that can be readily tested.   If an association is found, then the hypothesis can be extended to the molecular level of inquiry.

It should be noted that these developments make available an analysis of chromosome translocations at the molecular level for the first time in mammalian cells.   The molecular events of chromosomal translocation can now be described, because the *onc* gene sequences for which probes exist reside at the sites of translocation.   It will be of interest to know whether particular kinds of translocations, for example those that involve immunoglobulin sequences, represent a distinct class. These exchanges may make use of switch sequences that normally would be involved in splicing events involved in the maturation of the *Ig* loci. Will this mechanism extend to other translocations or will different classes of translocations be unique on mechanistic and/or structural ground? The approaches outlined here may provide an answer to this question.

The purpose of this chapter has been to illustrate the potential role of somatic cell genetics in the analysis of tumorigenesis in mammals—particularly humans. The system allows one to perform a direct analysis of genetic modifications relevant to the neoplastic process. The somatic cell genetic approach also potentiates Mendelian genetic studies based on the analysis of kindreds. One can now ask whether polymorphic variants of cellular oncogenes or sequences involved in chromosome rearrangements may carry a higher risk of tumor development. If such were the case, polymorphisms could be used as predictors for risk of neoplastic disease and possibly serve as the basis of a new preventive medicine approach to cancer.

REFERENCES

Berg, K., Evans, H. J., Hamerton, J. L., and Klinger, H. (eds.) (1981). *Birth Defects Orig. Artic. Ser. 18*, 341.
Bergman, D. G., Sanza, L. M., and Baluda, M. A. (1981). *J. Virol. 40*, 450.
Bessmer, P., Snyder, H. W., Jr., Murphy, J. E., Hardy, W. D., Jr., and Parodi, A. (1983). *J. Virol. 46*, 606-613.
Botstein, D., White, R. L., Skolnick, M., and Davis, R. W. (1980). *Am. J. Hum. Genet. 32*, 314.
Cohen, R. S., Wong, T. L., and Lai, M. M. C. (1981). *Virology 113*, 672.
Cooper, G. M. (1982). *Science (Washington, D.C.) 217*, 801.
Crews, S., Barth, R., Hood, L., Prehn, J., and Calome, K. (1982). *Science (Washington, D.C.) 218*, 1319.

Dalla-Favera, R., Granchini, G., Matinotti, S., Wong-Staal, Gallo, R. C., and Croce, C. (1982a). *Proc. Natl. Acad. Sci. USA 79*, 4714.

Dalla-Favera, R., Gallo, R. C., Giallongo, A., and Croce, C. (1982b). *Science (Washington D.C.) 218*, 686.

Dalla-Favera, R., Bregni, M., Erikson, J., Patterson, D., Gallo, R., and Croce, C. (1982c). *Proc. Natl. Acad. Sci. USA 79*, 7824.

de Klein, A., Guerts van Kessel, A., Grosveld, G., Bartram, C. R., Hagemeijer, A., Bootsma, D., Spurr, N. K., Heisterkamp, N., Groffen, J., and Stephenson, J. R. (1982). *Nature (London) 300.*

D'Eustachio, P., Pravtcheva, D., Marcu, K., and Ruddle, F. H. (1980). *J. Exp. Med. 151*, 1545.

Donner, L., Fedele, L. A., Jaron, C. F., Anderson, S. J., and Shen, C. J. (1982). *Virol. 41*, 489.

Goff, S., Tobin, C., Lee, R., Wang, J., D'Eustachio, P., Ruddle, F. H., and Baltimore, D. (1981). *In* "RNA Tumor Viruses" (J. Coffin and G. Van de Woude, eds.), p. 147. Cold Spring Harbor Lab., Cold Spring Harbor, New York.

Goff, S., D'Eustachio, P., Ruddle, F. H., and Baltimore, D. (1982). *Science (Washington, D.C.) 218*, 1317.

Harris, L. J., D'Eustachio, P., Ruddle, F. H., and Marcu, K. M. (1982). *Proc. Natl. Acad. Sci. USA 79*, 6622.

Heisterkamp, N., Groffen, J., Stephenson, J. R., Spurr, N., Goodfellow, P. N., Solomon, E., Carritt, B., and Bodmer, W. F. (1982). *Nature (London) 299*, 747.

Huttner, K. M., and Ruddle, F. H. (1982). *Natl. Cancer Inst. Monogr. 60*, 63.

Kirsch, I. R., Morton, C. C., Nakahara, K., and Leder, P. (1982). *Science (Washington, D.C.) 216*, 301.

Klein, G. (1981). *Nature (London) 294*, 313.

Li, Y., Magorion, C., and Stavnezer, E. (1982). *In* "RNA Tumor Viruses" (J. Coffin and G. Van de Woude), p. 21. Cold Spring Harbor Lab., Cold Spring Harbor, New York.

Malcolm, S., Barton, P., Murphy, C., Ferguson-Smith, M. A., Bentley, D. L., and Rabbitts, T. H. (1982). *Proc. Natl. Acad. Sci. USA 79*, 4957.

Marcu, K. B., Harris, L. J., Stanton, L. W., Erikson, J., Watt, R., and Croce, C. (1983). *Proc. Natl. Acad. Sci. USA.*

Martinville, de B., Giaclone, J., Shih, C., Weinberg, R. A., and Francke, U. (1983). *Science 219*, 487-501.

McBride, O. W., Swan, D. C., Santos, E., Barbacis, M., Tronick, S. R., and Aaronson, S. A. (1982). *Nature (London) 300*, 773.

Neel, G., Jhonwai, S. C., Gaghanti, R. S. K., and Hayward, W. S. (1982). *Proc. Natl. Acad. Sci. USA 79*, 7842.

Nowell, P. C., and Hungerford, D. A. (1960). *Science (Washington. D.C.) 132*, 1497.

O'Brien, S. J., Nash, W. G., Goodwin, J. L., Lowy, D. R., and Chang, E. H. (1983). *Nature (London) 302*, 839-842.

Ohno, S., Babonits, M., Wiener, F., Spira, J., and Klein, G. (1979). *Cell 18*, 1001.

Parada, L. F., Tabin, C. J., Shih, C., and Weinberg, R. A. (1982). *Nature (London) 297*, 474.

Prakash, K., McBride, O. W., Swan, D. C., Dvare, S. G., Tronick, S. R., and Aaronson, S. A. (1982). *Proc. Natl. Acad. Sci. USA 79*, 5210.

Roussel, M., Saule, S., Lagrou, C., Rommens, C., Beng, H., Graf, T., and Stehelin, D. (1979). *Nature (London) 281*, 452.

Rowley, J. (1982). *Science (Washinton, D.C.) 216*, 749.

Ruddle, F. H. (1981). *Nature (London) 294*, 115.

Ruddle, F. H., and Creagan, R. P. (1975). *Annu. Rev. Genet.* , 407.

Sakaguchi, A. Y., Naylor, S. L., Weinberg, R. A., and Shows, T. B. (1982). *Am. J. Hum. Genet. 34*B, 175A.

Santos, E., Tronick, S. R., Aaronson, S. A., Pulciani, S., and Barbacid, M. (1982). *Nature (London) 298*, 343.

Scangos, G., and Ruddle, F. H. (1981). *Gene 14*, 1.

Schmid, G. W., and Jelinek, W. R. (1982). *Science (Washington, D.C.) 216*, 1065.

Shen-Ong, G. L. C., Keath, E. J., Piccoli, S. P., and Cole, M. D. (1982). *Cell 31*, 443.

Shepard, J. S., Pettengill, O. S., Wurster-Hill, D. H., and Sorenson, G. D. (1974). *Cancer Res. 34*, 2852.

Shepard, J. S., Pettengill, O. S., Wurster-Hill, D. H., and Sorenson, G. D. (1978). *J. Natl. Cancer Inst. (US) 61*, 255.

Shibuya, M., Hanafusa, H., and Balduzzi, P. C. (1982). *J. Virol. 42*, 143.

Shimizu, K., Goldfarb, M., Suard, Y., Perucho, M., Li, Y., Kamato, T., Feramisco, J., Stavnezer, E., and Wigler, M. (1983). *Proc. Natl. Acad. Sci. USA*, in press.

Swan, D., D'Eustachio, P., Leinwand, L., Seidman, J., Keithley, D., and Ruddle, F. H. (1979). *Proc. Natl. Acad. Sci. USA 76*, 2735.

Taub, R., Kersch, I., Morton, C., Lenoir, G., Swan, D., Tronick, S., Aaronson, S., and Leder, P. (1982). *Proc. Natl. Acad. Sci. USA 79*, 7837.

VanNess, B. G., Shapiro, M., Kelley, D. E., Perry, R. P., Weigert, M., D'Eustachio, P., and Ruddle, F. H. (1983). *Proc. Natl. Acad. Sci. USA*, in press.

Wyman, A., and White, R. L. (1980). *Proc. Natl. Acad. Sci. USA 77*, 6754.

Weiss, R., Zeich, N., Varmus, H., and Coffin, J. (eds.) (1982). "RNA Tumor Viruses." Cold Spring Harbor Lab., Cold Spring Harbor, New York.

VII. Viral Oncogenesis

25

RETROVIRUSES, *onc* GENES, AND HUMAN CANCER

Stuart A. Aaronson, E. Premkumar Reddy,
Keith Robbins, Sushilkumar G. Devare,
David C. Swan, Jacalyn H. Pierce,
and Steven R. Tronick

Laboratory of Cellular and Molecular Biology
National Cancer Institute
Bethesda, Maryland

I. INTRODUCTION

Viruses have provided a means for scientists to study
fundamental cellular mechanisms, such as DNA replication and

gene regulation, in more readily dissectable ways than by
studying the more complex cell. Time and again, this concep-
tual approach has proved itself. Thus it was not without
precedence that many scientists, in efforts to learn more about
how normal cells become malignant, have turned their attention
to the study of tumor viruses.

For several years, our laboratory has been involved in
the investigation of RNA tumor viruses, designated type C
retroviruses. They consist of two major groups: chronic and
acute transforming retroviruses. The chronic viruses when
inoculated into susceptible animals cause tumors, mostly
leukemias, but only after a latent period of several months.
These viruses replicate in the absence of any apparent transforming effect on known assay cells in tissue culture. In
contrast, acute transforming viruses induce tumors within a
very short period of days to weeks. They cause a variety of
tumors, including sarcomas, hematopoietic tumors, and even
carcinomas. In tissue culture, these viruses generally induce
foci of transformation in appropriate assay cells. This
chapter documents how systematic investigation of these viruses
has led to important insights into mechanisms that lead normal
cells to become malignant. The knowledge gained from such
studies is now being applied directly to the understanding of
human oncogenesis.

II. THE RETROVIRUS GENOME

The chronic leukemia virus genome contains *gag*, *pol*, and
env genes, which code for internal structural proteins, reverse
transcriptase, and envelope proteins, respectively (Baltimore,
1974). The proviral genome also contains a repeat sequence of
anywhere from 300 to 600 bases at either terminus of the viral

genome (Fig. 1). These long terminal repeats (LTRs) contain
signals for the initiation and termination of transcription
and resemble prokaryotic transposable elements (Dhar *et al.*,
1980; Shimotohno *et al.*, 1980). Chronic leukemia viruses do
not appear to possess an additional discrete transforming gene,
and the mechanism of transformation by these agents is not as
yet resolved.

The mode of action of acute transforming viruses is
somewhat better understood and has become immediately relevant
to the understanding of naturally occurring malignancies. Our
ability to learn about these viruses has been immeasurably
aided by the development and application of modern molecular
biological techniques. It is apparent from observation of the
physical maps (Fig. 1) of three mouse-derived acute transforming retroviruses molecularly cloned in our laboratory (Tronick
et al., 1979; Andersen *et al.*, 1981; Srinivasan *et al.*, 1981)
why years ago we initially found that these viruses were
capable of transformation but were replication defective
(Aaronson and Rowe, 1970). In each case, the genome of the
acute transforming virus is smaller than that of the chronic
leukemia virus and contains a substitution of a discrete segment of nonviral-related information. In addition, each has
substituted a discrete segment of information. Thus, each of
these viruses lacks essential leukemia virus information required for its replication.

Of particular importance with respect to cancer research are
the discrete segments that are unrelated to the leukemia virus
genome. In the viruses shown (Fig. 1), each of these segments
differs from the other; however, when DNA probes are prepared
from these segments, they detect in normal mouse cell DNA not
multiple, but one or at most a few copies of related sequences.
Similar findings by a number of laboratories have led to the
understanding that acute transforming retroviruses have arisen

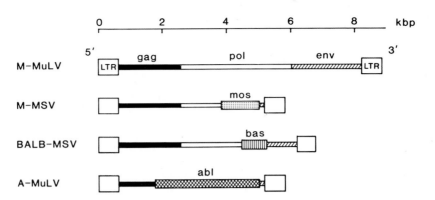

Fig. 1. Relationship of three murine transforming retroviral genomes to the chronic leukemia virus genome. The *onc*
gene of each retrovirus is indicated by a differently shaded
box to denote the different cellular origin of each. The viral
genomes were cloned and physically characterized as previously
reported (Tronick *et al*.., 1979; Srinivasan *et al*., 1981;
Andersen *et al*., 1981a).

in nature by recombination of leukemia viruses with cellular
genes.

III.   RETROVIRAL TRANSFORMING (*onc*) GENES

The cell-derived *onc* genes of transforming retroviruses
are required for viral transforming functions. This was initially demonstrated by classic genetic approaches with Rous
sarcoma virus, one of the few transforming viruses that
possesses both transforming and replication functions. Trans-
formation-defective mutants are spontaneously generated at
relatively high frequency, and these mutants were shown to
have specifically deleted the cell-derived *src* gene (for
review see Bishop, 1978; Wang, 1978).

An independent approach has utilized deletion analysis of
replication-defective transforming retroviral DNAs. This
approach can be illustrated by a molecular genetic analysis of

the cloned DNA of simian sarcoma virus (SSV), a primate-derived
acute transforming virus. In order to localize the region of
SSV required for transformation, we constructed a variety of
deletion mutants from a molecular clone of SSV DNA and tested
their ability to transform NIH/3T3 cells in a transfection
assay (Robbins *et al.*, 1983). As shown in Fig. 2, the intact
viral genome (pSSV-11) exhibited a transforming activity of
$10^{4.1}$ focus-forming units (ffu)/pmol viral DNA. A subgenomic
clone, pSSV 3/1, from which the 3' LTR was deleted, showed no
reduction in biological activity. In contrast, pSSV 3/2, a
subclone lacking the 3' LTR as well as all but 25 bp of *v-sis*,

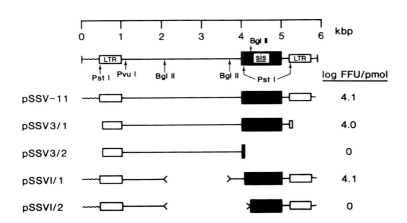

Fig. 2. Construction and biological analysis of SSV-
deletion mutants. The integrated form of SSV was excised from
λ-SSV-11 Cl 1 (Robbins *et al.*, 1983) and purified by elution
from a preparative agarose gel. pSSV 3/1 and 2 were constructed by cloning products of a reaction in which purified
SSV DNA was partially digested with PstI. pSSV-11 was obtained
by cloning the λ-SSV-11 Cl 1 insert at the *Eco*RI site of
pBR322. pSSV I/1 and 2 were constructed by limited *Bgl*II
digestion of pSSV-11 followed by religation. In each case,
the structure of individual deletion mutants was determined by
restriction enzyme and Southern blotting analysis. Transfection of NIH/3T3 cells with plasmids containing SSV wt or mutant
DNAs was performed by the calcium phosphate precipitation
technique (Graham and Van der Eb, 1973). Transformed foci were
scored at 14 to 21 days.

demonstrated no detectable transforming activity. These results strongly imply the essential nature of *v-sis* in SSV
transformation.

pSSV I/1, a mutant lacking an internal 1.8-kbp *Bgl*II
fragment (Fig. 2), transformed NIH/3T3 cells with an efficiency
of $10^{4.1}$ ffu/pmol viral DNA. However, a subclone, pSSV I/2,
which lacked an additional stretch of 245 bp of SSAV sequences
as well as the first 339 bp of *v-sis*, possessed no transforming
activity. These results localize the SSV-transforming gene to
a region encompassing *v-sis*, along with 254 and 302 bp of
flanking SSAV sequences, to the left and right of *v-sis*,
respectively (Robbins *et al.*, 1983). These and analogous
studies with other transforming retroviral DNAs have documented
that their *onc* genes are responsible for the induction and
maintenance of the virus-transformed state.

IV. *onc* GENES INCORPORATED BY RETROVIRUSES ARE LIMITED IN NUMBER

Analysis of independent isolates of transforming retroviruses has indicated that there are a limited number of
distinct cellular *onc* sequences with transforming potential
that such viruses have transduced. Table I summarizes the
known mammalian transforming retrovirus isolates and their
species of origin, as well as available information concerning
their transforming gene products. Of more than 20 independent
transforming retrovirus isolates, certain isolates of the same
species appear to contain the same or closely related *onc*
genes (Stehelin *et al.*, 1976; Donoghue *et al.*, 1979; Duesberg
and Vogt, 1979; Frankel *et al.*, 1979; Ellis *et al.*, 1981;
Ghysdael *et al.*, 1981; Andersen *et al.*, 1981b). For example,
Snyder-Theilen (ST-) and Gardner-Arnstein (GA-) FeSV isolates
appear to have independently incorporated the same gene

TABLE I.   Mammalian Retrovirus Transforming (*onc*) Genes

Virus	Origin	Gene	Protein	Function
Moloney-MSV	Mouse	*mos*	p37	—
Abelson-MuLV	Mouse	*abl*	p120	PK[a]
FBJ-MSV	Mouse	*fos*	—	—
FBR-MSV	Mouse	?	p78	—
BALB-MSV	Mouse	*bas*	p21	—
Harvey-MSV	Rat	*ras-H* (*has*)	p21	—
Ra-MSV	Rat	*ras-H* (*has*)	p29	—
Kirsten-MSV	Rat	*ras-K* (*kis*)	p21	—
ST-FeSV	Cat	*fes*	P85	PK
GA-FeSV	Cat	*fes*	P95	PK
SM-FeSV	Cat	*fms*	p180	(PK)
GR-FeSV	Cat	*fgr*	P70	PK
SSV	Woolly monkey	*sis*	p28	—

[a]*PK, protein kinase.*

(Table I).   Several studies have shown that the Fujinami sarcoma virus, an avian sarcoma virus, has also transduced the homologus avian cellular gene.   These findings have emerged from studies utilizing sarcoma virus-specific cDNA probes or antibodies capable of recognizing immunologically related sarcoma viral gene products (Shibuya *et al.*, 1980; Barbacid *et al.*, 1981; Beemon, 1981).

When we compared the molecularly cloned *onc* gene (*v-bas*) of BALB-MSV, a spontaneous mouse sarcoma virus isolate, with the *ras* gene of the rat-derived Harvey-MSV genome, a colinear 750-bp region of homology was observed.   Moreover, BALB-MSV transformants were found to express high levels of a 21,000-dalton protein, immunologically related to the *ras* gene product, p21

(Andersen *et al.*, 1981b). Thus, *bas* and *ras* represent the same cellular homolog independently transduced by mouse type C viruses from the genomes of rat and mouse species (Andersen *et al.*, 1981a) (Table I).

Comparison of the molecular structures of BALB-MSV and Harvey-MSV revealed that their *onc* genes are in very different locations. Whereas Harvey-MSV *ras* is near the 5' terminus of the genome, BALB-MSV *bas* is located toward the 3' end of the molecule. Ra-MSV is an independent rat-derived transforming virus isolate (Rasheed *et al.*, 1978) that contains *ras* sequences (Young *et al.*, 1979) (Table I). Its transforming gene product is synthesized as a larger polypeptide composed of rat helper viral *gag* and p21 products (Young *et al.*, 1981). This suggests that its gene sequence organization is different from that of either BALB- or Harvey-MSV. Thus, whatever function(s) helper viral sequences provide for replication and expression of this transforming gene, the gene can be localized with the viral genome in very different positions.

There is emerging evidence that *onc* genes incorporated by retroviruses may comprise an even smaller number of families of evolutionarily related genes. Kirsten-MSV (Table I) codes for a transforming protein immunologically related to those of BALB- and Harvey-MSV despite the fact that its *onc* sequences originate from a different cellular gene (Ellis *et al.*, 1981). Although there is little detectable nucleotide sequence homology between Kirsten-MSV *ras* and the *onc* genes of either BALB- or Harvey-MSV, nucleotide sequence analysis of these genes has revealed striking homology at the protein level (Dhar *et al.*, 1982; Tsuchida *et al.*, 1982; E. P. Reddy, *et al.*, unpublished). Such homology is likely to have resulted from divergence from a common ancestral gene.

The Rous sarcoma virus *src* gene product has been shown to be a protein kinase (Collet and Erickson, 1978; Levinson *et al.*,

1978) with rather unique specificity for phosphorylating tyro-
sine residues (Hunter and Sefton, 1980). Analogous functions
have been ascribed to the *onc* genes of several mammalian
transforming retroviruses (Table I). Rous sarcoma virus *src*,
Moloney-MSV *mos*, and the *onc* gene from an avian transforming
retrovirus, Y73, lack detectable relatedness by molecular
hybridization and possess extensive homology with different
cellular genes. However, these *onc* genes demonstrate varying
degrees of homology at the amino acid sequence level (Van
Beveren *et al.*, 1981; Kitamura *et al.*, 1982). There is accumulating evidence from nucleotide sequence studies that a number
of other transforming retroviruses with protein kinase activities (Table I) may also possess striking degrees of homology
with the Rous *src* protein. Thus, acute transforming viruses
have incorporated from a potential battery of thousands of
cellular genes only a very few. These findings strongly argue
that the number of cellular genes that can be altered or
activated to become transforming genes when incorporated within
the retrovirus genome is limited.

V. APPROACHES TOWARD DETECTING *onc* GENE PRODUCTS

In some cases, it has been possible to detect *onc* gene-
coded proteins by means of antisera prepared in animals bearing
tumors induced by these viruses. We have utilized another
strategy to obtain antisera capable of recognizing *onc* gene
products. As a result of the advances of recombinant DNA and
nucleotide sequencing, it is possible to prepare antisera to
peptides synthesized on the basis of a known nucleotide
sequence. By such an approach, it is hoped that the antiserum
will be capable of recognizing the entire translational product
of the gene in question.

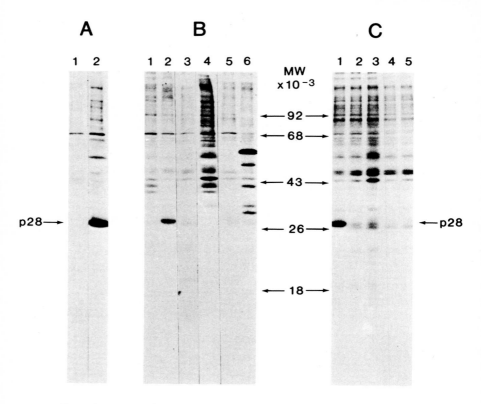

Fig. 3. *In vivo* detection of a *v-sis* translational
product by immunoprecipitation analysis (Robbins *et al.*, 1983).
Subconfluent cultures (around 10^7 cells/10-cm petri dish) were
labeled for 3 h at 37°C with 4 ml of methionine-free Dulbecco's
modified Eagle's minimal essential medium containing 100 µCi
[^{35}S]methionine (1200 Ci/nmol, Amersham)/ml. Radiolabeled
cells were lysed with 1 ml of a buffer containing 10 m*M* sodium
phosphate pH 7.5, 100 m*M* NaCl, 1% Triton X-10, 0.5% sodium
deoxycholate, and 0.1 m*M* phenylmethylsulfonyl fluoride per
petri dish, clarified at 100,000 *g* for 30 min, and divided into
four identical aliquots. Each aliquot was incubated with 4 µl
of antisera for 60 min at 4°C. Immunoprecipitates were recovered with the aid of *Staphylococcus aureus* protein A bound
to Sepharose beads (Pharmacia) and analyzed by electrophoresis
in sodium dodecyl sulfate–14% polyacrylamide gels as described
(Robbins *et al.*, 1983).   (A) Immunoprecipitation of labeled
extracts of SSV (SSAV)-transformed producer (lane 1) or uninfected (lane 2) marmoset cells with anti-SSV *sis* peptide serum.
(B) Immunoprecipitation of labeled extracts of SSV clone 11
transformed nonproducer NRK cells with preimmune rabbit serum
(lane 1), anti-*sis* peptide serum (lane 2), or anti-SSAV serum

The simian sarcoma virus *sis* gene, as well as several other *onc* genes sequenced by scientists in our laboratory, contain open reading frames that initiate in helper viral sequences within a few bases to the left of their cell-derived *onc* gene and continue for several hundred nucleotides into the *onc* genes themselves (Reddy *et al.*, 1981; Devare *et al.*, 1982; E. P. Reddy *et al.*, unpublished). A peptide composed of 15 amino acids from the N-terminal region of the predicted *sis* protein was used to immunize rabbits. As shown in Fig. 3, this antiserum detected a 28,000-MW protein in SSV-transformed cells that could not be precipitated with preimmune serum or detected by the antiserum in uninfected cells. Moreover, precipitation of this protein could be completely inhibited by preincubation with the peptide (Fig. 3) (Robbins *et al.*, 1983).

This protein corresponds in size to that predicted for the SSV-transforming protein from our sequence studies (Devare *et al.*, 1982), further indicating that we have indeed identified the SSV-transforming gene product in SSV-transformed cells. It is hoped that this approach will be useful not only in characterizing this protein but will help as well in identifying and characterizing the *onc* gene products of other acute transforming retroviruses.

VI.   CHROMOSOMAL MAPPING OF HUMAN *onc* GENE HOMOLOGS

Genes related to retroviral *onc* genes are well conserved in human DNA. It is possible to map these genes to specific

(Fig. 3 continued) (lane 6). Anti-*sis* peptide serum was also used to immunoprecipitate uninfected (lane 3) Moloney murine sarcoma virus-transformed nonproducer (lane 4) or SSAV-infected (lane 5) NRK cell extracts. (C) Immunoprecipitation of extracts of SSV clone 11 transformed nonproducer NRK cells with anti-*sis* peptide serum that was preincubated with 0, 0.1, 0.3, 1, or 10 μg (lanes 1-5, respectively) of *sis* peptide.

human chromosomes by testing for the presence of human DNA
fragments related to the *onc* gene in question in somatic cell
hybrids possessing varying numbers of human chromosomes as well
as in segregants of such hybrids. This strategy requires use
of a restriction endonuclease that yields different-sized DNA
fragments containing *onc*-related human and rodent sequences.
In some cases, it has been possible to utilize the cloned viral
onc gene as a probe, whereas in others we have utilized cloned
DNAs from the human *onc*-related locus itself. With human
probes, the signal intensity of the human *onc*-related DNA
fragment can be markedly enhanced over that of its rodent
homolog under appropriate hybridization conditions.

Table II summarizes the human chromosomal locations of
onc-related genes so far analyzed. By this approach *sis* has
been assigned to chromosome 22 (Swan *et al.*, 1982), whereas
mos (Prakash *et al.*, 1982) and MC-29 *myc* (Taub *et al.*, 1982)
are located on chromosome 8. BALB- and Harvey-MSV *onc* genes

TABLE II. Chromosomal Assignments of the Human Homologs of
            Retroviral *onc* Genes

onc gene	Chromosomal localization	Chromosomal aberration	Tumor[a]
sis	22	9:22 8:22	CML Burkitt lymphoma
myb	6	—	—
fes	15	—	—
mos; myc	8	8:14 8:22 2:8 8:21	Burkitt lymphoma Burkitt lymphoma Burkitt lymphoma AML
bas	11	del 11p	Wilms' tumor

[a]*Cancers with chromosomal aberrations affecting chromosomes to which onc gene homologs have been localized.*

and the AMV *onc* gene *myb* have been localized to human chromosome 11 (McBride *et al.*, 1982) and 6, respectively (Dalla-
Favera *et al.*, 1982; D. C. Swan *et al.*, unpublished). Finally,
Dalla-Favera *et al.* (1982) have assigned the human homolog of
fes to chromosome 15. Thus, it appears that *onc*-related human
genes are distributed throughout the human genome.

The chromosome to which *sis* has been assigned is known to
exhibit a highly reproducible translocation in chronic myelo-
genous leukemia (Rowley, 1980), whereas the chromosome to which
mos and *myc* are localized exhibits a specific translocation in
Burkitt lymphoma (Bernheim *et al.*, 1981). Klein (1981) has
speculated that chromosomal translocations may result in the
activation of *onc* genes. Very recent evidence has demonstrated
that *myc* and immunoglobulin heavy chain μ are rearranged in the
8:14 translocations observed in Burkitt lymphoma (Dalla-Favera
et al., 1982; Taub *et al.*, 1982). Studies are currently in
progress to resolve whether the specific activation of the *myc*
gene by such a mechanism plays a role in these tumors.

VII. HUMAN *onc* GENE HOMOLOGS ARE TRANSCRIBED IN HUMAN TUMOR CELLS

We sought to determine whether the human homologs of
retroviral *onc* genes are transcribed in human cells and whether
their expression could be in some way correlated with the
malignant state (Eva *et al.*, 1982; Westin *et al.*, 1982). We
analyzed polyadenylated RNAs from a large series of tumor cells
derived from different solid tumors and hematopoietic malignancies. The probes utilized were derived from the *onc* genes
of transforming retroviruses known to induce tumors of a wide
variety of tissue types. There was rather striking specificity
in the detection of transcripts related to certain *onc* genes
such as that of simian sarcoma virus (Eva *et al.*, 1982; Westin
et al., 1982).

Sis-related transcripts were found only in certain fibrosarcoma or glioblastoma cells but not in normal fibroblasts,
other solid tumors, or for the most part in any normal or
malignant hematopoietic cells analyzed. In contrast, we found
that certain *onc* genes detected related transcripts not only
in tumor cells but in normal cells as well (Eva *et al.*, 1982;
Westin *et al.*, 1982). Whatever their role in tumors, these
genes were likely to be functioning and thus important in
human cells.

VIII.   ISOLATION OF HUMAN ONCOGENES BY DNA-MEDIATED GENE TRANSFE

An independent approach to the identification of transforming genes has come from the application of DNA-mediated
gene transfer techniques. DNAs of a variety of tumors,
including some of human origin, have been shown to induce foci
of transformation upon transfection of suitable assay cells
(for review see Cooper, 1982). Several such dominant transforming genes have been partially isolated by molecular cloning
techniques. The first oncogene of human origin has been
obtained from EJ and T24 human bladder carcinoma cells
(Goldfarb *et al.*, 1982; Pulciani *et al.*, 1982; Shih and Weinberg
1982). The number of oncogenes detected by transfection
analysis also appears to be limited. For example, different
mammary carcinomas appear to possess the same activated cellular sequences, whereas many lung and colon carcinomas possess
another oncogene (Cooper, 1982).

IX.   RELATIONSHIP OF HUMAN ONCOGENES TO RETROVIRAL *onc* GENES

It was of interest to ascertain whether any of the newly
identified human oncogenes were related to the set of trans-

forming genes that have been transduced by retroviruses. We observed that the T24 human bladder tumor gene reciprocally hybridized to *v-bas*, the *onc* gene of BALB-MSV. A cloned 6.6-kbp *Bam*HI human DNA fragment harboring the T24 oncogene readily hybridized with a DNA probe containing 675 bp of *v-bas*, the *onc* gene of BALB-MSV. Moreover, *v-bas* DNA was detected with a probe composed of the T24 oncogene. Additional studies localized the *v-bas*-related sequences to a 3.0-kbp *Sac*I fragment of the T24 oncogene (Santos *et al.*, 1982). Two other laboratories have obtained analogous results utilizing *v-ras* as a molecular probe (Der *et al.*, 1982; Parada *et al.*, 1982).

To compare the T24 oncogene with normal human sequences related to *v-bas* [designated *c-bas*(human)], we isolated *c-bas*(human) from a library of normal human fetal liver DNA (Lawn *et al.*, 1978). A recombinant λ Charon 4A phage containing a 19-kbp *Eco*RI insert of human DNA exhibited a 6.4-kbp internal *Bam*HI segment that specifically hybridized with *v-bas*. This 6.4-kbp *Bam*HI fragment was subsequently subcloned in pBR322 and a representative plasmid, designated p344, used for restriction enzyme analysis. As shown in Fig. 4, the restriction map of this 6.4-kbp *Bam*HI fragment of normal human DNA closely matched that of the T24 oncogene. In fact, the only detectable difference between the two molecules was a 200-bp deletion that mapped between the *Sph*I and *Cla*I cleavage sites in *c-bas*(human) (Fig. 4). Note that this deletion maps outside the transforming sequences of the T24 oncogene, as well as outside the sequences related to *v-bas* (Fig. 4). These results established that *c-bas*(human) is an allele of the T24 bladder carcinoma oncogene.

The T24 oncogene has been shown to transform NIH/3T3 cells efficiently, with a specific activity of ~5 x 10^4 ffu/pmol (Goldfarb *et al.*, 1982; Pulciani *et al.*, 1982; Shih and Weinberg, 1982). It was of obvious interest to determine

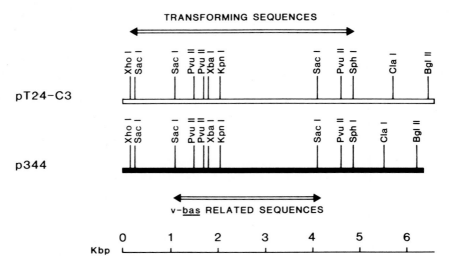

Fig. 4.   Comparative restriction maps of the T24 oncogene and *c-bas*(human). The diagram depicts the location of the cleavage sites for *Xho*I, *Sac*I, *Pvu*II, *Xba*I, *Kpn*I, *Sph*I, *Cla*I, and *Bgl*II restriction endonucleases within the subcloned *Bam*HI human DNA fragments containing the T24 oncogene (pT24-C3) and *c-bas*(human) (p344). The location of the transforming sequences of the T24 oncogene and its *c-bas*(human) related sequence are as indicated.

whether molecularly cloned *c-bas*(human) sequences exhibited similar biological activity. As much as 1 μg of *c-bas*(human) DNA demonstrated no detectable focus-forming activity, whereas in the same experiment, NIH/3T3 cells were readily transformed with as little as 1 ng of the T24 oncogene. These results, taken together, strongly imply that the acquisition of transforming activity by the T24 oncogene must be the result of subtle genetic alterations (Santos *et al.*, 1982).

Der *et al.* (1982) have reported that oncogenes associated with human lung and colon carcinomas are related to the *ras* gene of Kirsten-MSV. Similar results have been obtained in our own laboratory (Pulciani *et al.*, 1982). Thus, the homology detected between human oncogenes and retroviral *onc* genes is not likely to represent a few isolated examples. Whether the battery of available retroviral *onc* genes will be sufficient to identify all newly identified dominant transforming genes of human tumors remains to be determined. In any case, the distinctions between these two sets of transforming genes appear to be diminishing rapidly.

X. ROLE OF RETROVIRAL *onc*-RELATED GENES IN HUMAN CANCER

The role of activated or altered human homologs of retroviral *onc* genes in processes leading to human malignancy requires much further investigation. Nontheless, it is possible to make some speculations on the basis of the extensive information already available concerning the retroviral *onc* genes to which several human oncogenes are closely related. For example, it has been known for some time that Kirsten-MSV possesses the ability to induce a variety of tumors in animals (Kirsten and Mayer, 1967; Scher *et al.*, 1975) and even to induce morphological transformation of diploid human fibroblasts in culture (Aaronson and Todaro, 1970). Thus, transformation by human oncogenes related to the Kirsten-MSV *onc* gene may not be limited to the karotypically abnormal and continuous NIH/3T3 cell line.

BALB and Harvey murine sarcoma viruses, whose *onc* genes are related to the T24 oncogene, have been shown to transform a lymphoid precursor cell *in vivo* (Pierce and Aaronson, 1982). When we infected normal mouse bone marrow cultures with either of these viruses, we detected the rapid growth of colonies (Fig. 5A). Analysis of such colonies revealed them to be composed of lymphoblast cells (Fig. 5B), which could be continuously propagated in many cases. Such cells were malignant when inoculated into mice. Thus, the interaction of retroviral *onc* genes, closely related to the T24 human oncogene, with diploid

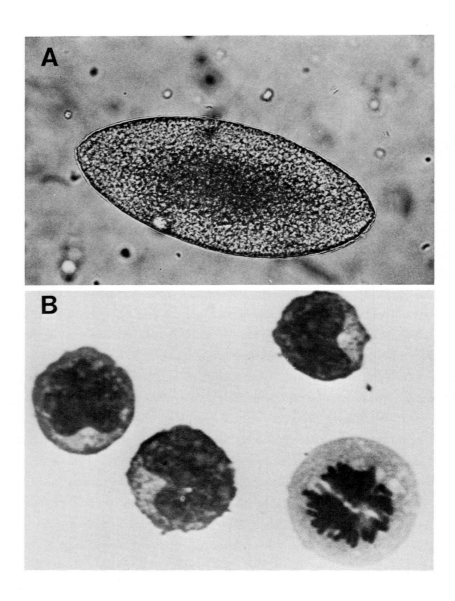

Fig. 5. Morphology of BALB-MSV-induced hematopoietic
colonies. (A) Colony growing in soft agar at 4 days post-
infection. (B) Wright-Giemsa stained preparations of cells
from a BALB-MSV-induced hematopoietic colony.

mouse bone marrow cells led rapidly to their acquisition of neoplastic properties. These results support the possibility that human counterparts of these *onc* genes could play an important and even primary role in inducing malignancy of the analogous human hematopoietic cell type.

There appears to be a strikingly high frequency at which transforming genes closely related to BALB-, Harvey- and Kirsten-MSV *onc* genes are activated in diverse human tumors. Studies within our laboratory have shown that these genes can be detected in sarcomas and hematopoietic tumors, as well as in carcinomas of different tissues (S. Pulciani, *et al.*, 1982; A. Eva *et al.*, in press). It is not yet certain why this is the case. However, retroviruses that contain these *onc* genes possess a wide spectrum of target cells for transformation *in vivo* and *in vitro*. In addition to their inducing sarcomas and tumors of immature lymphoid cells (Pierce and Aaronson, 1982), these viruses are able to stimulate the proliferation of erythroblasts (Hankins and Scolnick, 1981), and monocyte/macrophages (Greenberger, 1979). They can even induce alterations in the growth and differentiation of epithelial cells (B. Weissman and S. A. Aaronson, 1983). The wide array of tissue types that can be induced to proliferate abnormally by these *onc* genes may help to explain the high frequency of detection of their activated human homologs in diverse human tumors. If these genes can be definitively implicated in the dausation of such tumors, knowledge of their functions is likely to be crucial to the eventual understanding of human oncogenesis.

REFERENCES

Aaronson, S. A., and Rowe, W. P. (1970). *Virology 42*, 9-19.
Aaronson, S. A., and Todaro, G. J. (1970). *Nature (London)*
   225, 458-459.
Andersen, P. R., Devare, S. G., Tronick, S. R., Ellis, R. W.,
   Aaronson, S. A., and Scolnick, E. M. (1981a). *Cell 26*,
   129-134.
Andersen, P. R., Tronick, S. R., and Aaronson, S. A. (1981b).
   J. Virol. 40, 431-439.
Baltimore, D. (1974). *Cold Spring Harbor Symp. Quant. Biol.*
   39, 1187-1200.
Barbacid, M., Breitman, M. L., Lauver, A. L., Long, L. K., and
   Vogt, P. K. (1981). *Virology 110*, 411-419.
Beemon, K. (1981). *Cell 24*, 145-153.
Bernheim, A., Berger, R., and Lenoir, G. (1981). *Cancer Genet.*
   Cytogenet. 3, 307-315.
Bishop, J. M. (1978). *Annu. Rev. Biochem. 47*, 35-88.
Collet, M. S., and Erickson, R. L. (1978). *Proc. Natl. Acad.*
   Sci. USA 75, 2021-2024.
Cooper, G. M. (1982). *Science (Washington, D.C.) 217*, 801-806.
Dalla-Favera, R., Franchini, G., Martinotti, S., Wong-Staal,
   F., Gallo, R. C., and Croce, C. M. (1982). *Proc. Natl.*
   Acad. Sci. USA 79, 4714-4717.
Dalla-Favera, R., Bregni, M., Erickson, J., Patterson, D.,
   Gallo, R. C., and Croce, C. M. (1982). *Proc. Natl. Acad.*
   Sci. USA 79, 7824-7827.
Der, C. J., Krontiris, T. G., and Cooper, G. M. (1982). *Proc.*
   Natl. Acad. Sci. USA 79, 3637-3640.
Devare, S. G., Reddy, E. P., Robbins, K. C., Andersen, P. R.,
   Tronick, S. R., and Aaronson, S. A. (1982). *Proc. Natl.*
   Acad. Sci. USA 79, 3179-3182.
Dhar, R., McClements, W. L., Enquist, L. W., and Vande Woude,
   G. W. (1980). *Proc. Natl. Acad. Sci. USA 77*, 3937-3941.
Dhar, R., Ellis, R., Shih, T. Y., Oroszlan, S., Shapiro, B.,
   Maizel, J., Lowy, D., and Scolnick, E. (1982). *Science*
   (Washington, D.C.) 217, 934-937.
Donoghue, D. J., Sharp, P. J., and Weinberg, R. A. (1979). *J.*
   Virol. 32, 1015-1027.
Duesberg, P. H., and Vogt, P. K. (1979). *Proc. Natl. Acad.*
   Sci. USA 76, 1633-1637.
Ellis, R. W., DeFeo, D., Shih, T. Y., Gonda, M. A., Young, H.
   A., Tsuchida, N., Lowy, D. R., and Scolnick, E. M. (1981).
   Nature (London) 292, 506-511.
Eva, A., Robbins, K. C., Andersen, P. R., Srinivasan, A.,
   Tronick, S. R., Reddy, E. P., Ellmore, N. W., Galen, A. T.,
   Lautenberger, J. A., Papas, T. S., Westin, E. H., Wong-Staal,
   F., Gallo, R. C., and Aaronson, S. A. (1982). *Nature*
   (London) 295, 116-119.

Eva, A., Gol, R., Tronick, S. R., Pierce, J. H., and Aaronson, S. A. (1983). *Proc. Natl. Acad. Sci. USA*, in press.

Frankel, A. E., Gilbert, J. H., Porzig, K. J., Scolnick, E. M., and Aaronson, S. A. (1979). *J. Virol.* 30, 821-827.

Ghysdael, J., Neil, J. C., and Vogt, P. K. (1981). *Proc. Natl. Acad. Sci. USA* 78, 2611-2615.

Goldfarb, M., Shimizu, K., Perucho, M., and Wigler, M. (1982). *Nature (London)* 296, 404-409.

Graham, F. L., and van der Eb, A. J. (1973). *Virology* 52, 456-467.

Greenberger, J. S. (1979). *J. Natl. Cancer Inst. (US)* 62, 337-344.

Hankins, D. W., and Scolnick, E. M. (1981). *Cell* 26, 91-97.

Hunter, T., and Sefton, B. M. (1980). *Proc. Natl. Acad. Sci. USA* 77, 1311-1315.

Kirsten, W. H., and Mayer, L. A. (1967). *J. Natl. Cancer Inst. (US)* 39, 311-319.

Kitamura, N., Kitamura, A., Toyoshima, K., Hirayama, Y., and Yoshida, M. (1982). *Nature (London)* 297, 205-208.

Klein, G. (1981). *Nature (London)* 294, 313-318.

Lawn, R. M., Fritsch, E. F., Parker, R. C., Blake, G., and Maniatis, T. (1978). *Cell* 15, 1157-1174.

Levinson, A. D., Opperman, H., Levintow, L., Varmus, H. E., and Bishop, J. M. (1978). *Cell* 15, 561-572.

McBride, O. W., Swan, D. C., Santos, E., Barbacid, M., Tronick, S. R., and Aaronson, S. A. (1982). *Nature (London)* 300, 773-774.

Parada, L. F., Tabin, C. J., Shih, C., and Weinberg, R. A. (1982). *Nature (London)* 297, 474-478.

Pierce, J. H., and Aaronson, S. A. (1982). *J. Exp. Med.* 156, 873-887.

Prakash, K., McBride, O. W., Swan, D. C., Devare, S. G., Tronick, S. R., and Aaronson, S. A. (1982). *Proc. Natl. Acad. Sci. USA* 79, 5210-5214.

Pulciani, S., Santos, E., Lauver, A. V., Long, L. K., Robbins, K. C., and Barbacid, M. (1982). *Proc. Natl. Acad. Sci. USA* 79, 2845-2849.

Pulciani, S., Santos, E., Lauver, A. V., Long, L. K., Aaronson, S. A., and Barbacid, M. (1982). *Nature (London)* 300, 539-542.

Rasheed, S., Gardner, M. B., and Huebner, R. J. (1978). *Proc. Natl. Acad. Sci. USA* 75, 2972-2976.

Reddy, E. P., Smith, M. J., and Aaronson, S. A. (1981). *Science (Washington, D.C.)* 214, 445-450.

Robbins, K. C., Devare, S. G., and Aaronson, S. A. (1981). *Proc. Natl. Acad. Sci. USA* 78, 2918-2922.

Robbins, K. C., Devare, S. G., Reddy, E. P., and Aaronson, S. A. (1983). *Science (Washington, D.C.)* 218, 1131-1133.

Rowley, J. D. (1980). *Annu. Rev. Genet.* 14, 17-39.

Santos, E., Tronick, S. R., Aaronson, S. A., Pulciani, S., and Barbacid, M. (1982). *Nature (London) 298*, 343-347.

Scher, C. D., Scolnick, E. M., and Siegler, R. (1975). *Nature (London) 256*, 225-226.

Shibuya, M., Hanafusa, T., Hanafusa, H., and Stephenson, J. R. (1980). *Proc. Natl. Acad. Sci. USA 77*, 6536-6540.

Shih, C., and Weinberg, R. A. (1982). *Cell 29*, 161-169.

Shimotohno, K., Mizutani, S., and Temin, H. M. (1980). *Nature (London) 285*, 550-554.

Srinivasan, A., Reddy, E. P., and Aaronson, S. A. (1981). *Proc. Natl. Acad. Sci. USA 78*, 2077-2081.

Stehelin, D., Guntaka, R. V., Varmus, H. E., and Bishop, J. M. (1976). *J. Mol. Biol. 101*, 349-365.

Swan, D. C., McBride, O. W., Robbins, K. C., Keithley, D. A., Reddy, E. P., and Aaronson, S. A. (1982). *Proc. Natl. Acad. Sci. USA 79*, 4691-4695.

Taub, R., Kirsch, I., Morton, C., Lenoir, G., Swan, D., Tronick, S. R., Aaronson, S. A., and Leder, P. (1982). *Proc. Natl. Acad. Sci. USA 79*, 7837-7841.

Tronick, S. R., Robbins, K. C., Canaani, E., Devare, S., Andersen, P. R., and Aaronson, S. A. (1979). *Proc. Natl. Acad. Sci. USA 76*, 6314-6318.

Tsuchida, N., Ryder, T., and Ohtsubo, E. (1982). *Science (Washington, D.C.) 217*, 937-939.

Van Beveren, C., Galleshaw, J. A., Jonas, V., Berns, A. J. M., Doolittle, R. F., Donoghue, D. J., and Verma, I. M. (1981). *Nature (London) 289*, 258-262.

Wang, L. H. (1978). *Annu. Rev. Microbiol. 32*, 561-592.

Weissman, B., and Aaronson, S. A. (1983). *Cell 32*, 599-606.

Westin, E. H., Wong-Staal, F., Gelmann, E. P., Dalla-Favera, R., Papas, T. S., Lautenberger, J. A., Eva, A., Reddy, E. P., Tronick, S. R., Aaronson, S. A., and Gallo, R. C. (1982). *Proc. Natl. Acad. Sci. USA 79*, 2490-2494.

Young, H. A., Shih, T. Y., Scolnick, E. M., Rasheed, S., and Gardner, M. B. (1979). *Proc. Natl. Acad. Sci. USA 76*, 3523-3527.

Young, H. A., Rasheed, S., Sowder, R., Benton, C. V., and Hendersen, L. E. (1981). *J. Virol. 38*, 286-293.

26

STUDIES ON THE ROLE OF ADENOVIRUS E1 GENES IN TRANSFORMATION AND ONCOGENESIS

A. J. Van der Eb, R. Bernards, P. J. Van den Elsen, J. L. Bos, and P. I. Schrier

Department of Medical Biochemistry
Sylvius Laboratories
University of Leiden
Leiden, The Netherlands

I. INTRODUCTION

Human adenoviruses are divided into at least three subgroups on the basis of their oncogenicity in hamsters: subgroup A containing highly oncogenic viruses, subgroup B weakly oncogenic viruses, and subgroup C (most of the) nononcogenic viruses (see Flint, 1980). Despite these clear distinctions in oncogenic activity among the three sugroups, all human adenoviruses are capable of transforming cultured cells into tumor-like cells. Cells transformed by oncogenic adenoviruses are usually tumorigenic in syngeneic animals, whereas cells transformed by nononcogenic viruses are not. These results indicate that morphological transformation and tumorigenicity of cells are distinct properties that are not necessarily expressed together. DNA transfection studies and analysis of viral DNA sequences present in transformed cells have shown that both activities are functions of the leftmost 11% of the viral genomes (Graham *et al.*, 1974; Gallimore *et al.* 1974; Shiroki *et al.*, 1977; Sekikawa *et al.*, 1978; Dijkema *et al.*, 1979; Van der Eb *et al.*, 1979). This region correspond to early region 1 (E1), that is, one of the four or five regions of the viral genome expressed early in lytic infection (Tooze, 1981). The E1 region consists of two transcriptional units, E1a and E1b, that both specify a number of coterminal RNAs.

Transformation experiments with primary baby rat kidney (BRK) cells using DNA fragments comprising parts of region E1 have shown that such fragments also induce transformation in BRK cells but that the cells have an abnormal phenotype: For example, BRK cells transformed by the left-most 8% of adeno-virus type 12 (Ad12) (containing E1a and part of E1b) appear almost completely transformed but have lost their oncogenic potential in *nude* mice (Jochemsen *et al.*, 1982). Figure 1 shows that the missing E1b segment between 8 and 11.5% encodes the C-terminal part of the 55-kdalton protein, as a consequence of which this polypeptide is absent, or at least truncated, in cells transformed by the 8% segment. This would imply that the 55-kdalton protein is required for oncogenicity but not

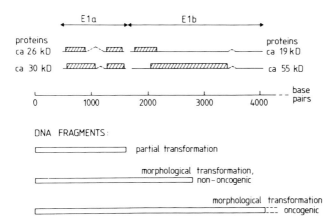

Fig. 1. Organization of early region 1 (E1) of human adenovirus type 5; the origanization of region E1 of adenovirus type 12 is basically similar. The solid lines with the hatched bars represent the major mRNAs expressed in transformed cells (introns are indicated as broken lines). The hatched bars represent the regions expressed into polypeptides. The open bars in the lower part of the figure represent DNA fragments that induce the indicated transformed phenotype.

for morphological transformation. The left-terminal 4.5% segment (containing region E1a only) induces a semitransformed phenotype, in the sense that the cells appear less transformed, are unable to grow to high saturation densities, are fibroblastic rather than epithelial, and are nononcogenic in *nude* mice. This suggests that the 19-kdalton protein and/or the N-terminal part of the 55-kdalton protein are required for induction of complete morphological transformation.

It is difficult to conclude from these results what the role is of region E1a in transformation and oncogenesis, except that its presence is essential: Preliminary results showed that E1b alone has no transforming activity, although the results just mentioned suggest that most of the transforming properties are located in this DNA segment. Apparently, one function of E1a is to convert cells with a limited *in vitro* life span (e.g., primary BRK cells) into an immortal cell type

(primary BRK cells have a very limited life span *in vitro*)
(Houweling *et al.*, 1980).

It has been shown that in lytic infection, region Ela is
required to induce expression of region Elb (Jones and Shenk,
1979; Berk *et al.*, 1979). Furthermore, experiments by Nevins
(1981) and by Persson *et al.* (1981) and Katze *et al.* (1981)
have suggested that regulation of Elb expression occurs either
indirectly at the level of transcription, by inactivating a
putative cellular repressor that normally blocks Elb transcription, or by stabilizing Elb transcripts, respectively.
Thus, the available data suggest that Ela may have at least
two different functions or effects: immortalization of primary
cells and regulation of Elb expression.

To obtain more insight into the mechanism of transformation by adenoviruses, we have carried out a series of experiments designed to answer the following questions: (1) Can we
obtain more information on the mechanism of regulation of Elb
expression by Ela in transformation, (2) Which functions (roles)
can be assigned to regions Ela and Elb in morphological transformation, and (3) What is the role of the two subregions in
oncogenesis?

II. MATERIAL AND METHODS

A. Cells and Transformation Assays

Assays of transforming activity of cloned viral DNA
fragments were carried out by means of the calcium phosphate
technique (Graham and Van der Eb, 1973; Van der Eb and Graham,
1980), with primary baby rat kidney cells from WAG RIJ rats
(an inbred rat strain obtained from the Radiobiological
Institute, Rijswijk, The Netherlands) or the established rat

rat cell line 3Yl (Shiroki *et al.*, 1977). Cell cultures were maintained in Eagle's minimum essential medium supplemented with 8% newborn calf serum.

B. Recombinant DNA Experiments

Viral DNA fragments were cloned in plasmid vectors a according to standard procedures, using *E.coli* HB101 as host cell. The construction of the various clones is described in the references given in section III, Results.

C. Immunoprecipitation of Viral T Antigens

Viral T antigens expressed in transformed cells were identified by means of immunoprecipitation as described by Schrier *et al.* (1979). The anti-T sera were obtained from hamsters or rats bearing adenovirus-induced tumors.

D. Tumorigenicity Tests

Tumorigenicity of transformed cells was tested by injection of 10^6-10^7 cells subcutaneously either into *nude* mice (6- to 12-week-old homozygous BALB/c *nude* males) or into 4- to 5-day-old WAG RIJ rats. The animals were checked for development of tumors twice weekly during a period of at least 6 months.

III. RESULTS

A. Regulation of Expression of Region E1b

It has been shown that expression of region E1b of human adenovirus 5 in lytic infection is controlled by region E1a, either at the level of transcription (Nevins, 1981) or at the

level of Elb RNA stabilization (Persson *et al.*, 1981; Katze
et al., 1981). In order to ivestigate whether this control
also occurs in a nonlytic infection (transformation) and, more
specifically, whether control is mediated through an interaction with the promoter region of Elb, we have constructed a
hybrid plasmid in which the Elb promoter of Ad12 is fused to
the protein-coding region of the herpesvirus thymidine kinase
gene (pElb-*tk*/-520; Bos *et al.*, 1983). An Ad12 DNA fragment
comprising the Elb cap site and the preceding 520 nucleotides
was used as the promoter segment (Fig. 2). Thus the mRNA
transcribed from the Elb-tk fusion product contained the complete coding sequence of the tk enzyme. The plasmid was
transfected into mouse L tk$^-$ cells, both in the presence and
the absence of plasmids carrying region Ela of Ad5 or Ad12,[1]
and tk$^+$ colonies were selected in HAT medium.

Table I shows that colony formation is (almost) entirely
dependent on the presence of region Ela. The Ela region of
Ad12 is less effective in stimulating the hybrid *tk* gene than
the Ela region of Ad5, in agreement with the results on morphological transformation obtained by Bernards *et al.* (1982) and
Van den Elsen *et al.* (1982). Nuclease *S1* analysis has indicated that RNA synthesis starts at the Ad12 Elb cap site
(not shown). We conclude, therefore, that expression of the
Elb region is indeed regulated by region Ela and that this
control occurs via an interaction with the Elb promoter. This
result does not exclude, however, the existence of other
control mechanisms.

---

[1]*Experiments by Van den Elsen et al. (1982) have demonstrated that the adenovirus subregions Ela and Elb can cause
normal transformation in cultured cells when they are transfected as separate DNA molecules, that is, without being
linked to each other.*

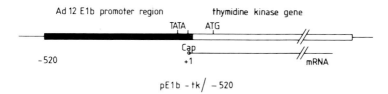

pE1b - tk/ - 520

Fig. 2. Structure of plasmid pE1b-tk/-520. The plasmid was constructed essentially by ligating the left-terminal Ad12 DNA segment (0-1534 bp), cloned in pAT153, to a 2275-bp fragment containing the herpes simplex virus thymidine kinase (*tk*) gene (*Bgl*II-*Bam*HI fragment). From the resulting clone the Ad12 DNA segment from nucleotide 0 to 1003 was removed, resulting in a plasmid in which the coding region of the thymidine kinase gene is preceded by the Ad12 DNA segment from nucleotide 1003 to 1534. This Ad12 fragment harbors the E1b promoter and the 3'-terminal part of region E1a. From J. L. Bos *et al.*, (unpublished).

In order to locate the DNA segment involved in regulation of E1b expression more precisely, we have removed increasingly longer segments from the left end of the Ad12 E1b promoter fragment (starting at -520 bp from the cap site; Bos *et al.*, 1983). The resulting plasmids were tested for tk expression in the presence of region E1a. Table II shows that full tk

TABLE I. Transformation of Mouse L tk⁻ Cells by Plasmid pE1b-tk/-520[a]

Plasmid	Colonies/dish
pE1b-tk/-520	1
pE1b-tk/-520 + E1a Ad12	19
pE1b-tk/-520 + E1a Ad5	119
pE1b-tk/-520 + HSV tk	196

[a] *Mouse L tk⁻ cells were transfected with 0.5 µg/dish of plasmid pE1b-tk/-520 in the presence or absence of 1 µg/dish of Ad5 or Ad12 region E1a DNA. tk-Positive colonies were selected by growing the cultures in HAT medium, starting 24 h after transfection. Colonies were counted 15 days later.*

TABLE II.   Transformation of Mouse L tk⁻ Cells by pElb-tk
            Plasmids[a]

Plasmid	Colonies/dish	
	−Ad5 Ela	+Ad5 Ela
pElb-tk/-520	1	119
pElb-tk/-135	0	133
pElb-tk/-102	1	0
pElb-tk/-83	0	0

[a]*Mouse L tk⁻ cells were transfected with different pElb-tk
plasmids in the presence or absence of Ad5 region Ela DNA, as
described in Table I.   The pElb-tk plasmids differ from each
other in the length of the Ad12 DNA segment preceding the cap
site at position +1 (see Fig. 2).*

activity is still obtained when 135 bp are left in front of

the cap site, but that tk expression is abolished when only

102 bp are left.   This shows that the Ad12 segment between

−135 and +11 bp from the cap site is important for Elb ex-

pression.   A more detailed analysis of the Elb promoter se-

quences involved in regulation by region Ela is in progress.

A comparison of the nucleotide sequences in the promoter area

of region Elb and other early regions of various adenovirus

serotypes revealed the presence of a common DNA sequence,

GGGPyG, approximately 50 bp in front of the cap site.   This

sequence might be part of a recognition signal involved in

regulation by Ela.

B.   Studies on the Role of Regions E1a and E1b
     in Cell Transformation

     Our previous experiments had suggested that induction of
morphological transformation by Ad5 is principally a function
of region E1b. The role in transformation of region E1a was
unclear, except that experiments with primary BRK cells had
suggested that immortalization might be one of the functions
supplied by E1a (Houweling et al., 1980). Repeated attempts
to induce transformation with region E1b alone had been unsuccessful, both in primary rat cells and in established rat
cell lines (Van den Elsen et al., 1982). Because it has become
clear that expression of E1b is dependent on a functional E1a
region, we have constructed E1b plasmids in which the promoter
region, presumably harboring the recognition site for regulation by E1a, is replaced by the SV40 early promoter + enhancer
sequences (Van den Elsen et al., 1983). It was expected that
this modified E1b region would be expressed, even in the absence of E1a. (The SV40 early region is expressed in mammalian
cells independent of other viral genes.)

     The structure of a number of the E1b-SV40pr plasmids
(pPDCs), in which increasingly larger DNA segments in front of
the E1b-coding region are deleted, is shown in Fig. 3. The
transforming activity of these clones was tested in primary
BRK cells and in the rat cell line 3Y1, both in the presence
and absence of region E1a plasmids. Table III (top) shows that
none of the clones is able to cause transformation in BRK cells
without region E1a, but that normal transformation is obtained
when the E1b clones are mixed with region E1a. Figure 4A
(lanes 2-5) shows that the major E1bT antigens are expressed
in these transformed cells, indicating that the E1b-SV40pr
plasmids are biologically active. A comparison of lanes 2, 3,
4, and 5 shows that the quantity of the 55-kdalton

TABLE III. Transforming Activity and T-Antigen Expression of
Ad5 Elb-SV40pr Plasmids and of Ad5 Region Elb in
Primary BRK Cells and in Rat 3Yl Cells

| | Primary BRK Cells[a] | | |
| | Morphological transformation | | Ad5 Elb Proteins detected |
Plasmid	-Ela	+Ela	+Ela
pPDC21	-	+	19- + 55-kdalton
pPDC26	-	+	19- + 55-kdalton
pPDCll	-	+	19- + 55-kdalton
p5*Sma*I F (Elb)	-	+	19- + 55-kdalton
—	-	+ (Atypical)	—

| | 3Yl cells, after cotransfection with pAG60 selection of G-418-resistant colonies[b] | | | |
| | Morphological transformation | | Ad5 Elb Proteins detected | |
Plasmid	-Ela	+Ela	-Ela	+Ela
pPDC21	-	+	19- + 55-kdalton	19- + 55-kdalton
pPDC26	-	+	19- + 55-kdalton	19- + 55-kdalton
pPDCll	-	+	19- + 55-kdalton	19- + 55-kdalton
p5*Sma*I F	-	+	—	19- + 55-kdalton
p5*Xho*I C	+	n.d.[c]	19- + 55-kdalton	n.d.
—	-	+ (Atypical)	—	—

[a]*Primary baby rat kidney cells were transfected with different p5Elb-SV40pr plasmids or plasmid p5SmaI F (region Elb), in the presence or absence of Ad5 region Ela DNA. Transformed foci were scored 3 weeks later, and isolated transformed cell lines were tested for production of Ad5 Elb-T antigens by immunoprecipitation with Ad5 anti-T sera.*

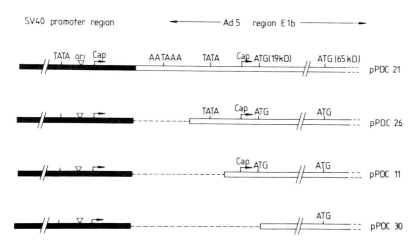

Fig. 3. Structure of four different Ad5 Elb-SV40pr plasmids. A DNA fragment containing the SV40 early promoter (*HpaII/BamHI*) was cloned into pAT153. The SV40 promoter fragment (*HpaII/StuI*) was subsequently ligated into plasmids containing also region Elb of Ad5. Prior to ligation, these plasmids were linearized and treated with nuclease *Bal*31, resulting in the removal of increasingly longer stretches of DNA from the Elb leader/promoter region, starting at nucleotide 1575.

(= 55 kdaltons) protein decreases and the relative amount of the 19-kdalton protein increases, as the distance between the SV40 promoter and the 19-kdalton gene becomes smaller. This phenomenon is probably related to the fact that the 5' ends of the Elb RNAs transcribed from the hybrid plasmids pPDC26 (lanes 3 and 4) and pPDCll (lane 5) are located at the SV40

(Table III continued)
[b]Rat 3Y1 cells were transfected with different p5Elb-SV40pr plasmids and pAG60, containing the neomycin-resistance gene, in the presence or absence of Ad5 region Ela DNA. Colonies expressing the neomycin-resistance gene were selected in medium containing 200 µg/ml G-418. The cultures were examined 14 days after transfection and were tested for expression of Ad5 region Elb proteins by immunoprecipitation.

[c]n.d., not done.

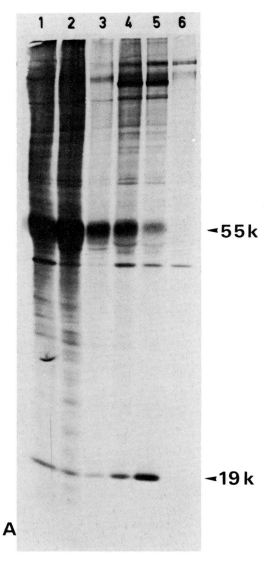

Fig. 4(A). Ad5 region Elb-specific proteins immunoprecipitated from BRK cells transformed by Ad5 fragment *Xho*I C
(region El) (lanes 1 and 6), Ad5 region Ela DNA plus the Elb-
SV40pr plasmid pPDC21 (lane 2), Ad5 Ela plus pPDC26 (lanes 3
and 4), or Ad5 Ela plus pPDC11 (lane 5). Immunoprecipitations
were carried out with hamster Ad5 anti-T serum (lanes 1-5) or
with nonimmune hamster serum (lane 6).

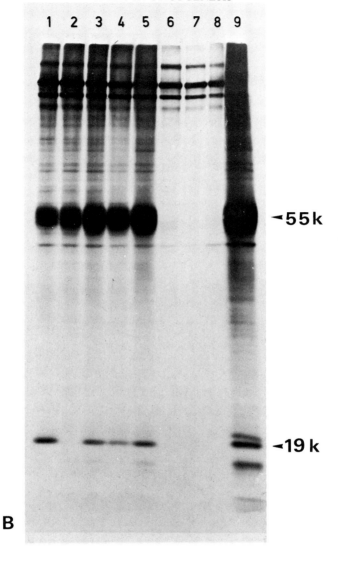

Fig. 4(B). Ad5 region Elb-specific proteins immunoprecipitated from 3Yl cells after transfection with plasmid pAG60
and selection for G-418-resistant colonies. The transfection
mixtures contained, in addition to pAG60, the plasmids pPDC11
(lane 1), pPDC12 (lane 2), pPDC21 (lane 3), pPDC26 (lane 4),
p5XhoI C (region E1; lane 5), p5SmaI F (region Elb; lane 6).
Lane 7 shows an extract from cells transfected with pAG60 only.
Lanes 8 and 9 are immunoprecipitations from Ad5 XhoI C-trans-
formed BRK cells. The proteins were precipitated with Ad5
hamster anti-T serum (lane 9) or nonimmune serum (lane 8).

early cap site. As a result, these mRNAs contain a longer 5'
untranslated region than the mRNAs starting at the Ad5 Elb
cap site (pPDC21), and this could result in a shift in the
ratio 19:55 kdaltons in favor of the 19-kdalton protein.

Transfection of 3Y1 cells with the Elb-SV40pr plasmids
similarly did not result in detectable transformation. Because
transformed foci are often difficult to distinguish in dense
cultures of 3Y1 cells, we have also selected "competent" cells
that have taken up DNA, by cotransfecting 3Y1 cultures with
Elb-SV40pr plasmids and pAG60, a clone harboring the neomycin-
resistance gene. Cells expressing the neomycin gene are
resistant to the antibiotic G-418 (Colbère-Garapin *et al.*,
1981). Table III (bottom) shows that G-418-resistant colonies
expressed the Elb T antigens, when co-transfected with Elb-
SV40pr plasmids, even in the absence of region Ela. Plasmids
carrying the Elb region containing the natural Elb promoter
are not expressed without region Ela. Figure 4B shows the Ad5
Elb proteins immunoprecipitated from 3Y1 cells transfected
with Elb-SV40pr plasmids and pAG60 (without Ela). The 19-
kdalton protein is not expressed in cells transfected with
clone pPDC30 (lane 2), because the 19-kdalton initiation codon
at position 1714 is deleted in this plasmid.

Inspection of the G-418-resistant colonies shows that the
cell clones expressing Ad5 Elb proteins in the absence of
region Ela are indistinguishable from those expressing pAG60
plus the SV40 promoter only (Fig. 5). In contrast, colonies
transfected with an intact region El of Ad5 (p*Xho*I C, containing region El) are clearly morphologically transformed (Fig. 5).
It was concluded that expression of region Elb alone does not
result in morphological transformation and, thus, that region
Ela must have a contribution in this process, in addition to
regulating expression of region Elb.

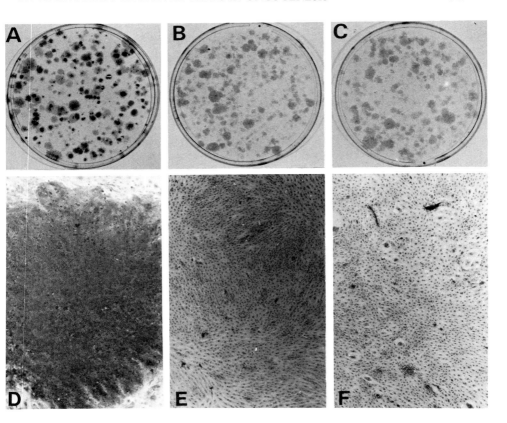

Fig. 5. Colonies obtained after cotransfection of rat 3Y1 cells with plasmids pAG60 and p*Xho*I C (Ad5 region E1) (A); pAG60 and pPDC11 (B); or pAG60 and pESV40pr (containing the early SV40 promoter segment) (C). G-418-resistant colonies were selected in medium containing 200 µg/ml G-418. (D, E, and F) Higher magnifications of colonies shown in A, B, and C, respectively.

C. The Contribution of Regions E1a and E1b in Oncogenicity

Our previous results had suggested that region E1b of Ad12, or at least the C-terminal portion of the 60-kdalton protein, is involved in oncogenicity in *nude* mice (Jochemsen *et al.*, 1982). In order to study this aspect in more detail and to answer the question which gene product(s) of the

TABLE IV. Transforming Activity and Oncogenicity of BRK Cells Transformed by Plasmids Containing Region E1 of Ad5 or Ad12 and by Plasmids Carrying Ad5/Ad12 Hybrid E1 Regions (pAd512 and pAd125)

Plasmid	Efficiency of transformation foci/µg genome equivalent	Expression in transformed cells		Oncogenicity (%) in:	
		E1a	E1b	*Nude mice*	Syngeneic rats
p5XhoI C	11.6	Ad5	Ad5	50 (15 of 31)	0 (0 of 51)
p12RIC	0.55	Ad12	Ad12	100 (23 of 23)	100 (18 of 18)
pAd512	7.6	Ad5	Ad12	95 (17 of 18)	0 (0 of 17)
pAd125	0.42	Ad12	Ad5	10 (2 of 19)	5 (1 of 22)

nononcogenic Ad5 causes this virus to be nononcogenic, we have
constructed hybrid region E1 plasmids consisting of E1a of Ad5
linked to E1b of Ad12 (pAd512), and vice versa (pAd125)
(Bernards et al., 1982). This approach appeared feasible,
because the overall organization of the E1 regions of Ad5 and
Ad12 is basically similar (Flint, 1980), and the regions are
even considerably homologous at the nucleotide level (Van
Ormondt et al., 1980; H. Van Ormondt et al., 1983). Table IV
shows that the two hybrid E1 regions are active in cell transformation, indicating that E1a and E1b of the two serotypes
are functionally compatible. Both subregions of each of the
two hybrid clones are expressed as was shown by nuclease S1
analysis of the RNA extracted from the transformed cells,
whereas immunoprecipitation experiments showed that the cells
synthesized the expected E1b T antigens (not shown). (The E1a
proteins are weakly immunogenic and hence are difficult to
detect.) Plasmids containing E1a of Ad5 have the same relatively high transforming activity as plasmids harboring an
intact Ad5 E1 region, whereas plasmids containing the E1a
region of Ad12 show a low activity in BRK cells, characteristic for E1 of Ad12. This suggests that the origin of the
E1a region determines the efficiency of transformation.

The results of the oncogenicity tests in nude mice are
also shown in Table IV. Cells transformed by intact region
E1 of Ad12 are oncogenic in 100% of the animals tested, whereas
those transformed by E1 of Ad5 are less oncogenic, causing
tumors in about 50% of the mice. Apparently, Ad5-transformed
cells do have an oncogenic potential that is detectable in
animals with a deficient immune system. In fact, earlier
observations have already shown that Ad5-transformed hamster
cells form tumors in hamsters (Graham et al., 1974). Furthermore, Table IV shows that cells transformed by the hybrid

plasmids are highly oncogenic in *nude* mice when Elb is derived from Ad12, and weakly oncogenic when Elb is derived from Ad5. This indicates that the property of high oncogenicity in *nude* mice segregates with the Elb region.

In order to identify the gene product(s) responsible for oncogenicity more precisely, two recombinant plasmids were constructed carrying hybrid Elb regions. These recombinants were obtained by cloning in the same plasmid vector an Ad5 El region in which the large Elb protein was mutated, as well as an Ad12 El region in which the small Elb protein was mutated (plasmid pLT12) and, vice versa, a plasmid containing an Ad5 El region with a mutated small Elb protein plus an Ad12 El region with a mutated large Elb protein (plasmid pST12). Both

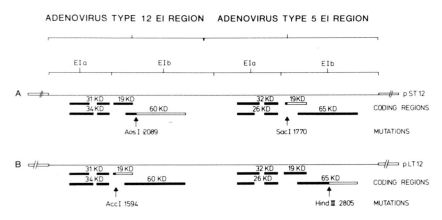

Fig. 6. Structure of Ad5/Ad12 Elb-hybrid plasmids. Two recombinant plasmids were constructed containing the El regions of both Ad5 and Ad12. In one plasmid, pST12, frameshift mutations had been introduced into the 19-kdalton Elb gene of Ad5 and the 55-kdalton Elb gene of Ad12 (here indicated as 60 kdaltons). The plasmid contains intact Ela regions of both Ad5 and Ad12. In the other plasmid, pLT12, frameshift mutations had been introduced into the 19-kdalton gene of Ad12 and the 55-kdalton gene of Ad5 (here indicated as 65 kdaltons). This plasmid also contains intact Ela regions of both Ad5 and Ad12.

constructions, therefore, contain an intact Ela region from
both serotypes (Fig. 6; Bernards *et al.*, 1983). BRK cells
transformed by these hybrid molecules were tested for their
oncogenic potential in *nude* mice. The results showed that
cells transformed by plasmid pLT12 are oncogenic in 100% of
the animals tested, whereas cells transformed by pST12 are
oncogenic in only 23% of the animals (Table V). The high
oncogenicity is therefore correlated with the presence of the
55-kdalton protein of Ad12 and not with that of the 19-kdalton
protein. That the 19-kdalton protein is nevertheless essential for oncogenicity is shown by the finding that cells transformed by plasmid p12dlAcc, in which the 19-kdalton protein is
almost completely deleted but the 55-kdalton protein is intact,
is nononcogenic, even in *nude* mice. Mutation of the 55-kdalton
protein without affecting the 19-kdalton protein also results
in a transformed cell type that is not oncogenic in *nude* mice
(Jochemsen *et al.*, 1982).

Because *nude* mice have a defective immune system, it was
of interest to test the oncogenicity of a number of hybrid-
transformed cells in immunocompetent animals as well. Table
IV shows the oncogenicity of the Ela/Elb hybrid-transformed
cells after injection into newborn syngeneic rats. As
expected, cells transformed by Ad5 region E1 (p5*Xho*I C) were
not oncogenic in rats, whereas Ad12 E1-transformed cells were
oncogenic in 100% of the animals. Surprisingly, pAd125-
transformed cells exhibited the same low oncogenic activity
in rats as in *nude* mice, whereas pAd512-transformed cells were
completely nononcogenic in rats although they were 100%
oncogenic in *nude* mice. This result indicates that region Ela
has a profound serotype-specific influence on tumorigenicity
in immunocompetent animals.

TABLE V. Oncogenicity in *Nude Mice* of BRK Cells Transformed by Plasmids Carrying Region El of Ad5 or Ad12, and Plasmids Carrying Hybrid Elb Regions or Region El of Ad12 in Which the Protein is Deleted, and of Ad12 *HindIII* G-Transformed Cells

Plasmid	Expression in transformed cells		Oncogenicity in *nude* mice (%)
	Ela	Elb	
p5XhoI C	Ad5	Ad5	50 (15 of 31)
p12RIC	Ad12	Ad12	100 (23 of 23)
pLT12[a]	Ad5 + Ad12	Ad5 19-kdalton Ad12 55-kdalton	100 (27 of 27)
pST12[a]	Ad5 + Ad12	Ad5 55-kdalton Ad12 19-kdalton	23 (5 of 22)
p12dℓAcc[b]	Ad12	Ad12 55-kdalton	0 (0 of 12)
Ad12 *HindIII* G	Ad12	Ad12 19-kdalton	0 (0 of 16)

[a] *Plasmids carrying hybrid Elb regions; see Fig. 6.*

[b] *Plasmids carrying region El of Ad12, in which 19-kdalton protein is deleted.*

Because oncogenicity of adenoviruses is defined as the ability to induce tumors in certain rodents (hamsters, rats) after infection of newborn animals with infectious virus, we have also constructed intact adenoviruses with hybrid-E1 regions. The viruses that have been isolated so far are an Ad5 virus in which E1a is replaced by E1a of Ad12 and a similar virus in which E1b is replaced by E1b of Ad12. Both viruses are fully viable and replicate efficiently in human embryonic kidney cells and KB cells. The biological properties of these viruses are presently being studied.

IV. DISCUSSION AND SUMMARY

In this chapter we report new results concerning the contribution of regions E1a and E1b of human adenovirus types 5 and 12 in transformation and oncogenesis.

By using recombinant plasmids in which the herpes simplex virus *tk* gene was brought under control of the adenovirus E1b promoter, we were able to show that expression of the *tk* gene is regulated by region E1a through an interaction with the E1b promoter. In agreement with this result is the finding that E1b can only be fully expressed in cultured cells in the absence of region E1a when its promoter is replaced by a heterologous promoter. From these results we conclude that activation of region E1b by E1a occurs at the level of an interaction with the E1b promoter region, although alternative modes of regulation cannot be excluded.

Whereas our previous data had suggested that the adenovirus-transformed phenotype is largely determined by E1b, our present results show that E1b alone has no detectable transforming effect in primary cells or cell lines, even under conditions where the E1b genes are fully expressed. We conclude, therefore, that morphological transformation apparently is not a major function of Elb and that region Ela must have an important role in this process. It cannot even be excluded that *in vitro* transformation is largely or exclusively a function of Ela. The fact that Ad5 Ela-transformed BRK cells show a semitransformed phenotype and differ clearly from El-transformed cells could well be explained by the extremely low concentration of Ela-specific RNA (Approximately 10-100 times lower than in El-transformed cells; Jochemsen *et al.*, 1982; P. J. Van den Elsen, unpublished). In the case of oncornaviruses, examples are known where a (viral) protein is nontransforming in low concentrations but strongly transforming at higher doses. Because the simultaneous presence of Ela and Elb results in increased transcription of Ela (Jochemsen *et al.*, 1982; P. J. Van den Elsen, unpublished), it is conceivable that the two regions in fact regulate their own expression. Clearly, more work is needed to clarify this point.

Although the role of region Elb in morphological transformation is uncertain and probably only indirect, our present results show that Elb does have an important function in tumorigenicity in *nude* mice. Both Elb proteins (19 and 55 kdaltons) appear to be strictly required for this property, because cells expressing only the 55-kdalton Elb gene (pl2dℓAcc) and cells expressing only the 19-kdalton Elb gene (fragment Adl2 *Hin*dIII G; Jochemsen *et al.*, 1982) are nontumorigenic even in *nude* mice. The contribution of the 55-kdalton protein is serotype specific, in the sense that oncogenicity is high (Adl2 specific) when the 55-kdalton protein is derived from Adl2, and low (Ad5 specific) when it is derived from Ad5. The 19-kdalton protein does not show this serotype specificity.

An unexpected result was that cells transformed by Ad5 Ela + Ad12 Elb, which are highly oncogenic in *nude* mice, are completely nononcogenic in syngeneic normal rats, whereas cells transformed by Ad12 Ela + Ad5 Elb are weakly oncogenic, both in *nude* mice and in rats. The latter result shows that the intrinsically low oncogenicity conferred by Ad5 Elb is expressed irrespective of whether the animal host is immunodefective or immunocompetent. Presumably, a product of region Ela of Ad12 somehow sllows the cells to escape the immune surveillance of the host. In the reverse situation (Ad5 Ela + Ad12 Elb), the cells are intrinsically highly oncogenic, that is, they have a strong tendency to grow *in vivo* (oncogenic in 100% of *nude* mice). The presence of region Ela of Ad5, however, apparently elicits such a strong T-cell response that the transformed cells are nononcogenic in immunocompetent rats.

In summary, the results reported in this chapter show that region Ela has the following properties (functions) in transformation and oncogenesis: (1) It regulates expression of Elb; (2) it has an important role in morphological transformation; (3) it causes immortalization of primary rat cells; and (4) it determines whether or not a transformed cell is recognized and rejected by the host immune system. The properties of Elb identified so far are as follows: (1) Both 19- and 55-kdalton Elb proteins have a role in oncogenicity as defined by the ability to grow autonomously in an animal (in this case the *nude* mouse); and (2) the 55-kdalton Elb protein determines the (serotype-specific) degree of oncogenicity.

Although considerable progress has been made in understanding the biology of adenoviruses, the actual mechanism of transformation by these viruses is still unknown. A more detailed understanding of this process will require knowledge of the biochemical functions of the E1 genes and their interaction with cellular components.

654 A. J. VAN DER EB *ET AL.*

ACKNOWLEDGMENTS

The authors wish to acknowledge the expert assistance by
Ada Houweling Sylvia de Pater and Heleen ten Wolde.

REFERENCES

Berk, A. J., Lee, F., Harrison, T., Williams, J., and Sharp,
    P. A. (1979). *Cell 17*, 935-944.
Bernards, R., Houweling, A., Schrier, P. I., Bos, J. L., and
    Van der Eb, A. J. (1982). *Virology 120*, 422-432.
Bernards, R., Schrier, P. I., Bos, J. L., and Van der Eb, A. J.
    (1983). *Virology 127*, 45-54.
Bos, J. L., and Ten Wolde-Kraamwinkel, H. C. (1983). *EMBO J.
    2*, 73-76.
Colbère-Garapin, F., Horodniceanu, F., Kourilsky, P., and
    Garapin, A.-C. (1981). *J. Mol. Biol. 150*, 1-14.
Dijkema, R., Dekker, B. M. M., Van der Feltz, M. J. M., and
    Van der Eb, A. J. (1979). *J. Virol. 32*, 943-950.
Flint, S. J. (1980). *In* "The Molecular Biology of Tumor
    Viruses" (J. Tooze, ed.), (Part 2, pp. 547-576). Cold
    Spring Harbor Lab., Cold Spring Harbor, New York.
Gallimore, P. H., Sharp, P. A., and Sambrook, J. (1974). *J.
    Mol. Biol. 89*, 49-72.
Graham, F. L., and Van der Eb, A. J. (1973). *Virology 54*,
    536-539.
Graham, F. L., Abrahams, P. J., Mulder, C., Heijneker, H. L.,
    Warnaar, S. O., de Vries, F. A. J., Fiers, W., and Van der
    Eb, A. J. (1974). *Cold Spring Harbor Symp. Quant. Biol.
    39*, 637-650.
Houweling, A., Van den Elsen, P. J., and Van der Eb, A. J.
    (1980). *Virology 105*, 537-550.
Jochemsen, H., Daniëls, G. S. G., Hertoghs, J. J. L., Schrier,
    P. I., Van den Elsen, P. J., and Van der Eb, A. J. (1982).
    Virology 121.
Jones, N., and Shenk, T. (1979). *Proc. Natl. Acad. Sci. USA
    76*, 3665-3669.
Katze, M. G., Persson, H., and Philipson, L. (1981). *Mol.
    Cell. Biol. 9*, 807-813.
Nevins, J. R. (1981). *Cell 26*, 213-220.
Persson, H., Monstein, H. J., Akusjärvi, G., and Philipson, L.
    (1981). *Cell 23*, 485-496.
Schrier, P. I., Van den Elsen, P. J., Hertoghs, J. J. L., and
    Van der Eb, A. J. (1979). *Virology 99*, 372-385.

Sekikawa, K., Shiroki, K., Shimojo, H., Ojima, S., and
    Fujinaga, K. (1978). *Virology 88*, 1-7.
Shiroki, K., Handa, H., Shimojo, H., Yano, H., Ojima, S., and
    Fujinaga, K. (1977). *Virology 82*, 462-472.
Van den Elsen, P. J., De Pater, S., Houweling, A., Van der
    Veer, J., and Van der Eb, A. J. (1982). *Gene 18*, 175-185.
Van den Elsen, P. J., Houweling, A., and Van der Eb, A. J.
    (1983). *Virology*, in press.
Van der Eb, A. J., Van Ormondt, H., Schrier, P. I., Lupker, J.
    J., Jochemsen, H., Van den Elsen, P. J., De Leys, J., Maat,
    J., Van Beveren, C. P., Dijkema, R., and De Waard, A.
    (1979). *Cold Spring Harbor Symp. Quant. Biol. 44*, 383-399.
Van der Eb, A. J., and Graham, F. L. (1980). *Methods Enzymol.
    65*, 826-839.
Van Ormondt, H., Maat, J., and Dijkema, R. (1980). *Gene 12*,
    63-76.
Van Ormondt, H., and Hesper, B. (1983). *Gene 21*, 217-226.

27

HUMAN RETROVIRUS (ATLV)
AND ITS GENOME STRUCTURE

*Mitsuaki Yoshida, Motoharu Seiki,
and Seisuke Hattori*

Department of Viral Oncology
Cancer Institute
Tokyo, Japan

I. INTRODUCTION

Molecular analyses of animal retroviruses have identified
a number of transforming genes that were acquired from cellular
counterparts (Bishop, 1982; Stehelin *et al.*, 1976) and the long
terminal repeats (LTRs) in the integrated provirus genome (Hsu
et al., 1978; Varmus, 1982) that could be involved in activation of cellular *onc*-related sequences (Hayward *et al.*, 1981).
From the accumulation of these observations, a retrovirus
involved in human carcinogenesis is expected to provide powerful information on the mechanism of malignant transformation
of human cells.

In 1980, a first isolation of human leukemia virus was
reported by Poiesz *et al.* (1980) from a patient with cutaneous
T-cell lymphoma, and Reitz *et al.* (1981) have characterized
the virus as new retrovirus HTLV (human T-cell leukemia virus).
Following these reports, Hinuma *et al.* (1981) described a
retrovirus-like particle in a cell line established from
Japanese adult T-cell leukemia (ATL), and Yoshida *et al.* (1982)
have isolated and characterized these particles as retroviruses,
thus calling them ATLV (adult T-cell leukemia virus). Adult
T-cell leukemia (ATL) is a new clinical entity of T-cell
malignancy proposed by Uchiyama *et al.* (1977) on the basis of
its characteristic clinical and hematological features. The
disease has also been called endemic adult leukemia/lymphoma
(ATLL) because of its leukemic lymphomatous nature and the

peculiar geographical distribution of the birth places of
patients, that is, clustering in the southwestern part of
Japan. ATLV has clearly been shown to be closely associated
with the leukemia ATL by the presence of provirus DNA in all
ATL patients tested so far, but not in healthy adults (Yoshida
et al., 1982), and also by antibody against ATLV protein p24
(Yoshida et al., 1982) in all sera from ATL patients tested.

In early stages of the studies, the diseases from which
the two viruses (HTLV and ATLV) were isolated, were thought to
be different; the relationship between the two isolates of the
viruses was of considerable interest. However, a disease
similar or identical to ATL has been found in the West Indies,
and HTLV was also isolated from those patients (Catovsky et al.,
1982). Furthermore, Gallo's group has detected HTLV-related
antigens and antibody in Japanese ATL patients (Robert-Guroff
et al., 1982). These studies from Gallo's laboratory clearly
showed that the two viruses, HTLV and ATLV, are related. In
order to study the nature and origin of the virus and also to
study the mechanisms of the leukemogenesis of this particular
ATL, we have molecularly cloned the integrated provirus of
ATLV and then analyzed the structure. In this chapter we
describe the detection of the provirus in the fresh leukemic
cells of the ATL patient and the terminal structure of the
provirus DNA.

II. MATERIALS AND METHODS

A. Cells

Two cell lines, MT-1 and MT-2, were supplied by I. Miyoshi.
The MT-1 cell line (Miyoshi et al., 1980) was derived from
leukemic cells of peripheral blood from a patient with ATL,
and the MT-2 cell line (Miyoshi et al., 1981) was established

from cord lymphocytes that had been co-cultivated with leukemic
cells from a patient with ATL. Cells were cultured in RPMI
1640 medium supplemented with 10% fetal calf serum.

B. Preparation of [^{32}P]cDNA

[^{32}P]cDNA complementary viral RNA was prepared similarly
to that described previously (Yoshida *et al.*, 1982). The
reaction mixture consisted of 50 mM Tris-HCl, pH 7.5, 5 mM DTT,
3 mM MgCl$_2$, 0.1 mM each of dATP, dGTP, and dTTP, 100 µCi of
[^{32}P]dCTP, 0.02-0.04% NP40, 50 µg/ml of actinomycin D, and an
appropriate amount of virions. The [^{32}P]cDNA$_{ATLV}$ synthesized
was treated with 0.1 M NaOH to remove RNA at 37°C for several
hours and separated from shorter products on a Sephadex G25
column.

C. Nucleic Acid Hybridization

DNA was digested with restriction endonucleases, separated
by agarose gel electrophoresis, and transferred onto a nitrocellulose membrane by a modified method (Yoshida *et al.*, 1980)
of the Southern procedure (Southern, 1975). The membrane
filters were hybridized with [^{32}P]cDNA$_{ATLV}$ at 68°C for 18 to
48 h in a solution of 4 x SSC (XXC = 0.15 M NaCl, 0.015 M
sodium citrate, pH 7.5), 0.02% bovine serum albumin, 0.02%
polyvinylpyrrolidone, 0.02% Ficoll 4000, 100 µg/ml sonicated
and heat-denatured *E. coli* DNA, and 1-3 x 10^6 cpm of
[^{32}P]cDNA$_{ATLV}$. After hybridization the filter was washed with
0.5 x SSC at 68°C and exposed to X-ray film.

D. DNA Cloning of Integrated Provirus of ATLV

High molecular weight DNA from cell line MT-1 (Miyoshi
et al., 1980), which produces ATLV although in low titer, was
digested with *Eco*RI, and DNA fragments of about 11 to 15 kbp
were separated by agarose gel electrophoresis. The DNA fragments were ligated to the arms of Charon 4A phage DNA
(Williams and Blattner, 1979) and subjected to *in vitro*
packaging as described by Blattner *et al.* (1978). About 5 x
10^5 plaques of the recombinant phages were screened with
$[^{32}P]$viral cDNA, and one recombinant phage λATM-1 was isolated.
The viral sequence had one cutting site for *Sal*I. The two
fragments produced were subcloned in pBR322, and pATM-1 and
pATM-3 were obtained (see Fig. 2). For further analysis, the
5- and 8-kbp insert DNAs in these clones were purified on
agarose gel after cleavages with *Eco*RI and *Sal*I.

E. Preparation of cDNA Clones of Viral RNA

ATLV RNA containing poly(A) was prepared from the virions
(Yoshida *et al.*, 1982) purified from MT-2 cell line (Miyoshi
et al., 1981). cDNA of the viral RNA was synthesized by
extending oligo(dT) primer at the 3' end of poly(A) with
reverse transcriptase. The second-strand DNA complementary to
cDNA was synthesized by the method described by Taniguchi *et al.*
(1978). Both ends of the molecules were tailed with poly(dC)
by use of terminal transferase and annealed to the oligo(dG)
tails at the *Pst*I site of pBR322. The recombinant plasmids
were used for transformation of the χ1776 strain of *E. coli*
K12 and two Tc^r clones, pATV-1 and pATV-2, containing the cDNA
fragment were selected by colony hybridization with viral
$[^{32}P]$cDNA.

F.   Nucleotide Sequence Analysis

DNA fragments from the recombinant plasmids were digested
with *Sma*I, *Pst*I, *Hinf*I, or *Hpa*II and were labeled either at
their 5' end by using [γ-^{32}P]ATP and polynucleotide kinase as
described by Maxam and Gilbert (1980), or at their 3' end by
using [α-^{32}P]dCTP and the Klenow fragment of polymerase I.
End-labeled DNA fragments were applied to gel for strand
separation or digested with an appropriate restriction endonuclease, and the nucleotide sequences of the reisolated fragments were determined by the procedure of Maxam and Gilbert
(1980).

G.   Synthesis of Strong-Stop cDNA

ATLV virions purified from MT-2 were incubated in a
mixture consisting of 50 mM Tris-HCl, pH 7.5, 10 mM MgCl$_2$,
10 mM DTT, 0.1 mM each of dATP, dGTP, and dTTP, various concentrations of [^{32}P]dCTP, 0.02-0.1% NP 40, and 50 µg/ml of
actinomycin D at 39°C for 30 min. The cDNA was purified by
digestion with proteinase K and phenol extraction followed by
alkaline treatment.

III.   RESULTS

A.   Detection of ATLV Proviral DNA in Fresh Lymphocytes
     from ATL Patients

Previously we have reported the isolation and characterization of retrovirus ATLV (Yoshida *et al.*, 1982) and also
shown by Southern blotting technique (Southern, 1975) that
provirus DNA is integrated in chromosomal DNA of cell lines
MT-1 and MT-2 (Yoshida *et al.*, 1982), which were established

from the leukemic cells of ATL patients by co-cultivating with normal cord lymphocytes (Miyoshi *et al.*, 1980, 1981).

To obtain more information on the association of ATLV with ATL, we tested for the presence of ATLV proviral DNA in cellular DNA of fresh peripheral lymphocytes from ATL patients and from healthy adults. DNA was extracted from fresh lymphocytes from the peripheral blood of five patients with ATL and analyzed by the Southern blotting procedure. As shown in Fig. 1, all five ATL patients showed discrete positive bands,

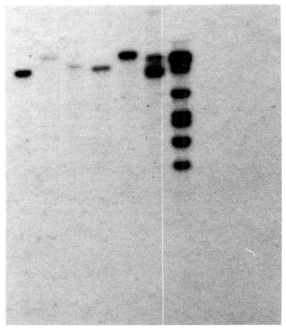

Fig. 1. Detection of proviral ATLV DNA sequences in leukemic cells from ATL patients. Total DNA was extracted from fresh lymphocytes in peripheral blood of ATL patients (a-e) and from those of healthy adults (h-j) and digested with *Eco*RI. The digests were analyzed Southern blotting technique (Southern, 1975). As positive controls, MT-1 and MT-2 cell DNAs (f and g) were also included.

indicating the presence of ATLV proviral DNA in their cellular
DNA. The presence of only one band of each DNA with different
sizes in different patients indicates differences in cellular
sites of integration of ATLV proviral DNA. This finding was
in agreement with the previous conclusion that ATLV is not a
widely distributed endogenous virus but is acquired only
locally.

DNA preparations of fresh lymphocytes from three healthy
adults in a nonendemic area did not contain the proviral DNA
sequences. This close association of ATLV proviral DNA with
ATL suggested the involvement of ATL in leukemogenesis in
human ATL.

B. Isolation of Provirus Clone and Strategy for Sequencing
    of LTR Regions

As described in the previous section, ATLV was shown to
be closely associated with the leukemia ATL. To get more
information on the nature of the virus, origin, and mode of
transmission, the provirus DNA ingrated in chromosomal DNA of
MT-1 was molecularly cloned into Charon 4A (Seiki *et al.*,
1982). The clone isolated, λATM-1, contained a 13-kbp insert.
A simple restriction map of molecularly cloned ATLV DNA λATM-1
was constructed (Fig. 2). To determine the location of the
possible LTR sequences, the fragments formed by *Sma*I digestion
were hybridized to strong-stop viral cDNA, which represents
the 5' end of the viral RNA. Two fragments, which were
separated by a sequence of about 8.0 kbp, were shown to
hybridize strongly to the probe (data not shown). For sequencing these regions separately, two *Sal*I fragments each
containing one of the hybridizable regions was subcloned in
pBR322, and pATM-1 and pATM-3 were obtained. Sequencing

strategy of the hybridizable regions in these clones were
indicated in Fig. 2, and the sequence is shown in Fig. 3A.

C. Sequence Organization of LTR Regions and Flanking Sequences

    The identical nucleotide sequences that were hybridizable
to viral strong-stop cDNA in the two clones pATM-1 and pATM-3
were defined as the long terminal repeats (LTR) regions of the
integrated provirus genome of ATLV (Fig. 3A). Each LTR consisted of 754 bp, and one terminus of each LTR was linked to a
directly repeated cellular 6-bp sequence, GCATTC, as illustrated in Fig. 3B. LTR had a terminal inverted repeat of 2 bp.
These structural features of the viral-cellular junction are
consistent with those found generally for other animal retroviruses (Temin, 1981) and are also similar to those of transposable elements in lower organisms (Shimotohno et al., 1980).

    In general, the LTR sequence consists of one copy each of
the 3' end (U3) and 5' end (U5) regions, and terminal repeats
(R) of the viral RNA. To determine the region of the 3' end
of viral RNA in LTR, we determined the nucleotide sequences of
two cDNA clones pATV-1 and pATV-2. These two clones contained
identical sequences adjacent to a long (dA) stretch, thus
indicating that these cDNA clones represented a sequence at
the 3' end of viral RNA, but not a sequence primed at a small
oligo(A) cluster within the viral genome. The nucleotide
sequence in the cDNA clones was also found to be identical to
that upstream from position 581 in LTR (Fig. 3A), except for
alterations of two bases (positions 572 and 581). Thus the
poly(A) site for viral RNA was identified at position 581,
defining 173 bases from this point to the end of LTR as U5.
Differences of 2 bases between LTR and cDNA clones could be

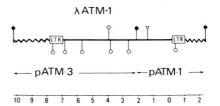

Fig. 2.   Restriction map of integrated provirus of ATLV in a clone λATM-1.   The regions contained in subclones pATM-1 and pATM-3 are also shown. ●, *Sal*I; ▽,*Xho*I; ♦, *Xba*I; O, *Sma*I.

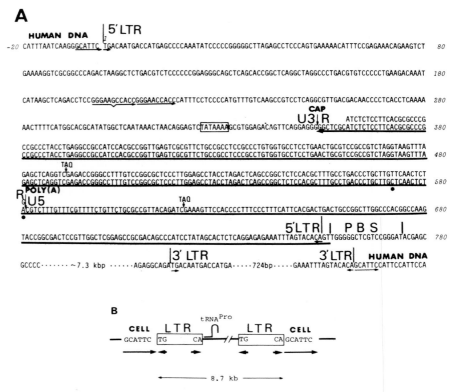

Fig. 3.   (A) Nucleotide sequences of 5' LTR in subclone pATM-3 and of cDNA clone pATV-1.   The sequence of the (+) strand (same sense as viral RNA) is presented.   The shorter sequence around the middle of LTR is that of cDNA clone pATV-1 containing the 3' end of viral RNA.   Numbering is from the beginning of the LTR.   Regions of interest are marked: U3 is the sequence from the 3' end of viral RNA also present at the 5' end of viral DNA; R is the sequence repeated at both ends

explained by point mutations among the different isolates of
ATLV: LTR clones were isolated from the MT-1 cell line, established from one patient with ATLV, whereas virion RNA for cDNA
clones was isolated from the MT-2 cell line, which was established from another and unrelated patient with ATL (Miyoshi
et al., 1980, 1981).

To determine the site of the 5' terminus of viral RNA, we
analyzed the strong-stop viral cDNA. Purified ATLV virions
were incubated under the conditions for general cDNA synthesis,
except that a higher concentration of dCTP and slightly higher
temperature (39°C) were used. In this way cDNA of a discrete
size was synthesized after a short reaction period (Fig. 4A).
The maximum size of the main product was 403 ± 1 nucleotides
and was not affected by the concentration of detergent or
substrates. Therefore, cDNA of 403 ± 1 bases was concluded to
be strong-stop viral cDNA, which had been primed by tRNA on
the genome RNA and stopped at the 5' end of the genome. Three
fragments of cDNA were obtained by digestion with TaqI, and
these were mapped as shown in Fig. 4B. For this mapping,
immature small products, which were synthesized with a low
concentration of dCTP as shown in Fig. 4A, lanes d-f, were
used. The sequences in LTR contained the identical map of TaqI
sites to that in cDNA, as indicated in Fig. 3A. Thus the
strong-stop cDNA was concluded to correspond to the region
shown with a thick underline in Fig. 3A. Therefore, the cap
site for the 5' terminus of viral RNA was identified at

(Fig. 3 continued) of viral RNA. U5 is the sequence from the
5' end of viral RNA between R and the primer (tRNA[pro]) binding
site. PBS is the 18-bp sequence identical to the tRNA[pro]
binding site in MuSV/MuLV, putative primer. The possible
promoter sequence is shown in a box. Horizontal arrows indicate the sequences of direct or inverted repeats. The long
thick underline represents strong-stop cDNA. TaqI sites are
shown by small vertical arrows. (B) Schematic illustration of
the arrangement of provirus DNA in λATM-1.

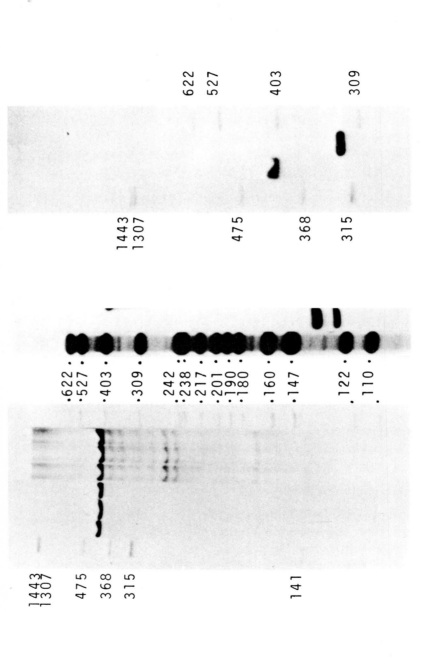

Fig. 4. (A) Analysis of strong-stop viral cDNA of ATLV and BLV and the physical map of TaqI sites. cDNA were synthesized as described in Section II with 0.1 mM [^{32}P]dCTP (lanes a–c) or with 0.005 mM [^{32}P]dCTP (lanes d–f) in the presence of various concentrations of Np 40; 0.02% for

B

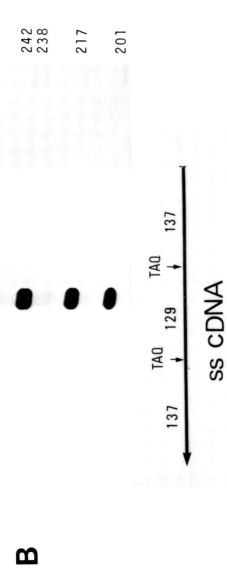

242
238

217

201

137 → TAQ 129 TAQ → 137

ss CDNA

(Fig. 4 continued) a and d; 0.05% for b and e; 0.1% for c and f. The reaction was carried out at 39°C for 30 min. The cDNA extracted from lane a was digested with *Taq*I and run in a separate gel (lane g). ATLV cDNA in lane a was compared with that of BLV strong-stop cDNA (lane h). The size markers of pBR322 fragments formed by *Taq*I (M-1) or *Hpa*II digestion (M-2) are also included, and the sizes are shown by nucleotide numbers. (B) The arrow in the map represents strong-stop cDNA (SS cDNA) and its direction of synthesis.

TABLE I.   Sizes of Various Regions in the LTR Sequence[a]

Virus	LTR	IR	R	R + U5	Primer tRNA
ATLV	754	2	228 ± 1	403 ± 1	Pro (?)
BLV	-750	—	—	320 ± 1	—
ALV/SV[b]	326-344	12	21	99	Trp
SNV[b]	543-615	3	79	174	Pro
MLV/SV[b]	515-588	11	60-68	136-151	Pro
MMTV[b]	1330	6	16	136	Lys

[a]*IR, inverted repeat at ends of LTR in integrated pro-virus; R, repeated sequence at both ends of viral RNA; R + U5, strong-stop viral cDNA.*

[b]*Numbers for these viruses are from the review by Temin (1981).*

position 353 ± 1, defining the upstream 353 ± 1 bases as U3 and the downstream 228 ± 1 bases as the terminal-repeat sequence (R) at the ends of viral RNA. This length of 228 ± 1 bases for R is much longer than those of other known retroviruses (see Table I).

IV.   DISCUSSION

A.   Provirus and the Integration Site

     RNA genome of retrovirus is reverse-transcribed into DNA, and the provirus DNA is integrated in the host chromosomal DNA for the viral replication and for the expression of the viral information. The integrated provirus DNA behaves as a host genome and is not easily removed or moved around. Therefore, the presence of the provirus DNA in cellular DNA is direct evidence for the infection of cells with retrovirus; furthermore, the structure of the integrated provirus and the site of the integration can suggest the mode of the viral infection and the possible activation of cellular gene (Hayward *et al.*, 1981). From this point of view, we have analyzed the integrated provirus DNA in fresh leukemic cells and cell lines.

The DNA preparations from fresh peripheral lymphocytes of all five patients with ATL contained the ATLV provirus DNA (Fig. 1). So far we have analyzed 16 patients, and all contained the provirus in the lymphocytes (data not shown). These findings indicate that the retrovirus ATLV is closely associated with human leukemia (ATL), because lymphocytes from normal adults did not contain the provirus. These observations suggest that the ATLV is exogenous for humans. In most of the cases, only a single band of proviral DNA was detected with each DNA of fresh lymphocytes from ATL patients when the DNA was digested with *Eco*RI, which does not cut viral genome, and the sizes varied in different patients. These results suggest that the cellular site of integration of ATLV provirus differs, thus implying that ATLV is not a widely distributed endogenous virus but is acquired locally.

B. General Features of Provirus and LTR Structures

The main functions of LTR in retroviruses are (1) reverse transcription of viral RNA, (2) integration of the provirus DNA into cellular DNA, and (3) regulation of the synthesis of viral RNA. The LTR of the ATLV provirus was shown to have the same structural organization as that of other animal retroviruses, that is, U3-R-U5. This structural organization suggests that this LTR has similar functions to other LTRs in viral replication.

LTR is bound by 2-base inverted repeats, TG and CA. Known inverted repeats in LTR are larger than 3 bp. Thus ATLV provides an example of minimum inverted repeats at the ends, which are thought to be important for integration of the provirus DNA. The viral sequence of about 8.7 kbp in λATM-1 had LTR sequences at both ends and was linked to cellular sequences by a 6-bp direct-repeat sequence of GCATTC. Clone λATM-1 seemed to contain the whole viral genome of ATLV, judging from the presence of two LTRs in the same direction and the total size.

Adjacent to 5'-LTR in pATM-3, after 2 bp there is a sequence of 18 bp identical to the tRNA^{pro} binding site in MuSV (Beveren *et al.*, 1981) (Fig. 3A). This sequence suggests that tRNA^{pro} is a primer for reverse transcription of the viral genome as MuLV/SV, although a sequence of tRNA^{pro} of human origin is not available.

All these structural features suggest that the mechanism of replication of ATLV is the same as that of other animal retroviruses, although the infectivity of ATLV is hard to demonstrate. The size of the viral sequence of about 9.0 kbp is consistent with the previous findings (Yoshida *et al.*, 1982) that the largest viral RNA in infected cell lines was 35S. This size is similar to that of animal lymphatic leukosis viruses, which do not contain a transforming gene.

C. Sequences Possibly Related to Transcriptional Control

As in other LTRs, a consensus sequence TATAAA, which is thought to be the signal for contributing to promote the transcriptional initiation of the proviral genome, was found at position 325-331. This sequence is located 29 ± 1 bp upstream of the cap site at position 354 ± 1, thus being consistent with the general features for sequence arrangements of

"TATAA" and initiation site (Corden *et al.*, 1980). Short
direct repeats of 10 bp were present at about 130 bp before
the "TATAA" box. This could be an enhancer signal for initiation of transcription, although the direct repeat is shorter
than those in the known viral LTRs (Shimotohno *et al.*, 1980;
Beveren *et al.*, 1981).

The end of R—that is, the poly(A) site—is TA at position
581. This TA was changed to TG in both the cDNA clones, pATV-1
and pATV-2. In any case, these ends of R are unique, because
all R sequences of other known retroviruses end with CA
(Temin, 1981). Furthermore, AATAAA, the so-called poly(A)
signal, was not present 10-30 bp upstream of the poly(A) site.
Without this signal sequence, ATLV viral RNA contained poly(A)
at the 3' end, although the sequence AATAAA is thought to be
required for polyadenylation (Proudfoot and Brownlee, 1976).
Almost all known eukaryotic mRNAs containing poly(A) have this
signal sequence, although a few exceptions have been reported,
namely, surface glycoprotein mRNA in Trypanosoma (Majumder
et al., 1981) and transcripts from the *cyc*-1 locus in yeast
(Zaret and Sherman, 1982). Our finding, together with these
previous exceptions, suggest that the consensus sequence AATAAA
is not absolutely required or other unknown factor, such as
secondary structure, is involved.

D. Unusual Structure of the ATLV LTR

The sequence R, which is repeated at both ends of viral
RNA, was 228 ± 1 bp. This was much longer than those of known
R sequences (Table I), among which 79 bp in spleen nephrosis
virus of chicken was the longest (Temin, 1981). This great
difference in the size of the R sequence suggests that ATLV is
a member of a different group from the known avian, mouse, or
primate retroviruses. This unusually long R sequence and the

absence of a poly(A) signal may be related to the inefficient
replicative nature of this virus. We also analyzed strong-stop
viral cDNA of bovine leukemia virus (BLV), which also replicates
inefficiently, and found it was 320 ± 1 bases (Table I, data
not shown). Although it was different from that of ATLV, it
was also unusually long.

These results suggest that ATLV and BLV should be classified in a distinct class of retroviruses from other known
retroviruses, because the LTR sequences were well conserved
among the related viruses (Lovinger and Schochetman, 1980).
This conclusion is supported by the preliminary finding that
strong-stop cDNA of BLV hybridizes significantly with the ATLV
LTR sequence under nonstringent conditions. The relatedness
of BLV with HTLV has been reported by Oroszlan *et al.* (1982),
showing that virion p24 of BLV and HTLV has a similar amino
acid sequence. Because similarities between ATLV and HTLV
were suggested from the immunological cross-reactivity of p24
or p19 (Robert-Guroff *et al.*, 1982), our conclusion from ATLV
genome analysis is consistent with that on HTLV by Oroszlan
et al. (1982). From these results ATLV and BLV are suggested
to be derived from a common ancestor of retroviruses.

V. SUMMARY

Adult T-cell leukemia virus (ATLV) is a human retrovirus
isolated from adult T-cell leukemia (ATL). The ATLV proviral
DNA was detected in fresh peripheral lymphocytes from all
patients with ATL tested so far, but not in those from healthy
adults, suggesting the possible involvement of the retrovirus
in leukemogenesis of human ATL. For structural analysis the
integrated provirus DNA and cDNA from virion RNA were molecularly cloned.

The clone (λATM-1) of an integrated provirus DNA in the MT-1 cell line, which had been established from ATL leukemic cells by co-cultivation with cord lymphocytes, contained about 13 kbp DNA as well as long terminal repeats (LTR) at both ends of the viral sequence that were about 9.0 kbp long. These two LTR sequences were linked to cellular sequences with direct repeats of 6 bp. Each LTR consisted of 754 bp including inverted repeats of 2 bp at the ends and the "TATAA" box, as characteristics in common with those of LTRs of other known retroviruses. Adjacent to the 5' LTR, there was a sequence identical to the tRNA^{pro} binding site in MuLV, suggesting that tRNA^{pro} is a primer for reverse transcription of the viral genome.

From these structural features, the mechanism of ATLV replication was suggested to be the same as that of other known animal retroviruses. However, the length of the small terminal repeats at the ends (R) of the RNA genome was 228 ± 1 bases which is much longer than the lengths of up to 79 bases of those in avian, mouse, or primate retroviruses so far analyzed. These findings suggest that ATLV should be classified in a distinct group of retroviruses with bovine leukemia virus, which was also shown to make unusually long strong-stop cDNA.

ACKNOWLEDGMENTS

The suthors thank Dr. H. Sugano for valuable discussion and encouragement during this work and also Ms. Y. Hirayama for excellent technical assistance. This work was partly supported by a Grant-in-Aid for Cancer Research from the Ministry of Education, Science and Culture of Japan.

REFERENCES

Beveren, C. V., Straaten, F. V., Galleshaw, J. A., and Verma,
    I. (1981). Cell 27, 97-108.
Bishop, J. M. (1982). Sci. Am. 246, 69-78.
Blattner, F. R., Blechl, A., Denniston-Thompson, K., Faber,
    H. E., Richards, J. E., Slightom, J. L., Tucker, P. W., and
    Smithies, O. (1978). Science (Washington, D.C.) 202,
    1279-1284.
Catovsky, D., Greaves, M. F., Rose, M., Galton, D. A. G.,
    Goolden, A. W. G., McCluskey, D. R., White, J. M., Lampert,
    I., Bourikas, G., Ireland, R., Brownell, A. I., Bridges, J.
    M., Blattner, W. A., and Gallo, R. C. (1982). Lancet,
    March 20, 639-643.
Corden, J., Wasylyk, B., Buckwalder, A., Sassone-Corsi, P.,
    Kedinger, C., and Chamborn, P. (1980). Science (Washington,
    D.C.) 209, 1406-1414.
Hayward, W. S., Neel, B. G., and Astrin, S. M. (1981). Nature
    (London) 290, 475-480.
Hinuma, Y., Nagata, K., Hanaoka, M., Nakai, M., Matsumoto, T.,
    Kinoshita, K., Shirakawa, S., and Miyoshi, I. (1981). Proc.
    Natl. Acad. Sci. USA 78, 6476-6480.
Hsu, T. W., Sabaran, J. L., Mark, G. E., Guntaka, R. V., and
    Taylor, J. M. (1978). J. Virol. 28, 810-818.
Lovinger, G. G., and Schochetman, G. (1980). Cell 20, 441-449.
Majumder, H. K., Boothroyd, J. C., and Weber, H. (1981).
    Nucleic Acids Res. 9, 4745-4753.
Maxam, A. M., and Gilbert, W. (1980). Methods Enzymol. 65,
    499-560.
Miyoshi, I., Kubonishi, I., Sumida, M., Hiraki, S., Tsubota,
    T., Kimura, I., Miyamoto, K., and Sato, J. (1980). Gann
    71, 155-156.
Miyoshi, I., Kubonishi, I., Yoshimoto, S., Akagi, T., Ohtsuki,
    Y., Shiraishi, Y., Nagata, Y., and Hinuma, Y. (1981).
    Nature (London) 294, 770-771.
Oroszlan, S., Sarngadharan, M. G., Copeland, T. D., Kalyanaramar
    V. S., Gilden, R. V., and Gallo, R. C. (1982). Proc. Natl.
    Acad. Sci. USA 79, 1291-1294.
Poiesz, B. J., Ruscetti, F. W., Gazdar, A. F., Bunn, P. A.,
    Minna, J. D., and Gallo, R. C. (1980). Proc. Natl. Acad.
    Sci. USA 77, 7415-7419.
Proudfoot, N. J., and Brownlee, G. G. (1976). Nature (London)
    263, 211-214.
Reitz, M. S., Poiesz, B. J., Ruscetti, F. W., and Gallo, R. C.
    (1981). Proc. Natl. Acad. Sci. USA 78, 1887-1891.
Robert-Guroff, M., Nakao, Y., Notake, K., Ito, Y., Sliski, A.,
    and Gallo, R. C. (1982). Science (Washington, D.C.) 215,
    975-978.

Seiki, M., Hattori, S., and Yoshida, M. (1982). *Proc. Natl. Acad. Sci. USA 79*, 6899-6902.

Shimotohno, K., Mizutani, S., and Temin, H. M. (1980). *Nature (London) 285*, 550-554.

Southern, E. M. (1975). *J. Mol. Biol. 98*, 503-517.

Stehelin, D., Varmus, H. E., Bishop, J. M., and Vogt, P. K. (1976). *Nature (London) 260*, 170-173.

Taniguchi, T., Palmieri, M., and Weisman, C. (1978). *Nature (London) 274*, 223-228.

Temin, H. M. (1981). *Cell 27*, 1-3.

Uchiyama, T., Yodoi, J., Sagawa, K., Takatsuki, K., and Uchino, H. (1977). *Blood 50*, 481-492.

Varmus, H. E. (1982). *Science (Washington, D.C.) 216*, 812-820.

Williams, B. G., and Blattner, F. R. (1979). *J. Virol. 29*, 555-575.

Yoshida, M., Kawai, S., and Toyoshima, K. (1980). *Nature (London) 287*, 653-654.

Yoshida, M., Miyoshi, I., and Hinuma, Y. (1982). *Proc. Natl. Acad. Sci. USA 79*, 2031-2035.

Zaret, K. S., and Sherman, F. (1982). *Cell 28*, 563-573.

28

HUMAN T-CELL LEUKEMIA VIRUS AND HUMAN LEUKEMOGENESIS

M. G. Sarngadharan and V. S. Kalyanaraman

Department of Cell Biology
Litton Bionetics, Inc.
Kensington, Maryland

M. Robert-Guroff, M. Popovic, J. Schuepbach,
M. S. Reitz, F. Wong-Staal, and R. C. Gallo

Laboratory of Tumor Cell Biology
National Cancer Institute
National Institutes of Health
Bethesda, Maryland

I. INTRODUCTION

Etiological association between retroviruses (RNA tumor viruses) and animal leukemias has been well established. Since Ellermann and Bang (1908) reported the transmission of leukemia in chicken with cell-free filtrates, and Rous (1911) identified a chicken sarcoma virus, retroviruses have been demonstrated in the natural incidence of leukemias and lymphomas of cats, cows, gibbon apes, and some wild mice (see Wong-Staal and Gallo, 1982). A similar viral etiology has been sought for human leukemias and lymphomas for decades but not until recent years with success. Some of the animal models just mentioned provide a few important insights for consideration of human leukemias.

Most virus-induced leukemias and lymphomas are associated with abundant replication of virus, but in bovine leukemia the causative agent, bovine leukemia virus (BLV), was not detected until the leukemic cells were cultured *in vitro* (see Miller and Van der Maaten, 1980). Obviously, human leukemias are not characterized by abundant replication of a virus, and it brings out the importance of careful and long-term culture of appropriate target cells for virus detection and isolation. Many virus-induced leukemias in animals are of T-cell origin (Kaplan, 1974), and yet, the ability to grow T cells in the laboratory has only recently been acquired.

In 1976, our laboratory, which has long been interested in long-term growth and differentiation of human hematopoietic cells, reported the discovery of a factor termed T-cell growth factor (TCGF) (Morgan et al., 1976). As a result, we were for the first time able to establish several neoplastic mature human T-cell lines on a routine basis and to systematically examine them for expression of retroviruses on the basis of use of partially purified TCGF (Mier and Gallo, 1980;

Poiesz *et al.*, 1980a). Several of these human neoplastic
T-cell lines have become producers of a type C retrovirus that
we have termed human T-cell leukemia virus (HTLV) (Poiesz
et al., 1980b, 1981; Gallo *et al.*, 1982a; Popovic *et al.*,
1983). These HTLV-producing cell lines have been derived from
leukemia/lymphoma patients from widely separated geographical
locations around the world. There are some similarities in
the clinical picture of many HTLV-positive patients. They
commonly include lymphadenopathy, visceral organ enlargement,
and poor survival (about 75% of cases to date). They frequently show skin involvement and hypercalcemia. The ultrastructure of the leukemic cell frequently shows convoluted
nuclei. In the following sections we describe the characteristics of the retrovirus expressed by these leukemic/lymphoma
patients including some of its biological properties and draw
some correlations between the virus and certain types of human
T-cell malignancies.

II.   CHARACTERIZATION OF HUMAN T-CELL LEUKEMIA VIRUS (HTLV)

A.   Relatedness to Other Retroviruses

    Morphologically, HTLV is a typical type C retrovirus as
seen by electronmicroscopy (Fig. 1). Like all retroviruses,
it contains a reverse transcriptase and a high molecular weight
RNA genome, and it buds from the cell membrane. The reverse
transcriptase of HTLV was not inhibited by antibodies raised
against several known animal retroviruses (Rho *et al.*, 1981).
By molecular hybridization using cDNA transcribed from the
viral genomic RNA, it was shown that HTLV was not substantially
related to any previously described animal retrovirus (Reitz
et al., 1981).

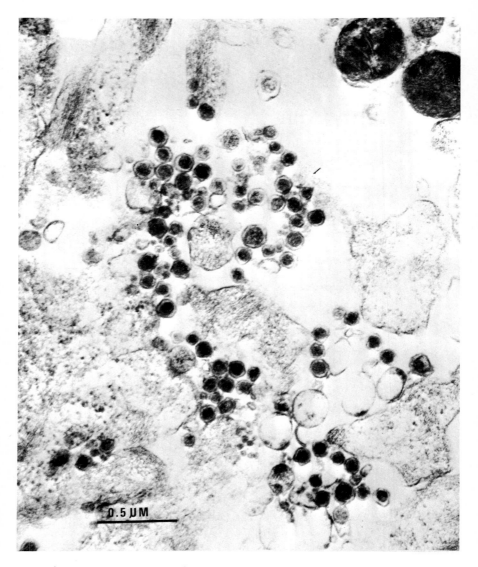

Fig. 1.   Electron micrograph showing extracellular HLTV particles.

Three *gag* gene proteins of HTLV have been identified and characterized. They are p24, p19, and p15. p24 is the major structural protein (Kalyanaraman *et al.*, 1981a), p19, the NH_2 terminal *gag* protein (S. Oroszlan, unpublished), and p15, the nucleic acid-binding protein. Amino acid sequence analysis of p24 and p15 revealed that they are the p30 and p10 (nucleic acid-binding protein) homologs, respectively, of HTLV. These sequences were specific and pointed to the uniqueness of HTLV. Comparison of the amino acid sequences of p24 and p15 to those of the homologous proteins of other retroviruses indicated a significant, but distant homology with the p24 and p12, respectively, of BLV, suggesting that these two sets of proteins may have evolved from common ancestral molecules (Oroszlan *et al.*, 1982; S. Oroszlan, unpublished). The extent of homology between HTLV proteins and BLV proteins, although statistically significant, was not sufficient to cause immunological cross-reactions in conventional radioimmunoassays. Thus, no cross-reactivities were detected between HTLV and other retroviruses including BLV in homologous radioimmunoassays using purified HTLV p24, p15, or p19 (Kalyanaraman *et al.*, 1981a; V. S. Kalyanaraman *et al.*, unpublished) or in a variety of heterologous radioimmunoassays capable of detecting most type B, type C, and type D animal retroviruses (Kalyanaraman *et al.*, 1981a).

HTLV nucleic acid sequences were not present in normal human DNA. Furthermore, even in a virus-positive patient (e.g., C. R., whose cells provided the first isolate of HTLV), the viral sequences were only present in the DNA from the T-cell lines, but were absent in the DNA from a normal B-cell line (Fig. 2) (Gallo *et al.*, 1982a). Therefore, HTLV is not an endogenous human retrovirus transmitted through the germ line. The virus must be acquired by a postzygotic infection.

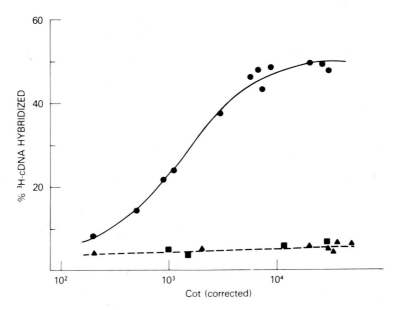

Fig. 2. HTLV proviral DNA in T- but not B-cell lines of patient C. R., [³H]HTLV cDNA was annealed to cellular DNA from C. R. T lymphocytes (●), C. R. B lymphocytes (▲), and PHA-stimulated normal human peripheral blood T lymphocytes (■).

B.   Natural Antibodies to HTLV in Human Sera

1. *In T-Cell Leukemia/Lymphoma Patients*

Natural HTLV infection frequently elicits serum antibodies to the viral antigens (Posner *et al.*, 1981; Kalyanaraman *et al.*, 1981b, 1982a; Robert-Guroff *et al.*, 1982). We have conducted extensive seroepidemiological surveys of T-cell leukemia patients and normal donors for antibodies to HTLV in order to determine the relationship of HTLV to particular human malignancies. Because the virus appeared from the initial series of results to be T-cell tropic, a large number of patients with a variety of T-cell malignancies were screened for evidence of HTLV infection. In the United States, HTLV-positive T-cell malignancies occur sporadically. There is a form of adult T-cell

leukemia (ATL) that is more common in Japan. Clinical epidemiology of Japanese ATL had indicated a geographical clustering in the southwestern islands of Kyushu and Shikoku and the
involvement of an infectious vector, possibly a virus in its
etiology (Takatsuki et al., 1977, 1979; Uchiyama et al., 1977).

Our studies have shown that nearly 90% of all Japanese
ATL patients have serum antibodies to HTLV (Robert-Guroff et
al., 1983), obviously indicating that HTLV is associated with
this disease (Table I). In addition, we have obtained three
retrovirus isolates from Japanese ATL patients, and all are
extremely similar to the original U.S. isolates of HTLV (see
Section III). Furthermore, a retrovirus was isolated from
Japanese ATL cells independently by Japanese workers (Miyoshi
et al., 1981) and has been characterized by Yoshida et al.
(1982). By immunological comparison of the structural proteins
and by nucleic acid hybridization studies, we have shown that
this isolate also belongs to the HTLV group (Popovic et al.,
1982).

The Caribbean basin has been found to be another area
where HTLV-associated malignancies appear to be endemic.
Antibodies to HTLV were found in 11 of 11 West Indian patients
(Blattner et al., 1982, 1983) (Table I) with T-cell lympho-
sarcoma cell leukemia (T-LCL) (Catovsky et al., 1982), an
aggressive malignant disease similar to Japanese ATL.

As indicated earlier, HTLV-associated T-cell malignancies
are only sporadically found in the United States, although
HTLV was first isolated from the T-cell lines developed from a
U.S. patient diagnosed with cutaneous T-cell lymphoma (CTCL),
a disease clinically somewhat different from the Japanese ATL
and the Caribbean T-LCL. Although natural antibodies to HTLV
have been detected in sera from some patients, most CTCL
patients surveyed lacked HTLV-specific antibodies (Gallo et al.,
1983). We postulate that a few of the HTLV-positive CTCL

TABLE I.   Prevalence of Natural Antibodies to HTLV in Sera of
           Patients with Malignancies of Mature T Cells, Their
           Healthy Relatives, and Random Normal Donors

	Antibodies to HTLV	
Serum donors	No. positive/No. tested	% Positive
Healthy relatives of U.S. patients with HTLV-associated malignancy	2/12	17
Unrelated healthy donors, Washington, D.C.	1/185	<1
Unrelated healthy donors, Georgia	3/158	2
Caribbean T-LCL patients	11/11	100
Healthy relatives of Caribbean patients	3/16	19
Random healthy donors, Caribbean	12/337	4
Japanese ATL patients	40/46	87
Healthy relatives of ATL patients	19/40	48
Random healthy donors, nonendemic area, Japan	9/600	2
Random healthy donors, endemic area, Japan	50/419	12

patients actually had a disease more akin to ATL, which is
rarely diagnosed in the United States. However, we do not
rule out an association of HTLV with CTCL. Antibody-negative
patients sometimes still possess unexpressed HTLV information
as integrated proviral sequences. This question remains open.

2. In Normal Population

Sera of random normal donors in the United States and Europe do not show antibodies to HTLV. In Japan where HTLV infection is endemic in certain parts, the prevalence of serum antibodies in the normal population varied considerably and correlated closely with the geographical distribution of ATL. Thus, the incidence was 15–16% in the Nagasaki and Kagoshima areas of Kyushu Island, and about 9% in the Uwajima area of Shikoku Island, but only about 2% on Honshu Island and even lower on Hokkaido Island (Robert-Guroff *et al.*, 1983). It is known that once an individual acquires serum antibodies to HTLV, that individual becomes an antibody carrier for a long period even without chances of frequent reexposure to the virus (Schuepbach *et al.*, 1983). Unlike in Japan, clustering of T-LCL in specific regions of the Caribbean basin has not been studied. About 4% of the normal Caribbean population screened showed antibodies to HTLV, indicating that HTLV infection may be generally widespread in these regions.

3. HTLV-Specific Antibodies in Sera of Healthy Relatives of T-Cell Leukemia/Lymphoma Patients

If HTLV is an infectious virus, close family members of virus-positive patients will be the most likely group to have a high incidence of serum antibodies to HTLV proteins. Therefore, we conducted a detailed and systematic screening of multiple healthy family members of a group of leukemia/lymphoma patients known to be associated with HTLV by virtue of having HTLV-specific serum antibodies or expressing HTLV antigens or intact viral particles in their cultured lymphocytes. These families were from the United States, the Caribbean basin, and Japan. The single significant group that is positive for HTLV-specific antibodies in the United States is the family members

of HTLV-positive patients (Table I). Four relatives each of
patients C. R., M. J., and W. A., all of whom were sources of
separate HTLV isolates (Poiesz *et al.*, 1980b; Gallo *et al.*,
1982a; Popovic *et al.*, 1983) were studied. The wife of C. R.
(Kalyanaraman *et al.*, 1981b; Schuepbach *et al.*, 1983; Robert-
Guroff *et al.*, 1982) and the mother of W. A. were found to be
positive for antibodies to HTLV p24 and p19 (Robert-Guroff
et al., 1983). Similarly, four Caribbean families were
screened, and 3 of 16 members were antibody positive.

By far the highest incidence noticed was among relatives
of Japanese ATL patients. Of 40 members studied belonging to
12 families, 19 individuals had antibodies to HTLV proteins.
One of the Japanese families studied in this group (S. K.) was
particularly significant. In this family, sera and peripheral
blood leukocytes were obtained from a 22-year-old male ATL
patient, his mother, father, and a fraternal twin brother and
sister. Antibodies to HTLV p24 and p19 were found in the sera
of the patient and both of his parents (Robert-Guroff *et al.*,
1983; Sarin *et al.*, 1983). Cultured T cells of all of these
antibody-positive family members and the patient produced
extracellular virus (Sarin *et al.*, 1983). In addition, there
was a low-level expression of HTLV p24 and p19 in the cultured
cells of the patient's brother, although his serum had not
shown antibodies to HTLV. The data indicate that he may have
been recently infected, and it is of interest to follow this
individual in time. The healthy mother of the patient S. K.
is also an interesting case. Some (7%) of her peripheral blood
lymphocytes histologically resemble neoplastic T cells typical
of HTLV infection and spontaneously synthesize DNA in culture
even though she is without symptoms of disease (Sarin *et al.*,
1983).

It should be remembered that in certain geographical locations, especially in Japan and in the Caribbean basin where HTLV infection has been found to be endemic, some of the healthy relatives of the virus-positive leukemia patients may have been infected with HTLV outside the family contacts just as were a significant proportion of the normal antibody-positive people in these same areas. However, in any given area family members of virus-positive patients exhibit a much higher incidence of infection than healthy donors not known to be related to HTLV-positive patients, as judged by serum antibodies to HTLV or the expression of virus antigens upon culturing their T cells. This is a further confirmation of the transmission of HTLV by horizontal infection.

4. Specificity of the Antibodies in Human Sera

The antibodies to HTLV detected in the sera of leukemia patients, their relatives, and normal individuals show strong specificity. Figure 3 shows the precipitation of well-characterized antigens of HTLV by an assortment of sera belonging to T-cell leukemia patients, some of their relatives, and some positive normal donors not known to be related to any HTLV-positive leukemia patients. The data indicate that the sera possess antibodies directed against p24, p19, and p15, all internal gag proteins of HTLV, and may mean that these individuals support at least a low level of virus replication. The immune precipitation seen in these experiments were highly specific and were blocked only by extracts of HTLV or cells producing HTLV. A large number of other animal retroviruses and cell lines not expressing HTLV had absolutely no effect on the immune reaction (Fig. 4). In addition, the precipitation was caused by separate and specific reactivities in the sera. This is demonstrated in the following experiment. Homogeneous

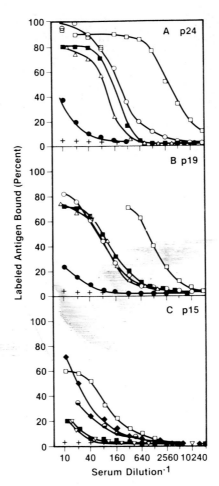

Fig. 3.   Representative radioimmunoprecipitations of
purified and labeled HTLV proteins p24 (A), p19 (B), and p15
(C) by serum samples of ATL patients (B-2, O; C-1, ●; D-1, Δ;
F, +), their family members (H, ■), and healthy individuals
from the Caribbean (V-4, □; M, ▽; N, ◆; O, ◓).   Serial dilutions of serum were incubated with 8000 to 10,000 cpm of the
labeled protein.   A 30-fold excess of goat anti-human IgG
antibody was added, and the percentage of labeled antigen bound
in the precipitation was determined.   From Schuepbach *et al.*
(1983).

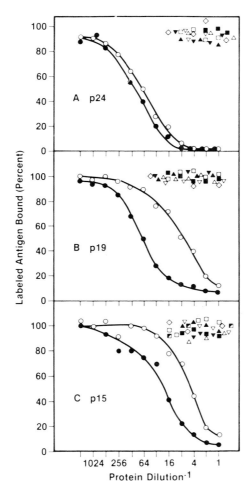

Fig. 4. Viral and cellular competition in the precipitation of HTLV proteins p24 (A), p19 (B), and p15 (C). Competition radioimmunoassays were performed with ^{125}I-labeled HTLV
p24, p19, or p15, and limiting dilution of the Caribbean normal
serum V-4. Serial dilutions of the unlabeled antigens,
starting with 100 ng of protein for viral and 50 µg of protein
for cellular extracts, were preincubated with the serum for 1 h
at 37°C. Labeled proteins (8000-10,000 cpm) were then added,
and precipitations were performed as described. O, HuT-102;
□, HuT-78; ■, normal human T cells; ●, HTLV; ▨, SSV; Δ,
BaEV-M7; ▲, BLV; ▽, MPMV; ▼, FeLV; ◇, R-MuLV. From Schuepbach
et al. (1983).

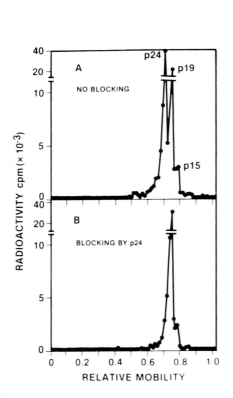

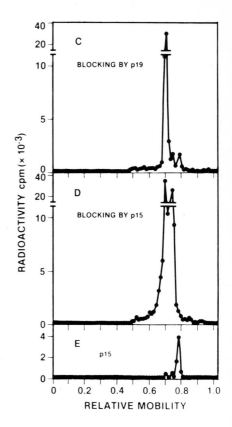

Fig. 5. SDS-polyacrylamide gel electrophoretic analysis of purified and labeled HTLV proteins precipitated by natural anti-HTLV serum. ^{125}I-labeled p24, p19, and p15 (100,000 cpm each) were mixed and incubated with 10 µl of serum V-4 (see legend to Fig. 3), and processed as described in the legend to Fig. 3. The precipitate was washed twice in 5 ml of buffer and analyzed by 12% SDS-polyacrylamide gel electrophoresis (A). To determine the specificity of individual human antibodies for p24, p19, or p15, the serum was also preabsorbed during 3 h at 37°C with 100 ng of purified unlabeled p24 (B), 500 ng of p19 (C), or 500 ng of p15 (D), before the mixture of the labeled proteins was added, and precipitations were performed and anlyzed as previously described. A separate precipitate of labeled p15 by 20 µl of serum V-4 was analyzed (E), to give additional proof for the existence of the p15 peak in A through D. From Schuepbach *et al.* (1983).

HTLV p24, p19, and p15 were labeled with ^{125}I, mixed together, and immunoprecipitated, and the precipitate analyzed by poly-acrylamide electrophoresis in the presence of SDS. Figure 5A shows labeled protein peaks representing p24, p19, and p15. When the precipitations just described were repeated in the presence of unlabeled p24, p19, or p15, the unlabeled protein specifically blocked the precipitation of the corresponding labeled protein (Fig. 5B-D). p24, p19, and p15 are therefore separate antigens capable of eliciting separate and exlusive immune responses in the infected individual.

III. MULTIPLE HTLV ISOLATES AND THEIR INTERRELATIONSHIP

A. Wide Geographical Distribution of HTLV

Although HTLV was initially repeatedly isolated from T-cell cultures of patient C. R., a U.S. patient with CTCL, finding of HTLV-positive T-cell malignancies in the United States is sporadic. However, serological screening did identify several antibody-positive patients in the United States. Many of these antibody-positive patients were kept on surveillance, and their T lymphocytes were cultured from time to time. Thus, T cells of patient M. J., who was one of the earliest CTCL patients found to carry serum antibodies to HTLV proteins (Kalyanaraman et al., 1981b), expressed HTLV particles upon culturing (Popovic et al., 1983). However, HTLV isolation was never more predictable than with cultured T cells of Japanese ATL or Caribbean T-LCL patients, probably a reflection of the wide-spread involvement of HTLV in ATL and T-LCL.

TABLE II. Comparison of Properties of HTLV Isolates[a]

Designation	Cell line	Geographical origin	RNA	p24	p19
HTLV-I$_{CR}$	HuT-102	United States	*	*	*
HTLV-I$_{MJ}$	M. J.	United States	++	++	++
HTLV-I$_{MB}$	CTCL-2	Caribbean	++	++	++
HTLV-I$_{MI}$	M. I.	Caribbean	++	++	++
HTLV-I$_{UK}$	U. K.	Israel	++	++	++
HTLV-I$_{SK}$	S. K.	Japan	n.d.	++	++
HTLV-I$_{TK}$	T. K.	Japan	n.d.	++	++
HTLV-I$_{HK}$	H. K.	Japan	n.d.	++	++
HTLV-I$_{SD}$	S. D.	Japan[b]	++	++	++
HTLV-I$_{MT-1}$ ("ATLV")	MT-1	Japan	++	++	++
HTLV-I$_{MT-2}$ ("ATLV")	MT-2	Japan	++	++	++
HTLV-II$_{MO}$	M. O.	United States	±	+	+

[a]*, prototype HTLV; ++, highly related to or indistinguishable from the prototype; ±, slightly or not significantly related; +, related and readily distinguishable; n.d., no data.

[b]A cell line developed from a 49-year-old female ATL patient who was born in Kyushu, Japan and emigrated to the United States at age 23. (Haynes et al., 1983.)

Alternatively, the Japanese ATL and the Caribbean T-LCL may be characterized by a greater replication of the virus than T-cell malignancies elsewhere. We have obtained three retrovirus isolates from cell cultures initiated from a Japanese ATL patient (S. K.) and his close relatives (T. K. and H. K.) (see Section II.B.3). With the availability of such multiple isolates from widely separated geographical locations (Table II), it was possible to make some comparisons, especially between HTLV isolated in the United States and the virus present in Japanese ATL. In addition to the Japanese isolates obtained in our own laboratory, two cell lines, MT-1 (Miyoshi et al., 1980) and MT-2 (Miyoshi et al., 1981), were also used as sources of the retrovirus of Japanese ATL. In preliminary analyses, competition radioimmunoassays (RIA) were performed using ^{125}I-labeled p24 of HTLV$_{CR}$ and a hyperimmune antibody against HTLV$_{CR}$ p24. In these experiments the retrovirus expressed by the cell lines MT-1 and MT-2, as well as S. K., T. K., and H. K., exhibited the same competion pattern as cell lines producing HTLV$_{CR}$, HTLV$_{MJ}$, HTLV$_{UK}$, and so on. (Popovic et al., 1982, 1983). Figure 6 shows a comparison of the

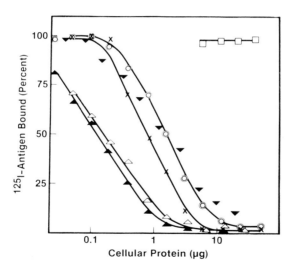

Fig. 6. Homologous competition radioimmunoassay for HTLV p24. The assay was set up using ^{125}I-labeled p24 of HTLV$_{CR}$ and a rabbit hyperimmune serum against HTLV$_{CR}$ as described in the legend to Fig. 4. Competing antigens were present in the extracts of the following cells: X——X, HuT-102 (produces HTLV$_{CR}$); O——O, M. J.; Δ——Δ, U. K.; ▲——▲, M. I.; ▼——▼, S. K.; □——□, normal human cultured peripheral blood T cells.

competition curves obtained with some of these isolates in the
RIA for p24. Similarly, hybridization curves were developed
between cDNA copy of the 70S RNA of $HTLV_{CR}$ and mRNA from cell
lines expressing the various isolates of HTLV (Fig. 7). Once
again there was no major difference in the patterns between
the Japanese ATL cell lines and those expressing $HTLV_{CR}$,
$HTLV_{MJ}$, $HTLV_{UK}$, and so on, suggesting that these different
isolates, including the Japanese isolates, belong to a closely
related group of human T-cell leukemia viruses. Fine structure
variations might still exist among the various isolates, and
these will not be known until amino acid sequencing of the
proteins and nucleic acid sequencing of the genes are done for
the individual isolates.

B. $HTLV_{MO}$, A New Subgroup of HTLV

We obtained a new HTLV isolate from a T-cell line established from an adult male (M. O.) with a hematopoietic malignancy described as a T-cell variant hairy-cell leukemia (Saxon
et al., 1978). This was substantially different from all other
HTLV isolates (Kalyanaraman *et al.*, 1982 b). In homologous
competition RIA for $HTLV_{CR}$ p24, $HTLV_{MO}$ did compete with $HTLV_{CR}$.
However, the pattern of competition indicated measurable differences between the two isolates (Fig. 8A). These differences
were not evident in a heterologous RIA using $HTLV_{CR}$ p24 and
the natural antibody in M. O. serum (Fig. 8B). Figure 8C shows
that an assay using the serum of another patient (M. J.), who
expresses a retrovirus indistinguishable from $HTLV_{CR}$ (see
Section III,A), once again brings out the differences in cross-
reactivity between $HTLV_{MO}$ and $HTLV_{CR}$. Further, we have found
that nucleic acid sequence homology between $HTLV_{CR}$ and $HTLV_{MO}$
can be detected only under very nonstringent hybridization

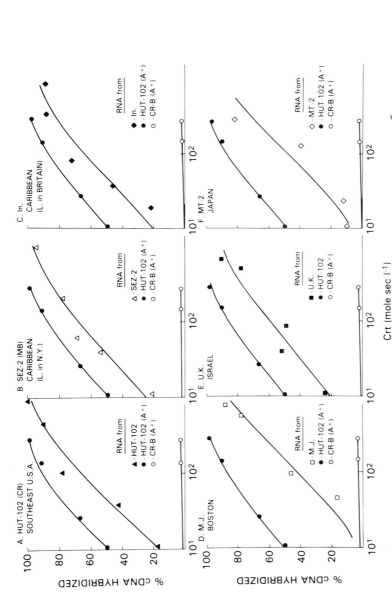

Fig. 7. Relationship of different HTLV isolates by RNA hybridization. [³H]HTLVCR cDNA was synthesized using calf thymus DNA primer (Reitz et al., 1981) and hybridized to cellular RNA from different HTLV-positive cell lines. Results with the controls with poly(A)-containing RNA from CR-T (HuT-102) and CR-B cells are superimposed on each panel for comparison with the others. From Reitz et al. (1983).

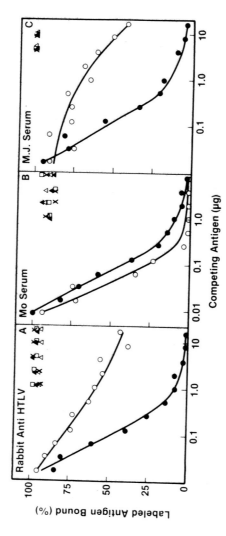

Fig. 8. Homologous and heterologous competition radioimmunoassays of HTLV p24. Assays were carried out as described (Kalyanaraman et al., 1981) using 125I-labeled HTLVCR p24 and a limiting dilution of hyperimmune rabbit antibody to HTLVCR or sera from patients M. O. and M. J. (A) Competition RIA using rabbit anti-HTLVCR; (B) competition RIA using M. O. serum; (C) competition RIA using M. J. serum. Virus extracts used for competition were as follows: ●——●, HTLVCR; ○——○, HTLVMO; X——X, Mason Pfizer monkey virus; △——△, bovine leukemia virus; □——□, Rauscher murine leukemia virus, and ▲——▲, simian sarcoma virus. From Kalyanaraman et al. (1982b). Copyright ©1982 by the American Association for the Advancement of Science.

conditions (Wong-Staal *et al.*, 1983). Therefore, HTLV$_{MO}$ forms a distinct subgroup in the HTLV family. We propose to group the prototype HTLV$_{CR}$ and the other isolates indistinguishable from it as HTLV-I, and HTLV$_{MO}$ as HTLV-II, and to identify the individual isolates as HTLV-I$_{CR}$, HTLV-I$_{MJ}$, HTLV-I$_{SK}$, and so on, and HTLV-II$_{MO}$ (Kalyanaraman *et al.*, 1982b) (Table II). Additional subgroups of HTLV may be identified in the future.

IV. BIOLOGICAL PROPERTIES OF HTLV

A. *In Vitro* Transmission of HTLV

Seroepidemiological data presented earlier leave no doubt that HTLV is an infectious agent and that it is transmitted horizontally. The same infectious nature has been demonstrated using tissue culture cells. Several of the HTLV isolates have been successfully transmitted to human cord blood lymphocytes by cocultivation (Popovic *et al.*, 1983). Virus-positive neoplastic cells used as donors were either treated with mitomycin-C or X irradiated before cocultivation with recipient cord blood lymphocytes. The cultures were analyzed for HTLV expression, karyotype, HLA type, and T-cell markers. Karyotype and HLA consistently matched those of the recipient cells. In a majority of cases the HTLV-producing T cells were of the helper/inducer phenotype, although some rare examples of cell lines consisting of both helper/inducer and suppressor/cytotoxic phenotypes have been observed (Gallo *et al.*, 1983a). However, none of the infected cell lines were found to express pure suppressor/cytotoxic phenotype. Unlike the HTLV-infected cord blood cells, phytohemagglutinin-stimulated (control) cells consist of 70% helper/inducer and 30% suppressor/cytotoxic

T cells.   These studies suggest that, as in natural disease, the target of HTLV infection in the tissue culture is a subset of mature T cells.

HTLV infection of the cord blood lymphocytes led to their reduced requirement of TCGF for growth.   In several cases the infection caused transformation of the cord blood T cells, and they grew without exogenously provided TCGF.   These cells show striking morphological, surface phenotype, and growth characteristics similar to primary HTLV-positive malignant cells obtained from patients.   In many cases the transformed secondary cultures expressed HTLV at high levels and therefore were of important practical value as large-scale sources of HTLV.

B.   Possible Mechanism of Transformation by HTLV

Pathogenic retroviruses are grouped into transforming viruses and nontransforming viruses.   The transforming viruses cause acute malignant transformation *in vivo* and carry a transforming gene, variously described as *src, onc, leuk,* and so on.   These genes are derived from normal host cell DNA in the past, presumably by recombination events between viral and host DNA.   The nontransforming retroviruses do not carry *onc* genes and usually do not transform cells *in vitro*.   They cause leukemias and lymphomas only after long latent periods.   Most naturally occurring animal leukemia viruses belong to this category.   Several of these "chronic" leukemia viruses are thought to induce leukemias by activating cellular *onc* genes as a result of provirus integration in the proximity of these cellular genes.   This is termed "downstream promotion" and has been suggested as the mechanism whereby avian retroviruses induce avian bursal lymphomas (Hayward *et al.*, 1981; Neel *et al.*, 1981).   Such integration may provide either a viral

"promoter" or an "enhancer" sequence for the expression of
these normally unexpressed host genes. It has been suggested
that HTLV infection might cause the downstream promotion of
the gene for TCGF and/or TCGF receptor, resulting in inappropriate T-cell expansion. Some of the available evidence favors
such a model (Gallo, 1982).

It is obvious that HTLV infection does not always cause
T-cell leukemia, because many normal people manifest persistent
HTLV infection, indicated by persistent serum antibodies
against HTLV internal proteins (Kalyanaraman et al., 1981 ,
1982 ; Robert-Guroff et al., 1982, 1983; Blattner et al., 1982)
and even harboring virus antigens in their peripheral blood
T cells (Robert-Guroff et al., 1983; Sarin et al., 1983). It
has been estimated that only about 1 in 2000 antibody-positive
persons in Japan develop ATL (Suchi and Tajima, 1982). Host-
specific environmental factors, age at first infection, repetitive infections, and route of infection may all be involved.
Although it is clear that HTLV is transmitted horizontally,
its precise mode of spread is not clear. If a substantial
portion of the normal population in an endemic region is
infected, there is no need for a nonhuman reservoir. HTLV
does not appear to be highly infectious, and it may need prolonged intimate contact for transmission; this is also suggested by the increased incidence of infection within families
of virus-positive patients. In the endemic areas, blood
transfusions or insect bites could be significant routes of
virus transmissions.

V. MOLECULAR BIOLOGY OF HTLV

We have cloned DNA sequences derived from approximately 1 kb of the 5' and 3' termini of the HTLV genome as well as a 4- or 5-kb defective HTLV provirus flanked by cellular sequences (Manzari *et al.*, 1983a). These sequences were used as probes to survey fresh leukemic cells and tumor tissues from patients with different lymphoid and myeloid malignancies for DNA sequences related to HTLV (Fig. 9) (Wong-Staal *et al.*, 1983). Several conclusions can be made from these studies:

1. Cells from some patients of mature T-cell malignancies, including all patients with ATL, contained one or few copies of HTLV provirus. Cells from other types of malignancies involving immature T cells, B cells, or myeloid cells are by and large negative.

2. The correlation of the surveys by molecular hybridization and by serology is not 100%. This could arise from lack of expression of HTLV genome in some virus-positive patients. In some cases, the ptients may be exposed to HTLV and therefore be positive for anti-HTLV antibodies, but their disease may not be linked to HTLV (Fig. 10).

3. The tumor cells are clonal expansions of single infected cells. Monoclonality is a common feature of tumors induced by the chronic leukemia viruses. Several of the neoplastic T cells producing HTLV contain a single-copy provirus of 8.5-9.0 kb with no suggestion of a second defective component.

Therefore, in spite of its capacity to transform cells *in vitro* (see Section IV.A), HTLV probably does not carry an *onc* gene. It has been speculated that chronic leukemia viruses, which represent most retroviruses associated with naturally occurring leukemias and lymphomas, induce diseases by activating specific

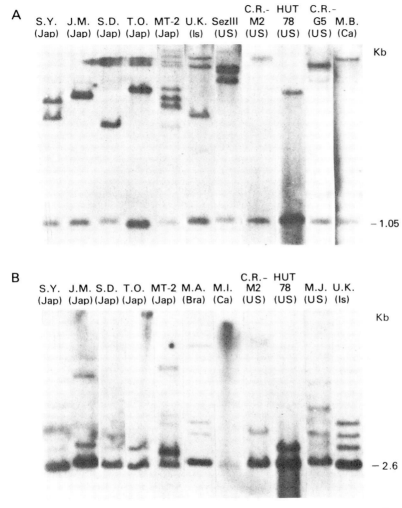

Fig. 9. Conservation of the HTLV genomes present in diverse geographical areas. DNA from fresh leukemic cells or cell lines from HTLV-positive patients from different areas of the world was digested with the restriction enzymes (A) *Bam*HI and (B) *Pst*I, which cut more than once within HTLV$_{CR}$ and blot hybridized to a cloned HTLV probe. Abbreviations for places of origin: Jap, Japan; Is, Israel; US, United States; Ca, Caribbean; Bra, Brazil.

Ab + Provirus +	Ab − Provirus +
ATL (mature)	ATL (mature) patients infected but not expressing HTLV Ag/Ab
Ab + Provirus − T-ALL (immature) 1 case Patient is HTLV carrier, but disease not due to HTLV	Ab − Provirus − Various malignancies

Fig. 10. Correlation of serology and detection of provirus of HLTV.

cellular genes in the vicinity of the provirus integration sites (see Section IV,B). We have evidence that HTLV integrates into the same immediate locus in several neoplastic T-cell samples derived from patients from the United States and Japan (Hahn *et al.*, 1983), although it is not known which, if any, gene(s) are transcriptionally activated as a result. Because HTLV specifically transforms mature T cells, it is likely to affect directly or indirectly expression of genes that are important in T-cell proliferation. Along this line, we have identified and isolated a gene that is expressed at high levels in all HTLV-positive neoplastic T cells and in normal cord blood T cells after infection with HTLV, but not in the uninfected counterparts (Manzari *et al.*, 1983b). Study of the pattern of expression of this gene in uninfected human hematopoietic cells suggests that its expression may be linked to TCGF production or response. It would be of interest to determine whether activation of this gene is a primary or secondary consequence of HTLV integration.

REFERENCES

Blattner, W. A., Kalyanaraman, V. S., Robert-Guroff, M., Lister,
T. A., Galton, D. A. G., Sarin, P., Crawford, M. H.,
Catovsky, D., Greaves, M., and Gallo, R. C. (1982). *Int.
J. Cancer 30*, 257-264.
Blattner, W. A., Blayney, D. W., Robert-Guroff, M., Sarngadharan,
M. G., Kalyanaraman, V. S., Sarin, P., Jaffe, E. S., and
Gallo, R. C. (1983). *J. Infect. Dis. 147*, 406-416.
Catovsky, D., Greaves, M., Rose, M., Galton, D. A. G., Goolden,
A. W. G., McCluskey, D. R., White, J. M., Lampert, I.,
Bourikas, G., Ireland, R., Bridges, J. M., Blattner, W. A.,
and Gallo, R. C. (1982). *Lancet 1*, 639-643.
Ellermann, V., and Bang, O. (1908). *Zentralbl. Bakteriol.
Parasitenkd. Infektionskr. 46*, 595-609.
Gallo, R. C. (1982). *In* "Viruses and Environment" (E. Kurstak
and K. Maramorosch, eds.), pp. 43-78. Academic Press,
New York.
Gallo, R. C., Mann, D., Broder, S., Ruscetti, F. W., Madea, M.,
Kalyanaraman, V. S., Robert-Guroff, M., and Reitz, M. S.
(1982a). *Proc. Natl. Acad. Sci. USA 79*, 5680-5683.
Gallo, R. C., Popovic, M., Sarin, P. S., Reitz, M. S.,
Kalyanaraman, V. S., Aoki, T., Sarngadharan, M. G., and
Wong-Staal, F. (1983a). *In* "Modern Trends in Human Leu-
kemia" (R. Neth *et al.*, eds.), Vol. 5, pp. 311-319.
Springer-Verlag, Berlin.
Gallo, R. C., *et al.* (1983b). *Cancer Res.*, in press.
Hahn, B., Manzari, V., Columbini, S., Franchini, G., Gallo, R.
C., and Wong-Staal, F. (1983). *303*, 253-256.
Haynes, B. F., Miller, S. E., Palker, T. J., Moore, J. O., Dunn,
P. H., Bolognesi, D. P., and Metzgar, R. S. (1983). *Proc.
Natl. Acad. Sci. USA 80*, 2054-2058.
Hayward, W. S., Neel, B. G., and Astrin, S. M. (1981). *Nature
(London) 290*, 475-480.
Kalyanaraman, V. S., Sarngadharan, M. G., Poiesz, B. J.,
Ruscetti, F. W., and Gallo, R. C. (1981a). *J. Virol. 38*,
906-915.
Kalyanaraman, V. S., Sarngadharan, M. G., Bunn, P. A., Minna,
J. D., and Gallo, R. C. (1981b). *Nature (London) 294*,
271-273.
Kalyanaraman, V. S., Sarngadharan, M. G., Nakao, Y., Ito, Y.,
Aoki, T., and Gallo, R. C. (1982a). *Proc. Natl. Acad. Sci.
USA 79*, 1653-1657.

Kalyanaraman, V. S., Sarngadharan, M. G., Robert-Guroff, M., Miyoshi, I., Blayney, D., Golde, D., and Gallo, R. C. (1982b). *Science (Washington, D.C.) 218*, 571-573.

Kaplan, H. (1974). *Ser. Haematol. 7*, 94-163.

Manzari, V., Wong-Staal, F., Franchini, G., Colombini, S., Gelmann, E. P., Oroszlan, S., Staal, S. P., and Gallo, R. C. (1983a). *Proc. Natl. Acad. Sci. USA 80*, 1574-1578.

Manzari, V., Gallo, R. C., Franchini, G., Westin, E., Ceccherin Nelli, L., Popovic, M., and Wong-Staal, F. (1983b). *Proc. Natl. Acad. Sci. USA 80*, 11-15.

Mier, J. W., and Gallo, R. C. (1980). *Proc. Natl. Acad. Sci. USA 77*, 6134-6138.

Miller, J. M., and Van der Maaten, M. J. (1980). *Cell Proliferation 7*, 901-910.

Miyoshi, I., Kubonishi, I., Sumida, M., Hiraki, S., Tsubota, T., Kimura, I., Miyamoto, K., and Sato, J. (1980). *Gann 71*, 155-156.

Miyoshi, I., Kubonishi, I., Yoshimoto, S., Akagi, T., Ohtsuki, Y., Shiraishi, Y., Nagata, K., and Hinuma, Y. (1981). *Nature (London) 294*, 770-771.

Morgan, D. A., Ruscetti, F. W., and Gallo, R. C. (1976). *Science (Washington, D.C.) 193*, 1007-1008.

Neel, B. G., Hayward, W. S., Robinson, H. L., Fang, J., and Astrin, S. M. (1981). *Cell 23*, 323-334.

Oroszlan, S., Sarngadharan, M. G., Copeland, T. D., Kalyanaraman, V. S., Gilden, R. V., and Gallo, R. C. (1982). *Proc. Natl. Acad. Sci. USA 79*, 1291-1294.

Poiesz, B. J., Ruscetti, F. W., Mier, J. W., Woods, A. M., and Gallo, R. C. (1980a). *Proc. Natl. Acad. Sci. USA 77*, 6815-6819.

Poiesz, B. J., Ruscetti, F. W., Gazdar, A. F., Bunn, P. A., Minna, J. D., and Gallo, R. C. (1980b). *Proc. Natl. Acad. Sci. USA 77*, 7415-7419.

Poiesz, B. J., Ruscetti, F. W., Reitz, M. S., Kalyanaraman, V. S., and Gallo, R. C. (1981). *Nature (London) 294*, 268-271.

Popovic, M., Reitz, M. S., Sarngadharan, M. G., Robert-Guroff, M., Kalyanaraman, V. S., Nakao, Y., Miyoshi, I., Minowada, J., Yoshida, M., Ito, Y., and Gallo, R. C. (1982). *Nature (London) 300*, 63-66.

Popovic, M., Sarin, P. S., Robert-Guroff, M., Kalyanaraman, V. S., Mann, D., Minowada, J., and Gallo, R. C. (1983). *Science (Washington, D.C.) 219*, 856-859.

Posner, L. E., Robert-Guroff, M., Kalyanaraman, V. S., Poiesz, B. J., Ruscetti, F. W., Bunn, P. A., Minna, J. D., and Gallo, R. C. (1981). *J. Exp. Med. 154*, 333-346.

Reitz, M. S., Poiesz, B. J., Ruscetti, F. W., and Gallo, R. C. (1981). *Proc. Natl. Acad. Sci. USA 78*, 1887-1891.

Reitz, M. S., Kalyanaraman, V. S., Robert-Guroff, M., Popovic, M., Sarngadharan, M. G., Sarin, P. S., and Gallo, R. C. (1983). *J. Infect. Dis. 147*, 399-405.

Rho, H. M., Poiesz, B. J., Ruscetti, F. W., and Gallo, R. C. (1981). *Virology 112*, 355-360.

Robert-Guroff, M., Nakao, Y., Notake, K., Ito, Y., Sliski, A., and Gallo, R. C. (1982). *Science (Washington, D.C.) 215*, 975-978.

Robert-Guroff, M., Kalyanaraman, V. S., Blattner, W. A., Popovic, Popovic, M., Sarngadharan, M. G., Maeda, M., Blayney, D., Catovsky, D., Bunn, P. A., Shibata, A., Nakao, Y., Ito, Y., Aoki, T., and Gallo, R. C. (1983). *J. Exp. Med.* , - .

Rous, P. (1911). *J. Exp. Med. 13*, 397-411.

Sarin, P. S., Aoki, T., Shibata, A., Ohnishi, Y., Aoyagi, Y., Miyakoshi, H., Emura, I., Kalyanaraman, V. S., Robert-Guroff, M., Popovic, M., Sarngadharan, M. G., Nowell, P. C., and Gallo, R. C. (1983). *Proc. Natl. Acad. Sci. USA 80*, in press.

Saxon, A., Stevens, R. H., and Golde, D. W. (1978). *Ann. Intern. Med. 88*, 323-326.

Schuepbach, J., Kalyanaraman, V. S., Sarngadharan, M. G., Blattner, W. A., and Gallo, R. C. (1983). *Cancer Res. 43*, 886-891.

Suchi, T., and Tajima, K. (1983). *In* "The Role of the Environment and Pathogenesis of Leukemias and Lymphomas" (I. T. McGrath, G. T. O'Conor, and B. Ramot, eds.), Raven, New York, in press.

Takatsuki, K., Uchiyama, T., Sagawa, K., and Yodoi, J. (1977). *Top. Hematol.*, pp. 73-77.

Takatsuki, K., Uchiyama, T., Ueshima, Y., and Hattori, T. (1979). *Jpn. J. Clin. Oncol. 9*, 317-324.

Uchiyama, T., Yodoi, J., Sagawa, K., Takatsuki, K., and Uchino, H. (1977). *Blood 50*, 481-492.

Wong-Staal, F., and Gallo, R. C. (1982). *In* "Leukemia" (F. Gunz, and E. Henderson, eds.), pp. 329-358. Grune & Stratton, New York.

Wong-Staal, F., Hahn, B., Manzari, V., Columbini, S., Franchini, G., Gelmann, E. P., and Gallo, R. C. (1983). *Nature (London) 302*, 626-628.

Yoshida, M., Miyoshi, I., and Hinuma, Y. (1982). *Proc. Natl. Acad. Sci. USA 79*, 2031-2035.

29

EPSTEIN–BARR VIRUS-INDUCED B-CELL LYMPHOMAS IN IMMUNE-DEFICIENT INDIVIDUALS [1]

David T. Purtilo, Shinji Harada, and Thomas Bechtold

Department of Pathology and Laboratory Medicine
University of Nebraska Medical Center
Omaha, Nebraska

Kiyoshi Sakamoto

IInd Department of Surgery
Kumamoto University Medical School
Kumamoto, Japan

Helen S. Maurer

Children's Memorial Hospital
Chicago, Illinois

[1] *This work was supported in part by a grant from the National Institutes for Health (CA 30196-01), American Cancer Society Rapid Development Grant, Nebraska Cigarette Tax Act, and the Lymphoproliferative Research Fund.*

I.   INTRODUCTION

Epidemiological studies by Denis Burkitt in Africa delineated a malignant lymphoma involving the jaw or visceral
organs of young children (Burkitt, 1958). Explanted tumor
grown in tissue culture by Epstein et al. (1964) was examined
by electron microscopy, and a unique herpesvirus was detected.
The Henles (1968) demonstrated that Epstein-Barr virus (EBV)
was the etiological agent of infectious mononucleosis (IM).
The virus has also been incriminated in nasopharyngeal carcinogenesis (Klein, 1975).

EBV has tropism for human B cells that results from the
presence of viral receptors (Henle et al., 1979). On entering
the cell, three antigens appear sequentially: EBV nuclear-
associated antigen (EBNA), early antigen (EA), and viral capsid antigen (VCA). The immune response to the antigens is
predictable and allows for assessment of the stage of the infection. Earliest antibody response is IgM anti-VCA, which is
transient. IgG anti-VCA appears shortly thereafter and persists throughout life. Anti-EA is transient and indicative of
active infection. Late appearing is anti-EBNA (Reedman et al.,
1973).

The description of Burkitt lymphoma and subsequent identification of EBV as the etiological agent of IM paved the way
to the recognition that immune-deficient individuals can develop a variety of life-threatening EBV-induced diseases. This
chapter summarizes the role of immune deficiency in EBV-induced
B-cell lymphomas and related diseases.

II.   MATERIALS AND METHODS

Our registries of X-linked lymphoproliferative syndrome,
fatal and chronic infectious mononucleosis, and familial lymphoproliferative malignancies were established to develop
diagnostic criteria and to investigate mechanisms of lymphomagenesis regarding immune deficiency, especially to EBV. Re-
ferrals of patients for study also include transplant recipients, male homosexuals with chronic lymphadenomegaly, and
various acquired and primary immune-deficiency syndromes.
Comprehensive clinical, immunological, virological, pathological, and genetic studies are possible because of collaborative
relationships. Cases summarized here were referred to our
registry and laboratory for study since 1978.

III.   RESULTS AND DISCUSSION

A.   X-Linked Lymphoproliferative Syndrome (XLP)

In 1969, one of us (D.T.P.) performed an autopsy on an
8-year-old boy who had succumbed to IM. Five other males in
the Duncan kindred had succumbed to related disorders. Study
of these six autopsies led to a description of X-linked recessive progressive combined variable immunodeficiency disease
(Duncan's disease) (Purtilo *et al.*, 1975). Subsequently, this

has been termed X-linked lymphoproliferative syndrome; this
generic name conveys the mode of inheritance and the major
phenotype.

The most frequent hematopathological findings of EBV-
induced lymphoproliferative diseases in immune-deficient XLP
patients include (1) presence of plasmacytoid lymphocytes in
peripheral blood smears, (2) elevated polyclonal Ig in serum,
and (3) a variety of B-cell lymphomas. Findings 1 and 2 are
seen in the fatal infectious mononucleosis (IM) phenotype of
XLP. Lymphoproliferative phenotypes range from monoclonal
malignancies, such as American Burkitt lymphoma, to polyclonal
fatal IM. In the agammaglobulinemia phenotype, extensive
necrosis of lymph nodes can be seen (Purtilo, 1980b). Aplastic
anemia can also be found associated with the IM phenotype.
This combination was always lethal.

Autopsy studies have revealed dynamic time-dependent
changes in the thymus gland. The thymus gland and peripheral
lymphoid tissues become hyperplastic for approximately 3 weeks
following onset of IM in patients with XLP. After about 3
weeks, destructive events often occur in the thymus gland:
multinucleated giant cells can be seen destroying Hassall's
epithelium. The finding of multinucleated giant cells in thymus raises the important question as to whether the destruction
of thymic epithelium is a virologically mediated or an immunologically mediated phenomenon. We think that virological me-
diation is unlikely to be involved: We have failed to infect
cultured thymic epithelium with EBV. Moreover, the normal thymus lacks receptors for Epstein-Barr virus (D. Volsky and
D. T. Purtilo, unpublished). After about 3 or 4 weeks of active IM, involution of the thymus gland and thymic-dependent
zones in the lymph nodes and spleen are observed. At autopsy,
after 3 weeks of illness, marked depletion of thymocytes is
found. Frequently, Hassall's epithelium may not be observed,
or calcified remnants may persist (Purtilo, 1980b).

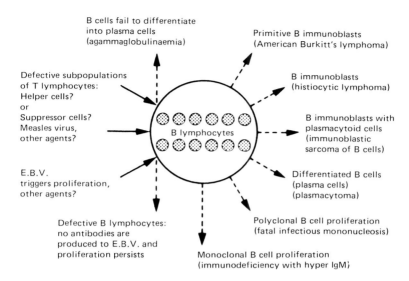

Fig. 1. Hypothesis regarding phenotypes and pathogenesis of X-linked lymphoproliferative syndrome. Epstein-Barr virus (EBV), on infecting males with X-linked lymphoproliferative syndrome (XLP), developed a variety of aproliferative or lymphoproliferative phenotypes depending on the functions of subpopulations of T-suppressor or helper cells. Published with permission of Lancet (Purtilo, 1976).

B. Hypothesis of Immunopathogenesis of Diverse Phenotypes of XLP following EBV Infection

In 1976 one of us (D.T.P.) had postulated that the pathogenesis and phenotypes of XLP could be explained by variable immune responses due to the defective lymphoproliferative control genetic focus on a maternal X chromosome (Purtilo, 1976). EBV was thought to trigger B-cell proliferation and to activate subpopulations of T cells. The individuals developing agammaglobulinemia were thought to develop this phenotype as a result of increased activity of suppressor T cells or lack of helper cells. In contrast, individuals developing the lymphoproliferative phenotypes were thought to have uncontrolled B-cell proliferation due to failure of suppression by T cells and lack

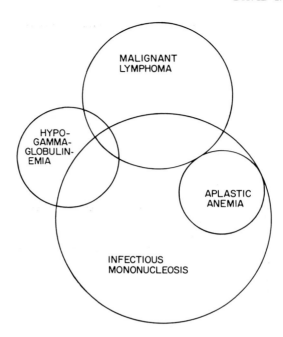

Fig. 2. Venn diagram illustrating the relative frequency
of phenotypes of X-linked lymphoproliferative syndrome. Note
that the relationship between infectious mononucleosis and
malignant lymphoma and between infectious mononucleosis and
hypogammaglobulinemia appears to be bidirectional. The hypogammaglobulinemia and aplastic anemia appear to be mutually
exclusive, suggesting different immunopathological mechanisms.
Published with the permission of Yorke publishers (Purtilo
et al., 1983).

of antibody production against EBV-specific antibodies
(Fig. 1).

Opportunities to test this hypothesis became possible when
the National Cancer Institute funded an international registry
of XLP. Figure 2 summarizes the phenotypes seen in the initial
100 cases (Purtilo *et al.*, 1982). The concordance of phenotypes offers clues to the pathogenesis of the phenotypes.
Eighty-two percent of the 100 individuals have succumbed. We
have extensively studied most of the surviving individuals.
Approximately two-thirds of the 100 cases have had life-

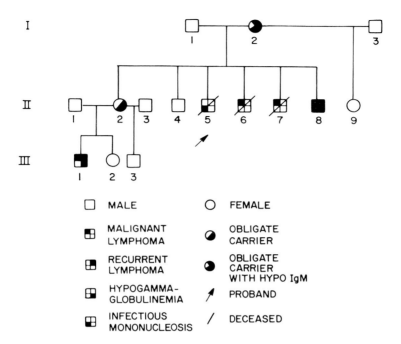

Fig. 3. Pedigree (phenotypic expressions) of family with X-linked lymphoproliferative syndrome. Various phenotypes have occurred in the patients with XLP. Two of the males survived and one of the mothers showed partial hypo-IgM (Maurer *et al.*, 1976).

threatening IM. Seventeen of individuals with IM have developed aplastic anemia, and all died. Nineteen individuals had hypogammaglobulinemia or agammaglobulinemia. This phenotype occurred following IM or may have preceded IM in a few cases. Approximately two thirds of the hypogammaglobulinemia cases occurred without an antecedent documented IM. Malignant lymphoma developed in 35 individuals, including 26 involving the terminal ileum. Other lymphomas were in extranodal sites as well. Nine of the cases appeared to have developed from chronic IM. The remaining cases showed no antecedent IM. The B-cell neoplasias ranged from American Burkitt lymphoma to plasmacytoma. In no instance was Hodgkin's disease found (Purtilo *et al.*, 1983).

Figure 3 depicts the current status of a kindred described by
Maurer *et al.* (1976), wherein three brothers and a maternally
related nephew had ML. In addition, another brother, summarized in the following section, had allegedly died of viral
hepatitis.

C. Typical Family Study: Case A

    This 18-year-old white male (Fig. 3, pedigree K4-II-5)
was admitted to a military hospital with cough, fever, malaise,
anorexia, and persistent vomiting for 1 week. He was treated
with penicillin and antiemetics without response. Past history
revealed severe measles with pneumonitis at 2, infections of
the eye at 8, and pneumonia at 14 and 17. The episode at 17
had occurred while in military training camp. Three brothers
and a nephew had ML (Fig. 3, pedigrees K4-II-6, II-7, II-8,
and III-1).

    He was well nourished, temperature 38°C, heart rate
108 beats/min, and blood pressure 120/70 mm Hg. His pharynx
was inflamed, and cervical lymphadenomegaly was noted. Neither
jaundice nor hepatosplenomegaly was detected.

    White blood count (WBC) was 9800/µl, hematocrit (Hct) 43%,
neutrophils 58%, lymphocytes 34%, eosinophils 3%, and monocytes
5%. Serum glutamic oxalacetic transaminase (SGOT) was 104 IU/
liter (slightly increased), and total bilirubin 4.4 with direct
reacting 2.0 mg/dl. Heterophile was 1:20. Three days later
WBC was 12,100/µl, with neutrophils 30%, lymphocytes 70%; 30%
were atypical, including plasma cells. Heterophile was 1:28,
total serum protein 6.7, and gammaglobulin 2.9 µg/dl.

    Chest X ray revealed interstitial pneumonitis. *Staphylo-
coccus aureus* was isolated from sputum and blood. Progressive
hepatosplenomegaly was noted. IM was not diagnosed, presumably
because the heterophile titer was only 1:28. He developed

mental confusion and jaundice. CSF contained a few atypical lymphocytes. On Day 11, Hct was 34% with 2.5% reticulocytes, SGOT 3600 IU/liter, and total bilirubin 16 with direct reacting 10 mg/dl. Exchange blood transfusions were to no avail; he expired on Day 20 of illness. Necropsy revealed generalized lymphadenomegaly with numerous immunoblasts, plasma cells, and focal necrosis. Thymus gland was not evaluated. Spleen weighed 550 g (160 g normal). The periarterial lymphoid sheath was necrotic, and immunoblastic proliferation with plasma cell differentiation was noted. The wrinkled, purple-gray liver weighed 1100 g (low normal). Intense periportal lymphoid infiltration was associated with massive hepatocytic necrosis. Numerous small lymphocytes and atypical lymphocytes invaded hepatic sinuses adjacent to necrotic cells. A prominent peribronchial lymphoid infiltration accounted for the interstitial pneumonitis.

Both the prosector and consultant pathologist attributed death to "acute viral hepatitis" (Maurer *et al.*, 1976). The prosector suggested malignant lymphoma (ML) as a primary diagnosis, whereas one consultant regarded immune deficiency as a factor. The family was studied for RNA tumor virus in 1974, but none was identified. Figure 1 and Table I summarizes the phenotypes of XLP, EBV-specific serology, and immune responses of family members. Normal values are as follows: serum IgG (750-2000 mg/dl), IgM (63-250 mg/dl), and IgA (84-462 mg/dl); mean antibody-dependent cellular cytotoxicity (ADDC) titer for normal persons is 1:1920, respectively. Other normal values in our laboratory include anti-VCA IgG 1:100, anti-EA <1:5, and anti-EBNA 1:54 (Sakamoto *et al.*, 1980; Purtilo, 1981).

Patient (II-8) had ML of the ileum at age 7 years in 1967 and recurrences at 11 and at 15 in abdominal lymph nodes (Table I). Treatment was successful with vincristine, cyclo-

TABLE I.

Pedigree number and date	Phenotype or disease	Age and sex	Serum Ig (mg/dl)		
			IgM	IgG	IgA
M.S. 1-2:					
10/20/71	Obligate	45 F	28	1170	218
1/28/79	carrier with		66	1085	180
2/14/80	hypo-IgM		69	1640	162
10/23/80		54	74	790	138
S.K. II-2:					
3/26/72	Obligate XLP	24 F	120	760	136
1/25/79	carrier		141	990	187
2/14/80			165	1305	249
II-4:					
1/20/79	Unaffected	29 M	220	840	210
F.P. II-5:					
6/17/71	Fatal IM	19 M+	n.d.	n.d.	n.d.
J.P. II-6:					
5/1/62	Malignant lymphoma, ileum, kidney, liver	3½	n.d.	n.d.	n.d.
II-7:					
4/6/66	Malignant lymphoma, liver, kidney, GI tract	6 M+	n.d.	n.d.	n.d.
C.P. II-8:					
12/14/67	Malignant lymphoma, ileum	7 M+			
	Recurrent ileal lymphoma	11	180	1275	300
	Recurrent lymphoma, testis, abdominal lymph nodes	15	48	850	108
	Chronic IM	18			
	Chronic bronchitis	19	26	640	82

| EBV-specific antibodies (GMT) | | | | | | | |
| VCA | | | EA | | | | |
IgM	IgG	IgA	DR	D	EBNA	ADCC	Comments
n.d.	n.d.	n.d.	n.d.	n.d.	n.d.	n.d.	Partial expression
<2	1280	160	40	40	40	3840	of XLP, hypo-IgM;
<2	2560	160	160	160	40	7680	active EBV infection,
<2	2560	80	160	160	20	n.d.	chronic bronchitis, smokes cigarettes
n.d.	n.d.	n.d.	n.d.	n.d.	n.d.	n.d.	Asymptomatic, partial
<2	160	5	<10	<10	80	960	expression of XLP,
<2	640	20	10	<10	40	3840	active EBV infection, chronic bronchitis, smokes cigarettes
<2	160	<2	<10	<10	40	n.d.	Normal male
n.d.	Heterophile 1:28, atypical lympho-cytosis						Thymus depletion, B-cell proliferation, massive hepatic necrosis
n.d.	Recurrent fever, died within one						
n.d.	Disseminated malignant lymphoma and peritonitis at autopsy						
							Treated with surgival removal, radiation, and chemotherapy
n.d.							
n.d.	1:2048	n.d.	n.d.	n.d.	n.d.	n.d.	Monospot positive, transient agranulo-cytosis
<2	320	<2	<10	<10	<2	2880	Is acquiring hypo-gammaglobulinemia

Table 1 (Continued)

Pedigree number and date	Phenotype or disease	Age and sex	Serum Ig (mg/dl)		
			IgM	IgG	IgA
R.P. II-9:					
3/26/72	At risk for being XLP carrier female	5 F	40	560	52
10/23/80		14	79	1030	108
F.P. III-1:					
6/15/69	Malignant lymphoma, ileum	2 M	n.d.	--	--
9/16/69	Malignant lymphoma, tonsil	2	n.d.	--	--
3/6/72	Pneumonia	4	18	<100	16
1/25/79	Agammaglobu-	11	20	150	14
2/14/80	linemia				
10/27/80					
D.P. III-2:					
3/6/72	At risk for	3 F	64	440	36
1/25/79	being car-	10			
10/23/80	rier 10 of XLP		68	1220	132
G.K. III-3:					
10/8/79	At risk for	6 mo.			
2/14/80	XLP	10 mo.			
10/22/80		M			

aAbbreviations: XLP, X-linked lymphoproliferative syndrome; F, female; M, male; EBV, Epstein-Barr virus; n.d., not done; VCA, viral capsid antigen; EA, early antigen; DR, diffuse and restricted patterns; EBNA, EB nuclear-associated antigen; +, death; IM, infectious mononucleosis.

| EBV-specific antibodies (GMT) | | | | | | | |
| VCA | | | EA | | | | |
IgM	IgG	IgA	DR	D	EBNA	ADCC	Comments
n.d.							Asymptomatic
n.d.							Treatment begun with
<2	80	<2	<10	<10	2	960	gammaglobulin
<2	40	<2	<10	<10	5		
n.d.							
<2	320	<2	<10	<10	n.d.		
<2	640	<2	<10	<10	320		
<2	40	<2	<10	<10	n.d.		Persisting maternal
<2	10	<2	<10	<10	<2		antibody?
<2	<5	<2	<10	<10	<2		Asymptomatic

phosphamide, methotrexate, cytosine arabinoside, and prednisone. However, fever, pharyngitis, cough, and weight loss had occurred for a 3-month period when he was 17. WBC was 86000/µl with neutrophils 10%, lymphocytes 88%, and 2% atypical lymphocytes. Heterophile screen test was positive, and anti-VCA IgG was markedly elevated to 1:2048. On July 28, 1978, WBC was reduced to 2800/µl with neutrophils 3% and lymphocytes 97%. The episodes of illness persisted for a year and then subsided.

Blood obtained on January 24, 1980 revealed slight reduction of T cells with 47% E rosettes, whereas normal numbers of B cells were present with 13% EAC rosettes, 5% surface IgM, and 4% IgD-bearing B cells. Natural killing at an effector:K562 target cell ratio of 50:1 was 30% (normal 25-75%).

A maternally related nephew (Fig. 3, pedigree K-4-III-1) had ML of the ileum treated with surgical resection at 2 in 1969. Details of the case are reported elsewhere (Maurer et al., 1976). Agammaglobulinemia was detected at 5 in 1972. Plasma therapy and antibiotics have maintained him. At age 2, malignant lymphoma of tonsils was diagnosed. The tonsillar mass showed immunoblastic proliferation with plasma cell differentiation and marked necrosis. He refused therapy, and gradually the tonsillar mass subsided. He exhibits active infection with EBV determined by spontaneous lymphoblastoid B-cell line formation of peripheral blood in vitro (Table I). Blood obtained on 24 January 1980, while he was asymptomatic, revealed 76% E rosettes, 13% EAC rosettes, and 5% surface IgM and 12% surface IgD-bearing cells. In vitro responses to phytohemagglutinin (PHA), streptolysin O, and mixed leukocyte responses were low. Natural killer of K562 was 27%. Both carrier mothers (Fig. 3, pedigrees K-4-I-2 and II-2, Table I) showed chronic active EBV infection with elevated anti-EA levels. This is probably a result of their having a partial immune defect of XLP (Sakamoto et al., 1982). Supporting this

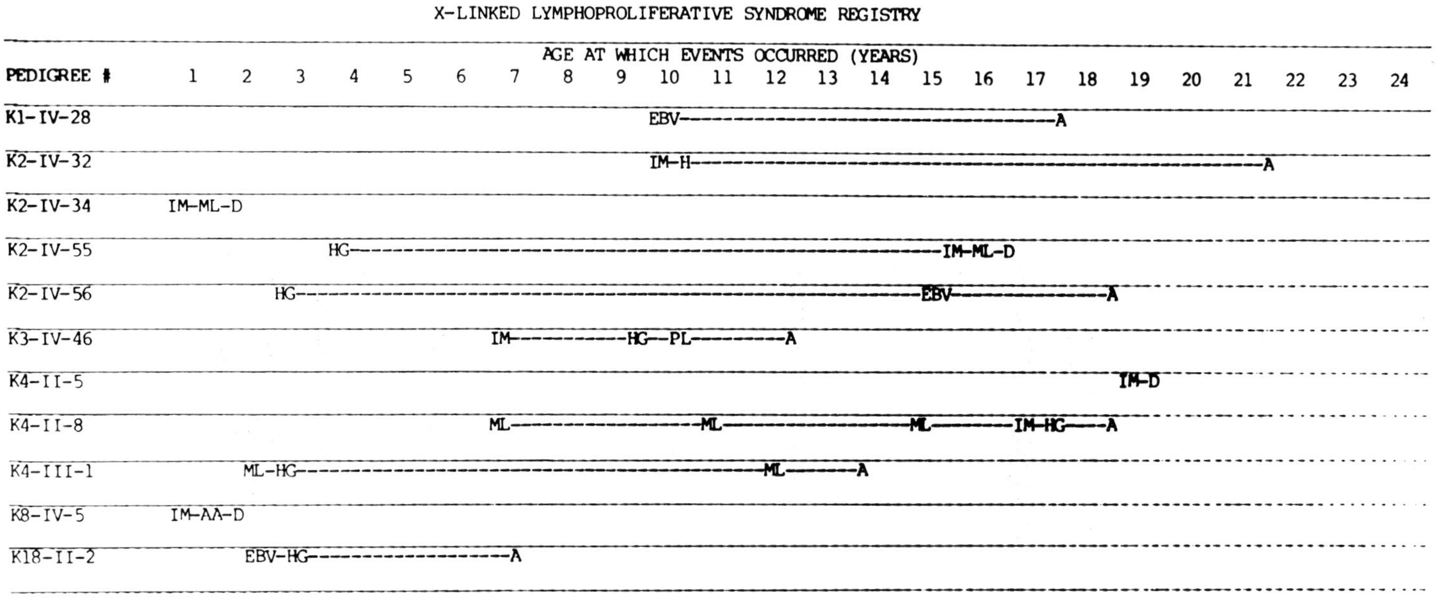

X-LINKED LYMPHOPROLIFERATIVE SYNDROME REGISTRY

Fig. 4. Chronological events in representative patients with X-linked lymphoproliferative syndrome from the Registry of XLP. K, kindred; EBV, Epstein-Barr virus; IM, infectious mononucleosis; HG, hypogammaglobulinemia; ML, malignant lymphoma; AA, aplastic anemia; PL, pseudolymphoma; D, death; A, alive; ?, status unknown. Published with the permission of Yorke publishers (Purtilo et al., 1983).

view, one mother (pedigree I-2) has partial IgM deficiency and low normal natural killing activity. The sole surviving brother (Fig. 3, pedigree K-4-II-4) is asymptomatic and has normal anti-EBNA and immunoglobulin levels.

The XLP registry includes 27 kindreds with more than 108 affected males (Portilo *et al.,* 1982).

Figure 4 summarizes several individuals in the XLP registry and their chronological events that have been documented. The clinical expressions of XLP probably depend on the individuals' immune competence to EBV during specific periods. For example, individual K1-IV-28 (Fig. 4) became infected by EBV in 1974 at age 10 years. Smoldering, but essentially asymptomatic EBV infection was present until age 18. Dramatically, he developed red cell aplasia. He was treated with gammaglobulin and red cell transfusion. One month after the onset of this episode, he developed generalized lymphadenomegaly, positive monospot test, and lymphocytosis. He showed marked activation of suppressor T cells, and gradually his immunity subdued EBV into latency again. Then he developed agammaglobulinemia, and red cell aplasia abated (not shown in Fig. 4) (D. T. Purtilo, unpublished).

Individual K2-V-19 had Burkitt lymphoma diagnosed involving his liver. His brother had succumbed to Burkitt lymphoma. The surviving brother developed fatal infectious mononucleosis many years after Burkitt lymphoma.

IV. NORMAL AND DEFICIENT IMMUNE RESPONSES TO EBV

Figure 5 summarizes the normal immune responses to EBV (Purtilo, 1981). This virus is estimated to have been present for millions of years. It probably arose from a common herpesvirus progenitor. The virus adapted to the C3d receptor on

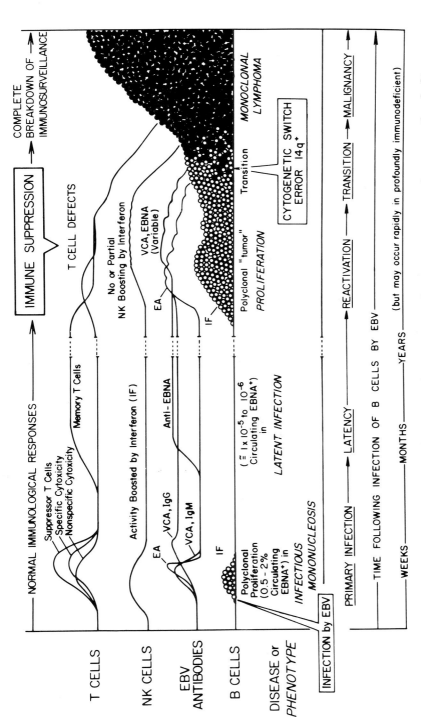

Fig. 5. Immune responses to Epstein–Barr virus. Normal responses are shown on the left, responses in immune-deficient individuals on the right. It is postulated that a cytogenetic error can convert polyclonal proliferation to monoclonal proliferation in individuals surviving subacute or chronic EBV infection with sustained B-cell proliferation. Published with permission of Academic Press.

human B cells or a nearby receptor on the lymphocyte. EBV
lives in relative harmony with humans and certain nonhuman
primates. Multiple fail-safe immune mechanisms have evolved
genetically under Darwinian evolutionary pressures to prevent
life-threatening diseases from occurring.

First-line defense against EBV infection is probably provided by natural killer cells (NK) (Fig. 5). Activity of these
cells is boosted by interferon (IF) *in vitro*, and IF is liberated *in vivo* by infected B cells. Suppressor T cells are activated and also suppress B-cell proliferation. Simultaneously, antibodies against EBV, EA, VCA, and membrane antigens develop. Late appearing are memory T cells and anti-EBNA antibodies, which persist throughout life. The virus persists in
latency throughout life.

Individuals with acquired or inherited immune suppression
may run the risk of developing life-threatening polyclonal
B-cell proliferation. The right side of the diagram of Fig. 5
shows events that may transpire in immune-deficient patients.
Individuals with severe immune defects will often succumb to a
polyclonal IM-like illness as a result of infiltration of vital
organs by infected B cells and responding lymphoid cells. In
contrast, individuals with more vigorous immunity may develop
indolent lymphoproliferation that with time could convert to a
monoclonal lymphoma vis-à-vis a cytogenetic error (Purtilo,
1981).

V. DOCUMENTATION OF EBV-INDUCED LYMPHOPROLIFERATIVE DISEASES
    IN IMMUNE-DEFICIENT PATIENTS

Failure to document that EBV could be responsible for lymphoproliferative diseases in immune-deficient patients resulted
from reliance on classical criteria for recognizing IM. Indi-

TABLE II. Documentation of Epstein-Barr Virus in Immune-
           Deficient Patients[a]

---

1. Polyclonal elevation of serum immunoglobulin

2. Atypical lymphocytosis especially with plasmacytoid forms

3. Positive monospot or heterophile of low titer

4. IgM anti-VCA (with acute infection) and anti-EBNA (lacking
    in severely immune-deficient children)

5. Too high or too low or limited range of EBV-specific anti-
    bodies

6. Spontaneous lymphoblastoid transformation of EBV-infected
    B cells in blood or tissues

7. EBNA staining of touch imprints of tissues

8. *In situ* EBV-DNA hybridization in tissue

9. EBV vDNA-DNA cRNA-DNA molecular hybridization of tissue

---

[a]*See ref.*

viduals with immune deficiency may not show the normal heterophile or monospot reactivity. Thus, specialized virological
and immunological studies are needed for diagnosis. Listed in
Table II are some of the findings (Purtilo, 1981).

In 1976 we postulated that individuals with XLP would show
deficient antibody production (Fig. 1) to the virus (Purtilo,
1976). Our studies have confirmed this postulate (Sakamoto *et
al.*, 1980, 1982). Males with XLP lack the capacity to produce
anti-EBNA. Anti-EBNA requires T-cell competence (Henle *et al.*,
1979). This finding has been useful in screening for males
with XLP. Thus far, no male at risk in a family with XLP who
has been capable of mounting an anti-EBNA titer of >1:10 has
developed the disease. Similarly, the finding of paradoxical
elevation of anti-EBV specific antigens in obligate carrier females has been useful in screening for carrier females (Sakamoto
et al., 1982) and for providing genetic counseling. The carrier females frequently show a moderate elevation IgG anti-VCA;

TABLE III.   Immune Findings of Patients with the X-Linked Lym-
            phoproliferative Syndrome

Defects

1. Incomplete EBV-specific antibody production: no anti-
    EBNA (mothers show elevated VCA, EA titers)

2. Poor development of EBV-specific memory T cells

3. Abnormal levels and ratios of OKT4 and OKT8 cells

4. Poor polyclonal Ig production *in vitro*

5. Deficient secondary response to OX174 *in vivo*:
    no IgM → IgG switch

6. Low NK cell activity (acquired defect)

7. Thymic epithelial destruction post-EBV infection

Normal

1. Normal WBC differential count when not acutely infected

2. Normal levels of OKT3-positive, Ia-positive, and surface
    Ig-positive cells

3. Normal proliferative responses to mitogens (PHA, PWM,
    EBV)

4. Normal primary response to OX174 *in vivo*

5. Normal IgM production by EBV-transformed B-cell lines

---

they also show persistent IgA anti-VCA, and many show anti-EA
(Table III).

    A second major facet of our hypothesis (Purtilo, 1976) re-
garding the pathogenesis of phenotypes of XLP was that an immunoregulatory defect was responsible for the various expressions following EBV infection. Evaluation of lymphocytes from
blood using routine cell surface markers of lymphocytes of 15
surviving males with XLP has failed to show abnormalities. For
example, the surviving males show normal numbers of sheep
erythrocyte rosetting cells, and the B cells show normal numbers containing IgM and IgD markers. However, using monoclonal
OKT antibodies reveals significant abnormalities in numbers of

subpopulations of T cells (Seeley *et al.,* 1981). Noteworthy is the increased proportion of lytic/suppressor OKT 8-bearing cells. The surviving males after EBV infection have shown a decreased T4 helper/inducer to T8 suppressor/lytic populations (Fig. 6).

Functional assays including responses to PHA show diminished proliferative responses in the affected males (Table III). Similarly, responses to pokeweek mitogen (PWM) showed impaired proliferative responses. When EBV is used as a mitogen, a slight depression in proliferative responses is found. IgG synthesis *in vitro* by lymphocytes from the patients with XLP showed more marked defects, especially in response to PWM. Response to PWM requires T-cell help for production of IgG. The lymphoblastoid cell lines of the patient show normal production of immunoglobulins, thus suggesting that T-cell factors influence the production of Ig *in vitro* from fresh whole blood (D. T. Purtilo *et al.,* unpublished).

NK cells are thought to be a major deterrent against viral infection, and some investigators have proposed that they provide immune surveillance against tumors. Our initial assessment of NK activity in 13 males with XLP revealed that 80% showed diminished cytotoxicity, and boosting by interferon was minimal (Sullivan *et al.,* 1980). Despite these NK defects, these males were asymptomatic at the time of study. This finding suggests that NK activity may not be vital in controlling lymphoproliferation.

Prospective studies of males at risk for XLP suggests that an immunoregulatory defect occurs prior to EBV infection. This immunoregulatory defect is probably responsible for their failure to control B-cell proliferation. EBV is unique in that it infects the immune system and relies on normal immunoregulatory responses to control the proliferation of B cells. Individuals with immunoregulatory disturbances may be at a great risk for

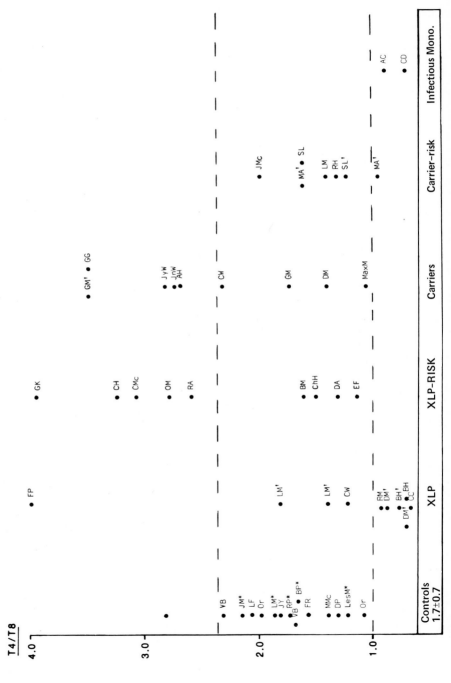

Fig. 6. Ratio of OKT4 helper/inducer to KT8 suppressor/lytic positive lymphocytes in XLP family members and controls. Dots indicate individual donors; circled dots indicate family members; other symbols represent individual values of donors tested more than once. The area between the two horizontal lines represents ±2 S.D. from the mean of the control group.

life-threatening diseases following infection.   The NK defect appears to be acquired (Table III) (Seeley et al., 1982). Males with XLP also show defective T-cell cytotoxicity when assessed by measuring their immune T-cell responses to autologous EBV-infected B cells in an outgrowth assay (Harada et al., 1983).   XLP is an X-linked recessive progressive combined variable immunodeficiency disease (Purtilo et al., 1975).

VI.   PRIMARY IMMUNODEFICIENCY DISORDERS AND LYMPHOMAGENESIS

The immunodeficiency-Cancer Registry (Spector et al., 1978) now contains more than 300 cases with immune deficiency and cancer.   Approximately 60% of the cases are lymphoproliferative malignancies.   Hodgkin's disease is markedly underrepresented, as are carcinomas found commonly in the general population.   The lymphoproliferative malignancies include a spectrum ranging from Burkitt lymphoma through histiocytic lymphoma. Noteworthy is the relative lack of malignancy in individuals with X-linked agammaglobulinemia.   Perhaps the reason for this is that their cells lack receptors for EBV and are not thereby capable of being transformed by the virus (Purtilo, 1981).

None of the primary immune-deficiency patients listed in the WHO classification have been reported to succumb to IM. However, they are at high risk for developing B-cell neoplasia. Our preliminary studies measuring EBV-specific antibody titers in 100 patients with primary immune deficiency reveal various immune defects (D. T. Purtilo et al., unpublished).   For example, individuals with severe combined immune deficiency may completely lack antibody response to the virus.   Individuals with combined immune defects such as ataxia telangiectasia or Wiskott-Aldrich syndrome may show elevated titers.

Comprehensive studies to assess the role of EBV by using multiple techniques have revealed EBV genome in lymphoproliferative disorders in patients with XLP, ataxia telangiectasia (Saemundsen *et al.*, 1982), severe combined immunodeficiency following thymic epithelial transplant (Reece *et al.*, 1981), IgM deficiency (Purtilo *et al.*, 1982), and common variable immunodeficiency (Purtilo, 1981a).

Perhaps the reason that individuals with XLP are more vulnerable to life-threatening lymphoproliferative diseases as compared to other individuals with primary immune deficiency is that immunoregulatory defects are more profound in XLP. Nearly all males having the XLP locus will manifest one of the phenotypes of the syndrome. This includes approximately two thirds with IM phenotypes and 35% with malignant lymphoma. In contrast, approximately 4% of individuals with other immunodeficiency disorders show malignant lymphoproliferative diseases (Spector *et al.*, 1978), and none has exhibited fatal IM.

VII. MALIGNANCIES IN ORGAN TRANSPLANT RECIPIENTS

Beginning in the late 1960s, Penn and Starzl began to report increased frequency of cancer in renal transplant recipients (RTR). Four types of cancers occur at increased frequency in this population: (1) carcinoma of skin and lips, (2) B-cell lymphoma, (3) carcinoma of uterine cervix, and (4) Kaposi's sarcoma (Purtilo, 1981). All of these malignancies can potentially be due to ubiquitous viruses. One of us (D.T.P.) has speculated that defects in the immune surveillance may allow viruses to be opportunistic and to induce the malignancies.

EBV-induced lymphoproliferative diseases in renal transplant recipients occur in approximately 1 in 100 patients

TABLE IV.   Epstein-Barr Virus-Induced Lymphoproliferative
            Diseases in Renal Transplant Recipients

---

1. 1 in 100 patients develop "lymphoma" or IM

2. Hodgkin's diseases underrepresented

3. Located extranodal, CNS

4. Incubation brief (weeks) disseminated versus long (years) localized

5. EBNA, EBV genome positive

6. Polyclonal, usually

7. Cytogenetics, generally diploid

8. Survival dismal

9. Therapy acyclovir, interferon, serum

10. Other cancers overrepresented including Kaposi's sarcoma, squamous cell carcinoma, and uterine cervical carcinoma

---

(Hanto *et al.,* 1981) (Table IV).   Hodgkin's disease is under-represented in this group.   The malignant lymphomas tend to be located in extranodal sites and in the central nervous system. The incubation period following renal transplantation may be brief (weeks) in the disseminated forms versus long (years) in the localized malignancies (Hanto *et al.,* 1981).   The young RTR tends to develop disseminated IM-like disease in response to primary EBV infection, whereas the older age RTRs develop solid lymphomatous masses.   The lymphoproliferation will contain EBNA, and EBV genome was found in all of the cases we have examined (Saemundsen *et al.,* 1981).   Generally the cases have been polyclonal; however, two have appeared to be in transition to monoclonality.   The survival rate is dismal in these individuals.

In addition to renal transplant patients, cardiac homograft recipients (G. Klein, personal communication) and one bone marrow transplant recipient (Schubach *et al.,* 1983) have exhibited EBV-carrying lymphoproliferative malignancies. Also, two patients receiving therapy for acute lymphoblastic leukemia have been shown to have EBV-associated lymphoproliferative diseases (Look *et al.*, 1981; D. T. Purtilo *et al.*, unpublished).

VIII. LYMPHOMAGENESIS IN THE ACQUIRED IMMUNE DEFICIENCY SYNDROME (AIDS)

Promiscuous male homosecuals have displayed AIDS. Opportunistic infections, Kaposi's sarcoma, and malignant B-cell lymphomas are occurring at an alarming rate. EBV genome has been isolated from several of the lymphomas (Marmor *et al.*, 1982).[2] Female prostitutes may be protected from similar consequences because of the immunological superiority of females as compared to males (Purtilo and Sullivan, 1979). Drawing on our experience in studying EBV in patients with life-threatening EBV-induced lymphoproliferative diseases, we propose that acquired defects in immunity to EBV are responsible for some of the lymphomas in men with AIDS. We have observed multiple immune defects including inversion of T4:T8 ratios and EBV-specific defects in 145 males with AIDS (J. Sonnabend, D. Abrams, and D. T. Purtilo, unpublished).

The findings of EBV-induced lymphoproliferative diseases in individuals with primary and acquired immunodeficiency suggest to us that the immune competence of an individual determines the outcome of EBV infections (Purtilo *et al.*, 1981b). This phenomenon may also be important in the pathogenesis of Burkitt lymphomagenesis.

---

[2] *AIDS has received much attention in the press. For example, see Science 217, 618 (1982) "New Disease Baffles Medical Community."*

IX.   HYPOTHESIS OF BURKITT LYMPHOMAGENESIS

        Two major hypotheses attempt to explain the role of EBV
in Burkitt lymphoma. One hypothesis proposes that the virus
is simply a passenger that enters B cells following transformation by some other agent. An alternative hypothesis considers that an immune defect, either genetically or environmentally induced, allows escape of EBV-infected B cells from
immune surveillance. We favor the latter hypothesis.

        Several empirical observations suggest to us that immune
deficiency could render an individual susceptible to Burkitt
lymphomagenesis (Purtilo, 1980a). For example, the African
child becomes infected with EBV within months following disappearance of maternal antibodies; in other words, between 6 and
9 months of age, approximately 80% seroconvert. Second, the
individuals at risk are often immunosuppressed by malaria,
malnutrition, and parasites, and they usually are males. The
males show less immune competence than do females (Purtilo and
Sullivan, 1979). The findings of EBV-induced lymphoproliferative diseases in the immuno-deficient renal transplant patients
and individuals with primary immune deficiency also suggest
that immune surveillance is an important deterrent to Burkitt
lymphomagenesis and other EBV-induced lymphoproliferative
diseases. The cotton-topped marmoset is relatively immune deficient to EBV and is the experimental model for Burkitt lymphomagenesis. These animals lack antibody responses, and their
lymphoproliferative diseases mimic those found in XLP (Purtilo,
1981). Finally, the spectrum of diseases induced by EBV in
XLP, ranging from IM to Burkitt lymphoma, suggest that the host
immune response is important in determining the outcome of EBV
infection.

        George Klein (1979) has considered three steps in the
pathogenesis of Burkitt lymphoma in Africa: (1) EBV transforms

B cells and immortalizes them at an arrested stage of development; (2) an environmental factor (i.e., holoendemic malaria) promotes proliferation of the B cells; and (3) a cytogenetic error (i.e., 14q+) emerges randomly and endows the cell with advantages of survival over the normal diploid cells. We concur with Klein's postulates, except that we regard immune deficiency as an important cofactor in allowing the infected B cells to continue proliferating. Moreover, we consider that there is a continuous spectrum of EBV-induced lymphoproliferative diseases ranging from IM to Burkitt lymphoma. The cytogenetic events and the host T-cell responses are responsible for the differences in the clinical and laboratory manifestations of the infection. The immunoglobulin phenotype of Burkitt lymphoma is determined by the location of the breakpoint and translocation where the Ig locus resides (Rowley, 1982).

The precise role of individual variability of immune responses to EBV, and of genetic and environmental factors, which are important in determining whether EBV infection produces nasopharyngeal carcinoma, Burkitt lymphoma, or infectious mononucleosis, need to be further elaborated by prospective studies. Figure 7 summarizes expressions of EBV virus infection that seems to be determined by age, social class, and immune competence (Purtilo and Sakamoto, 1982).

X. THERAPY FOR EBV-INDUCED LYMPHOPROLIFERATIVE DISEASES IN
    IMMUNE-DEFICIENT PATIENTS

Prevention of life-threatening EBV-induced diseases can be achieved by genetic counseling of individuals at risk for primary immunodeficiency. A rational basis for treatment of individuals with immunodeficiency and severe EBV infection is by

FACTORS WHICH DETERMINE
EPSTEIN-BARR VIRUS-INDUCED
DISEASES:

Normal, physiologic immunosuppression of pregnancy
reactivates virus, anti-
bodies become elevated and
virus is excreted in saliva.
Infants in low social class,
multisib families become
infected early and higher
class, small sibship
families are infected
later in childhood or
during early adulthood.

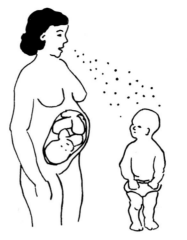
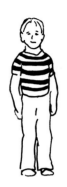

PERIOD OF LIFE CYCLE (AGE):

PERCENT SEROPOSITIVE:
IMMUNOCOMPETENT PERSONS:

IMMUNODEFICIENT PATIENTS:

	IN-UTERO	6-60 MOS	6-10 YEARS
	60-85%	0-60%	30-70%
	Elevated maternal antibodies protect fetus & newborn.	Vulnerable to silent primary infection from pregnant mother or others.	Relatively resistent to infectious mononucleosis.
	Rarely, in-utero infection or infected in sero-negative mothers late in pregnancy causes birth defects?	Fatal infectious mononucleosis, acquired agammaglobulinemia or malignant B cell lymphoma.	Fatal infectious mononucleosis, malignant lymphoma or acquired agammaglobulinemia.

Fig. 7. Hypothesis regarding the impact of age, immune
competence, and social class in the outcome of EBV-related
diseases. Published with the permission of Medical Hypothesis
(Purtilo and Sakamoto, 1982).

enhancing immunity and providing antiviral therapy; for example,
high-titer gammaglobulin may be of value. Burkitt lymphoma and
phenotypes of XLP do not occur before 4 or 5 months of age,
presumably because of neutralizing antibodies from maternal
blood. Immunotherapy with interferon would be of potential
value by boosting NK activity, interfering with viral replica-

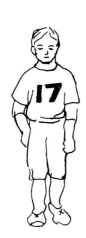 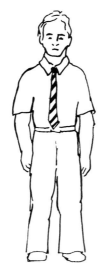 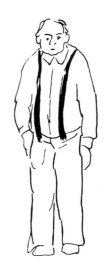

II-I7 YEARS

50-75%
Vulnerable to
infectious mono-
nucleosis if sero
negative.

Malignant lymph-
oma or fatal in-
fectious mono-
nucleosis.

18-35 YEARS

60-80%
Vulnerable to
infectious mono-
nucleosis if sero-
negative.

Hodgkin's Disease?
B cell lymphomas
relatively less
common.

36-85 YEARS

85-90%
Lifelong immunity
is protective.

Acquired immuno-
deficiency (i.e.,
renal transplant)
polyclonal B cell
lymphoma, Hodgkin's
disease is uncommon.

tion, and preventing lymphoproliferation. Antiviral therapy
with Acycloguanosine has been disappointing thus far (Hanto
et al., 1982b; Sullivan *et al.*, 1982). Development of immuno-
suppressive agents for homograft transplantation that will not
allow EBV and other viruses to reactivate is needed to prevent
life-threatening viral infections. The correction of the im-

mune defect in children with inherited immune deficiency may become possible by transplantation of bone marrow or thymus. Insertion of genes to correct mutant immune response genes may also eventually be employed to correct defects permanently in individuals with inherited immune deficiency.

Study of patients with immunodeficiency for opportunistic viral oncogenesis by ubiquitous viruses has been useful in elucidating the role of viruses in oncogenesis and the mechanisms responsible for expression of these disorders. For example, we have recognized a continuous spectrum of EBV-induced diseases in immune-deficient individuals ranging from benign to malignant. Similarly, one might anticipate that other ubiquitous viruses may produce a comparable spectrum of diseases. We are optimistic that many of the diseases including the malignancies caused by viruses may be preventable in the near future.

REFERENCES

Burkitt, D. P. (1958). *Br. J. Surg. 46,* 218-223.
Epstein, M. A., Achong, B. G., and Barr, Y. M. (1964). *Lancet i,* 702-703.
Hanto, D. W., Sakamoto, K., Purtilo, D. T., Simmons, R. L., and Najarian, J. S. (1981). *Surgery 90,* 204-213.
Hanto, D. W., Sakamoto, K., Sullivan, J. L., Simmons, R. L., and Najarian, J. S. (1981). *Cancer Res. 41,* 4253-4261.
Hanto, D., Frizzera, G., Gajl-Peczalska, K. J., Sakamoto, K., Purtilo, D. T., Balfour, H. H., Simmons, R. L., and Najarian, J. S. (1982). *N. Engl. J. Med. 306,* 913-918.
Harada, S., Sakamoto, K., Seeley, J. K., and Purtilo, D. T. (1983). *Int. J. Cancer 216,* 739-744.
Henle, W., Henle, G., and Lennette, E. L. (1979). *Sci. Am. 241,* 48-59.
Klein, G. (1975). *N. Engl. J. Med. 293,* 1353-1357.
Klein, G. (1979). *Proc. Natl. Acad. Sci. USA 76,* 2442-2446.
Look, A. T., Naegele, R. F., Calihan, T., Herrod, H. G., and Henle, W. (1981). *Cancer Res. 41,* 4280-4283.

Marmor, M., Labenstein, L., William, D. C., Friedman-Kien, A.
E., Byrum, R. D., D'Onofrio, S., and Dubin, N. (1982).
Lancer i, 1083-1088.
Maurer, H. S., Gotoff, S. P., Allen, L., and Bolan, J. (1976).
Cancer (Amsterdam) 37, 2224-2231.
Purtilo, D. T. (1976). *Lancet ii*, 882-885.
Purtilo, D. T. (1980a). *Lancet i*, 300-303.
Purtilo, D. T. (1980b). *Pathol. Annu.* , - .
Purtilo, D. T. (1981). *Adv. Cancer Res. 34*, 279-312.
Purtilo, D. T., and Sakamoto, K. (1981). *Hum. Pathol. 13*,
43-46.
Purtilo, D. T., and Sakamoto, K. (1982). *Med. Hypotheses 8*,
401-408.
Purtilo, D. T., and Sullivan, J. L. (1979). *Am. J. Dis. Child.
133*, 1251-1253.
Purtilo, D. T., Cassel, C., Yang, J. P. S., Stephenson, S. R.,
Harper, R., Landing, G. H., and Vawter, G. F. (1975).
Lancet i, 935-941.
Purtilo, D. T., Sakamoto, K., Saemundsen, A. K., Sullivan,
J. L., Synnerholm, A. C., Anvret, M., Pritchard, J.,
Sloper, C., Sieff, C., Pincott, J., Pachman, L., Rich, K.,
Cruzi, F., Cornet, J., Collins, R., Barnes, N., Knight, J.,
Sandstedt, B., and Klein, G. (1981a). *Cancer Res. 41*,
4226-4236.
Purtilo, D. T., Liao, S. A., Sakamoto, K., Snyder, L. M.,
DeFlorio, D., Bhawan, J., Paquin, L., Yang, J. P. S.,
Hutt-Fletcher, L. M., Muralidharan, K., Raffa, P.,
Saemundsen, A. K., and Klein, G. (1981b). *Cancer Res. 41*,
4248-4252.
Purtilo, D. T., Sakamoto, K., Barnabei, V., Seeley, J. K.,
Bechtold, T., Rogers, G., Yetz, J., and Harada, S. (1982).
Am. J. Med. 73, 49-56.
Reece, E. R., Gartner, J. G., Seemayer, T. A., Joncas, J. H.,
and Pagano, J. S. (1981). *Cancer Res. 41*, 4243-4247.
Reedman, A. M., and Klein, G. (1973). *Int. J. Cancer 11*,
499-500.
Rowley, J. D. (1982). *Science (Washington, D.C.) 216*, 749-751.
Saemundsen, A. K., Purtilo, D. T., Sakamoto, K., Sullivan, J.
L., Synnerholm, A. C., Hanto, D., Simmons, R., Anvret, M.,
Collins, R., and Klein, G. (1981). *Cancer Res. 41*, 4237-
4242.
Sakamoto, K., Freed, H., and Purtilo, D. T. (1980). *J. Im-
munol. 125*, 921-925.
Sakamoto, K., Seeley, J. K., Lindsten, T., Sexton, J., Yetz, J.,
Ballow, M., and Purtilo, D. T. (1982). *J. Immunol. 128*,
904-907.
Schubach, W. H., Hackman, R., Neiman, P. E., Miller, G., and
Thomas, E. D. (1983). *Blood,* in press.

Seeley, J. K., Sakamoto, K., Ip, S. H., Hansen, P. W., and
      Purtilo, D. T. (1981). *J. Immunol. 127,* 2618-2620.
Seeley, J. K., Bechtold, T., Lindsten, T., and Purtilo, D. T.
      (1982). *In* "Natural Cell Mediated Immunity" (R. Herberman,
      ed.), Vol. 2, pp. 1211-1218. Academic Press, New York.
Spector, B., Perry, G., and Kersey, J. (1978). *Clin. Immunol.
      Immunopathol. 11,* 12-2.
Sullivan, J. L., Byron, K., Brewster, F., and Purtilo, D. T.
      (1980). *Science (Washington, D.C.) 210,* 543-545.
Sullivan, J. L., Byron, K. S., Brewster, F. E., Sakamoto, K.,
      Shaw, J. E., and Pagano, J. J. (1982). *Am. J. Med. July
      20,* 262-266.

30

THE RELATIONSHIP OF HEPATITIS B AND RELATED VIRUSES (HEPADNA VIRUSES) TO HEPATOCELLULAR CARCINOMA

*William S. Robinson, Roger H. Miller,
and Patricia L. Marion*

Stanford University School of Medicine
Stanford, California

I.   INTRODUCTION

Hepatitis B virus (HBV) is one of the most common and interesting human hepatitis viruses. Investigation of HBV during
the 1970s revealed unique antigenic, ultrastructural, molecular, and biological features that distinguished it from members
of all of the recognized virus groups. One of the most notable
features of this virus was its DNA structure. Virions contain
small circular DNA molecules (Robinson *et al.*, 1974) that are
partly single-stranded (Summers *et al.*, 1975; Landers *et al.*,

1977; Hruska *et al.*, 1977), and a DNA polymerase in the virion
(Kaplan *et al.*, 1973; Robinson and Greenman, 1974) can repair
the DNA to make it fully double-stranded (Summers *et al.*, 1975;
Landers *et al.*, 1977). Among the unique biological features
are its liver tropism (Murphy *et al.*, 1975) and the common occurrence of persistent infection with viral antigen and infectious virus in high concentrations in the blood (Barker and
Murray, 1972; Barker *et al.*, 1975; Shikata *et al.*, 1977;
Scullard *et al.*, 1982) continuously for years. This pattern
of infection accounts for the common transmission of HBV by
percutaneous transfer of serum and serum-containing material.
Several disease syndromes in addition to acute hepatitis may
occur during acute and chronic HBV infection. Included are a
serum sickness-like syndrome, membranous glomerulonephritis,
and necrotizing vasculitis (polyarteritis), all probably related to viral antigen-antibody complex-mediated tissue injury
(Gocke, 1975). In addition, persistent infection can be associated with near normal liver or with chronic hepatitis. The
latter may be severe and progressive, and lead to cirrhosis
and in some cases hepatocellular carcinoma (Szmuness, 1978).
Its narrow host range (confined to humans and a few higher
primates) and failure so far to infect tissue culture cells
have made it difficult to investigate some questions about HBV.

    Although for several years HBV was considered to be a
unique virus, similar viruses have been found in three different animal species. The first, woodchuck hepatitis virus
(WHV), discovered in 1978 in sera of eastern woodchucks
(*Marmota monax*), a member of the Sciuridae or squirrel family,
by Summers, Smolec, and Snyder (1978b), after Snyder had observed that the most frequent cause of death in captive woodchucks in the Philadelphia Zoo was hepatocellular carcinoma accompanied by chronic hepatitis. The third member of this virus
family, ground squirrel hepatitis virus (GSHV), was found in

the Beechey ground squirrel (*Spermophilus beecheyi*), another
genus of the Sciuridae family by Marion *et al.* (1980b). The
observation of frequent hepatomas in a species of domestic
ducks in the People's Republic of China led to the discovery
of the fourth member of this virus family, now called duck
hepatitis B virus (DHBV), in sera from ducks in China by
Summers, London, Sun, Blumberg *et al.* (unpublished). A similar
virus has been found in Pekin ducks (*Anas domesticus*) in the
United States (Mason *et al.*, 1980). HBV and the three related
viruses of lower animals share unique ultrastructural, molecular, antigenic, and biological features, and this virus
family has been called the hepadna virus group (Robinson, 1980).
The evidence for a relationship between infection with these
viruses and hepatocellular carcinoma (HCC) will be reviewed
here. The antigenic, molecular, and ultrastructure of these
viruses and their biological properties have been reviewed in
detail elsewhere (Marion and Robinson, 1983).

II. EPIDEMIOLOGICAL ASSOCIATION OF HEPADNA VIRUS INFECTION
    AND HEPATOCELLULAR CARCINOMA (HCC)

HCC in humans has a worldwide distribution and numerically
is one of the major cancers in the world today. Although HCC
is rare in many parts of the world, it occurs commonly in sub-
Saharan Africa, eastern Asia, Japan, Oceania, Greece, and Italy.
In certain areas of Asia and Africa, it is the most common cancer. Geographical areas with the highest incidence of HCC are
also areas where persistent HBV infections occur at the highest
known frequencies. Within the limits of the data available,
there appears to be a good correlation between geographical
distribution of HCC and active HBV infection, with the highest
frequency of both being sub-Saharan Africa and eastern Asia

(Szmuness, 1978). In addition, hepatitis B surface antigen
(HBsAg), a marker of active HBV infection, has been found four
to six times more frequently in serum of patients with HCC than
in tumor-negative controls in both high-HCC incidence and low-
HCC incidence geographical areas (Szmuness, 1978). An ongoing
prospective study of 22,707 male government workers in Taiwan,
15% of whom were HBsAg positive, revealed the incidence of HCC
to be more than 300 times higher in HBsAg-positive than in
HBsAg-negative individuals (Beasley *et al.*, 1981). Three percent of HBsAg-positive patients 50 years or older developed HCC
per year, and 43% of all deaths in HBsAg carriers 40 years or
older were due to HCC.

The high incidence of persistent HBV infection in mothers
of HCC patients, in contrast to that in fathers (Larouze *et
al.*, 1976), suggests that transmission from mothers to newborn
or infant children may be a frequent mode and may be the time
of HBV infection in HCC patients. The finding of low HBsAg
titers, together with the rare occurrence of HB core antigen
(HBcAg) and HB e-antigen (HBeAg) in most patients (Nishioka
et al., 1973; Szmuness, 1978) also suggests that the persistent
infections in HCC patients are of long duration. If HBV infection does occur frequently at very early ages in HCC patients,
the age distribution of patients when the tumors were clinically recognized in high-incidence areas (Steiner, 1960) would
suggest that tumors appear after a mean duration of approximately 35 to 40 years of HBV infection. Very few cases of HCC occur in children (Steiner, 1960). Between 60 and 90% of HCC patients have coexisting cirrhosis (Steiner, 1960; Trichopoulos
et al., 1975; Peters, 1976; Beasley *et al.*, 1981) suggesting
that this lesion in association with persistent HBV infection
may predispose to HCC, although clearly the presence of cirrhosis is not an absolute requirement. Epidemiological data de-

fining the association of HCC and persistent HBV infection have been reviewed in detail (Szmuness, 1978; Kew, 1978), and these data represent strong evidence for an important role of HBV in HCC formation in humans.

HCC appears to occur even more frequently in WHC-infected captive woodchucks (Summers *et al.*, 1978b). In two colonies of woodchucks in the United States, approximately one third of animals persistently infected with WHV have been observed to develop HCC per year. All such animals have histological findings of moderately severe active hepatitis and moderately high levels of DNA-containing virions and WHsAg in their serum. No hepatomas have developed in uninfected animals.

GSHV-infected ground squirrels have a dramatically different disease response. Although the rate of persistent infection is very high in endemic areas (up to 52%), and levels of DNA-containing virions and GSHsAg in serum are always unusually high (Marion *et al.*, 1980b), little or no hepatitis and no HCC have been observed in infected animals (Marion and Robinson, 1983b).

III. THE OCCURRENCE AND STATE OF HBV IN HCC TISSUE

Immunofluorescent and immunoperoxidase staining of tumor tissue has demonstrated that in patients with HBsAg and/or HBcAg, tumor cells appear most often to be negative, although some studies have reported small numbers of positive cells in some tumors (reviewed by Kew, 1978). HBsAg has also been reported to have been detected infrequently by immunoperoxidase staining in tumors of patients without HBsAg in the blood (Peters *et al.*, 1977).

Viral DNA has also been found in HCC tissue. Lutwick and Robinson (1977) found viral DNA base sequences in DNA extracted from tumor tissue of a single patient in the United States with HBsAg in the blood (although significantly less than in nontumorous tissue of infected patients) and no viral DNA base sequences in the DNAs of two HCCs from HBsAg-negative patients. Summers *et al.* (1978a) found HBV DNA base sequences in the DNAs extracted from 9 of 10 African HCC patients with HBsAg in the blood and in one of four tumors of patients who were HBsAg negative.

With the development of methods to cleave DNAs at specific sites with restriction endonucleases, separate the resulting DNA fragments by gel electrophoresis, and transfer them to nitrocellulose or other solid media for hybridization with radiolabeled DNA probes (Southern, 1975), and to clone specific DNA fragments in bacterial cells, more definitive analysis of the state of viral DNA in HCC tissue has been possible. In addition to free or episomal unit length HBV DNA in HCC tissue from some HBsAg-positive patients, evidence for viral DNA sequences integrated in tumor cell DNA has also been found by several investigators (Brechot *et al.*, 1980, 1981; Chakraborty *et al.*, 1980; Edman *et al.*, 1980; Koshy *et al.*, 1981; Marion *et al.*, 1980a; Shafritz *et al.*, 1981; Twist *et al.*, 1980). Evidence for this is the finding of one or more DNA fragments containing viral DNA sequences that are larger than unit length viral DNA (3200 bp) after but not before digestion of cell DNA with a restriction enzyme (e.g., *Hind*III) for which no recognition sites exist in the viral DNA.

Similar findings of viral sequences have also been reported for some tumors in cirrhotic patients who were HBsAg negative (Brechot *et al.*, 1982). The sizes of the large DNA fragments containing viral sequences are different in different tumors, indicating that the integration sites are different and no single integration sites common to all tumors is apparent. Such evidence for integration of HBV DNA is not unique to HCC, because similar high molecular weight *Hind*III fragments with viral sequences have been detected in DNA of chronically infected nontumorous liver (Brechot et al., 1982; Chen et al., 1982; Shafritz, 1982). Again, the specific high molecular weight *Hind*III DNA fragments containing viral sequences were different in different patients.

The ability to detect such a DNA fragment by Southern blotting has been interpreted to mean that viral DNA is integrated in the same site in many different cells of the liver of each patient, but the site is different in different patients. The complete meaning of these findings is not clear, however; integration of other viral DNAs (e.g., retroviruses) appears to be random, so that specific integration sites are not detected in tissue DNA by the experimental strategy just described unless the cells are of clonal origin (e.g., as are cells in most viral-induced tumors). More direct evidence that these high molecular weight DNA fragments from infected liver and HCC actually represent cellular DNA covalently attached to viral DNA is needed. For example, isolation of these fragments by molecular cloning in bacterial cells would permit more definitive characterization of them. High molecular weight DNA forms containing viral sequences without cellular sequences have been detected in infected woodchuck (Rogler and Summers, 1983) and ground squirrel (Marion et al., 1982) liver. These appear not to represent integrated viral DNA but could be confused with integrated sequences when analyzed only by Southern blotting.

Similar findings suggesting viral DNA integrations have been made in HCC from woodchucks infected with WHV. Not only has Southern blot analysis of woodchuck HCC DNA restricted with *Hind*III revealed high molecular weight DNA fragments containing HBV sequences (Mitamura et al., 1982), but such fragments have been cloned in bacterial cells using lambdoid

vectors and shown to contain viral DNA sequences covalently attached to cellular DNA (Ogston *et al.,* 1981). The viral DNA
showed gross rearrangements and deletions. Thus many HCCs in
humans and woodchucks contain viral DNA sequences, and these
appear to be integrated in cellular DNA.

IV. THE STATE OF HBV IN TISSUE CULTURE CELL LINES ISOLATED
     FROM HUMAN HCC

A tissue culture cell line PLC/PRF/5 PLC cells) isolated
in 1975 from HCC tissue of an African man with persistent HBV
infection has been shown to produce HBsAg continuously in culture (Macnab *et al.,* 1976). The cells produce no detectable
HBcAg, whole virions, or infectious HBV (Macnab *et al.,* 1976;
Marion *et al.,* 1979). HBV DNA sequences appear to be present
exclusively in an integrated form, and no unit length free or
episomal viral DNA has been detected (Brechot *et al.,* 1980;
Chakraborty *et al.,* 1980; Edman *et al.,* 1980; Marion *et al.,*
1980a). The amount of viral DNA corresponds to only a few
(<10) copies of viral DNA per cell. Sequences in all regions
of the viral DNA are represented, suggesting that all of the
viral DNA is present (Marion *et al.,* 1980a). Restriction endonuclease *Hind*III (an enzyme that does not cleave HBV DNA) digestion of PLC/PRF/5 cell DNA produces at least eight specific
DNA fragments containing integrated HBV DNA and flanking cell
DNA sequences (Miller and Robinson, 1983). The *Hind*III fragments containing HBV DNA sequences have electrophoretic mobili-
ties of linear DNA fragments with sizes of 40,000, 38,000,
24,000, 17,200, 11,700, 6,600, 4,800, and 1,900 Kb (Miller
and Robinson, 1983). These results suggest that there are at
least eight sites in PLC cell DNA in which HBV DNA is integrated.
Viral-specific RNAs corresponding to extensive regions of the

viral DNA have been demonstrated in the cell (Marion *et al.*, 1980a; Edman *et al.*, 1980).

The observation that only HBsAg and not HBsAg is expressed. in these cells, although the DNA sequences within both genes are present, raises the question of mechanisms controlling viral gene expression. Because methylation of some herpes simplex virus and adenovirus genes appears to turn off their expression in infected cells, methylation of the HBsAg and HBcAg genes in PLC cells has been studied in this laboratory (Miller and Robinson, 1983). The methylation of various hepatitis B virus (HBV) DNA sequences was examined using the restriction endonucleases *Hpa*II and *Msp*I. Although both enzymes recognize the DNA sequence 5'-CCGG-3', *Hpa*II will not cleave the DNA if the internal cytosine is methylated. HBV DNA from Dane particles and virus-infected liver tissue (nontumor) was digested with *Hpa*II or *Msp*I, fractionated by electrophoresis in agarose gels, and the restriction enzyme cleavage pattern examined by Southern blot analysis. No methylation of the 5'-CCGG-3' recognition sequence was detected in either virion DNA or HBV DNA from infected liver tissue. However, digestion of PLC/PRF/5 DNA with *Hpa*II and *Msp*I showed that the integrated HBV DNA sequences were methylated. Further analysis using probes specific for various regions of the HBV genome demonstrated that some of the hepatitis B viral DNA sequences, including those specifying the major surface antigen polypeptide, were methylated infrequently or not at all. In contrast, the viral DNA sequences coding for the major core polypeptide were extensively methylated. Because surface antigen is expressed in these cells, whereas the core antigen is not, the results indicate that DNA methylation could account for the selective expression of HBV genes in this hepatoma cell line.

V. CONCLUSIONS

Epidemiological studies clearly show that persistent HBV infection is strongly associated with the occurrence of HCC in humans in both high- and low-prevalence geographical areas of the world. The incidence of HCC in WHV-infected woodchucks is even higher than in HCC in HBV-infected humans.

Viral DNA is frequently found in an integrated state in HCC tissue of infected patients and woodchucks. The presence of viral genes in tumors is a necessary condition for tumor induction by the mechanisms known for the recognized tumor viruses that have been studied extensively in animal systems. HBV DNA has also been found to be present exclusively in an integrated state and in multiple sites in a cell line isolated from human HCC tissue. Although all of viral DNA sequences are apparently present in these cells, only the gene for the HBsAg polypeptide (the viral envelope protein) and not for the internal HBcAg polypeptide is expressed. The regulation of viral gene expression in these cells may involve selective methylation of viral genes.

The exact role of HBV and WHV in HCC formation is not understood at the molecular level at this time, but it is of interest that at least superficially these viruses appear to share some features with retroviruses. Among these features are similarities in genome structure, although the nucleic acid type in virions is different for the two viruses, that is, DNA in the case of hepadna viruses and RNA in retroviruses. Separation and repair of the cohesive ends of hepadna virus DNAs results in linear molecules with inverted, repeat terminal sequences of approximately 300 bp (Sattler and Robinson, 1979), similar to those of retroviruses.

In both viruses all of the viral messenger RNAs appear to be transcribed from the same DNA strand and thus in the same direction. In addition, it has been suggested (Summers and Mason, 1982) that at least the duck virus DNA may replicate through an RNA intermediate utilizing a reverse transcriptase, a mechanism with some analogy to retrovirus replication. A third similarity is that viruses of both groups appear to integrate readily in cellular DNA. However, it has yet to be shown that hepadna virus DNA integration is a regular and integral event in virus replication, that the viral genome in the integrated state retains its organization, that integration occurs at a specific site in the viral DNA, or that integration is essential to the mechanism of cell transformation--all of which appear to be features of retroviruses.

A fourth similarity is that when exclusively integrated in the DNA of infected cells, both hepadna virus (Marion *et al.*, 1979, 1980a) and retroviruses (Robinson *et al.*, 1981) may express only the gene for their envelope protein. A fifth similarity is tumor formation during infection by at least some members of each virus group. The clear association between HBV and WHV infections and hepatocellular carcinoma is among the more intriguing features of these viruses, and it will be of great interest to investigate in more detail their role in formation of these tumors. It will be important to determine whether they may integrate in sites adjacent to oncogenes and function as retroviruses are thought to function in cell transformation and tumor induction (Hayward *et al.*, 1981).

Although the different hepadna viruses all share many unique features, and at least HBV and WHV infections are associated with HCC formation, there are interesting differences. The highest rates of HCC formation in humans appear to occur only after infection for prolonged periods of time (e.g., 30 years or more), at a time when the virus infection has largely subsided to a low level of virus replication, so that frequently only very low titers of incomplete HBsAg forms and no

complete virus remain in the blood.   Cirrhosis is a common but
not an indispensable accompanying factor.

Woodchucks, in contrast, develop HCC after a shorter period
of infection, and they regularly have high concentrations of
both complete virus and incomplete surface antigen forms in the
blood, and have coexisting active hepatitis but never cirrhosis.
Finally, chronically infected ground squirrels have little or no
hepatitis or other liver disease, and they have the highest concentrations of complete virus and incomplete surface antigen
forms in the blood.   Yet infected animals develop HCC, if at
all, at a much lower frequency than do infected woodchucks.   The
relationship of DHBV to HCC in ducks is not yet clear.   The differences in liver disease, including HCC associated with infection with these very similar viruses, is very intriguing and
would appear to offer an opportunity to identify factors that
are important in pathogenesis of HCC.   Further investigations
much consider differences in pathogenicity of the viruses,
genetic or other differences in their respective hosts, and environmental factors.

REFERENCES

Barker, L. F., and Murray, R. (1972).   *Am. J. Med. Sci. 263,*
    27-29.
Barker, L. F., Maynard, J. E., and Purcell, R. H. (1975).   *J.*
    Infect. Dis. 132, 451-456.
Beasley, R. P., Hwang, L.-Y., Lin, C.-C., and Chien, C.-S.
    (1981).   *Lancet 2,* 1129-1133.
Brechot, C., Pourcel, C., Louise, A., Rain, B., and Tiollais,
    P. (1980).   *Nature (London) 286,* 533-535.
Brechot, C., Hadchouel, M., Scotto, J., Fonck, M., Potet, F.,
    Vyas, G. N., and Tiollais, P. (1981).   *Proc. Natl. Acad.*
    Sci. USA 78, 3906-3910.
Brechot, C., Pourcel, C., Hadchouel, M., Dejean, A., Louise,
    A., Scotto, J., and Tiollais, P. (1982).   *Hepatology*
    (Baltimore) 2, 27S-34S.

Chakraborty, P. R., Rinz-Opazo, N., Shouval, D., and Shafritz, D. A. (1980). *Nature (London) 286,* 531-533.

Chen, D. S., Hoyer, B., Nelson, J., Purcell, R. H., and Gerin, J. L. (1982). *Hepatology (Baltimore) 2,* 42S-46S.

Edman, J., Gray, P., Valenzuela, P., Rall, L. B., and Rutter, W. J. (1980). *Nature (London) 286,* 535-537.

Gocke, D. J. (1975). *J. Virol. 36,* 787-791.

Hayward, W., Neel, B. G., and Astrin, S. (1981). *Nature (London) 290,* 475-476.

Hruska, J. F., Clayton, D. A., Rubenstein, J. L. R., and Robinson, W. S. (1977). *J. Virol. 21,* 666-671.

Kaplan, P. M., Greenman, R. L., and Gerin, J. L. (1973). *J. Virol. 11,* 995-1001.

Kew, D. M. (1978). *In* "Viral Hepatitis: A Contemporary Assessment of Etiology, Epidemiology, Pathogenesis and Prevention" (G. N. Vyas, S. N. Cohen, and R. Schmid, eds.), pp. 439-449. Franklin Inst. Press, Philadelphia, Pennsylvania.

Koshy, R., Maupas, P., and Muller, R. (1981). *J. Gen. Virol. 57,* 95-101.

Landers, T., Greenberg, H. B., and Robinson, W. S. (1977). *J. Virol. 23,* 368-374.

Larouze, B., London, W. T., Saimot, B., Werner, B. G., Lustbader, E. D., Payet, M., and Blumberger, B. S. (1976). *Lancet 2,* 534-538.

Lutwick, L. I., and Robinson, W. S. (1977). *J. Virol. 21,* 96-101.

Macnab, G. M., Alexander, J. J., Lecatsas, G., Bey, E. M., and Urbanowicz, J. M. (1976). *Br. J. Cancer 34,* 509-515.

Marion, P. L., and Robinson, W. S. (1983). Hepadna Viruses: Hepatitis B and Related Viruses. *Current Topics in Microbiology and Immunology,* Vol. 25, in press.

Marion, P. L., Salazar, F. H., Alexander, J. J., and Robinson, W. S. (1979). *J. Virol. 32,* 796-802.

Marion, P. L., Salazar, F. H., Alexander, J. J., and Robinson, W. S. (1980a). *J. Virol. 33,* 795-806.

Marion, P. L., Oshiro, L. S., Regnery, D. C., Scullard, G. H., and Robinson, W. S. (1980b). *Proc. Natl. Acad. Sci. USA 77,* 2941-2945.

Marion, P. L., Robinson, W. S., Rogler, C. E., and Summers, J. (1982). *J. Cell. Biochem. (Suppl.) 6,* 203.

Mason, W. S., Seal, G., and Summers, J. (1980). *J. Virol. 36,* 829-835.

Miller, R., and Robinson, W. S. (1983). *Proc. Natl. Acad. Sci. USA 80,* 2534-2538.

Mitamura, K., Hoyer, B. H., Ponzetto, A., Nelson, J., Purcell, R. H., and Gerin, J. L. (1982). *Hepatology (Baltimore) 2,* 47S-51S.

Murphy, B. L., Petersen, J. M., and Ebert, J. W. (1975). *Intervirology 6,* 207-214.

Nishioka, K., Hirayama, T., and Sekine, T. (1973). *Gann Monogr. Cancer Res. 14,* 167-179.

Ogston, C. W., Jonak, G. J., and Tyler, G. V. (1981). *Proc. Symp. Viral Hepatitis 1981,* pp. 809-810.

Peters, R. L. (1976). *In* "Hepatocellular Carcinoma" (K. Okuda and R. L. Peters, eds.), pp. 107-117. Wiley, New York.

Peters, R. L., Afroudakis, A. P., and Tatter, D. (1977). *Am. J. Clin. Pathol. 68,* 1-13.

Robinson, H. L., Astrin, S. M., Senior, A. M., and Salazar, F. H. (1981). *J. Virol. 40,* 745-751.

Robinson, W. S. (1980). *Ann. N.Y. Acad. Sci. 354,* 371-381.

Robinson, W. S., and Greenman, R. L. (1974). *J. Virol. 13,* 1231-1238.

Robinson, W. S., Clayton, D. N., and Greenman, R. L. (1974). *J. Virol. 14,* 384-392.

Rogler, H., and Summers, J. (1982). *J. Virol. 44,* 852-862.

Sattler, F., and Robinson, W. S. (1979). *J. Virol. 32,* 226-233.

Scullard, G., Greenberg, H. B., Smith, J. L., Gregory, P. B., Merigan, T. C., and Robinson, W. S. (1982). *Hepatology (Baltimore) 2,* 39-49.

Shafritz, D. (1982). *Hepatology (Baltimore) 2,* 35S-41S.

Shafritz, D., Shouval, D., Sherman, H., Hadziyannis, S. J., and Kew, M. C. (1981). *N. Engl. J. Med. 305,* 1067-1073.

Shikata, T., Karasawa, K., Abe, T., Uzawa, T., Suzuki, H., Oda, T., Imai, M., Mayumi, M., and Moritsugu, Y. (1977). *J. Infect. Dis. 136,* 571-576.

Southern, E. M. (1975). *J. Mol. Biol. 98,* 503-520.

Steiner, P. E. (1960). *Cancer 13,* 1085-1092.

Summers, J., and Mason, W. S. (1982). *Prog. Med. Virol. 24,* 40-55.

Summers, J., O'Connell, A., and Millman, I. (1975). *Proc. Natl. Acad. Sci. USA 72,* 4597-4601.

Summers, J., O'Connell, A., Maupas, P., Goudeau, A., Coursaget, P., and Drucker, J. (1978a). *J. Med. Virol. 2,* 207-214.

Summers, J., Smolec, J. M., and Snyder, R. (1978b). *Proc. Natl. Acad. Sci. USA 75,* 4533-4537.

Szmuness, W. (1978). *Prog. Med. Virol. 24,* 40-69.

Trichopoulos, D., Violaki, M., Sparros, L., and Xirouchaki, E. (1975). *Lancet 2,* 1038-1039.

Twist, E. M., Clar, H. F., and Aden, D. P. (1980). *J. Virol. 32,* 796-802.

31

STUDIES ON HUMAN LIVER CARCINOGENESIS

Sun Tsung-tang

Department of Immunology
Cancer Institute
Chinese Academy of Medical Sciences
Beijing, China

Wang Neng-jin

Pathology Section
Qidong Liver Cancer Institute
Jiangsu, China

I.   INTRODUCTION

Significant progress has been achieved in research on possible etiological factors and mechanisms of their actions in liver cancer development as a result of both epidemiologi-

cal and laboratory studies. Liver cell cancer, the predominant type of primary liver neoplasm, constitutes one of the
major human cancers in the world. Crude estimates indicate
that probably more than 200,000 people die of this cancer each
year. It appears to be a global health problem, especially
when the closely associated chronic hepatitis is also taken
into account (Sun, 1983). Studies have narrowed down the
search for causative factors and have identified the hepatitis
B virus (Blumberg, 1982) and the mycotoxins (Linsell, 1980),
especially the former, to be the major candidates as etiological agents for human liver cancer.

The importance of host factors influencing the course of
cancer development has also been stressed (Sun et al., 1981).
Progress in the molecular biology of HBV infection (Robinson
et al., Chapter 30) and the metabolic activation of mycotoxins
(Wogan et al., 1982), as well as the development of relatively
long-term human epithelial tissue and cell culture techniques
(Harris et al., 1980) and also the animal model systems (Summers et al., 1978; Wang et al., 1980), have greatly facilitated
the more straightforward analysis of the carcinogenic mechanism
of the individual factors as well as their possible interactions.

On the basis of research progress achieved in this field,
prevention strategy aiming at the ultimate control of liver
cell cancer has been taking shape (Sun, 1983) and well-based
preventive trials have already been started in the high-
incidence field. The very close association of field and laboratory studies, and the integration of carcinogenesis investigation and prevention trials, as shown in the case of liver
cancer, may constitute the appropriate approach to controlling
some of the major human cancers. In the present chapter, the
natural history and carcinogenesis of human liver cell cancer
will be reviewed mainly on the basis of field studies; in ad-

dition, some experimental systems that might be useful for analyzing carcinogenesis mechanisms in humans will be presented.

II. NATURAL HISTORY OF LIVER CANCER DEVELOPMENT

Early-detection trials using the liver cell differentiation antigen AFP as the marker in the high-incidence field Qidong of China have identified many patients with liver cell cancer at its early stages of development and more patients with precancerous hepatic lesions highly at risk for subsequent malignant change (Sun and Chu, 1981). The relatively long-term follow-up of these patients, many of whom received surgical treatment, offered unique opportunities to watch closely the natural course of development of human liver cancers. On the basis of such studies, its natural history of evolution was summarized and is schematically shown in Fig. 1. Under the influence of various carcinogenic and cocarcinogenic factors, a stage of persistent liver cell hyperplasia as an important component of chronic hepatitis is induced. The increased turnover results in an expanded population of hepatic cells at the differentiation stage capable of secreting AFP into the circulation. This period may extend for many years. Under the continued action of increased exposure to environmental carcinogens interacting with host factors, a clone of malignant cells might grow up at any point in the hepatic mass. Being localized mostly in earlier stages, intrahepatic dissemination to the extent beyond surgical resection usually occurred before the appearance of any characteristic symptom or sign. Therefore, patients commonly seen in the clinics are mostly in the late stages of development.

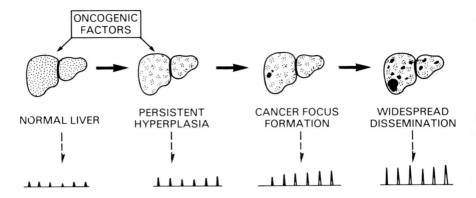

Fig. 1. A block diagram showing the natural history of development of human liver cell cancer. The level of α-feto-protein was determined by radio-rocket immunoelectrophoresis.

Two main features shown in Fig. 1 need further emphasis. First, the occurrence of liver cancer was mostly preceded by chronic hepatitis characterized by prominent hyperplasia per-sisting for many years. An analysis of the pathological data from 100 consecutive surgical cases of liver cell cancer demon-strated that although there was a spectrum in the severity of hepatic pathology, liver cell hyperplasia was found to be uni-versally present among all cases examined (N. J. Wang and Z. T. Sun, unpublished). This series included the 27 5-year survivals detected early in the subclinical stage through sero surveys. Obviously, hepatitis, causing prominent hyperplasia, forms the pathological background on which liver cancer de-velops (Sun *et al.*, 1979).

Other lines of evidence have also accumulated in the pros-pective studies on the groups of people found in serosurveys to exhibit a low-level fluctuating pattern of serum AFP, re-flecting active hepatic hyperplasia. These people were highly at risk for developing liver cancer in subsequent years (Sun and Chu, 1981). For example, among 25 patients having the characteristic AFP pattern, 7 of them developed liver cancer randomly in the 7 years of follow-up, reaching an average incidence of 4% per annum. This is an extension of our previous observation (Ji *et al.*, 1979). Similar results have also been obtained by other groups in larger series both in Shangai and some other areas of higher incidence (Xu *et al.*, 1980; Chu, 1981).

A report analyzing the follow-up data of 2,470 cases seen in the hepatology clinics in Qidong showed that the average incidence rate of those patients having a low-level fluctuating pattern of serum AFP, usually accompanied by some other biochemical abnormalities, reached a level of around 2% per annum in the subsequent 2-4 years of follow-up, being 15 times more at risk than the larger group having no or some biochemical abnormalities but without AFP expression (Chu *et al.*, 1982). These facts all indicated that in the complex of chronic liver disease, persistent and severe hepatic hyperplasia having significantly increased population of liver cells at the less differentiated stage appeared to be essential in the pathogenesis of human liver cancer, at least in areas of higher prevalence. Malignant change in such hyperplastic cells with their AFP genes still being expressed results in the formation of AFP-positive liver cancer, which happens in over 90% of hepatoma cases in the high-incidence field. Human liver carcinogenesis, whether caused by viral and/or chemical factors, should be characterized by a relatively long period of hepatic hyperplasia, this being an essential component of the chronic liver disease background. The process observed in humans is consistent with findings obtained in the animal systems, demonstrating that increased proliferation of hepatic cells also increased their susceptibility to chemical carcinogens and that liver cancer foci usually occurred on the background of hyperplastic nodules (Craddock, 1976; Farber, 1978).

Another feature shown in Fig. 1 illustrates the localized
growth in liver cancer at early stages of development, probably
as a result of a unifocal origin of growth. The conventional
concept of multifocal origins of liver cancer was based on the
observations made in clinical and autopsy cases. Such an impression was also obtained from experimental systems where
multiple scattered hepatoma nodules were usually seen in animals fed with various chemical carcinogens. However, explora-
tory laparotomy on patients detected in subclinical stages
through mass screenings demonstrated that, in contrast to the
situations seen in the advanced cases, usually single or a few
nodules in close proximity were encountered among such patients.
Because the majority of the hepatic tissues were conserved after limited resection in these early cases, new liver cancer
might quickly develop from the major background if the tumors
were multifocal in origin and thus occurred randomly in the
liver mass. However, limited resection resulted in 40% 6-year
survivals of the surgical series detected early through AFP
serology (Sun and Huang, 1982). Taking together those cases
in the same series that were inoperable due to unfavorable location of the tumors or to the poor liver background, liver
cancers in a localized state were found in the majority of
cases. The impression of unifocal origin of the liver cancer
is also consistent with the estimation of the probability of
concomitant occurrence of two or more tumors in the same individual, being well below 5%. Therefore, liver cancer formation from the pool of the vast number of hepatic cells in a
hyperplastic state appears to be a very rare biological event.

III. CAUSATIVE FACTORS OF LIVER CARCINOGENESIS IN HUMANS

The pattern of very uneven distribution of liver cancer on a worldwide scale and the analytical epidemiological studies thus followed had yielded valuable clues to its causation. Whereas many factors had been either excluded or not found to play any important role, hepatitis B virus and probably also some mycotoxins were identified as the highly probable etiological factors of human liver cell cancer. Encouragingly, preventive measures aiming at the ultimate control of this fatal disease appear to be emerging on the horizon. The two factors having major etiological significance will be discussed separately in the succeeding paragraphs.

A. Hepatitis B Virus

Liver cell cancer has long been known to be closely associated with chronic liver disease. Since the discovery of Australian antigen by Blumberg and the subsequent identification of the relevant virion, the relationship between B virus-associated hepatitis and the hepatoma was quickly established. A substantial body of evidence has now been accumulated that consistently supports the hypothesis that persistent infection with HBV is required for the development of most cases of liver cell cancer and that the association appears to be a causal one. This subject has been reviewed by many researchers (Sun *et al.*, 1981; Blumberg, 1982, Robinson *et al.*, Chapter 30).

Three lines of epidemiological studies and also laboratory findings of HBV integration into the cellular genome have strongly supported the suggestion that HBV is very likely the major carcinogenic factor of human liver cell cancers.

1. There is a close correlation in the geographical distribution of liver cancer and HBV infections (Szmuness, 1978).

Liver cancer occurs more in the regions where chronic carriers are also prevalent. In China, the high-incidence areas of liver cancer have a high carrier rate of HBsAg, reaching a level of around 15%, or even higher in some townships (Lu *et al.*, 1983).

2. Serological and immunohistochemical evidence of persistent HBV infection were much more commonly seen in liver cancer patients than in either normal people or nonhepatic malignancies (Blumberg, 1982). As many as 80% or more of the liver cancer patients had coexisting HBV infection. Such observations made in various parts of the world have yielded consistent results. Because these studies were done mainly on patients in late stages of liver cancer, increased chance of infection during the course of cancer development might account for the findings. However, the causal nature of such an association was further supported by studies done on patients having either subclinical cancers or premalignant lesions detected through AFP serology. They were apparently asymptomatic and had no history of receiving repeated venous punctures. Most of these patients, however, were also found to be HBV infected when examined by various serological and immunohistochemical means (Sun *et al.*, 1979, 1980).

3. Strong evidence demonstrating that HBV infection preceded the occurrence of liver cancer and that this association was probably of causal nature was obtained in three independent prospective studies carried out since 1975 or 1976 in Taiwan (Beasley *et al.*, 1981), in Japan (Sakuma *et al.*, 1982), and in Qidong, China (Lu *et al.*, 1983). These studies showed consistent results that liver cancers predominantly occurred in the apparently healthy carriers during the subsequent years of follow-up. Thus, in the Qidong series extending over 5½ years, 33 liver cancers occurred among 2560 carriers having an average incidence rate of 234 per 10^5. Only 9 liver cancers were

observed in the seronegative control group of 12,134 people with an average incidence of 13.5 per 10^5. The difference will be even more striking if the RPHA assays of serum HBsAg are replaced by the more sensitive RIA techniques. Because the period of observation in this study had far exceeded the probable time course of liver cancer development, which was estimated to be around 3 years on the basis of the doubling time of serum AFP in early liver cancer patients in the same area (Sun and Huang, 1982), it could be concluded that liver cancer predominantly developed on the background of preexisting HBV infection.

Several laboratory studies have obtained consistent findings that HBV genome was incorporated into the DNA of hepatoma cells in culture (Marion et al., 1980; Edman et al., 1980; Chakraborty et al., 1980; Brechot et al., 1980) as well as in the specimens of human hepatocellular carcinoma (Brechot et al., 1980; Shafritz and Kew, 1981). Integrated HBV nucleotide sequence was also found in the nontumorous liver tissue of the cancer patients and in liver biopsies from long-term carriers (Shafritz et al., 1981). It is interesting to note that among 20 patients with alcoholic cirrhosis and hepatocellular carcinoma, it was reported that 9 of the 16 tested had serological markers of HBV infection, but all 20 had HBV DNA integrated into the genome of the neoplastic liver cells (Brechot et al., 1982). These data, if confirmed in extended series, imply that HBV might play a carcinogenic role even in those having no serological markers of any kind detectable by sensitive RIA assays. The consistent identification of HBV sequences in hepatoma cells using molecular hybridization techniques further substantiated the causal relationship of HBV with liver cell cancer and indicated the direct oncogenic potential of this DNA virus.

The strong association between HBV infection and liver cancer found throughout the world and the very high risk factor

wherever calculated justifies conducting primary prevention
trials among the high-risk groups to control HBV infection.
Consistent results in vaccination trials had clearly demonstrated the protective nature of anti-HBsAg antibodies and the
high protection rate in the high-risk adults (Szmuness et al.,
1980), in children (Maupas et al., 1981), and also in newborn
infants of HBeAg-positive mothers (K. Nishioka et al., personal
communication, 1982). Because early horizontal transmission
was found to be important for HBV infection in the high-
incidence area, our collaborative study on immunization of all
newborn infants in the defined hot spot has been started. The
integration of carcinogenesis study with prevention trial offers the unique opportunity to identify definitely the major
causative factor of human liver cancer, and also the rational
approach to cancer control.

In spite of significant progress achieved in the field
mentioned, the possible mechanism of HBV oncogenesis still remains largely hypothetical. HBV might act as a promoter, inducing a stage of persistent hepatic hyperplasia following
cell injury in the infection process. HBV might also act as
an initiator following integration of the viral sequence to
cause perturbations at the gene level in the host cells. The
two possibilities are not mutually exclusive, and alternative
mechanisms might also be operative. The possible interaction
with chemical carcinogens and host factors needs to be explored. It may be expected that the field of liver carcinogenesis will progress rapidly following the development of molecular biology in the coming years.

B. Aflatoxins

Although the accumulated evidence strongly suggests that
HBV is the predominant etiological factor of human liver cell
cancer, epidemiological data also indicate the importance of

other environmental factors. For example, the liver cancer incidence in Qidong is 6 times that of Beijing, whereas the ratio of their carrier rate is about 2.5-fold. The HBsAg-positive carriers in Qidong are 2.5 times more at risk to develop liver cancers than their counterparts in Beijing. The incidence of liver cancer among the HBsAg-negative population is also severalfold higher in the hot area. These observations suggest that other factors may be operative in conferring the additional risk (Sun et al., 1980).

Among environmental substances having carcinogenic potential, aflatoxins are the most frequently encountered family and possess the highest hepatotoxicity, especially the B_1 member. Aflatoxin B_1 is a potent carcinogen in rats, but it may also induce hepatic injury and hepatoma in a wide species range, including nonhuman primates, though with varying susceptibility (Wogan, 1976; Adamson et al., 1976). Its wide spectrum of animal hepatocarcinogenicity indicates that humans might not be an exception.

Possible increases of human exposure to aflatoxins in high-incidence fields of liver cancer in China have been summarized, demonstrating the increased content of AFB_1 both in corn and also in the domestic foods randomly selected for analysis (Chen et al., 1980; Yeh et al., 1982). Close association between the estimated amount of aflatoxin ingestion and the incidence of liver cancer was demonstrated consistently in field studies carried out in Thailand, Kenya, Mozambique, Swaizerland, and China (Linsell and Peers, 1977; Yeh et al., 1982). The approximately linear relationship, resembling the dose-effect curve in animal experiments, provided strong support to the hypothesis that aflatoxins may be one of the important causative factors of liver cancer in areas of higher incidence. However, a necessary further step is the reliable quantitation of minute amounts of aflatoxin metabolites in the

biological fluid, which will reflect the level of intake on individual basis and will also serve as a guide to monitor intervention trials. Studies along these lines are under way.

What is the possible mechanism of human liver carcinogenesis induced by the potential carcinogen AFB_1. It may act
as an initiator, by altering the DNA structure through adduction. Animal studies have demonstrated that a metabolically
activated intermediate of aflatoxin, probably an epoxide, can
bind with the guanine moiety of the DNA molecule to form an
AFB_1-DNA adduct, and that the carcinogenicity is proportional
by the extent of such *in vivo* binding (Essigmann *et al.*, 1977;
Garner, 1978). Qualitatively similar DNA adduction was also
observed in cultured human tissues and cells (Autrup, 1982).
That such a reaction could happen in intact humans has been
demonstrated by the identification of AFB_1-guanine adducts in
the urine of African natives who had consumed foods heavily
contaminated with aflatoxins (H. Autrup, personal communication). These potential carcinogens can also act as promoters.
They may induce persistent hyperplasia of liver cells following toxic injuries. The cells in increased turnover are more
susceptible to various carcinogenic factors, including the
mycotoxin itself. The facts observed are encouraging; however,
the elucidation of the mechanism of carcinogenesis still requires much further study.

IV. MODEL SYSTEMS OF HUMAN LIVER CARCINOGENESIS

Even in the endemic areas where exposure to potential oncogenic factors such as HBV and aflatoxins are severe, only a
very small proportion of the population develops liver cancer.
Host factors expressed through various mechanisms might explain
the difference in individual susceptibility (Sun *et al.*, 1981).

Obviously, human liver cancer is most likely the result of multifactorial interactions. Accordingly, relevant model systems that will facilitate the delineation of the various facets of liver carcinogenesis in humans should be sought.

A. Duck Hepatoma

It has long been known that in the high-incidence areas of human liver cancer, hepatomas and chronic liver disease identified on the basis of pathological findings were also prevalent in ducks (Chang, 1973). We had confirmed these observations and found 6 primary hepatomas among 56 adult ducks randomly selected from the same local area of Qidong, having an average age around 2.5 years

The high incidence of duck hepatomas was formerly attributed to the increased exposure of mycotoxins, especially aflatoxin B_1. It was known that duck is a species that is highly sensitive to AFB_1. Feeding young ducks with local domestic corn contaminated with aflatoxins regularly induced much higher incidences of hepatic cancers than the control groups (Qian et al., 1976). There appears to be no doubt that aflatoxin B_1 plays an important role in the causation of these local duck hepatomas in areas of much increased exposure.

However, the morphological pattern of the presence of chronic hepatitis observed in the noncancerous portion of hepatic tissue in the local ducks, resembling that commonly seen in human liver cancer patients, suggested the possible existence of some infectious agent(s). Electron-microscopic examination of the pelleted material following ultracentrifugation of the duck sera revealed the presence of virus-like particles in 10 of the 17 samples tested. They resembled Dane particles, but showed no measurable cross-reactivity with HBsAg using sensitive assay (Wang et al., 1980). DNA polymerase activity was

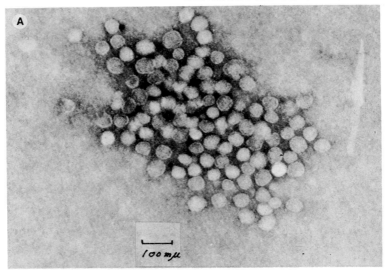

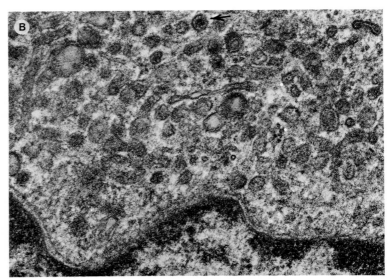

Fig. 2.   Virus-like particles in ducks from the high-
incidence area of human liver cell cancer.   (A) TEM of VLP in
duck serum after isopycnic banding in CsCl.   Buoyant density
= 1.195 (negative staining).   (B) TEM of VLP in the cytoplasm
of duck hepatoma cell (×60,000).

also found to be associated with such particles (Zhou *et al.*,
1980).   Clearer structure of the virus particles could be seen

after isopycnic centrifugation. As shown in Fig. 2A, the particle has an outer coat and an inner core, mostly in the range of 40 to 50 nm. Their bouyant density centers around 1.195 in the CsCl gradient.

Numerous morphologically similar virus-like particles in close relation with the endoplasmic reticulum were also observed in the hepatoma cells under the electron microscope (Fig. 2B). They were seen in different stages of maturation (Wang et al., 1983). Similar virus particles were also present in the noncancerous hepatic cells, having a pathological picture of chronic hepatitis. In all those ducks where viremia had been identified, moderate to severe hepatic pathology consistent with chronic hepatitis was also present. As shown in Table I, among six ducks with hepatoma that were observed, the presence of virus and chronic liver disease were also demonstrated. The close association of virus, hepatitis, and hepatoma suggested their probable causal relationship in the ducks studied.

However, chronic liver disease of varying extent was also observed in those ducks where the virus-like particles had not been identified in the sera. Because the antigenic system of the duck virus described has not been defined as yet, the magnitude of risk that could be solely attributed to the relevant virus in morphologically characterized hepatitis and hepatoma development cannot be assessed at present. It should be noted that in experiments of feeding ducks locally with AFB_1-contaminated food, the control group fed with a normal diet had a very low incidence of liver cancer, in striking contrast to the experimental group (Qian et al., 1976). This is consistent with the observations that an HBV-like virus could be found in a significant percentage of domestic ducks in U.S. flocks introduced early from China; liver pathology of only amyloidosis, but not hepatitis, was reported (Mason et al., 1981). The virus

TABLE I. Association of Virus, Hepatitis, and Hepatoma in
          Ducks from the High-Incidence Area of Human Liver
          Cell Cancer

Duck number	Serum VLP[a]	Hepatitis pathology	VLP in cancer cell	Liver cancer
11	+++	+++	n.d.[b]	Present
15	+	+++	++	Present
29	++	++	++	Present
38	+++	+++	+++	Present
39	++	++	++	Present
48	++	++	++	Present

[a]VLP, virus-like particles.
[b]n.d., not done.

was found to be valuable in analyzing the replication mechanism
of this virus family (Summers and Mason, 1982); its role in
liver carcinogenesis, probably as a result of multifactorial
interaction, will need further investigation.

B. Human Fetal Liver Cultures

    Improvements in culturing human epithelial tissues and
cells for relatively long periods of time have provided cancer
researchers with very important tools to study the many facets
of carcinogenesis directly in the epithelial sites of most common human cancers, bridging the gap between animal experiments
in model systems and clinical observations on intact humans
(Harris et al., 1982). Such an approach may provide insight
into the mechanisms of interaction of various factors at the
molecular, cellular, and tissue levels of biological organization. This is particularly pertinent to liver cancer research,
where the major carcinogenic factors have been better defined.
However, human liver tissue and cell cultures are still at an
early stage of development. This is due partly to the difficulties in maintaining the highly metabolizing hepatic cells *in*

vitro and partly to the lower availability of good hepatic tissues in sufficient amounts for studies. The use of fetal livers may offer an attractive alternative that will provide fresh and sterile materials in adequate quantity and will have inherent capacity to grow and differentiate. In populated areas where birth control has been actively managed, adequate sources of fetal materials suitable for *in vitro* culture studies could be sought and maintained.

Fetal livers having relatively short periods of anoxia were obtained following abortion by water balloon inflation procedure. The freshness of liver samples, an important determinant of the outcome of culture, could be identified by the general appearance of the organ as well as by the percentage of viability of thymocytes. Conditions for culturing fetal liver tissues and cells, and also the organ's capacity to metabolize chemical carcinogens, were studied in collaboration with Dr. C. C. Harris and colleagues of the NCI. In organ cultures, fresh slices cut in 1×2-mm pieces in L-15 medium were transferred onto the Gelfoam® cushions soaked in 199 medium supplemented with 10% FBS, 2 mM glutamine, 0.2 µg/ml hydrocortisone, 5 µg/ml insulin, 20 mM Hepes, and some antibiotics. The culture dishes were maintained on a rocking platform in an atmosphere of 50% O_2, 5% CO_2, and 45% N_2 at 37°C. Culture media were changed every 2 days.

It was found that in the majority of cases, liver tissues could be maintained in culture for over 2 to 3 weeks, still remaining viable and retaining structural integrity. As shown in Fig. 3A, hepatic cells are closely packed, and in some nuclei of these cells [³H]thymidine was heavily incorporated after pulse labeling. The liver cells continued to grow during culture, forming islands at the periphery of the explants and usually penetrating into the meshes of the underlying Gelfoam. Electron micrographs of the cells after 2 weeks of culture

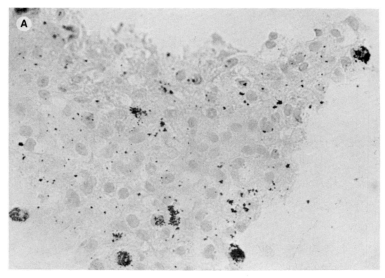

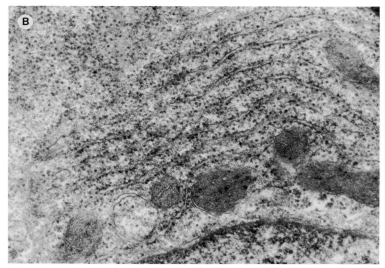

Fig. 3. Organ culture of human fetal liver. (A) Radio-
autograph after 14 days of culture, 6-month gestation female
fetus (light HE staining, ×160). (B) TEM of the same culture
after 14 days (×28,000).

showed parallel structure of endoplasmic reticulum, abundance
of glycogen granules, and other features of hepatic cells (Fig.
3B). The functional status of these hepatic cells was demon-

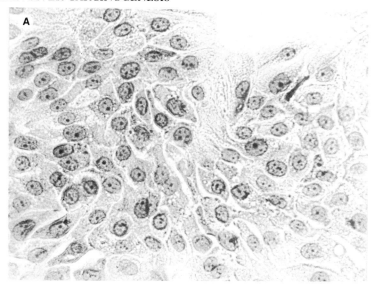

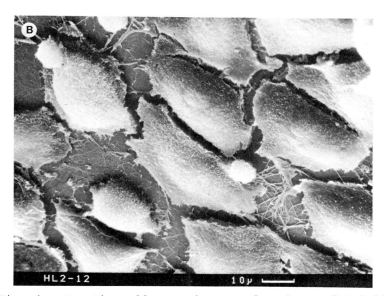

Fig. 4. Hepatic cells growing out from human fetal liver explant. (A) Epithelial cells under light microscope, 27 days after two transfers of the explant since the start of culture from a male 6-month-old fetus (Giemsa stain, ×400). (B) SEM of the epithelial cells from the same culture, 12 days after culture.

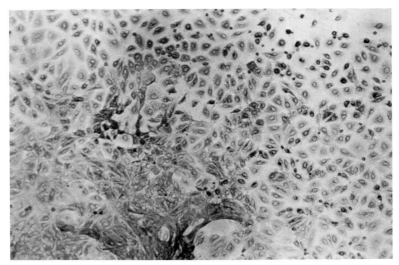

Fig. 5. Immunoperoxidase staining of human albumin in cells near the fetal liver explant. Deep staining of the cytoplasm of the epithelial cells was observed; 9 days after starting the culture from a 6-month male fetus (light microscope, ×80).

strated by the presence of human albumin in their cytoplasm through immunoperoxidase staining. Fetal liver explants were also cultured directly on the surface of a plastic dish coated with serum or fibronectin. They were regularly fed with 199 medium having a reduced concentration of calcium. The medium was supplemented with 1.25% FBS, 0.2 µg/ml hydrocortisone, 5 µg/ml insulin, 5 µg/ml epidermal growth factor, some trace elements, and 20 mM Hepes. The cultures were maintained in the same atmosphere as mentioned before. Usually after 10 to 14 days, mainly epithelial-like cells grew out from the periphery of most explants. These cells were polygonal in shape, having conspicuous nucleoli and many cytoplasmic processes (Figs. 4A and B). They were shown to be rich in glycogen by histochemical means. Immunoperoxidase staining had also demonstrated the presence of human albumin in relatively high content in the cytoplasm of most cells (Fig. 5), indicating their

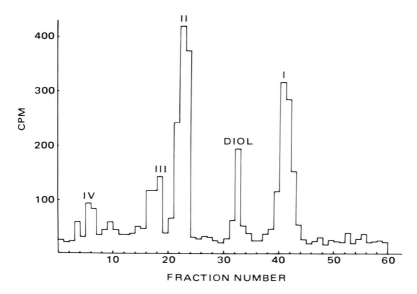

Fig. 6. HPLC profile of AFB$_1$-modified bases in DNA isolated from human fetal liver culture. The hydrolyzed sample was analyzed on a 4 × 300-mm µBondapak C$_{18}$ column using 18% ethanol with 0.02 M ammonium formate as the mobile phase at a flow rate of 1 ml/min. Fractions of 0.5 ml were collected for counting radioactivity.

cellular nature and differentiation status. Such explants could be transferred for several times over a period of 2 months, still providing the growth of hepatic cells at their periphery. The details of the conditions and characterization of hepatic cultures will be reported elsewhere (T. T. Sun *et al.*, unpublished).

The possible value of using fetal liver culture for human carcinogenesis studies would partly depend on whether the available liver tissues can metabolically activate chemical carcinogens, especially the aflatoxins. This has been found to be the case (H. Autrup *et al.*, unpublished). When tritiated AFB$_1$ was added to the fetal liver explants in short-term experiments, significant levels of binding to the DNA of the hepatic tissue

could be measured. HPLC profile of the hydrolyzed DNA revealed
that the major peaks of radioactivity (peaks II and I in Fig.
6) coincided with the positions of the ring-opened and ring-
closed forms of AFB_1-N^7-guanine adducts, respectively. These
facts indicated that the enzyme system responsible for the activation of aflatoxins has already developed at 5 to 6 months
of ontogenesis in hepatic cells. Possible intoxication during
fetal life might partly explain the very early occurrence of
liver cell cancer in a few children from the area where mycotoxin exposure was known to be increased.

Human fetal liver cultures are now being used for *in vitro*
carcinogenesis studies. Further investigations will show
whether such an approach might be a promising one.

REFERENCES

Adamson, R. H., Correa, P., Sieber, S. M., McIntire, K. R., and
    Dalgard, D. W. (1976). *J. Natl. Cancer Inst. (U.S.) 57,*
    67-78.
Autrup, H. (1982). *Drug Metab. Rev. 13,* 603-646.
Beasley, R. P., Lin, C. C., Hwang, L. Y., and Chien, C. S.
    (1981). *In* "Viral Hepatitis" (W. Szmuness, H. J. Alter,
    and J. E. Maynard, eds.), pp. 261-270. Franklin Inst.
    Press, Philadelphia, Pennsylvania.
Blumberg, B. S. (1982). *Proc. Int. Cancer Congr. 13th,* p. 11.
Brechot, C., Pourcel, C., Louise, A., Rain, B., and Tiollais,
    P. (1980). *Nature (London) 286,* 533-535.
Brechot, C., Nalpas, B., Courouce, A. M., Duhamel, C., Callard,
    P., Carnot, F., Tiollais, P., and Berthelot, P. (1982).
    N. Engl. J. Med. 306, 1384-1387.
Chakraborty, P. R., Ruiz-Opano, N., Shouval, D., and Shafritz,
    D. A. (1980). *Nature (London) 286,* 531-533.
Chang, L. Y. (1973). *Qidong Liver Cancer Res. Report* (in
    Chinese).
Chen, C. Y. (1980). *Qidong Liver Cancer Res.*   , pp. 32-37
    (in Chinese).
Chu, Y. Y. (1981). *Chin. J. Oncol. 3,* 35-38 (in Chinese).
Chu, Y. Y., Shi, P. F., Hwang, Q. S., and Ku, Y. Z. (1982).
    Jiangsu Med. J. 8, 55-57 (in Chinese).
Craddock, V. M. (1976). *In* "Liver Cell Cancer" (H. M. Cameron,

D. A. Linsell, and G. P. Warwick, eds.), pp. 153-201. Elsevier, Amsterdam.

Edman, J. C., Gray, P., Valenzuela, P., Rakkm, L. B., and Rutter, W. J. (1980). *Nature (London) 286,* 535-538.

Essigmann, J. M., Croy, R. G., Nadzan, A. M., Busby, W. F., Reinhold, V. N., Buchi, G., and Wogan, G. N. (1977). *Proc. Natl. Acad. Sci. USA 74,* 1870-1874.

Farber, E. (1978). *In* "Primary Liver Tumors" (H. Remmer, H. M. Bolt, P. Bannasch, and H. Popper, eds.), pp. 357-375. MTP Press, Lancaster.

Garner, R. C. (1978). *In* "Primary Liver Tumors" (H. Remmer, H. M. Bolt, P. Bannasch, and H. Popper, eds.), pp. 295-303. MTP Press, Lancaster.

Harris, C. C., Trump, B. F., and Stoner, G. D. (1980). *Methods Cell Biol. 21.*

Harris, C. C., Trump, B. F., Grafstrom, R. C., and Autrup, H. (1982). *In* "Mechanisms of Chemical Carcinogenesis" (C. C. Harris and P. Cerutti, eds.), pp. 289-298. Alan Liss, New York.

Ji, Z., Sun, Z. T., Wang, L. Q., Ding, K. S., Chu, P. P., and Li, F. M. (1979). *Chin. J. Oncol. 1,* 96-100 (in Chinese).

Linsell, A. (1980). *Ann. Acad. Med. Singapore 9,* 188-189.

Linsell, C. A., and Peers, F. G. (1977). *In* "Origins of Human Cancer" (H. H. Hiatt, J. D. Watson, and J. A. Winsten, eds.), pp. 549-556. Cold Spring Harbor Lab., Cold Spring Harbor, New York.

Lu, J. H., Li, W. K., Jian, Z. E., Hwang, F., and Ni, C. P. (1983). *Chin. J. Oncology 5*(6), in press. (In Chinese).

Marion, P. L., Salazar, F. H., Alexander, J. J., and Robinson, W. S. (1980). *J. Virol. 33,* 795-806.

Mason, W. S., Taylor, J. M., Seal, G., and Summers, J. (1981). *In* "Viral Hepatitis" (W. Szumness, H. J. Alter, and J. E. Maynard, eds.), pp. 107-116. Franklin Inst. Press, Philadelphia, Pennsylvania.

Maupas, P., Chiron, J. P., Barin, F., Coursaget, P., Goudeau, A., Perrin, J., Denis, F., and Diop Mar, I. (1981). *Lancet 1,* 289-292.

Qian, G. S., Xu, G. S., and Liu, Y. F. (1976). *Qidong Liver Cancer Res.,* pp. 68-76.

Sakuma, K., Takahara, T., Okuda, K., Tsuda, F., and Mayumi, M. (1982). *Gastroenterology 83,* 114-117.

Shafritz, D. A., and Kew, M. C. (1981). *Hepatology (Baltimore) 1,* 1-8.

Shafritz, D. A., Shouval, D., Sherman, H. I., Hadziyannis, S. J., and Kew, M. C. (1981). *N. Engl. J. Med. 305,* 1067-1073.

Summers, J., and Mason, W. S. (1982). *Cell 29,* 403-415.
Summers, J., Smolec, J. M., and Snyder, R. (1978). *Proc. Natl. Acad. Sci. USA 75,* 4533-4537.
Sun, T. T. (1983). *In* "Prevention Strategies of Cancer." World Health Organization, in press.
Sun, T. T., and Chu, Y. Y. (1981). *In* "Cancer" (J. H. Burchenal H. F. Oettgen, eds.), Vol. 1, pp. 651-658. Grunne & Stratton, New York.
Sun, T. T., and Huang, X. Y. (1982). *Proc. Int. Cancer Congr. 13th,* p. 11.
Sun, T. T., Tang, Z. Y., and Chu, Y. Y. (1981). *In* "Gastrointestinal Cancer" (J. J. DeCosse and P. Sherlock, eds.), Vol. 1, pp. 387-411. Nijhoff, The Hague.
Sun, Z. T., Wang, N., Xia, Q., Wang, L., and Zhang, Y. (1979). *Chin. J. Oncol. 1,* 13-19 (in Chinese).
Sun, Z. T., Chu, Y. Y., Wang, L., Xia, Q., Wang, N., and Zhang, Y. (1980). *Cold Spring Harbor Conf. Cell Proliferation 7,* 471-480.
Szmuness, W. (1978). *Prog. Med. Virol. 24,* 40-69.
Szmuness, W., Stevens, C. E., Harley, E. J., Zang, E. A., Oleszko, W. R., William, D. C., Sadovsky, R., Morrison, J. M., and Kellner, A. (1980). *N. Engl. J. Med. 303,* 833-841.
Wang, N. J., Sun, Z. T., Pang, Q. F., Zhu, Y. R., and Xia, Q. C. (1980). *Chin. J. Oncol. 2,* 174-176 (in Chinese).
Wang, Y. Y., Hsia, C. C., Wang, N. J., and Sun, T. T. (1983). *Acta Acad. Med. Sinica,* in press.
Wogan, G. N. (1976). *In* "Liver Cell Cancer" (H. M. Cameron, D. A. Linsell, and G. P. Warwick, eds.), pp. 212-152. Elsevier, Amsterdam.
Wogan, G. N., Croy, R., Essigmann, J., and Bennett, R. (1982). *Proc. Int. Cancer Congr. 13th,* p. 503.
Xu, K., Li, M., Guan, S., Yu, E., Song, M., and Shen, Y. (1980). *Chin. J. Oncol. 2,* 45-49 (in Chinese).
Yeh, F. S., Yan, R. C., Mor, C. C., Liu, Y. K., and Yang, K. C. (1982). *Proc. Int. Cancer Congr. 13th,* p. 340.
Zhou, Y. Z., Kou, P. Y., and Shao, L. Q. (1980). *Shanghai Med. 3,* 1 (in Chinese).

VIII. Laboratory Epidemiology Studies

32

THE INTERRELATIONSHIP OF EPIDEMIOLOGICAL AND LABORATORY SCIENCES: COLON CANCER

Ernst L. Wynder and Ruth M. Kay

American Health Foundation
New York, New York

Bandaru S. Reddy, Clara L. Horn, and John H. Weisburger

American Health Foundation
Naylor Dana Institute for Disease Prevention
Valhalla, New York

I. INTRODUCTION

Cancer researchers are striving toward the prevention of cancer and, should this not be possible, the early detection and, if this is failing, the successful treatment of cancer.

Those of us engaged in epidemiology have as our prime interest the primary prevention of neoplastic diseases.

Initial observations by alert clinicians and subsequent contributions by experts in epidemiological techniques have demonstrated that many types of human cancers relate to identifiable causes, many of which are man-made, and thus should be susceptible to human intervention (Wynder and Gori, 1977; Doll and Peto, 1981; Higginson and Muir, 1982) (Figs. 1 and 2). The epidemiologist, in fact, can identify causative factors for cancer, can suggest successful preventive measures even without having a detailed knowledge of the mechanism whereby the factor operates, and can monitor the definitive proof of causation--a reduction in the incidence of disease after the factor has been removed.

The laboratory scientist can significantly contribute to the primary prevention of cancer either by identifying a carcinogenic source that might not have been recognized by the epidemiologist or by explaining the mechanisms whereby a suspected factor enhances carcinogenesis, thus strengthening the epidemiological observations. Epidemiologists and laboratory scientists obviously are mutually supportive and flourish best when functioning side by side in an interdisciplinary working environment (Fig. 2). Laboratory science can make particularly pertinent contributions to the human cancer problem if it deals with questions derived from epidemiological observations. The laboratory scientist can conduct basic research on factors suspected or established to relate to the development of human cancer that is just as exciting as that done on factors that appear to have no such human basis.

Using colon cancer as an example, the following will describe, by an analysis of the factors associated with colon cancer causation, what a close interrelationship between epidemiology and laboratory science can accomplish. Involved in

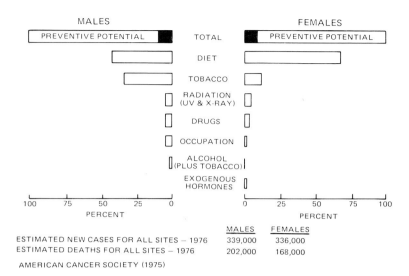

Fig. 1. Percentage of cancer incidence in the United States attributable to specific environmental factors. From Wynder and Gori (1977).

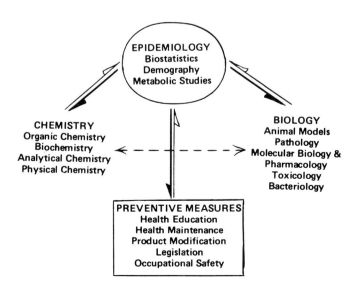

Fig. 2. Interdisciplinary approach to cancer prevention. From Wynder and Reddy (1977).

this analysis is the effect of nutrition on cancer of the
colon, particularly the nutritional effect on the production
and concentration of bile acids. Epidemiology and laboratory
sciences have well established that bile acids are effective
tumor enhancers but not complete carcinogens. It is important
to recognize that tumor enhancers, be they cocarcinogens or
tumor promoters, play an essential role in human carcinogenesis and may be particularly susceptible for use as a tool to
accomplish primary prevention, because they act only in relatively large concentrations and their action is reversible
(Hecker *et al.*, 1982; Weisburger and Horn, 1982).

II.   DESCRIPTIVE EPIDEMIOLOGY

The rarity of colon cancer noted in the societies of developing countries indicates that cancer of the colon is not
an inevitable consequence of aging. Although the diagnosis of
colon cancer in such societies may not always be adequately
made, careful autopsy studies from certain such populations do
support the rarity of colon cancer in these populations
(Burkitt, 1980). There are, in addition, industrialized societies where colon cancer is also relatively rare, such as
Japan, where clinical diagnoses and vital statistics are at
least on par with those of western countries (Wynder and Hirayama, 1977; Hirayama, 1979).

Two specific sets of data support a role for dietary fat
in the etiology of cancer of the colon. There is a high correlation between the per capita consumption of fat and the
death rate from colon cancer in various countries (Fig. 3).
Although such correlations do not prove causation, it is evident that in the absence of such correlation a causative association would be unlikely. These population data are supported

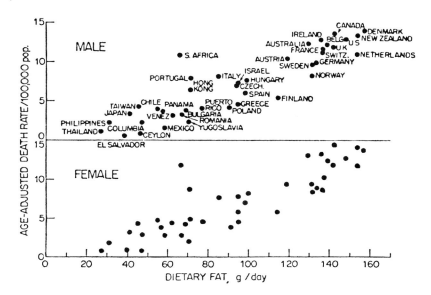

Fig. 3. Positive correlation between intake of dietary fat and age-adjusted mortality from cancer of the intestine (except rectum). From Carroll and Khor (1975).

by what we consider particularly powerful evidence, namely, that the rate of colon cancer increases in the first genera- tion as the low-risk Japanese migrate to Hawaii (Haenszel, 1975; Schottenfeld and Fraumeni, 1982) (Fig. 4). This increase parallels an increase in the intake of dietary fat, and, in turn, an increase in coronary heart disease among the migrating population is also seen (Haenszel, 1975; Wynder and Hirayama, 1977; Hirayama, 1979). The fact that the increase in the in- cidence of colon cancer is noted in the first generation of immigrants suggests that the dietary effect is principally that of tumor promotion. In recent years there has been some in- crease in the incidence of colon cancer in Japan itself--an increase concomitant with an increase in total fat consumption from 10 to over 20% of total calories (Hirayama, 1979).

An interesting epidemiological outlier (as appears on Fig. 3) is Finland. In spite of a high dietary fat intake and

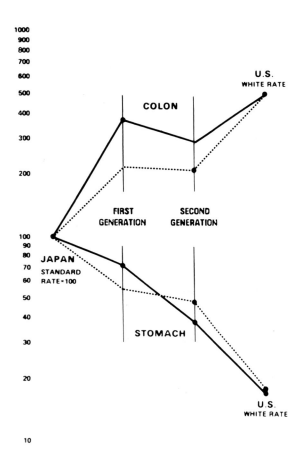

Fig. 4. Mortality trends of Japanese migrants to the
United States, showing changing rates for colon and stomach
cancer. There is a relatively rapid increase of the risk of
colon cancer, even in the first generation, and progressive
decrease of the risk for stomach cancer. ●——● , male;
●---● , female. From Wynder *et al.* (1981a).

a parallel high incidence of coronary heart disease, the inci-

dence of colon cancer is relatively low. In Finland, the fat

consumed is largely saturated fat, but importantly, the Finns

also consume a diet high in fiber. A number of retrospective

colon cancer studies have attempted to study the dietary intake

of colon cancer patients against controls, with relatively inconsistent results (Graham, 1981; Harper and Nichaman, 1982). This one would expect because of the relatively similar dietary patterns among Western populations in terms of the fat intake and also because of the inadequacy of dietary surveys (Harper and Nichaman, 1982). The problems inherent in dietary recall appear so large as to preclude usefulness, particularly when dietary habits of two or three decades ago are involved.

Although a correlation between dietary fat intake and colon cancer does exist along the lines described, such a correlation is much weaker for cancer of the rectum. It is important to stress that the epidemiology of cancer of the rectum--from the point of view of its distribution between the sexes, its socio-economic distribution, and its occurrence in developing countries--is quite different from that of cancer of the colon (Weisburger et al., 1975; Correa and Haenszel, 1978). More research needs to be carried out on the epidemiology and etiology of rectal cancer.

III. METABOLIC EPIDEMIOLOGY

A. Effects of Diet on the Enterohepatic Circulation and Fecal Excretion of Bile Acids

The biliary excretion and intestinal reabsorption of bile acids is normally subject to control mechanisms that rigidly curtail the amount of acid sterol escaping into the large bowel. Under specific dietary, anatomical, or metabolic conditions, the dynamics of the enterohepatic circulation may be altered such that biliary secretion is enhanced or reabsorption reduced, with a resultant increase in fecal bile acid concentration and excretion. The two dietary variables with the greatest effect on this process are fat intake and dietary fiber (Fig. 6).

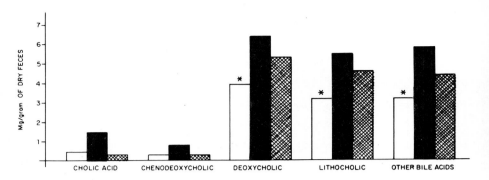

Fig. 5. Fecal bile acids in patients with colon cancer and patients at high risk. □, Controls (*N* = 30); ■, colon cancer (*N* = 30); ▨, polyps (*N* = 10); *, *p* < .05.

The concentration of bile acids in contact with the colonic mucosa is normally minor in individuals with an intact entero-hepatic circulation, when the fat intake is less than 20% of calories and the fiber intake is sufficient to provide a stool output greater than 200 g/day. Populations existing on a low-fat and/or high-fiber diet exhibit fecal bile acid (FBA) concentrations on the order of 4 to 5 mg or even less per gram dry weight of stool (Reddy *et al.*, 1980). Under these conditions, large-bowel neoplasms (both benign and malignant) are relatively infrequent.

1. *Dietary Fat*

Aries *et al.* (1969) noted that the amount of dietary fat determined the levels of intestinal bile acids as well as the composition of the gut microflora. Our group found that the level of dietary fat controlling the secretion of bile acids into the gut also modified the activity of gut microflora, so as to enhance the formation of secondary bile acids in the colon (Reddy *et al.*, 1980; Reddy, 1981a,b; Reddy and Ohmori, 1981).

Dietary fat enhances the biliary secretion of bile acids in humans (Lewis, 1958) and in animals (Redinger *et al.*, 1972;

Reddy et al., 1977a). This effect is apparently greatest for polyunsaturated fats and least for medium-chain triglycerides (Redinger et al., 1972). Because the fractional reabsorption of bile acids in the terminal ileum is relatively constant, dietary fat has a direct effect on total fecal bile acid concentration and output. Cummings et al. (1978) demonstrated that an increase in dietary fat from 62 (20% calories) to 152 g/day resulted in a corresponding increase in fecal bile acid output from 140 to 320, respectively. Similar results were obtained by Reddy (1981b). However, addition of further dietary fat to diets already containing 100 g or more of lipid appears to have relatively little effect on bile acid loss (Moore et al., 1968). This suggests that mean fat intakes of more than 20% of calories are required to modify total fecal bile acid excretion significantly.

Studies on the excretion of bile acids in the stools of populations at high and low risk for colon cancer development were carried out in our laboratory and elsewhere in an effort to determine whether changes in the diet in terms of fat and fiber could alter the concentration of colonic bile acids (Reddy and Wynder, 1973; Cummings et al., 1978; Reddy, 1981b). The results indicated that populations with a high risk for colon cancer have an increased amount of colonic secondary bile acids, namely, deoxycholic acid and lithocholic acid (Fig. 5), and increased metabolic activity of gut microflora measured by certain enzyme activities. In addition, individuals on a high-fat diet appear to have a higher level of fecal secondary bile acids and gut microbial activity compared to those on a low-fat diet.

We compared fecal bile acids between Seventh-Day Adventists (SDA), who are lacto-ovo-vegetarians, and age- and sex-matched non-SDAs consuming a high-fat, mixed Western diet (Reddy, 1981a). The fat intake was 28% lower and fiber intake was 2.5-fold

higher in vegetarian SDAs, but the total protein and calorie
consumption was similar between the two groups. The fecal excretion of deoxycholic acid and lithocholic acid was significantly lower in SDAs as compared with non-SDAs, 42 and 49%,
respectively.

2. *Dietary Fiber*

Dietary fiber also affects the enterohepatic circulation
and colonic concentration of bile acids. Certain types of
fiber such as pectin (Kay and Truswell, 1977b), lignin
(Rotstein *et al.*, 1981), and oat bran (Kirby *et al.*, 1981) directly adsorb bile acids in the upper intestine or colon, resulting in a reduction in bile acid reabsorption and an increase in total fecal bile acid output. Because these fibers
have relatively little stool-bulking capacity, colonic and
hence fecal bile acid concentration is correspondingly increased. Most common sources of dietary fiber (wheat bran,
whole-grain cereals, fruits, and vegetables) are rich in cellulose and hemicelluloses. These fibers have relatively minor
bile acid adsorption capacity but do effectively increase stool
bulk (Kay, 1982). Hence total bile acid output is unchanged,
but the colonic concentration of bile acids in direct contact
with the mucosal wall is reduced. Dietary fiber intake may
thus be an important variable affecting risk for large-bowel
cancer in the presence of a fat-rich diet.

We have studied the fecal bile acid excretion in healthy
controls in Kuopio (Finland), a low-risk population for colon
cancer development (Reddy *et al.*, 1978). The dietary histories
indicated that the total fat and protein consumption in Kuopio
is quite similar to the New York population, but the consumption of fiber, mainly on the cereal type, was threefold higher
in Kuopio compared to New York. The daily output of feces was
three times greater in Kuopio than that of healthy individuals

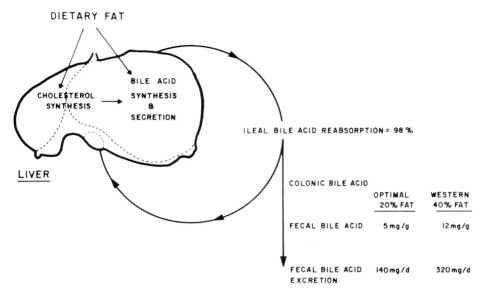

Fig. 6. Effects of dietary fat intake on the enterohepatic circulation and colonic concentration of bile acids. Dietary lipid increases bile acid secretion via direct effects and indirectly by increasing cholesterol and/or bile acid synthesis. Because the fraction of secreted bile acids reabsorbed in the distal ileum is relatively constant (∿98%), enhanced secretion is accompanied by an increase in fecal excretion and hence, unless dietary fiber is also increased, results in a greater concentration of bile acids in contact with the colonic mucosa. An optimal diet (20% fat) results in a fecal bile acid (FBA) concentration of 5 mg/g or less as compared to 12 mg/g in individuals on a typical Western diet.

in the United States. Hence the concentration of fecal secondary bile acids, deoxycholic acid and lithocholic acid, was decreased in Kuopio because of high fecal bulk, but the daily output remained equivalent in the two groups, as would be expected on the basis of similar intakes of dietary fat (Reddy et al., 1978) (Fig. 7). Total fecal bile acid concentration was significantly less in the Finnish population (4-6 mg/g stool) ingesting a high-fiber diet than in the American population consuming a lower fiber diet (11.7 mg/day). These differ-

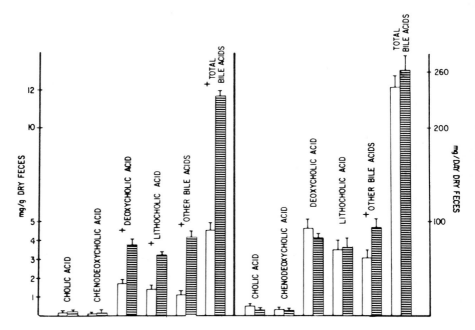

Fig. 7. Major fecal bile acid pattern of healthy controls
from rural Kuopio, Finland, and New York Metropolitan area.
☐, Kuopio (15); ▤, New York (20); +, *p* < .05. From Reddy
et al. (1978).

ences may reflect the corresponding disparity in colon cancer
incidence.

Cummings *et al.* (1978) and Kay and Truswell (1977a) reported that an increase in wheat bran intake increased the fecal weight and diluted the fecal bile acids (Kay, 1982). This
suggests that fecal bulk is an important factor regulating the
concentration of carcinogens and promoters in direct contact
with large-bowel mucosa.

B.   Genotoxic Carcinogens

Until recently, there was little information on the nature
of the genotoxic carcinogens associated with the etiology of
colon cancer. The question of the presence of carcinogenic

polycyclic aromatic hydrocarbons was raised many years ago
(Higginson, 1966). Charcoal-broiled meats were shown to contain such compounds (Lijinsky and Shubik, 1964), but in a careful analytical study Hecht et al. (1979) noted that the lower
large bowel and stools had no detectable benzo[a]pyrene after a
meal of broiled meat containing appreciable amounts of this and
probably related polycyclic carcinogens. Sugimura (see 1982)
discovered powerful mutagens on the surface of fried meat.
Weisburger et al. (1980) proposed that these mutagens may be
active colonic carcinogens. Several of the mutagens found in
fried meat are similar in chemical structure and metabolism to
the aromatic amines related to 3,2'-dimethyl-4-aminobiphenyl
(DMAB), which is an experimental colon carcinogen in animal
models. However, the question of the carcinogenic activity of
these mutagens for the colon in appropriate models remains to
be resolved (Weisburger and Horn, 1982).

Bruce et al. (1977) has discovered mutagenic activity in
the stool of some individuals. The search for mutagenic activity in the feces has been stimulated by the need to understand the nature of the genotoxic compounds that may be relevant to colon cancer. These studies demonstrate that the populations who are at high risk for colon cancer are consuming a
high-fat and/or low-fiber diet and excrete increased amounts of
fecal mutagens compared to low-risk populations (Bruce et al.,
1977; Reddy et al., 1978; Ehrich et al., 1979; Kuhnlein et al.,
1981; Mower et al., 1982). Studies are in progress in several
laboratories to isolate and further identify these fecal mutagens and to determine their carcinogenic activity. Hirai et
al. (1982) have proposed a chemical structure for such mutagens.
Of course we also need to consider the possibility that the colon carcinogens for humans are blood borne and thus do not enter
the luminal flow and the feces (Fiala, 1977).

TABLE I.   Current Concepts on Colon Cancer Causation and
          Development[a]

Risk factors: Diets high in fat, cholesterol, fried foods,
               and low in fiber

Postulated mechanisms

  High fat → High cholesterol biosynthesis → High gut bile
           High dietary cholesterol   acid levels

  Low fiber → High concentration of gut
             bile acids (low dilution
             through lack of bulk)

  High bile acid concentration → Promoting effect in colon
                                carcinogenesis

Mechanisms under study

  Fried food → Mutagens → Colon carcinogens?

  Role of micronutrients (vitamins and minerals) and different
   types of fiber in production and metabolism of carcinogens,
   bile acids, promoters?

Mechanisms of promotion?

---

   [a]*From Weisburger and Horn (1982).*

On the basis of the information just described, the following mechanisms have been suggested. The extent of the carcinogenic effect from exogenous sources is probably rather
weak, and thus the overall effect may depend on promoting action. Endogenously, a high-fat diet alters the concentration
of bile acids and the activity of the gut microflora, which,
in turn, may produce tumor-promoting substances from bile acids
in the lumen of the colon (Goldin and Gorbach, 1976; Reddy *et
al*., 1977b). In addition, certain dietary fibers not only directly sequester tumorigenic compounds in the gut, but also reduce the concentration of mutagens and promoters, so that their
effect on the colonic mucosa is attenuated. Dietary fat, fiber, and certain vegetables may modify the intestinal mucosal

and hepatic microsomal enzyme activity, so as to alter the capacity of the organism to metabolize tumorigenic compounds (Conney et al., 1980; Graham, 1981; Wattenberg and Lam, 1981) (Table I).

IV. EXPERIMENTAL STUDIES

Studies on the mechanisms of colon carcinogenesis have been assisted by the discovery of several animal models in which chemically induced colon tumors are histologically similar to lesions observed in humans (Pozharisski et al., 1979). Animal models are now being used effectively to study the multiple environmental factors involved in the pathogenesis of colon cancer.

Nigro (1981) induced intestinal tumors in male Sprague-Dawley rats by subcutaneous administration of azoxymethane (AOM) and compared animals fed Purina chow with 35% beef fat to those fed Purina chow containing 5% fat. Animals fed the high-fat diet developed more intestinal tumors and more metastases into abdominal cavity, lungs, and liver than the rats fed the low-fat diet. In another study, W/Fu rats fed a 20% lard diet had an increased number of 1,2-dimethylhydrazine (DMH)-induced colon tumors compared to the animals fed a standard low-fat diet (Bansal et al., 1978). Rats fed a diet high in beef fat (28%) with enough corn oil (2%) to prevent essential fatty acid deficiency, or a diet marginally deficient in lipotropes but high in fat were significantly more susceptible to DMH-induced colon tumors than those fed a low-fat diet (Rogers and Newberne, 1973). These results indicate total dietary fat to have an important role in the pathogenesis of experimentally induced colon cancer.

Our group (Reddy et al., 1980) carried out experiments to study the effect of type and amount of dietary fat on colon

TABLE II.   Colon Tumor Incidence in Rats Fed Diets High in Fat
            and Treated with Colon Carcinogens[a]

Dietary fat (%)	Protein as casein (%)	Carcinogen	Rats with colon tumors (%)
Lard			
5	25	DMH[b]	17
20	25	DMH	67
Corn oil			
5	25	DMH[b]	36
20	25	DMH	64
Beef fat			
5	22	DMH[c]	27
20	22	DMH	60
5	22	MNU[d]	33
20	22	MNU	73
5	22	MAM acetate[e]	45
20	22	MAM acetate	80
5	20	DMAB[f]	26
20	20	DMAB	74

[a]*From Reddy (1981a).*

[b]*Female F344 rats, at 7 weeks of age, were given DMH sc at a weekly dose rate of 10 mg/kg body weight for 20 weeks, and autopsied 10 weeks later.*

[c]*Male F344 rats, at 7 weeks of age, were given a single sc dose of DMH, 150 mg/kg body weight, and autopsied 30 weeks later.*

[d]*Male F344 rats, at 7 weeks of age, were given MNU ir, 2.5 mg/rat, twice a week for 2 weeks, and autopsied 30 weeks later.*

[e]*Male F344 rats, at 7 weeks of age, were given a single ip dose of MAM acetate, 35 mg/kg body weight, and autopsied 30 weeks later.*

[f]*Male F344 rats, at 7 weeks of age, were given DMAB sc at a weekly dose rate of 50 mg/kg body weight for 20 weeks, and autopsied 20 weeks later.*

carcinogenesis. Animals were fed specific diets for two generations before carcinogen exposure to mimic the traditional
dietary customs in high- and low-risk areas (Reddy *et al.*,
1976). Animals fed the diets containing 20% lard or 20% corn
oil were more susceptible to colon tumor induction by DMH than

those fed 5% lard or 5% corn oil (Table II). Broitman *et al.* (1977) showed that rats fed a 20% safflower oil diet had more DMH-induced large-bowel tumors than the animals fed either 5 or 20% coconut oil diets. These studies indicate that at high dietary fat levels, the source of dietary fat is relatively un-important. However, at low levels of fat intake, diets includ-ing polyunsaturated fats are more effective tumor promoters than diets containing saturated fats, irrespective of the source of the saturated fat. The underlying mechanisms are not yet clear but may relate to prostaglandin metabolism and intracel-lular control systems.

Investigations aimed at testing the effect of the dietary fat level on colon tumor induction by a variety of carcinogens-- DMH, methylazoxymethanol acetate (MAM), DMAB, or methylnitro-sourea (MNU)--that not only differ in metabolic activation but also represent a broad spectrum of possible exogenous carcino-gens, showed that, irrespective of the colon carcinogen used, animals fed a 20% fat diet had a greater incidence of colon tumors than did rats fed a diet containing 5% fat (Reddy, 1981a; Weisburger and Fiala, 1982) (Table II). Several reviews deal with this area (Weisburger, 1979; Reddy *et al.*, 1980; Fink and Kritchevsky, 1981).

The suggestion that promotion may be involved in intestinal cancer has been supported by the observation that the carcino-genic response to a variety of intestinal carcinogens is en-hanced by dietary fat. The enhanced tumorigenesis in animals fed a high-fat diet is due to promotional effects (Bull *et al.*, 1979). For example, ingestion of a high-fat diet increased the intestinal tumor incidence when fed after AOM administration but not when fed during or before AOM treatment (Nigro, 1981). Therefore, the high-fat diet in this model exhibited the proper-ties of a promoting agent. The carcinogenic process in humans may have similar characteristics. The possibility that colon-specific carcinogens are present at low concentrations suggests that promoting factors may have a preponderant influence on the eventual outcome of the neoplastic process in humans. This may also be true for events associated with breast and prostate cancer (Weisburger and Horn, 1982).

The relationship between dietary fiber consumption and colon cancer has been studied extensively in experimental animals (Nigro *et al.*, 1979; Freeman, 1982; Reddy, 1982). The results indicate that the protective effect of dietary fiber in colon carcinogenesis depends on the type of carcinogen and the source, type, and degree of milling of dietary fiber. Of the many fibers tested, wheat bran, dehydrated citrus fiber, pectin, and cellulose have been found to inhibit colon carcinogenesis in animal models.

V.   OPTIMAL BILE ACID CONCENTRATIONS

We tend to accept what we see. "Our theories are the mirrors in which we see ourselves [p. 179]" (Heidelberger, 1959). If adults in the Western world have average serum cholesterol levels of 225 mg/dl, we deem such levels to be normal; yet such levels are associated with undesirable risks for coronary artery disease. Thus, clearly this is not a normal level. A workshop concluded that optimal blood cholesterol levels for minimal heart disease risk are 160 mg/dl for adults (Blackburn *et al.*, 1979).

The dictionary defines *normal* as "agreeing with regular and established type," while defining *optimal* as "the best or most favorable." In line with this discussion, what is the optimal bile acid concentration per gram of stool? What is the optimal stool output by weight per day? We suggest that for both factors the Western levels are abnormal. Too high a level of bile acid production overwhelms the mechanism of their proper absorption from the small intestine, thereby abnormally increasing bile acid levels in the lower bowel and in the feces, and thus, the level of bile acids being absorbed through the wall of the colon. Metabolic overload results and with it the consequences of disease risk.

The question of an ideal fecal bile acid concentration has not been formally addressed. However, if we examine data derived from populations with a low incidence of colonic neoplasms such as Central Africa (Burkitt, 1980) and Finland or Japan (Reddy and Wynder, 1973; Reddy et al., 1978), a mean figure on the order of 4 mg bile acids/g dry weight of stool may be obtained. In contrast, the average concentration of fecal bile acids in subjects ingesting a typical North American (Reddy and Wynder, 1973; Reddy et al., 1978) or British (Cummings et al., 1978) diet is approximately 12 mg/g.

Metabolic ward studies suggest that manipulation of the current American diet (40% fat calories, 20 g/day dietary fiber) by reduction of dietary fat to 20% fat calories could be expected to reduce fecal bile acid concentration to about 7 to 8 mg/g. Addition of 20 g/day of dietary fiber from cereal sources such as wheat bran could be expected to double stool output and further reduce bile acid concentration to about 4 mg/g, a level commensurate with a low risk for large-bowel cancer. Studies in high-risk populations are required to test the efficacy of such dietary measures.

Thus it would seem that effective control and balance of dietary fat (20% of calories) and complex cereal fibers (to yield a wet stool weight of 200 g or more per day), plus a good supply of micronutrients from vegetables, might provide "optimal" bile acid concentrations commensurate with minimal colon cancer risk.

TABLE III.   Public Health Implications of Dietary Manipulation
in Disease Prevention

Average diet by country	Epidemiology	Public health action
Low fat--Japan	Low risk for MI and colon cancer	--
High fat, high fiber--Finland	High risk for MI and low risk for colon cancer	Lower total fat and maintain high complex fiber intake
High fat, low fiber--United States	High risk for MI and high risk for colon cancer	Lower total fat and increase complex fiber intake

VI.   PUBLIC HEALTH DECISION

To paraphrase the German philosopher, Kant, "Often in life
we have sufficient evidence for action but insufficient to
satisfy our intellect." When we in public health make a decision, we need to consider whether such a decision might have
negative effects in addition to having a possible beneficial
effect. We also need to recognize that if we make no decision
and thus keep a status quo, we have made a decision, nonethe-
less.

In terms of nutrition and colon cancer, a decision to decrease our intake of fat and to increase dietary fibers has potential beneficial effects and no apparent negative effects.
As we noted, the beneficial effects go beyond colon cancer in
that a reduction in fat intake might also influence the risk
for other diet-related cancers and, in particular, could reduce
the rate of the leading cause of early death, coronary heart
diseases (Table III).

We therefore recommend to the public, as was also done by
a committee from the National Academy of Sciences (1982), to

TABLE IV. American Health Foundation Food Plan[a]

Calories based on maintenance of ideal weight	1000 per day		1200 per day		1500 per day		1800 per day		2000 per day	
Content	% Total calories[b]	Calories	% Total calories[b]	Calories	% Total calories[b]	Calories	% Total calories[b]	Calories	% Total calories[b]	Calories
Protein (with an increase in vegetable protein)	12	120	12	144	12	180	12	216	12	240
Fat	25–30	250	25–30	300–360	25–30	375–450	25–30	450–540	25–30	500–600
Saturated fat	8–10	80	8–10	100–120	8–10	125–150	8–10	149–180	8–10	166–200
Monounsaturated fat	8–10	80	8–10	100–120	8–10	125–150	8–10	149–180	8–10	166–200
Polyunsaturated fat	8–10	80	8–10	100–120	8–10	125–150	8–10	149–180	8–10	166–200
Carbohydrate (with an increase in complex carbohydrate)	63	630	58–63	690–756	58–63	870–945	58–63	1044–1134	58–63	1160–1260
Other dietary components										
Dietary fiber	35 g/day		35 g/day		35 g/day		35 g/day		35 g/day	
Salt	3–5 g/day		3–5 g/day		3–5 g/day		3–5 g/day		3–5 g/day	
Cholesterol	200 mg/day		200 mg/day		200 mg/day		200 mg/day		200 mg/day	

[a]From Wynder et al. (1981b).
[b]Due to rounding off, figures may not add up to 100%.

reduce the fat intake and increase the fiber consumption of
their diet. The specifics of the American Health Foundation
Food Plan are shown in Table IV.

Simultaneously, we would recommend to the food manufacturers to produce foods that meet their guidelines (Livingston
et al., 1982). At present, it is premature to address the
question of the frying of meats as a possible source of carcinogens for humans, even though some methods are being developed to lower the formation of mutagens during frying
(Wang *et al.*, 1982). However, from the point of view of fat
consumption as such, it is advisable to modify the manner of
food preparation so as to avoid large amounts of fat in
cooking or baking. We stress the words *food plan* because they
represent what we should generally eat day by day. This is
not a diet, which we generally adopt as an emergency measure
after we have indulged in nutritional excesses, but rather a
continuing lifelong, low-risk, yet pleasant, tasteful, and
nutritious food plan. From the public health point of view,
therefore, the time to make nutritional declarations to
Western populations is now. The epidemiologist will have the
opportunity to monitor the success of such nutritional change.
We have come full circle: science discovers and evaluates
the impact. The epidemiologist and the experimentalist have
taken us this far. They cannot rest until we have succeeded
in making colon cancer as rare as nature intended.

REFERENCES

Aries, V., Crowther, J. S., Drasar, B. S., Hill, M. J., and
    Williams, R. E. O. (1969). *Gut 10,* 334-335.
Bansal, B. R., Rhoads, J. E., Jr., and Bansal, S. C. (1978).
    Cancer Res. 38, 3293-3303.
Blackburn, H., Lewis, B., and Wissler, R. W. (1979). *Prev.
    Med. 8,* 609-759.

Broitman, S. A., Vitale, J. J., Vavrouske-Jakuba, E., and
    Gottlieb, L. S. (1977). *Cancer (Philadelphia) 40*,
    2455-2463.
Bruce, W. R., Varghese, A. J., Furrer, R., and Land, P. C.
    (1977). *In* "Origins of Human Cancer" (H. H. Hiatt, J. D.
    Watson, and J. A. Winston, eds.), pp. 1641-1646. Cold
    Spring Harbor Lab., Cold Spring Harbor, New York.
Bull, A. W., Soullier, B. K., Wilson, P. S., Hayden, M. T.,
    and Nigro, N. D. (1979). *Cancer Res. 39*, 4956-4959.
Burkitt, D. P. (1980). *In* "Colorectal Cancer: Prevention,
    Epidemiology, and Screening" (S. J. Winawer, D. Schotten-
    feld, and P. Sherlock, eds.), pp. 13-18. Raven, New York.
Carroll, K. K., and Khor, H. T. (1975). *Prog. Biochem. Phar-
    macol. 10*, 308-353.
Conney, A. H., Buening, M. K., Pantuck, E. J., Pantuck, C. B.,
    Fortner, J. G., Anerson, K. E., and Kappas, A. (1980).
    Ciba Foundation Symp. 76, 147-161.
Correa, P., and Haenszel, W. (1978). *Adv. Cancer Res. 26*,
    2-142.
Cummings, J. H., Wiggins, H. S., Jenkins, D. J. A., Houston,
    H., Jivray, T., Drasar, B. S., and Hill, M. J. (1978).
    J. Clin. Invest. 61, 953-955.
Doll, R., and Peto, R. (1981). *J. Natl. Cancer Inst. (U.S.)
    66*, 1191-1308.
Ehrich, M., Ashell, J. E., Van Tassell, R. L., Wilins, T. D.,
    Walker, A. R. P., and Richardson, N. J. (1979). *Mutat.
    Res. 64*, 231-240.
Fiala, E. S. (1977). *Cancer (Philadelphia) 40*, 2436-2441.
Fink, D. J., and Kritchevsky, D. (1981). *Cancer Res. 41*,
    3641-3825.
Freeman, H. J. (1982). *In* "Dietary Fiber in Health and Disease"
    (G. V. Vahouny and D. Kritchevsky, eds.), pp. 287-295.
    Plenum, New York.
Goldin, B. R., and Gorbach, S. L. (1976). *J. Natl. Cancer
    Inst. (U.S.) 57*, 371-376.
Graham, S. (1981). *Banbury Rept.* No. 7, 395-408.
Haenszel, W. (1975). *In* "Persons at High Risk of Cancer"
    (J. F. Fraumeni, Jr., ed.), pp. 361-372. Academic Press,
    New York.
Harper, A. E., and Nichaman, M. Z. (1982). *Am. J. Clin. Nutr.
    35*, 1241-1291.
Hecht, S. S., Grabowski, W., and Groth, K. (1979). *Food
    Cosmet. Toxicol. 17*, 223-227.
Hecker, E., Fusenig, N., Marles, F., and Kunz, W. (eds.) (1982).
    "Cocarcinogenesis and the Biological Effects of Tumor
    Promoters." Raven, New York.
Heidelberger, C. (1959). In *"Ciba Foundation Symp. on
    Carcinogenesis,"* 179-96.

Higginson, J. L. (1966). *J. Natl. Cancer Inst. (U.S.) 37,*
    527-545.
Higginson, J. L., and Muir, C. S. (1982). *In* "Cancer Medicine"
    (J. F. Holland and E. Frei, III, eds.), 2nd ed., pp. 257-
    328. Lea & Febiger, Philadelphia, Pennsylvania.
Hirai, N., Kingston, D. G. I., Van Tassell, R. L., and Wilkins,
    T. D. (1982). *J. Am. Chem. Soc. 104,* 6149-6150.
Hirayama, T. (1979). *Nutr. Cancer 1,* 67-78.
Kay, R. M. (1982). *J. Lipid Res. 23,* 221-242.
Kay, R. M., and Truswell, A. S. (1977a). *Br. J. Nutr. 37,* 227.
Kay, R. M., and Truswell, A. S. (1977b). *Am. J. Clin. Nutr.
    30,* 171-175.
Kirby, R. W., Anderson, J. W., Sieling, B., Rees, E. D., Chen,
    W. J. L., Miller, R. E., and Kay, R. M. (1981). *Am. J.
    Clin. Nutr. 34,* 824-829.
Kuhnlein, U., Bergstrom, D., and Kuhnlein, H. (1981). *Mutat.
    Res. 85,* 1-12.
Lewis, B. (1958). *Lancet 1,* 1090-1092.
Lijinsky, W., and Shubik, P. (1964). *Science (Washington, D.C.)
    145,* 53-55.
Livingston, G. E., Moshy, R. J., and Chang, C. M. (1982).
    "The Role of Food Product Development in Implementing
    Dietary Guidelines." Food & Nutrition Press, Westport,
    Connecticut.
Moore, R. B., Anderson, J. T., Taylor, H. L., Keys, A., and
    Frantz, I. D. (1968). *J. Clin. Invest. 47,* 1517-1534.
Mower, H. F., Ichinotsubo, D., Wang, L. W., Mandel, M.,
    Stemmerman, C., Nomura, A., and Heilburn, L. (1982).
    Cancer Res. 42, 1164-1167.
National Academy Sciences (1982). "Diet, Nutrition and Cancer."
    Nat. Academy Press, Washington, D.C.
Nigro, N. D. (1981). *Cancer Res. 41,* 3769-3770.
Nigro, N. D., Bull, A. W., Klopfer, B. A., Pak, M. S., and
    Campbell, R. L. (1979). *J. Natl. Cancer Inst. (U.S.) 62,*
    1097-1102.
Pozharisski, K. M., Likhachev, A. J., Klimashevski, V. F., and
    Shaposhnikov, J. D. (1979). *Adv. Cancer Res. 30,* 166-238.
Reddy, B. S. (1981a). *Cancer Res. 41,* 3700-3705.
Reddy, B. S. (1981b). *Cancer Res. 41,* 3766-3768.
Reddy, B. S. (1982). *In* "Dietary Fiber in Health and Disease"
    (G. V. Vahouny and D. Kritchevsky, eds.), pp. 265-274.
    Plenum, New York.
Reddy, B. S., and Ohmori, T. (1981). *Cancer Res. 41,* 1363-1365.
Reddy, B. S., and Wynder, E. L. (1973). *J. Natl. Cancer Inst.
    (U.S.) 50,* 1437-1442.
Reddy, B. S., Narisawa, T., Vukusich, D., Weisburger, J. H., and
    Wynder, E. L. (1976). *Proc. Soc. Exp. Biol. Med. 151,*
    237-239.

Reddy, B. S., Mangat, S., Sheinfel, A., Weisburger, J. H., and
Wynder, E. L. (1977a). *Cancer Res. 37*, 2132-2137.
Reddy, B. S., Mangat, S., Weisburger, J. H., and Wynder, E. L.
(1977b). *Cancer Res. 37*, 3533-3536.
Reddy, B. S., Hedges, A. R., Laakso, K., and Wynder, E. L.
(1978). *Cancer (Philadelphia) 42*, 2832-2838.
Reddy, B. S., Cohen, L. A., McCoy, G. D., Hill, P., Weisburger,
J. H., and Wynder, E. L. (1980). *Adv. Cancer Res. 32*,
237-345.
Redinger, R. N., Hermann, A. H., and Small, D. M. (1972).
Gastroenterology 64, 610-621.
Rogers, A. E., and Newberne, P. M. (1973). *Nature (London)*
246, 491-492.
Rotstein, O. D., Kay, R. M., Wayman, M., and Strasberg, S. M.
(1981). *Gastroenterology 81*, 1099-1103.
Schottenfeld, D., and Fraumeni, J. F., Jr. (1982). "Cancer
Epidemiology, and Prevention." Saunders, Philadelphia,
Pennsylvania.
Sugimura, T. (1982). *Cancer (Philadelphia) 49*, 1970-1984.
Wang, Y. Y., Vuolo, L. L., Spingarn, N. E., and Weisburger,
J. H. (1982). *Cancer Lett. (Shannon, Irel.) 16*, 179-189.
Wattenberg, L. W., and Lam, L. K. T. (1981). *In* "Inhibition
of Tumor Induction and Development" (M. S. Zedeck and
M. Lipkin, eds.), pp. 1-22. Plenum, New York.
Weisburger, J. H. (1979). *Cancer (Philadelphia) 43*, 1987-
1995.
Weisburger, J. H., and Fiala, E. S. (1982). *In* Experimental
Colon Carcinogenesis" (H. Autrup and G. Williams, eds.),
pp. 27-50. CRC Press, Boca Raton, Florida.
Weisburger, J. H., and Horn, C. L. (1982). *Bull. N.Y. Acad.*
Med. 58, 296-312.
Weisburger, J. H., Reddy, B. S., and Joftes, D. L. (1975).
"Colo-Rectal Cancer." UICC, Geneva.
Weisburger, J. H., Reddy, B. S., Spingarn, N. E., and Wynder,
E. L. (1980). *In* "Colorectal Cancer: Prevention, Epi-
demiology and Screening" (S. Winawer, D. Schottenfeld,
and P. Sherlock, eds.), pp. 19-41. Raven, New York.
Wynder, E. L., and Gori, G. B. (1977). *J. Natl. Cancer Inst.*
(U.S.) 58, 825-832.
Wynder, E. L., and Wirayama, T. (1977). *Prev. Med. 6*, 567-594.
Wynder, E. L., and Reddy, B. S. (1977). *Cancer (Philadelphia)*
40, 2565-2571.
Wynder, E. L., McCoy, G. D., Reddy, B. S., Cohen, L. A., Hill,
P., Spingarn, N. E., and Weisburger, J. H. (1981a). *In*
"Nutrition and Cancer: Etiology and Treatment" (G. R.
Newell and N. M. Ellison, eds.), pp. 11-48. Raven, New
York.
Wynder, E. L., Hertzberg, S., and Parker, E. (1981b). "The
Book of Health." Franklin Watts, New York.

33

TOBACCO CARCINOGENESIS: METABOLIC STUDIES IN HUMANS

Dietrich Hoffmann, Stephen S. Hecht, Nancy J. Haley,
Klaus D. Brunnemann, John D. Adams, and Ernst L. Wynder

American Health Foundation
Naylor Dana Institute for Disease Prevention
Valhalla, New York

I.   INTRODUCTION

The association of tobacco usage with cancer at various sites suggests several approaches to metabolic studies in humans that would help to delineate mechanisms of tobacco carcinogenesis. Bioassays in laboratory animals have identified tumor initiators, tumor promoters, and organ-specific carcinogens in tobacco and its smoke (Wynder and Hoffmann, 1967; US Department of Health and Human Services, 1982). However, because nicotine has been incriminated as the major habituating agent in tobacco and tobacco smoke (Jarvik, 1977; U.S. Department of Health and Human Services, 1982), and because it

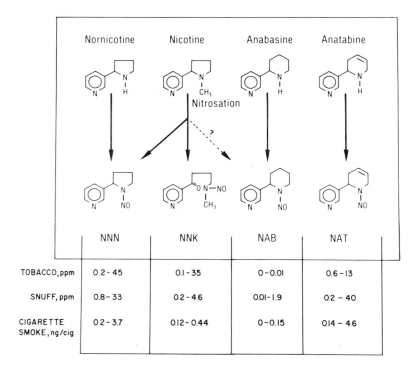

Fig. 1.   Formation of tobacco-specific nitrosamines (TSNA).

gives rise to carcinogenic *N*-nitrosamines, major research efforts have been placed on studying its fate during tobacco
processing and usage, as well as on its uptake and metabolism in
chewers and in active and passive smokers.   This presentation
will focus on metabolic studies relating to nicotine- and
alkaloid-derived carcinogens.

A.   Snuff Dipping

        Depending on the tobacco variety and stalk position, to-
bacco leaves contain between 0.5 and 3.0% of nicotine and as
much as 3.5% of nitrate (Tso, 1972).   Snuff is prepared from
specific Burley tobacco varieties that have been fire-cured,
powdered, mixed with sugars, and enriched with flavors (Wynder

and Hoffmann, 1967). Depending on the tobacco mixture and the amounts of additives, the final snuff products contain 0.5-3.1% of nicotine and as much as 3% of nitrate (Hecht et al., 1975; Hoffmann and Adams, 1981; Brunnemann et al., 1982).

During tobacco processing, the absolute amounts of nicotine in the leaves decrease. However, at the same time some of the nicotine and of the minor Nicotiana alkaloids are forming carcinogenic tobacco-specific N-nitrosamines (TSNA; Fig. 1). Concentrations of the TSNA in snuff exceed by at least two orders of magnitude those of N-nitrosamines found in other nonoccupational environments (Table I). In mice, rats, and Syrian golden hamsters, 4-(methylnitrosamino)-1-(3-pyridyl)-1-butanone (NNK) is a strong carcinogen, N'-nitrosonornicotine (NNN) is a moderately active carcinogen, and N'-nitrosoanatabine (NAT) and N'-nitrosoanabasine (NAB) are weakly carcinogenic (Table II) (Boyland et al., 1964a,b; Hoffmann et al., 1975, 1981; Singer and Taylor, 1976; Hilfrich et al., 1977; Hecht et al., 1978, 1980; Castonguay et al., 1982, 1983; D. Hoffmann, A. Rivenson, and S. S. Hecht, unpublished). These N-nitrosamines are not only organ-specific carcinogens but can also be local carcinogens. In Fischer rats, for example, NNN induces primarily cancer of the nasal cavity when given subcutaneously but evokes mainly cancer of the esophagus along with a moderate incidence of cancers of the nasal cavity when administered with the drinking water (Hoffmann et al.., 1975; Hecht et al., 1980a).

The observation that the TSNA can be active as local carcinogens is of major significance. Winn et al. (1981a,b) published a case-control study involving 255 women with oral and pharyngeal cancer in North Carolina.

The authors calculated a relative risk of 4.2 for oral cancer for the snuff dippers among white nonsmokers. For chronic snuff dippers this risk approached a 50-fold increase for cancer of the gum and buccal mucosa. In a retrospective

TABLE I.   Tobacco-Specific *N*-Nitrosamines in Snuff

Snuff brand	Tobacco-specific *N*-nitrosamines[a] (ng/g)			
	NNN	NNK	NAT	NAB
United States				
I	2200	600	1700	100
II	19000	2400	19000	800
III	33000	4600	40000	1900
IV	20000	8300	9100	500
V	830	210	240	10
Sweden				
I	5700	1700	900	140
II	6100	1000	2200	80
III	5300	1400	2400	70
IV	4000	610	1400	80
V	2000	800	1400	40

[a]*NNN, N'-nitrosonornicotine; NNK, 4-(methylnitrosamino)-1-(3-pyridyl)-1-butanone; NAT, N'-nitrosoanatabine; NAB, N'-nitrosoanabasine.*

study on oral cancer from Sweden, which included 33 cases of snuff users, Axéll *et al.* (1978) have shown that snuff dipping increases the risk of cancer at the site of direct contact with snuff five- to sixfold.

   In vitro and *in vivo* studies with mice, rats, and Syrian golden hamsters have shown that the tobacco-specific *N*-nitrosamines are metabolically activated by α-hydroxylation (Fig. 2; Hoffmann *et al.*, 1981; Castonguay *et al.*, 1982b; Hecht *et al.*, 1980b, 1982b). *In vitro* studies with human tissues, including tissues from the buccal mucosa, esophagus, bronchus, lung, and liver, have documented that NNN and NNK metabolism in humans follows routes of activation very similar to those in rodents (Hecht *et al.*, 1979; Castonguay *et al.*, 1982a).

   Several other observations also support the concept that TSNA are associated with an increased risk for cancer of the

TABLE II. Carcinogenic Activity of Tobacco-Specific
Nitrosamines

Compounds	Species	Application	Principal organs affected
NNN	Mouse	ip	Lung (adenoma, adenocarcinoma); salivary glands(?)
	Rat	sc	Nasal cavity (carcinoma)
		po (water)	Esophagus (papilloma, carcinoma), pharynx (papilloma), nasal cavity (carcinoma)
	Hamster	sc	Trachea (papilloma), nasal cavity (carcinoma)
NNK	Mouse	ip	Lung (adenoma, adenocarcinoma)
	Rat	sc	Nasal cavity (carcinoma), liver, lung (adenoma, carcinoma)
	Hamster	sc	Lung (adenoma, adenocarcinoma), trachea (papilloma, nasal cavity (carcinoma)
NAT	Rat	sc	Study not completed
NAB	Rat	po (water)	Esophagus (papilloma, carcinoma), pharynx (papilloma)
	Hamster	sc	inactive(?)

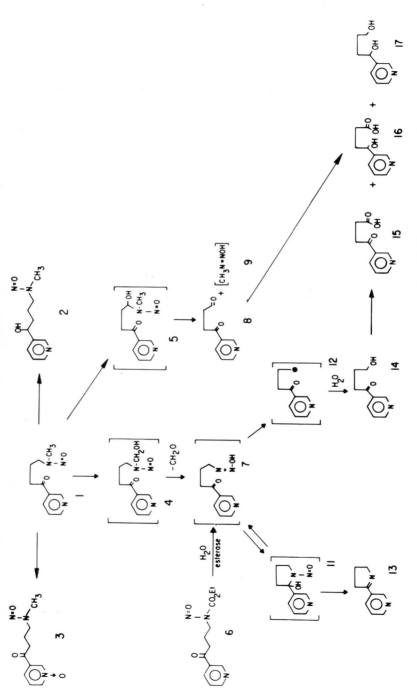

Fig. 2. Metabolism of NNK in the F344 rat. Compounds 2, 3, 8, 13, and 14 were detected *in vitro*; 8 may also be converted to 14 under the incubation conditions. Compounds 2, 3, 15, 16, and 17 were detected in the urine. Brackets represent hypothetical intermediates. From Hecht *et al.* (1980b).

TABLE III.   Analysis of Saliva of Snuff-Dipping Women

Snuff dipper[a]	Age (years)	Day of sampling	Saliva[b,c]				
			Nicotine (ppm)	NNN (ppb)	NNK (ppb)	NAT (ppb)	NNN:Nicotine ratio
1	41	1	189	140	26.2	210	1:1350
		2	448	106	21.0	470	1:4200
2	37	1	73	30	13	17.3	1:2400
		2	430	132	<10	51	1:3250
3	44	1	1150	420	96	370	1:2600
		2	1560	323	62	320	1:4900
4	52	1	210	25.9	10.6	12.5	1:8150
		2	430	56.8	22.5	45.9	1:7570

[a]The women were long-term snuff dippers (>10 years).
[b]Each volunteer used her specific snuff sample on 2 different days for the saliva analysis.
[c]Saliva of three non-snuff-dipping women (controls) was free of nicotine and tobacco-specific N-nitrosamines.

oral cavity in snuff dippers. First, saliva of snuff users contains relatively high concentrations of TSNA, ranging from 60 to 900 ppb (Table III; Hoffmann and Adams, 1981); moreover, additional amounts of these carcinogens are formed in the oral cavity during snuff dipping (Hecht et al., 1975; Hoffmann et al., 1981). Second, the N-nitrosamines are the only known organic carcinogens in snuff, which has induced preneoplastic lesions in the oral mucosa of rats (Hirsch and Thylander, 1981).

Finally, dose-response studies with N-nitrosamines in laboratory animals substantiate the risk association. The large-scale BIBRA study from England with rats has shown that administration of 1 ppm of N-nitrosodimethylamine (NDMA) or N-nitrosodiethylamine (NDEA) in the drinking water causes liver neoplasms in 23 and 42% of the rats, respectively. In addition, 1 ppm NDEA also caused esophageal tumors in 27% of the male rats (Peto et al., 1982). The total lifetime dose applied was

about 37 mg/kg for male rats and 64 mg/kg for female rats.
For the three most popular brands of U.S. snuff, we calculated
that the "average snuff dipper's" ($\sim$10 g snuff/day) exposure
during 30 years amounts to 270 mg of NNK ($\sim$3.9 mg/kg), 900 mg
of NNN ($\sim$13 mg/kg), 800 mg of NAT ($\sim$11.4 mg/kg), and 56 mg of
NAB ($\sim$0.8 mg/kg). Furthermore, a snuff dipper is also cumula-
tively exposed to trace amounts of NDMA, *N*-nitrosopyrrolidine,
N-nitrosodiethanolamine, and *N*-nitrosomorpholine. These considerations, taken together with the results of the BIBRA
study, suggest that the levels of nitrosamines in snuff are
sufficient to induce cancer.

Research on the elucidation of the mechanism(s) leading
to cancer of the oral cavity in snuff dippers needs to be continued. However, the evidence at hand should suffice to encourage regulatory agencies and manufacturers alike to undertake efforts toward reducing the carcinogenic *N*-nitrosamines
in all snuff brands. This request is underlined by the facts
that there are 2 million snuff dippers in the United States
alone and that snuff dipping is becoming increasingly popular,
especially among young people, in the United States and in
Sweden (Modéer *et al.*, 1980; Christen and Glover, 1981). The
feasibility of drastic reduction of *N*-nitrosamines in snuff
products has been well documented by the introduction of new
snuff brands in the United States and in Sweden (Table I;
Brunnemann *et al.*, 1982).

B.   Uptake of Nicotine by Smokers

It is now well known that cigarette smokers adjust their
smoking behavior in order to maintain a plasma nicotine level
characteristic of the individual candidate (Russell *et al.*,
1975; Russell, 1978, 1980; Schachter, 1978; Hill and Marquardt,
1980; Herning *et al.*, 1981; Hill *et al.*, 1983; N. J. Haley and

TABLE IV. Plasma and Urinary Cotinine and Nicotine in Smokers Smoking Different Brands of Cigarettes[a,b]

Subject	Brand	Nicotine per cigarette (mg)	Number of cigarettes per day	Plasma Nicotine (ng/ml)	Plasma Cotinine (ng/ml)	Urine Nicotine (mg/24 h)	Urine Cotinine (mg/24 h)
1	N	0.38	43	14	215	2.0	3.7
	C	0.81	24	20	204	2.8	3.1
	D	0.60	30	22	214	2.3	3.1
2	O	1.57	25	29	581	1.7	7.8
	C	0.81	39	30	613	1.0	8.2
	E[c]	0.15	40	9	260	1.2	2.6
3	R	1.62	30	25	407	2.6	6.9
	C	0.81	30	19	434	1.9	4.3
	D	0.60	40	15	401	2.9	5.4
4	O	0.60	24	5	196	1.2	2.2
	C	0.81	20	10	221	1.0	2.7
	D	0.60	24	9	180	1.3	2.6
5	N	0.38	20	8	76	0.7	1.2
	C	0.81	15	8	95	1.1	1.9
	D	0.60	15	6	81	0.6	1.5

[a] From Hill and Marquardt (1980).
[b] Plasma values average of two blood samples taken at 9:00 and 9:30 am on consecutive days: 24-h urine collection taken between blood samplings; no smoking was permitted for 30 min before blood sampling.
[c] Brand E, 0.15 mg nicotine to 1.5 mg tar and 2.6 mg CO.

P. Hill, unpublished). Data in Table IV support the concept
that smokers who change from their customary brand to a filter
cigarette with different nicotine delivery will adjust their
smoking intensity in order to reach their individual plasma
nicotine level as long as the change does not occur from a very
high nicotine level cigarette to a very low nicotine level cigarette (Hill and Marquardt, 1980). The adjustment is made
either by smoking more or fewer cigarettes and/or by smoking
more or less intensely. The smoking intensity can be increased
by taking puffs more frequently, by drawing a greater volume
per given puff duration, which is generally 2 sec (Herning *et
al.,* 1981), or by smoking to a shorter butt length and/or by
inhaling more deeply.

These changes result in greater nicotine delivery per cigarette than is generated by machine smoking under standard
conditions (Pillsbury *et al.,* 1969). It is important to recognize that more intense smoking results not only in higher nicotine yield but produces also higher yields of carbon monoxide
and of the carcinogenic smoke factors, namely "tar" and the
tobacco-specific *N*-nitrosamines (Wynder and Hoffmann, 1967;
US Department of Health and Human Services, 1982). Although
two case-control studies (Wynder and Stellman, 1979; Kunze and
Vutuc, 1980) and a prospective study (Hammond *et al.,* 1977)
have shown that the long-term filter cigarette smoker has a
lower risk for cancer of the lung and larynx than the smoker
of plain cigarettes, we cannot be certain whether we will see
a similar reduction of cancer in long-term smokers of low tar-
low nicotine cigarettes, because these smokers tend to smoke
much more intensely.

An ultralight cigarette with 0.94 mg of tar, 0.13 mg of
nicotine, and 1.1 mg of carbon monoxide has been introduced on
the U.S. market. This cigarette features a new filter design
with four longitudinal air channels at the periphery of the

TABLE V. Low-Yield Cigarettes: FTC-Tar, Nicotine, and Carbon Monoxide in Smoke of Cigarettes with Compressed Filter Tip[a]

| Filter cigarette brand (85 mm) | Mouthpiece (i.d. 7.00 mm) | | | | Doubled 7.00 mm tubing | | | | | | | |
| | | | | | Compressed mouthpiece (i.d. 6.82 mm) | | | | Compressed mouthpiece (i.d. 6.35 mm) | | | |
	RTD (mm H$_2$O)	Tar (mg)	Nicotine (mg)	CO (mg)	RTD (mm H$_2$O) (% change)	Tar (mg)	Nicotine (mg)	CO (mg)	RTD (mm H$_2$O) (% change)	Tar (mg) (% change)	Nicotine (mg) (% change)	CO (mg) (% change)
A	100	0.86	0.12	1.40	108 (−1)	0.91 (+6)	0.10 (−16)	1.25 (−11)	100 (−9)	1.20 (+40)	0.10 (−16)	1.45 (+4)
B	18	0.94	0.13	1.10	22 (+22)	1.29 (+37)	0.18 (+38)	1.97 (+80)	29 (+61)	2.75 (+193)	0.28 (+115)	2.81 (+155)
C	105	1.44	0.16	2.19	108 (+3)	1.23 (−15)	0.16 (0)	2.26 (+3)	116 (+10)	1.67 (+16)	0.18 (+13)	2.24 (+2)
D	64	5.45	0.42	8.03	67 (+5)	5.65 (+4)	0.45 (+7)	7.34 (−9)	65 (+2)	5.69 (+4)	0.39 (−7)	6.84 (−15)
E	96	5.94	0.52	5.57	98 (+2)	5.33 (−10)	0.52 (0)	5.52 (0)	99 (+3)	5.69 (−3)	0.44 (−15)	5.18 (−7)
F	131	8.37	0.70	9.04	130 (0)	8.10 (−3)	0.68 (−3)	8.7 (−4)	133 (+2)	8.09 (−3)	0.67 (−4)	8.19 (−9)
G	123	10.3	0.74	11.3	123 (0)	9.32 (−10)	0.72 (−3)	11.1 (−2)	127 (+3)	8.76 (−15)	0.69 (−7)	10.54 (−6)

[a] Smoking conditions: 1 puff/min, 35 ml, 2 sec duration. Average values for 24 cigarettes for each test. Tar was determined by the FTC method, nicotine by GC, and CO by GC with 3 clearing puffs. The values given for the standard smoking conditions were ±5% and for the smoking with a compressed mouthpiece, ±8%. RTD, resistance to draw.

TABLE VI.   Biochemical Measurements of Cigarette Constituent
             Absorption

	Cigarettes with Perforated Filter		Cigarettes with Longitudinal Air Channel Filter	
Number of cigarettes per day	24.5 ± 1.2		21.7 ± 1.3	
Plasma cotinine (ng/ml)	151 ± 17		256 ± 27	
	Baseline	+1 min[a]	Baseline	±1 min
After first cigarette				
Plasma nicotine (ng/ml)	0.35 ± 0.25	2.6 ± 0.8	0.40 ± 0.20	21.2 ± 6.1
COHb (%)	2.5 ± 0.3	2.9 ± 0.4	1.4 ± 0.3	1.8 ± 0.1
After 2 weeks				
Plasma nicotine (ng/ml)	1.0 ± 0.3	7.6 ± 1.8	1.0 ± 0.3	27.1 ± 7.9
COHb (%)	2.6 ± 0.2	3.3 ± 0.3	2.8 ± 0.3	3.4 ± 0.2

   [a]*+1 min samples were drawn 1 min after completion of the
cigarette and generally reflect the point of maximum nicotine
absorption.*

filter tip. Upon exerting minor pressure on the filter tip,
as may occur by the lips of a smoker during puffing, the yields
for tar, nicotine, and CO in the mainstream smoke rise significantly. We demonstrated this by smoking the cigarettes under
standard machine smoking conditions with and without compres-
sing the mouthpiece. For these tests the filter tips were inserted into cigarette holders with an inner diameter (i.d.) of
7.00, 6.82, or 6.35 mm, respectively. The smoke deliveries of
a cigarette with a conventional filter tip but with similar tar,
nicotine, and CO values were only insignificantly increased
upon filter compression (Table V). The closing of the longitudinal air channels by insertion of a metal ring into the holder,

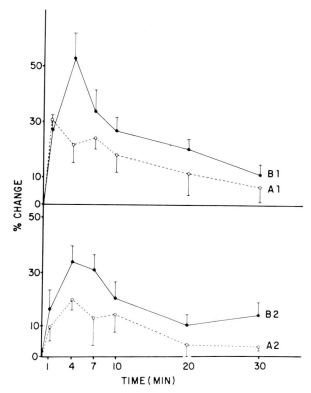

Fig. 3. Increase in pulse rate. (A) Conventional filter cigarette; (B) filter cigarette with air channels. (1) Initial measurements; (2) 2 weeks after smoking of these cigarettes.

simulating puff-drawing by a smoker, effected an inrease of the tar yield by 51%, nicotine by 69%, and CO by 147%; the same arrangement with a conventional filter cigarette increased the smoke yields only insignificantly.

A study on four smokers of low-nicotine cigarettes (<0.6 mg according to the FTC method) who were asked to switch to the filter cigarette with the longitudinal air channels, resulted in a significant increase in plasma nicotine without measurable rise in carboxyhemoglobin (COHb) 1 min after smoking the new cigarette for the first time and even after smoking this brand

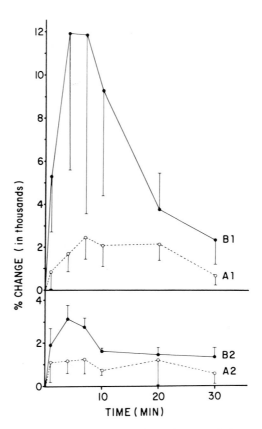

Fig. 4.   Increase in serum nicotine.   (A) Conventional filter cigarette; (B) filter cigarette with air channels. (1) Initial measurements; (2) 2 weeks after smoking these cigarettes.

for 2 weeks (Table VI).   The change in pulse rate was significantly higher for the smoker of this new type of filter cigarette than for the smoker of a conventional filter cigarette with similar (FTC) tar, nicotine, and CO delivery (Fig. 3). The change in plasma nicotine was even more pronounced for the smoker of the new filter cigarette (Fig. 4).   These findings indicate that the FTC data from machine smoking are misleading the consumer of the new type of filter cigarettes and may even be dangerous for some smokers.

C. *In vivo* Formation of *N*-Nitrosamines in Smokers

Our awareness of compensation techniques practices by
smokers of low-tar cigarettes leads to the recognition that
uptake of carcinogenic tar and *N*-nitrosamines is also much
greater than one would infer from the FTC data that are generated by machine smoking. Furthermore, the higher uptake of
all inhaled smoke constituents furnishes also greater amounts
of the precursors that will lead to *in vivo* formation of carcinogenic *N*-nitrosamines upon inhalation. These precursors
are nitrogen oxides and amines, especially nicotine and other
alkaloids, which constitute the most abundant amines in tobacco smoke.

Analytical sensitivity for *N*-nitrosamines with the gas
chromatography-thermal energy analyzer (GC-TEA) method is quite
high at a detection limit of about 0.1 ng/ml (Adams *et al.*,
1982); however, the concentration of nitrosamines in blood serum
after smoke inhalation is still too low for accurate measurements. This is primarily because of kinetics of the metabolism
of tobacco-specific *N*-nitrosamines (Hecht *et al.*, 1982a). However, occurrence of *N*-nitrosation may be monitored by an indicator for the endogenous formation of *N*-nitrosamines. A study
by Ohshima and Bartsch (1981) indicated that nitrosoproline
(NPRO) can be formed *in vivo* from proline with endogenic and/or
exogenic *N*-nitrosating agents. NPRO is safe as a monitoring
agent, because it is not carcinogenic in the laboratory animal and is not mutagenic in the Ames test with *Salmonella
typhimurium* TA 1535 or in the X-linked recessive lethal assay
in *Drosophila melanogaster* (Rostron, 1982). Furthermore, NPRO
is excreted in the urine in unchanged form (Ohshima and Bartsch,
1981).

Dailey *et al.* (1978) found that [^{14}C]NPRO was rapidly absorbed and excreted by fasted rats; about 98% was recovered as

unchanged NPRO in the urine within 24 h, and 1-2% appeared in
the feces after 24 to 48 h. Rats on an unrestricted feeding
schedule excreted 71-76% NPRO in the urine and 17-20% in the
feces 4-7 days after dosing, and exhaled about 2% of the
β-activity of the applied [^{14}C]NPRO as CO_2 (Dailey *et al.*,
1978). Chu and Magee (1981) reported in a detailed study on
rats that only 0.45-0.66% of the label of *N*-[*carboxy*-^{14}C]ni-
trosoproline is exhaled as $^{14}CO_2$ and that the remainder of the
compound appeared unchanged in the urine. The authors also
demonstrated in an *in vivo* experiment a lack of significant
binding to rat liver DNA.

On the basis of these data we initiated a study of NPRO
in the urine of 5 cigarette smokers and 5 nonsmokers. For the
assay all 10 volunteers were placed for 3 days on the same control diet. On Day 3 we collected the urine and determined NPRO
and, for control purposes, creatinine and total protein in these
urine specimens. In assay series II the same 10 volunteers were
again placed on the standard diet for 3 days; however, they received in addition 300 mg of proline each on Days 1, 2, and 3.
Urine was again collected on Day 3. In series III of this study
the same 10 probands received the standard diet and 300 mg proline, and at the same time also 1000 mg each of ascorbic acid on
Days 1, 2, and 3 followed by urine collection on Day 3.

In order to determine NPRO, we utilized a modified version
of the method by Ohshima and Bartsch (1981). Urine specimens
(24-h excretion) were collected in 2-liter polyethylene bottles
containing 10 ml of a 20% AS solution (ammonium sulfamate in
3.6 *N* sulfuric acid). Total excreted volume was recorded, an
aliquot (30 ml) was taken and mixed with 6 ml AS solution, 10 g
sodium chloride, and with 1 ml of 0.23 ppm nitrosopipecolic
acid (NPICA) in EtOAc as an internal standard. Elution through
Prep-tubes, concentrating of the organic layers (EtOAc), and
methylating with methanol and BF$_3$ reagent at 60°C for 1 h fol-

TABLE VII. *N*-Nitrosoproline in Urine of Smokers and Nonsmokers[a]

Urine (ml/24 h)	Cigarettes smoked		*N*-Nitrosoproline[c]	
	Average no./day	Type (mg tar/nico-tine/CO)[b]	ppb	µg/24 h
Smokers				
1 1100	20	F (7.8/0.6/9.6)	7.7	8.5
2 1780	10	F (11.0/0.87/12.3)	1.8	3.3
3 1090	20	F (14.2/1.05/16.2)	3.1	3.4
4 1450	15	F (3.6/0.38/3.2)	1.8	2.6
5 870	20	NF (24.0/1.46/17.0)	1.2	1.1[d]
Nonsmokers				
6 1170	–	–	1.4	1.6
7 620	–	–	3.6	2.3
8 1090	–	–	4.1	4.5
9 1940	–	–	5.3	9.3
10 1040	–	–	4.2	4.4
	$\bar{x}$ Smokers 4.5 µg/24 h			
	$\bar{x}$ Nonsmokers 4.6 µg/24 h			

[a]*Smokers and nonsmokers were on the same diet; urine collection was on Day 3.*
[b]*FTC Data, Dec. 1981. Federal Trade Commission (1981).*
F, cigarette with filter tip; NF, cigarette without filter tip.
[c]*Average of three analyses.*
[d]*The creatinine value was below the standard range of 1.0-2.0 g/24 h with 0.67 g/24 h; value excluded from calculation of average value.*

lowed. The reaction mixture was extracted with DCM-H_2O (1:4 ml), and the DCM layer was transferred into a serum vial with ∿100 mg anhydrous Na_2SO_4. A 5-µl aliquot was analyzed by GC-TEA to determine the NPRO as the methyl ester. GC conditions were as follows: a 12-ft (3.66 m), 2-mm i.d. glass column, packed with 10% Carbowax 20 *M* on Chromosorb W (80-100 mesh), oven temperature 185°C, injection port 210°C, Argon flow 30 ml/min. Retention times of the methyl esters of NPICA and NPRO were 8.3 and 9.1 min, respectively. Procedural losses and inaccuracies from volume changes were compensated for by using the ratio of NPRO and NPICA for both, standard and samples.

TABLE VIII. *N*-Nitrosoproline in Urine of Volunteers on a
Standard Diet Plus 300 mg Proline/Day

| Urine (ml/24 h) | Cigarettes smoked | | *N*-Nitrosoproline[b] | |
	Average no./day	Type (mg tar/nico- tine/CO)[a]	ppb	µg/24 h
Smokers				
1 950	20	F (7.8/0.6/9/6)	4.7	4.4
2 1720	10	F (11.0/0.87/12.3)	15.0	25.8
3 820	20	F (14.2/1.05/16.2)	3.7	3.0
4 1240	15	F (3.6/0.38/3.2)	40.0	49.9
5 1000	20	NF (24.0/1.46/17.0)	2.0	2.0
Nonsmokers				
6 1900	–	–	2.3	4.4
7 1500	–	–	4.0	5.9
8 840	–	–	5.4	4.5
9 1590	–	–	2.8	4.6
10 740	–	–	4.3	3.2
	$\bar{x}$ Smokers 17.0 µg/24 h			
	$\bar{x}$ Nonsmokers 4.5 µg/24 h			

[a]*FTC Data, Dec. 1981. Federal Trade Commission (1981).*
[b]*Average of three determinations.*

II. RESULTS

Table VII presents our findings for NPRO in urine of five
smokers and five nonsmokers who adhered to the same standard
diet for 3 days. Urine was collected from these subjects on
the fourth day. On the basis of these limited data, it appears
that under conditions of dietary control the endogenous levels
of NPRO were not affected by smoking.

In another assay we gave the volunteers, in addition to
the standard diet, a daily dose of 300 mg of proline, and we
analyzed the urine on Day 3. Table VIII suggests an increased
formation of NPRO in cigarette smokers but not in nonsmokers.
However, this conclusion may be misleading, because only two of
five cigarette smokers had significantly higher NPRO excretion.

TABLE IX. N-Nitrosoproline in Urine of Volunteers on a
Standard Diet Plus 300 mg Proline and 1000 mg
Ascorbic Acid/Day

Urine (ml/24 h)	Cigarettes smoked		N-Nitrosoproline[a]	
	Average no./day	Type (mg tar/nico-tine/CO)[b]	ppb	µg/24 h
Smokers				
1 1090	20	F (7.8/0.6/9.6)	3.6	3.9
2 1840	10	F (11.0/0.87/12.3)	2.9	5.4
3 1640	17	F (14.2/1.05/16.2)	n.d.	n.d.
4 1490	15	F (3.6/0.38/3.2)	5.7	8.2
5 2100	20	NF (24.0/1.46/17.0)	0.4	0.7
Nonsmokers				
6 1840	–	–	1.7	3.1
7 780	–	–	6.0	4.7
8 730	–	–	6.5	4.8
9 1920	–	–	3.4	6.4
10 620	–	–	11.6	7.2
	$\bar{x}$ Smokers 3.6 µg/24 h (4.5 g/24 h)			
	$\bar{x}$ Nonsmokers 5.2 µg/24 h (4.6 g/24 h)			

[a]Average of three analyses.
[b]FTC Data, Dec. 1981. Federal Trade Commission (1981).
[c]n.d., Not detected.

This tentative result requires confirmation with larger groups
of volunteers.

Finally, we explored the possibility that concurrent application of proline (300 mg/day) and ascorbic acid (1000 mg/
day) would demonstrate inhibition of NPRO formation in vivo.
Results in Table IX confirm that the in vivo formation of NPRO
from proline added to the diet is in fact inhibited by the co-
application of ascorbic acid, a known inhibitor of N-nitrosation.

Concurrently we are engaged in a detailed study of the endogenous formation of NPRO and other N-nitrosamines in smokers
and nonsmokers. It is our goal to estimate the total burden

of carcinogenic *N*-nitrosamines by inhalation of cigarette smoke
and by their *in vivo* formation from cigarette smoke precursors.
We consider this research program to be of special importance
for an understanding of the mechanisms involved in the increased
risk of cigarette smokers especially for cancer of the esophagus, pancreas, kidney, and urinary bladder. On the basis of
our present knowledge, the induction of tumors in these organs
is possibly associated with the exposure to *N*-nitrosamines.

III.   SUMMARY

   This discussion focuses on the habituating agent of tobacco products, nicotine, and its role in carcinogenesis. The
fate of this predominant tobacco alkaloid in tobacco users is
of major concern because of the compound's potential to form
N-nitrosamines, which are organ-specific as well as local carcinogens. Epidemiological evidence in men and women and laboratory studies with rodents have documented the carcinogenicity
of snuff, a finely ground tobacco product, most frequently
used as a chewing plug. Chemical analyses have identified the
alkaloid-derived *N*-nitrosamines 4-(methylnitrosamino)-1-(3-
pyridyl)-1-butanone (NNK), *N*'-nitrosonornicotine (NNN), *N*'-
nitrosoanatabine (NAT), and *N*'-nitrosoanabasine (NAB), all of
which have demonstrated strong to moderate activity as organ-
specific carcinogens and/or as local carcinogens.
   The metabolic activation of these cyclic *N*-nitrosamines
to their ultimate carcinogenic forms occurs via α-hydroxylation, as was shown by *in vitro* and *in vivo* studies with mice,
rats, and hamsters. More importantly, this route of activation
occurs also in human tissues such as buccal mucosa, esophagus,
bronchus, lung, and liver. It is deduced from dose-response
studies in laboratory animals and from estimates of human ex-

posure that the levels of *N*-nitrosamines in snuff suffice to induce cancer. Feasibility of *N*-nitrosamine reduction in snuff and chewing tobaccos has been demonstrated, and regulatory action for consumer protection is urged.

The role of nicotine as a precursor of *N*-nitrosamines in smoking tobaccos stresses the importance of the availability of low-tar, low-nicotine cigarettes for those individuals who choose to smoke. Dosimetry studies of mainstream smoke delivery versus uptake of nicotine and other smoke components by smokers point to the need for a review of the procedures used by the FTC to develop consumer guidance for tar and nicotine yields of U.S. cigarettes. The consumer needs to be made aware of the range of nicotine delivery in the mainstream smoke of any given cigarette, because this range depends on individual smoking intensity.

We have discussed the *in vivo* N-nitrosation potential of inhaled tobacco smoke for amines in a model study with volunteers on a standardized diet, using proline, which is converted *in vivo* to *N*-nitrosoproline. This noncarcinogenic *N*-nitrosamine is relatively stable and is excreted mainly in the urine and feces. Smokers and nonsmokers adhered to the standard diet with proline for 3 days. Urinalysis suggested increased formation of NPRO in cigarette smokers. This result requires confirmation by tests with a larger group of volunteers. However, our initial data confirmed also that the *in vivo* formation of NPRO from proline can be inhibited by coadministration of ascorbic acid.

ACKNOWLEDGMENTS

The authors are grateful for the assistance of Mrs. Ilse Hoffmann and Mrs. Bertha Stadler in the preparation of this manuscript. Our tobacco research program is supported by NCI grant 1P01-CA29580.

REFERENCES

Adams, J. D., Brunnemann, K. D., and Hoffmann, D. (1982). *J. Chromatogr. 256*, 347-351.
Assembly of Life Sciences (1981). "The Health Effects of Nitrate, Nitrite, and N-Nitroso Compounds," Part 1. Nat. Acad. Press, Washington, D.C.
Axéll, T., Mörnstad, H., and Sundström, B. (1978). *Laekartidningen (Med. News) 75*, 2224-2226.
Boyland, E., Roe, F. J. C., and Gorrod, J. W. (1964a). *Nature (London) 202,* 1126.
Boyland, E., Roe, F. J. C., Gorrod, J. W., and Mitchley, B. C. V. (1964b). *Br. J. Cancer 18,* 265-270.
Brunnemann, K. D., Scott, J. C., and Hoffmann, D. (1982). *Carcinogenesis 3,* 693-696.
Castonguay, A., Hecht, S. S., Hoffmann, D., Stoner, G. D., and Schut, H. A. J. (1982). *Proc. Am. Assoc. Cancer Res. 23*, 85.
Castonguay, A., Lin, D., Stoner, G. D., Radok, P., Furuya, K., Hecht, S. S., Schut, H. A. J., and Klauning, J. E. (1983). *Cancer Res. 43*, 1223-1229.
Christen, A. G., and Glover, E. D. (1981). *World Smoking Health 6,* 20-24.
Chu, C., and Magee, P. N. (1981). *Cancer Res. 41,* 3653-3657.
Dailey, R. E., Braunberg, R. C., and Blaschka, A. M. (1978). *Toxicology 3,* 23-28.
Federal Trade Commission (1981). "Report of 'Tar', Nicotine and Carbon Monoxide of the Smoke of 200 Varieties of Cigarettes." U.S. Govt. Printing Office, Washington, D.C.
Hammond, E. C., Garfinkel, L., Seidman, H., and Lew, E. A. (1977). *Cold Spring Harbor Conf. Cell Proliferation 4,* 101-112.
Hecht, S. S., Ornaf, R. M., and Hoffmann, D. (1975). *J. Natl. Cancer Inst. (U.S.) 54,* 1237-1244.
Hecht, S. S., Chen, C. B., Hirota, N., Ornaf, R. M., Tso, T. C., and Hoffmann, D. (1978). *J. Natl. Cancer Inst. (U.S.) 60,* 819-824.
Hecht, S. S., Chen, C. B., McCoy, G. D., Hoffmann, D., and Domellöf, L. (1979). *Cancer Lett. (Shannon, Irel.) 8,* 35-41.
Hecht, S. S., Chen, C. B., Ohmori, T., and Hoffmann, D. (1980a). *Cancer Res. 40*, 298-302.
Hecht, S. S., Young, R., and Chen, C. B. (1980b). *Cancer Res. 40*, 4144-4150.
Hecht, S. S., Castonguay, A., Chung, F. L., and Hoffmann, D. (1982a). *Banbury Rep. No. 12*, 103-120.

Hecht, S. S., Reiss, B., Lin, D., and Williams, G. M. (1982b). *Carcinogenesis 3,* 452-456.

Herning, R. I., Jones, R. T., Bachman, J., and Mines, A. H. (1981). *Br. Med. J. 283,* 187-189.

Hilfrich, J., Hecht, S. S., and Hoffmann, D. (1977). *Cancer Lett. (Shannon, Irel.) 2,* 165-175.

Hill, P., and Marquardt, H. (1980). *Clin. Pharmacol. Ther. 27,* 652-658.

Hill, P., Haley, N. J., and Wynder, E. L. (1983). *J. Chronic Dis.,* in press.

Hirsch, J. M., and Thylander, H. (1981). *J. Oral Pathol. 10,* 342-353.

Hoffmann, D., and Adams, J. D. (1981). *Cancer Res. 41,* 4305-4308.

Hoffmann, D., Raineri, R., Hecht, S. S., Maronpot, R., and Wynder, E. L. (1975). *J. Natl. Cancer Inst. (U.S.) 55,* 977-981.

Hoffmann, D., Castonguay, A., Rivenson, A., and Hecht, S. S. (1981). *Cancer Res. 41,* 2386-2393.

Jarvik, M. R. (1977). *In* "Research on Smoking Behavior" (M. E. Jarvik, J. W. Cullen, E. R. Gritz, T. M. Vogt, and L. J. West, eds.), pp. 122-146. HEW Publ. No. (ADM) 78-581. U.S. Govt. Printing Office, Washington, D.C.

Kunze, M., and Vutuc, C. (1980). *In* "A Safe Cigarette?" (G. B. Gori and F. G. Bock, eds.), pp. 29-36, *Banbury Rep.* No. 3. Cold Spring Harbor Lab., Cold Spring Harbor, New York.

Modéer, T., Lavstedt, S., and Ahlund, C. (1980). *Acta Odontol. Scand. 38,* 223-227.

Ohshima, H., and Bartsch, H. (1981). *Cancer Res. 41,* 3658-3662.

Peto, R., Gray, R., Branton, P., and Grasso, P. (1982). "The BIBRA Study on Nitrosamines." Br. Industrial Biological Res. Assoc., Carshalton, Surrey and Imperial Cancer Res. Fund Cancer Studies Unit, Oxford.

Pillsbury, H. C., Bright, C. C., O'Connor, K. J., and Irish, F. W. (1969). *J. Assoc. Off. Anal. Chem. 52,* 458-462.

Rostron, C. (1982). *Food Chem. Toxicol. 20,* 332-333.

Russell, M. A. H. (1978). *In* "Behavioral Effects of Nicotine" (K. Bättig, ed.), pp. 108-122. Karger, Basel.

Russell, M. A. H. (1980). *Banbury Rep.* No. 3, 297-310.

Russell, M. A. H., Wilson, C., Patel, V. A., Feyerabend, C., and Cole, P. V. (1975). *Br. Med. J. 2,* 414-416.

Schachter, S. (1978). *Ann. Intern. Med. 88,* 104-114.

Singer, G. M., and Taylor, H. W. (1976). *J. Natl. Cancer Inst. (U.S.) 57,* 1275-1276.

Tso, T. C. (1972). "Physiology and Biochemistry of Tobacco Plants." Dowden, Hutchinson & Ross, Stroudsburg, Pennsylvania.

U.S. Department of Health and Human Services (1982). "The
     Health Consequences of Smoking--Cancer, a Report of the
     Surgeon General, " Publ. No. DHHS (PHS) 82-50179. U.S.
     Govt. Printing Office, Washington, D.C.
Winn, D. M., Blot, W. J., Shy, C. M., Pickle, L. W., Toledo, A.
     and Fraumeni, J. R., Jr. (1981a). *New Engl. J. Med. 304,*
     745-749.
Winn, D. M., Blot, W. J., and Fraumeni, J. F., Jr. (1981b).
     New Engl. J. Med. 305, 2 30-231.
Wynder, E. L., and Hoffmann, D. (1967). "Tobacco and Tobacco
     Smoke--Studies in Experimental Carcinogenesis." Academic
     Press, New York.
Wynder, E. L., and Stellman, S. D. (1979). *J. Natl. Cancer
     Inst. (U.S.) 62,* 471-477.

34

MEASUREMENT OF ENDOGENOUS NITROSATION IN HUMANS: POTENTIAL APPLICATIONS OF A NEW METHOD AND INITIAL RESULTS

H. Bartsch, H. Ohshima, and N. Muñoz

International Agency for Research on Cancer
Lyon, France

M. Crespi

The Regina Elena Institute for the Study
and Therapy of Tumours
Rome, Italy

S. H. Lu

Cancer Institute
Chinese Academy of Medical Sciences
Beijing, People's Republic of China

Copyright © 1983 by Academic Press, Inc.
All rights of reproduction in any form reserved.
ISBN 0-12-327660-8

I. INTRODUCTION

Human exposure to carcinogenic *N*-nitroso compounds may
result from ingestion or inhalation of preformed compounds in
the environment or from nitrosation of amino precursors in the
body. Although limited data exist to quantitate human exposure, endogenous formation of *N*-nitroso compounds from ingested
precursors may be the largest single source of exposure to
these compounds for the general population (Coordinating Committee for Scientific and Technical Assessment of Environmental Pollutants, 1978).

Any nitrosation reaction, however, is influenced by many
factors such as pH, amounts of precursors involved, basicity
of the nitrosatable amine, and the presence of catalysts or
inhibitors. Although these factors have been studied in *in
vitro* systems, the lack of suitable methods for estimating endogenous nitrosation has hampered attempts to investigate them
under *in vivo* conditions.

For all these reasons, we have developed a simple and sensitive method for the quantitative estimation of nitrosation
reaction occurring *in vivo* (Ohshima and Bartsch, 1981a;
Ohshima *et al.*, 1982a). It is based on our findings and reports in the literature (Dailey *et al.*, 1975; Chu and Magee,
1981) that certain *N*-nitrosamino acids, such as *N*-nitrosoproline
(NPRO), are excreted unchanged almost quantitatively in the
urine and feces.

Results obtained from the application of this method to
study a number of factors affecting the nitrosation *in vivo* in
humans, after administration of nitrosatable amino acids and
nitrosating agents, are described. Initial results from clinical and field (pilot) studies in human subjects at high risk
for stomach and esophageal cancer are briefly presented.

II.   MATERIALS AND METHODS

A.   Precancerous Conditions of the Stomach and Study Subjects

It has been postulated that the achlorhydric environment
of the stomach provides a suitable milieu for intragastric formation of *N*-nitroso compounds. On the basis of this assumption, four groups of subjects have been included in our pilot
studies--that is, individuals with chronic atrophic gastritis,
pernicious anemia, those who underwent partial gastrectomy, and
subjects with different gastric secretory function (for more
details see Section III). All the study subjects have been
selected from those attending the gastroenterology department
of collaborating hospitals and on whom endoscopies have been
performed as part of a preestablished routine examination. Informed consent was requested for inclusion in the study.

Whenever possible, the following procedures (1-5) are
being followed for each study subject:

1. A questionnaire is completed containing basic demographic information as well as questions on smoking and drinking
habits and clinical symptoms.

2. Gastroscopy is performed, and the findings are recorded
on a special form. Localization of all lesions is indicated on
a diagram.

3. Fasting gastric juice is collected; the pH is measured
by a glass electrode, and an aliquot is frozen for bacteriologi-
cal studies and for analysis of total nitroso compounds (Walters
et al., 1978) (in collaboration with Dr. C. L. Walters, Leather-
head, United Kingdom).

4. For diagnostic purposes, during gastroscopy, at least
three biopsies are taken: the first from the greater curvature,
5 cm from the pylorus, the second from the greater curvature,
10 cm from the pylorus, and the third from the angular region of

the lesser curvature. The biopsies are fixed on 10% formalin.
All biopsies or unstained serial sections are sent to the IARC
for evaluation. In the histopathological evaluation, the following lesions are being considered: superficial gastritis,
chronic atrophic gastritis, and intestinal metaplasia, hyperplasia, and dysplasia.

    5. The *N*-nitrosoproline test: After endoscopy, subjects
are given 200 ml beetroot juice (containing 1300 mg of nitrate/
liter) as a source of nitrate, followed 30 min later by 10 ml
of an aqueous solution containing 500 mg *L*-proline. The subjects are asked to fast for an additional 2 h after ingestion
of proline; water is taken at libitum. During collection of
urine samples, the subjects are instructed to avoid foodstuffs
rich in nitrate and those presumed to contain preformed NPRO,
such as cured meat, smoked fish products, and beer.

    Urine samples are collected over 24 h after ingestion of
proline. To prevent artifactual formation of NPRO during collection, storage, and transport of the samples, specimens are
collected in a plastic bottle containing 10 g NaOH. The urine
collected in this way is thoroughly mixed and the volume recorded. An aliquot of the 24-h urine is then transferred into
a 100-ml plastic bottle and stored at -20°C prior to analysis.
Under these conditions, NPRO, NSAR (*N*-nitrososarcosine), and
nitrate/nitrite are stable, and artifactual formation or degradation of these compounds is negligible for at least
3 months.

B. Precancerous Lesions of the Esophagus and Study Subjects

    Previous studies in high-risk populations for esophageal
cancer in Iran and China (Crespi *et al.*, 1979; Muñoz *et al.*,
1982) suggest that the natural history of this tumor commences
with esophagitis, accompanied later by epithelial atrophy and

dysplasia. N-Nitroso compounds NO_3^-/NO_2^- have been suspected to be associated with this cancer in China (Coordination Group for Research on Etiology of Esophageal Cancer in North China, 1975; Yang, 1980). On the basis of observations, some collaborative pilot studies have been implemented on subjects living in Linxian, Jioaxian, and Fanxian counties (People's Republic of China). Excretion of N-nitroso compounds (pattern and amount) and NO_3^- in the urine was compared in subjects living in high-risk versus low-risk areas. Comparisons were also made among individuals with various degrees of precancerous lesions of the esophagus. Whenever possible, the following procedure was followed for each subject from Linxian and Jioaxian counties:

1. A questionnaire was completed containing demographic information and details on smoking and drinking habits, clinical symptoms, and foodstuffs consumed during urine collection.

2. Esophagoscopy was performed, and localization of all lesions was recorded on a special diagram.

3. Biopsies were taken from the middle and lower thirds and from any macroscopic lesion. They were evaluated for the presence of chronic esophagitis (classified as mild, moderate, or severe), epithelial atrophy, dysplasia, and clear cell acanthosis.

4. Twenty-four-hour urine specimens were collected to determine the background levels of NPRO, NSAR, and nitrate. To prevent artifactual formation of N-nitroso compounds, the urine samples were stabilized using 10 g of NaOH, as described earlier.

C. Analysis of Urinary N-Nitroso Compounds, Nitrate, and Nitrite

Urine samples were spiked with N-nitrosopipecolic acid (NPIC) as internal standard, and analysis for NPRO was carried out according to a published procedure (Ohshima and Bartsch,

1981a; Ohshima *et al.*, 1982a) after conversion of the nitrosamines to their methyl esters by means of diazomethane (Kawabata,
1974).

A Tracor 550 gas chromatograph (Austin, Texas) was used
with argon carrier gas (20 ml/min) and interfaced to a thermal
energy analyzer (TEA 502, Thermo Electron Corp., Waltham, Massachusetts). The average recoveries of NPRO and NSAR added to
the urine samples at a concentration of 20 µg/liter were 85 and
82%, respectively, with minimum detectable levels of 0.5 and
0.1 µg/liter, respectively. Under these conditions, the peaks
of the methyl esters of NSAR, NPRO, and NPIC were well resolved,
and no interfering peaks appeared on the chromatogram.

Nitrate and nitrite in urine samples were determined according to the method of Sen and Donaldson (1978). Nitrite was
determined colorimetrically with a modified Gries reagent. Nitrate was reduced to nitrite by cadmium reducing powder obtained
from Wako Pure Chemicals (Osaka, Japan).

III.   RESULTS AND DISCUSSION

A.   Kinetic Studies on the Endogenous Nitrosation of Proline in
     a Human Subject

In the absence of adverse biological effects of NPRO (IARC
Monographs on the Evaluation of the Carcinogenic Risk of Chemicals to Humans, 1978; Mirvish *et al.*, 1980), a number of kinetic
studies were previously carried out on the formation of NPRO *in
vivo* in a human volunteer who had ingested vegetable juice (as
a source of nitrate, 0-325 mg) and 30 min later an aqueous solution of proline (0-500 mg), and monitored urinary excretion of
NPRO (Ohshima and Bartsch, 1981a). The formation of NPRO *in
vivo* was found to be strongly dependent on nitrate intake. When
less than 195 mg nitrate were ingested, a marginal or in most

cases no increase in urinary NPRO was observed, as compared
with that in a control experiment (no nitrate intake). However, when >260 mg nitrate were consumed, the excretion of
NPRO increased exponentially with the dose of nitrate ingested.

The formation *in vivo* of NPRO was shown to be proportional
to the dose of proline ingested. These experiments show that
in a healthy human subject, with the highest doses of nitrate
(325 mg) and proline (500 mg) ingested, formation of NPRO
ranged from 16.6 to 30.0 µg (mean 23.3) per 24 h per person,
corresponding to 0.002 and 0.004% of the ingested amounts of
nitrate and proline, respectively.

Considering our results as a whole, the mechanism for NPRO
formation in humans appears to be as follows: The nitrate ingested in vegetable juice is resecreted in the saliva, starting
about 30 min after its ingestion, reaching a maximum after 1 to
2 h (Ishiwata *et al.*, 1975; Spiegelhalder *et al.*, 1976; Tannenbaum *et al.*, 1976). The resecreted nitrate is reduced to nitrite by the oral microflora. Proline ingested 30 min after
intake of vegetable juice probably reacts with salivary nitrite
to give NPRO under the acidic conditions prevailing in the
stomach.

B. Inhibition of Endogenous Nitrosation by Ascorbic Acid
    (Vitamin C) and α-Tocopherol (Vitamin E)

The inhibition of endogenous nitrosation by vitamins C and
E was previously assessed quantitatively in experiments on a
human subject (Ohshima and Bartsch, 1981a,b). The amounts of
NPRO excreted in the urine after ingestion of 325 mg of nitrate
and 250 mg of proline ranged from 14.0 to 15.9 µg/24 h, with a
mean value of 14.9 µg; the excretion rate was 5-7.5 times
higher than that in control experiments in which either nitrate
or proline alone were ingested. Intake of ascorbic acid (1 g)
simultaneously with the precursors was found to inhibit totally

the nitrosation of proline *in vivo*, and the amounts of NPRO
detected were the same as those in the controls. α-Tocopherol
(500 mg) was less effective and inhibited nitrosation *in vivo*
only by about 50%. Similar effects were observed in rats
(Ohshima *et al.*, 1982a).

C. Application of the NPRO Test in Clinical and Field Studies

1. Rationale of the NPRO Test and Practical Aspects

There is strong evidence to support the notion that in the
human body carcinogenic *N*-nitroso compounds can be formed by
the interaction of nitrosatable amino compounds and nitrosating
agents (Correa *et al.*, 1975; Ruddell *et al.*, 1976; Fine *et al.*,
1977; Tannenbaum *et al.*, 1979; Schlag *et al.*, 1980; Ohshima and
Bartsch, 1981a). The question that now requires clarification
is whether the amounts of *N*-nitroso compounds formed endogenously correlate with an increased incidence of specific types of
human cancer. However, the lack of suitable methods to estimate
endogenous nitrosation in humans has hindered attempts to obtain such data. Monitoring NPRO excreted in the urine appears
to be a useful method to estimate the extent of nitrosation *in*
vivo in high-risk populations or human individuals.

The rationale for applying this procedure in field or clinical studies is based on the following observations:

1. NPRO has been reported not to be carcinogenic and mutagenic (IARC Monographs on the Evaluation of the Carcinogenic
Risk of Chemicals to Humans, 1978; Mirvish *et al.*, 1980).

2. After gavage of rats with [^{14}C]NPRO, the ^{14}CO$_2$ production and DNA alkylation were negligible (Chu and Magee, 1981),
but urinary excretion of NPRO (as the unchanged compound) was
rapid and almost complete (Dailey *et al.*, 1975; Chu and Magee,
1981; Ohshima *et al.*, 1982a.

3. Urinary levels of NPRO in rats gavaged with proline

and nitrite reflected well endogenous nitrosation of proline (Ohshima et al., 1982a).

4. In humans, preformed NPRO ingested in the aqueous extract of broiled dried squids was also rapidly and almost quantitatively eliminated in the urine within 24 h after ingestion (Ohshima et al., 1982b).

Thus, the amount of NPRO excreted in the 24-h urine was an indicator of daily endogenous nitrosation (Ohshima and Bartsch, 1981a).

The application of the NPRO method to human subjects, to the best of our knowledge, therefore, does not involve a risk for their health, because when ingesting beetroot juice (as a source of nitrate) and proline: (1) The experiments involve only an increased intake of commonly occurring food ingredients at dose ranges that are considered as normal daily intake; (2) the absence of carcinogenic and mutagenic effects of NPRO is established; and (3) the natural occurrence of low levels of NPRO in many foodstuffs and in the urine of humans is known.

The method just outlined is now being explored to estimate the extent of endogenous nitrosation in individuals (groups of subjects) at high cancer risk in whom endogenously formed N-nitroso compounds are suspected to be associated, as described in the following section.

2. Evaluation of Human Exposure to N-Nitroso Compounds and Nitrate in High-Risk Areas for Esophageal Cancer

Epidemiological studies have associated an increased risk of esophageal and stomach cancer with an elevated exposure to nitrate (Armijo and Coulson, 1975; Coordination Group for Research on Etiology of Esophageal Cancer in North China, 1975; Cuello et al., 1976; Fraser et al., 1980; Yang, 1980). For

example, in some provinces in northern China esophageal cancer
is a prevalent disease, and a positive correlation has been reported between the cancer risk and the levels of nitrate/nitrite
in the drinking water, or the intakes of pickled vegetables and
moldy foods (Coordination Group for Research on Etiology of
Esophageal Cancer in North China, 1975; Yang, 1980). In order
to measure individual exposure to nitrate (nitrite) by monitoring excreted NPRO under conditions and dietary habits that may
prevail in this high-incidence area in China, a series of experiments have just been conducted in a human subject (Ohshima
and Bartsch, 1982); on the basis of the results (see later),
some (pilot) field studies were implemented.

   *a.   Endogenous NPRO formation in a human subject after
intake of nitrate-containing vegetables or after multiple precursor doses.*   Endogenous formation of NPRO was observed to occur in a human subject who ingested 100 g of pickled vegetables
(Chinese cabbage prepared in France) as a source of nitrate and
nitrite, followed 1 h later by 100 mg of proline. The pickled
vegetable ingested (one sample) contained about 750 ppm (mg/kg)
sodium nitrate and 4.5 ppm sodium nitrite. Preformed NPRO was
also detected in the pickled vegetable at a concentration of
35 ppb (µg/kg). Therefore, intake of the vegetable alone led
to an increase in urinary NPRO. However, when 100 mg proline
were ingested 1 h after intake of 100 g of the vegetable, the
urinary level of NPRO was further increased. These results
support the notion that *N*-nitroso compounds can be formed in
the body after simultaneous ingestion of nitrate/nitrite-
containing vegetables and nitrosatable precursors, which can
be present in foodstuffs or in the stomach.

   In high-incidence areas for esophageal cancer such as
exist in China, human subjects are more likely to be continuously exposed to nitrate/nitrite, which may be present in foodstuffs and drinking water or formed endogenously in the body.

In order to investigate experimentally such a situation, where chronic exposure is involved, the following four series of experiments were conducted in one male volunteer:

1. Three times a day, 100 mg proline were taken 1 h after each meal (consisting of a low-nitrate diet), following which only trace amounts of NPRO were excreted in the urine (1.7 μg/24 h/person).

2. Nitrate-rich meals (low-nitrate diet + 100 ml beetroot juice containing 130 mg NO_3^-) were taken three times a day together with three doses of proline; as a result, an increased amount of NPRO was excreted in the urine (13.4 μg/24 h).

3. The intake of three nitrate-rich meals without proline did not significantly increase the urinary NPRO, as compared to experiment 1 (2.9 μg/24 h).

4. When orange juice (a possible source of vitamin C) was taken at the end of each nitrate-rich meal, followed by proline, urinary excretion of NPRO was markedly suppressed (4.0 versus 13.4 μg/24 h in experiment 2).

The results obtained from these experiments indicate that endogenous nitrosation may occur continuously in the body following chronic nitrate exposure. However, even when the amount of ingested nitrate was high enough to give rise to the formation of *N*-nitroso compounds in the human body, the presence of dietary vitamin C effectively inhibited nitrosation. These results suggest that nitrosation *in vivo* may be modified by many factors, such as the presence of catalysts or inhibitors in foods (Ohshima *et al.*, 1982a; Pignatelli *et al.*, 1982). Thus, in addition to data on individual exposure to nitrate, assessing of the extent of endogenous nitrosation is required to establish a possible causal relationship between the amounts of *N*-nitroso compounds formed and an increased incidence of specific types of human cancers.

b. Excretion of N-nitroso compounds and nitrate in the urine of subjects living in high-risk and low-risk areas for esophageal cancer. The subjects were selected from those included in the IARC endoscopy surveys carried out in Linxian (high-risk area) by Muñoz *et al.* (1982) and in Jioaxian (low-risk area) in May 1981. In Linxian 43 subjects over 20 years of age were selected and 46 in Jioaxian.

In a feasibility study the background levels of NPRO, NSAR, and nitrate excreted in the 24-h urines of subjects living in these two areas were determined. In all the urine specimens, nitrite content was below detection limits (0.1 mg/liter).

The relationship between the daily amounts of NPRO and those of nitrate excreted in the 24-h urine is shown for subjects living in Linxian (Fig. 1a) and Jioaxian (Fig. 2), respectively. The relationship between the daily amounts of NSAR and those of nitrate of subjects in Linxian is presented in Fig. 1b. A positive correlation was observed only between the amounts of nitrate and NPRO excreted by the Linxian subjects ($r = .5$; $p < .01$, $n = 43$; Fig. 1a), but no apparent correlation was found between the urinary levels of nitrate and of NPRO in the Jioaxian subjects (Fig. 2). The scattering of our data points (Figs. 1b, 2) could be explained by the following: (1) A proportion of NPRO and NSAR excreted in the urine may be derived from ingestion of preformed NPRO and NSAR, and (2) modulators (catalysts and inhibitors) of *in vivo* nitrosation may have occurred in the body or were ingested in foodstuffs.

Fig. 1. A plot of the amount of urinary nitrate versus that of NPRO (a) and NSAR (b) excreted per 24 h by subjects living in Linxian county (People's Republic of China). For further details, see Section II and text.

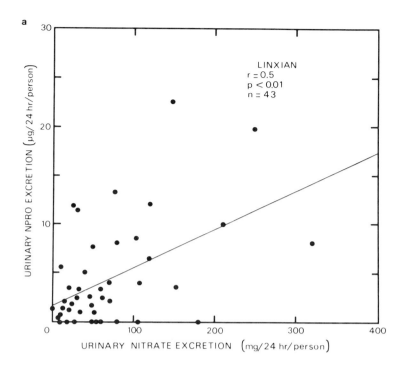

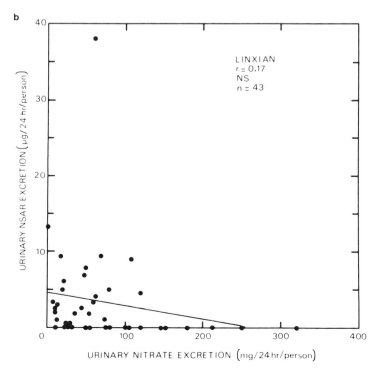

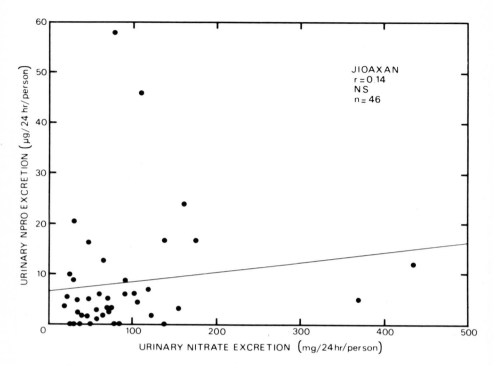

Fig. 2. A plot of the amount of urinary nitrate versus that of NPRO excreted per 24 h by subjects living in Jioaxian county (People's Republic of China). For further details, see Section II and text.

In Figs. 3 and 4, the frequency distribution of NPRO and NSAR concentrations that were detected in these urine samples is plotted. Daily exposure to *N*-nitroso compounds (estimated from the total amount of NPRO and NSAR excreted in the 24-h urine) ranged in Linxian from trace amounts to 38 µg (average ±SD: 7.8 ± 7.1; n = 43) and in Jioaxian from trace amounts to 58 µg per person (8.31 ± 11.0, n = 46). Amounts of nitrate excreted by subjects in Linxian ranged from traces to 321 mg/person (71 ± 68; n = 43) and from traces to 435 mg/person (89 ± 82; n = 41) in Jioaxian. Thus, the levels of NPRO and nitrate detected in the 24-h urines did not significantly differ in these two areas. However, higher levels of NSAR (a weakly active esophageal carcinogen in experimental animals) were

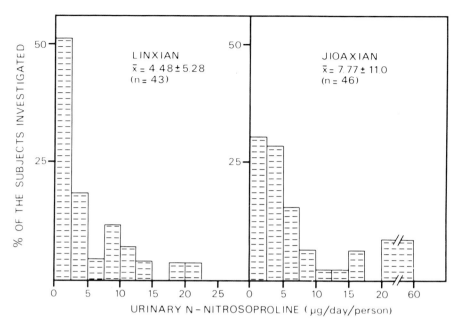

Fig. 3. Frequency distribution of urinary NPRO (μg/24 h/
person) excreted by subjects living in Linxian and Jioaxian
counties (People's Republic of China).

detected more frequently in Linxian than in Jioaxian, although
the difference is not statistically significant (Fig. 4).

Studies on the occurrence of *N*-nitroso compounds and their
precursors in water and food samples collected in high-
incidence areas for esophageal cancer in northern China (Coordination Group for Research on Etiology of Esophageal Cancer
in North China, 1975; Yang, 1980), show positive correlations
between the incidence rate of esophageal cancer and the levels
of nitrate/nitrite in drinking water or intake of pickled
vegetables and moldy foods. Our preliminary results for these
two counties could not provide a clear correlation between the
urinary levels of nitrate, NPRO, and NSAR, and the risk of cancer. In addition, no apparent relationship was found between
the occurrence or degree of precancerous lesions of the esopha-

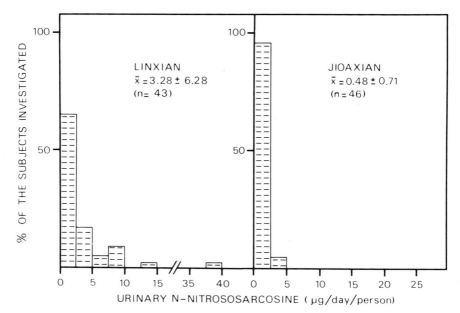

Fig. 4. Frequency distribution of urinary NSAR (µg/24 h/person) excreted by subjects living in Linxian and Jioaxian counties (People's Republic of China).

gus in Linxian subjects and the urinary levels of these compounds (data not shown); however, the number of subjects investigated so far in this feasibility study was too small to allow appropriate statistical analyses. It should further be noted that Jioaxian, selected as a low-incidence area for esophageal cancer, has a high incidence rate for stomach cancer. This fact complicated the interpretation of our results.

    In order to expand these studies, in the beginning of 1982, 250 urine samples were collected in Linxian county (high-risk area) and in Fanxian county (a low-risk area for both esophageal and stomach cancer). Specimens were collected according to three different protocols: (1) undosed subjects, (2) subjects who had ingested three times a day 100 mg *L*-proline after each meal, and (3) subjects who had ingested three times

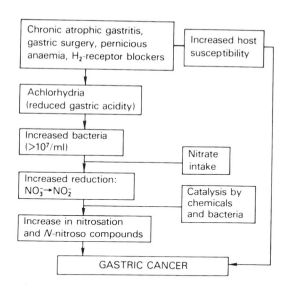

Fig. 5. Hypothetical flow diagram linking intragastric nitrosation, precursor lesions, and induction of gastric cancer. The scheme is collated from proposals made earlier in the literature (Correa *et al.*, 1975; Reed *et al.*, 1981).

a day 100 mg proline together with 100 mg vitamin C. The analyses for urinary nitrate and *N*-nitroso compounds are currently under way.

3. Monitoring of Endogenous Nitrosation in Human Subjects at High Risk for Stomach Cancer

Endogenous formation of *N*-nitroso compounds has been associated with an increased risk of stomach cancer. For example, an elevated risk for stomach cancer has been observed in patients with chronic atrophic gastritis or pernicious anemia, and in patients who have undergone gastric surgery such as Billroth-II gastrectomy (Blackburn *et al.*, 1968; Stalsberg and Taksdal, 1971; Cuello *et al.*, 1976). It has been postulated (see hypothetical flow diagram, Fig. 5) that the achlorhydric stomach found in such patients may provide a suitable milieu for intragastric formation of *N*-nitroso compounds by the

presence of a large number of bacteria, which may be involved
in the conversion of nitrate to nitrite and subsequent nitrosation *in vivo* (Correa *et al.*, 1975; Ruddell *et al.*, 1976;
Schlag *et al.*, 1980; Reed *et al.*, 1981). In fact, higher
levels of *N*-nitroso compounds were more frequently found in
fasting gastric juice samples of such patients than in those
of normal subjects (Reed *et al.*, 1981). However, the extent
of endogenous nitrosation occurring in these individuals at
high risk for stomach cancer has not been determined, but can
now be estimated using the NPRO test (see Section II). In
collaborative clinical studies, it is currently being applied
to study subjects belonging to the four groups indicated next.

   a. Gastric secretory function. Sixty male subjects aged
40-59 without localized gastric pathology such as polyps or
ulcers are being included in this study. The histopathological
evaluation of the gastric mucosa will be complemented by an
evaluation of the secretory function after stimulation with
pentagastrin. These subjects have been selected from the gastroenterology department of the Hôpital Edouard-Herriot, Lyons,
France (in collaboration with R. Lambert and Y. Minaire).

   b. Pernicious anemia. Thirty patients with pernicious
anemia and 30 control subjects with normal gastric mucosa or
with superficial gastritis have been selected from various departments of the University of Turku, Finland (in collaboration
with A. Lehtonen and M. Inberg).

   c. Postgastrectomy. Two hundred male subjects are being
selected from those who underwent partial gastrectomy in 1950-
1952 and who have agreed to participate in an ongoing screening
program for gastric cancer in Iceland (in collaboration with
H. Tulinius and G. Arnthorsson).

   d. Chronic atrophic gastritis (CAG). Fifty male individuals (20-49 years old) with various degrees of histologically
proven CAG, with and without intestinal metaplasia (IM) have

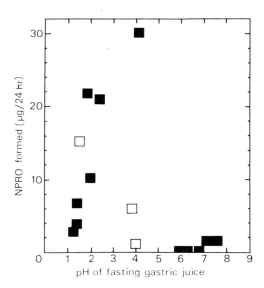

Fig. 6. A plot of the urinary NPRO excreted by subjects after ingestion of beetroot juice and proline versus the pH of the fasting gastric juice of the same individual (interim results). Control subjects (□) and patients with precancerous lesions (CAG) (■) of the stomach are shown. For further details, see Section II.

been selected. The results obtained in this group will be compared with those obtained in a control group of the same sex and age who have been found to have a histologically normal stomach or with superficial gastritis. These subjects have been selected from the gastroenterology department of the Regina Elena Institute of Rome.

Some interim results are presently available for study subjects in group d. The amount of NPRO excreted in the 24-h urine of 12 patients with chronic atrophic gastritis and 3 subjects with normal gastric mucosa is shown in Fig. 6. In the graph, the excretion of NPRO (μg/person/24 h) is plotted against the pH of fasting gastric juice obtained from the same subject. After ingestion of nitrate (260 mg) and proline (500 mg), the yield of NPRO in the urine of these subjects ranged from trace

amounts to 30 µg/24 h/person. It appeared to be dependent on
the pH of the gastric juice, as the highest values for NPRO
were seen at pH ≈ 2-2.5, which coincides with the optimum value
reported for nitrosation of proline *in vitro* (Mirvish *et al.*,
1973).

Because there were only three cases in the control group
(subjects with normal stomach mucosa), a comparison of endogenous nitrosation in subjects with or without precancerous
lesions or conditions of the stomach is pending until more
data (presently being collected) are available. In addition,
the levels of total nitroso compounds (measured by the method
of Walters *et al.*, 1978) and bacteria count in fasting gastric
juice obtained from each subject are being determined. These
results will be compared with those of the NPRO test.

4. *Occurrence of Nonidentified N-Nitroso Compounds in Human*
    Urine Samples

In addition to NPRO and NSAR, whose occurrence has been
reported here, urine samples from subjects receiving no precursor treatment frequently contained some unknown nonvolatile
compounds that gave a positive response with the *N*-nitroso
compound-specific detector; a typical chromatogram obtained by
gas chromatography-thermal energy analyzer (GC-TEA) analysis of
human urine extracts is shown in Fig. 7. These compounds, unidentified so far, are putatively characterized as nitrosamino
acids carrying a carboxyl group(s) in their molecule, because
they can be detected by gas chromatography only after esterification with diazomethane. Isolation and identification of
these unknown compounds in human urine as well as investigations on their origin are currently in progress.

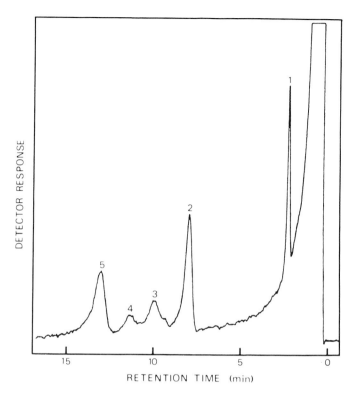

Fig. 7. A typical GC-TEA chromatogram of human urine extract (after esterification with diazomethane). Human urine extract was prepared as described earlier. Ohshima and Bartsch (1981a). GC conditions were as follows: 2 m × 3 mm i.d. glass column containing 5% FFAP on Chromosorb W-HP (80-100 mesh); temperature of column, 170°C, and of injection port, 220°C; carrier gas, argon (20 ml/min). Peak 1 was identified as NSAR, peak 2 as NPRO, and peaks 3, 4, and 5 are unknown compounds.

IV. CONCLUSIONS

Results obtained so far indicate that the NPRO method is simple, sensitive, and reproducible. Data from animal experiments and from pilot studies in human subjects support the notion that:

1. NPRO excreted in 24 h is an index for the rate of endogenous nitrosation.

2. The method can be satisfactorily applied to human subjects in clinical and field studies.

3. Because nitrosation *in vivo* was shown to be modified by inhibitors in the food (e.g., vitamin C), assessing of the extent of endogenous nitrosation in individual human subjects seems essential to establish a possible causal relationship between the levels of N-nitroso compounds found and an increased incidence of specific types of cancer.

4. Studies are in progress or being planned to use the NPRO method to estimate the potential of *in vivo* nitrosation in (a) subjects with precancerous lesions of the esophagus and stomach and in subjects without these lesions, and (b) asymptomatic subjects from high- and low-risk areas for cancers of the esophagus and stomach, and subjects with different dietary habits, especially those with contrasting intake of nitrates.

5. Vitamin C was shown to compete efficiently with the nitrosatable amine for the available nitrite *in vivo*. Therefore, should it be demonstrated that N-nitroso compounds formed in the human body are causative factors in certain human cancers, vitamin C would then appear to be effective in blocking N-nitrosation *in vivo* and thus play an important role from the point of view of primary cancer prevention.

NOTE ADDED IN PROOF

During the preparation of this manuscript, the unknown N-nitroso compounds (Fig. 7, peaks 3 and 4) have been identified as *trans*- and *cis*-epimers of N-nitroso-2-methylthiazolidin 4-carboxylic acid, respectively, and peak 5 as N-nitroso-thiazolidine 4-carboxylic acid.

ACKNOWLEDGMENTS

    We wish to thank Mrs. M. M. Courcier for secretarial help, and Mr. J. C. Bereziat, Mlle J. Michelon, and Mlle M. C. Bourgade for technical assistance. The TEA detector was provided on loan by the National Cancer Institute, Bethesda, Maryland, under contract No. NOI CP-55717.

REFERENCES

Armijo, R., and Coulson, A. H. (1975). *Int. J. Epidemiol. 4,* 301-309.
Blackburn, E. K., Callender, S. T., Dacie, J. V., Doll, R., Girdwood, R. H., Mollin, D. L., Saracci, R., Stafford, J., Thompson, R. B., Varadi, S., and Wetherly-Mein, G. (1968). *Int. J. Cancer 3,* 163-170.
Chu, C., and Magee, P. (1981). *Cancer Res. 41,* 3653-3657.
Coordinating Committee for Scientific and Technical Assessment of Environmental Pollutants (1978). *In* "Nitrates: An Environmental Assessment," pp. 435-484. Nat. Acad. Sci., Washington, D.C.
Coordination Group for Research on Etiology of Esophageal Cancer in North China (1975). *Chung-hua I Hsueh Tsa Chih (Peking) (Chin. Med. J.) 1,* 167-183.
Correa, P., Haenszel, W., Cuello, C., Tannenbaum, S., and Archer, M. (1975). *Lancet ii,* 58-59.
Crespi, M., Muñoz, N., Grassi, A., Aramesh, B., Amiri, G., and Mojtabai, A. (1979). *Lancet ii,* 217-221.
Cuello, C., Correa, P., Haenszel, W., Gordillo, G., Brown, C., Archer, M., and Tannenbaum, S. (1976). *J. Natl. Cancer Inst. (U.S.) 57,* 1015-1020.
Dailey, R. E., Braunberg, R. C., and Blaschka, A. M. (1975). *Toxicology 3,* 23-28.
Fine, D. H., Ross, R., Rounbehler, D. P., Silvergleid, A., and Song, L. (1977). *Nature (London) 265,* 753-755.
Fraser, P., Chilvers, C., Beral, V., and Hill, M. J. (1980). *Int. J. Epidemiol. 9,* 3-11.
IARC Monogr. Eval. Carcinog. Risk Chem. Humans, Vol. 17 (1978), pp. 303-311.
Ishiwata, H., Boriboon, P., Nakamura, Y., Harada, M., Tanimura, A., and Ishidate, M. (1975). *Shokuhin Eiseigaku Zasshi (J. Food Hyg. Soc. Jpn.) 16,* 19-24.
Kawabata, T. (1974). *IARC Sci. Publ.* No. 9, 154-158.
Mirvish, S. S., Sams, J., Fran, T. Y., and Tannenbaum, S. R. (1973). *J. Natl. Cancer Inst. (U.S.) 51,* 1833-1839.

Mirvish, S. S., Bulay, O., Runge, R. G., and Patil, K. (1980). *J. Natl. Cancer Inst. (U.S.) 64,* 1435-1442.

Muñoz, N., Crespi, M., Grassi, A., Qing, W. G., Qiong, S., and Cai, L. Z. (1982). *Lancet i,* 876-879.

Ohshima, H., and Bartsch, H. (1981a). *Cancer Res. 41,* 3658-3662.

Ohshima, H., and Bartsch, H. (1981b). *In* "Vitamin C (Ascorbic Acid)" (J. N. Counsell and D. H. Hornig, eds.), pp. 215-224. Applied Science, London and Englewood, New Jersey.

Ohshima, H., and Bartsch, H. (1982). *In* "Environmental Mutagens and Carcinogens" (T. Sugimura, S. Kondo, and H. Takebe, eds.), pp. 577-585. Univ. of Tokyo Press, Tokyo; Liss, New York.

Ohshima, H., Bereziat, J. C., and Bartsch, H. (1982a). *Carcinogenesis 3,* 115-120.

Ohshima, H., Bereziat, J. C., and Bartsch, H. (1982b). *IARC Sci. Publ.* No. 41, 397-411.

Pignatelli, B., Bereziat, J. C., O'Neill, I. K., and Bartsch, H. (1982). *IARC Sci. Publ.* No. 41, 413-423.

Reed, P. I., Smith, P. L. R., Haines, K., House, F. R., and Walters, C. (1981). *Lancet i,* 550-555.

Ruddell, W. S. J., Bone, E. S., Hill, M. J., Blendis, L. M., and Walters, C. (1976). *Lancet i,* 1037-1039.

Schlag, P., Bockler, R., Ulrich, H., Peter, M., Merkle, P., and Herfarth, C. (1980). *Lancet i,* 727-729.

Sen, N. P., and Donaldson, B. (1978). *J. Assoc. Off. Anal. Chem. 61,* 1389-1394.

Spiegelhalder, B., Eisenbrand, G., and Preussmann, R. (1976). *Food Cosmet. Toxicol. 14,* 545-548.

Stalsberg, H., and Taksdal, S. (1971). *Lancet ii,* 1175-1177.

Tannenbaum, S. R., Weisman, M., and Fett, D. (1976). *Food Cosmet. Toxicol. 14,* 549-552.

Tannenbaum, S. R., Moran, D., Rand, W., Cuelo, C., and Correa, P. (1979). *J. Natl. Cancer Inst. (U.S.) 62,* 9-12.

Walters, C. L., Downes, L. J., Edwards, L. W., and Smith, P. L. R. (1978). *Analyst (London) 103,* 1127-1133.

Yang, C. S. (1980). *Cancer Res.* 40, 2633- 2644.

35

PROBING GENETICALLY VARIABLE CARCINOGEN METABOLISM USING DRUGS

Jeffrey R. Idle and James C. Ritchie

Department of Pharmacology,
St. Mary's Hospital Medical School
London, England

I.   INTRODUCTION

A.   Cancer Etiology: A Role for Pharmacogenetics?

    The study of the chain of events linking chemical car-
cinogen exposure with appearance of tumors has little directly
to do with the subject of pharmacology. Nevertheless, the
former may draw fruitfully or the principles of the latter. In
the analogous model, drug may be a cocktail of potentially active substances (e.g., cigarette smoke) or simply a single
carcinogen such as aflatoxin B_1. In the same way that drugs
may exert their overall effects via a combination of events at
several types of high-affinity macromolecular receptors, carcinogens too have multiple effects at discrete peri- and intracellular sites. Finally, the organ distribution, metabolism,
and excretion of chemical carcinogens and their metabolites
can rationally be explained on the basis of pharmacokinetic
considerations that might apply to any administered or covert-
ly absorbed exogenous chemical.

    This parallel, however, contains some essential flaws.
First, the dose of a carcinogen, unlike a drug, is poorly controlled, and by necessity its assessment in humans is often
speculative. Second, whereas the effects of drugs are usually
transient and almost always reversible, those of carcinogens
and cocarcinogens are patently not so. Thus the application
of pharmacological principles such as dose-response relationships and pharmacokinetics, outside tightly controlled laboratory investigations, is not without great difficulties.

    Nevertheless, we believe that, in search of identifiable
and stable host factors that may give clues to the origins of
individual susceptibility to environmental chemical carcinogens, consideration of some of the developments in human pharmacogenetics may be of value.

B. Cytochromes *P*-450

An enormous accumulated body of evidence leaves us in little doubt as to the importance of the cytochromes *P*-450 in the metabolic activation and detoxication of many known carcinogens. For the purposes of this chapter, we will make no attempt to cite the plethora of references relating to this former statement but merely direct the reader to some of the many reviews of this topic (Miller and Miller, 1977; Evered and Lawrenson, 1980; Conney, 1981).

Many isoenzymic forms of cytochrome *P*-450 have now been isolated and purified from rat, rabbit, and even humans (Lu and West, 1980). Isolation of most of these cytochromes has been facilitated after chronic treatment of the animals with enzyme-inducing agents in order to produce a large number of copies of a few predominant forms of cytochrome, the presence of some of which it is difficult to demonstrate in the uninduced animal. Accordingly, relatively little is known about the nature of native cytochromes *P*-450. Hepatic parenchymal cells probably have the highest basal levels of cytochromes *P*-450, with concentrations of 0.22 to 0.92 and 0.26 to 1.02 nmol/mg microsomal protein for rat and humans, respectively (Vainio and Hietanen, 1980). Direct investigation of the nature of human *P*-450 is therefore difficult for living subjects, because only conservative biopsy of the liver can be performed. Interestingly, though, the quantitative variation in both rat and human *P*-450 is quite small (fourfold), and because most metabolic oxidations of drugs *in vivo* proceed in a first-order manner, as a result of the low tissue concentrations that they achieve relative to the K_m of the metabolizing system, the wide intersubject variation in human drug oxidation cannot be explained by such a fourfold variation (see later). Obviously, genetic polymorphic (qualitative) differences between subjects,

where the cytochromes in one person have different substrate
affinities and/or capacities from those in another, are
plausible explanations of the wide intersubject variation in
drug oxidation and carcinogen oxidation and activation by the
P-450 system.

C. Genetics of Metabolic Oxidation

By far the biggest contribution to our understanding of
the genetic regulation of cytochrome P-450 synthesis has been
made by Nebert and colleagues at the NIH, working on the murine Ah cluster. Wild mice and the majority of laboratory inbred strains so far tested, when treated with such agents as
20-methylcholanthrene, benzo[a]pyrene, or 2,3,7,8-tetrachloro-
dibenzo-p-dioxin, respond by increasing their synthesis of cytochrome P_1-450 [polycyclic aromatic-induced aryl hydrocarbon
(benzo[a]pyrene) hydroxylase (AHH; E.C. 1.14.14.2)] and thus
increase their *in vitro* metabolism of around 20 substrates
(Nebert, 1979; Nebert and Jensen, 1979). The prototype strain
is C57BL/6, whose trait of P_1-450 induction is an autosomal
dominant. The prototype nonresponsive recessive is the DBA/2
strain. At least two loci and a minimum of six alleles are
thought to regulate P_1-450 synthesis in the mouse (Robinson *et
al.*, 1974).

Evidence for polymorphism in the P-450 structural genes
of mouse, rat, and rabbit is only now emerging with the application of the new generation of genetic engineering techniques.
In fact, drawing on some of these data, Nebert has speculated
that any individual mammal has the genetic ability to produce
as many as several thousand unique P-450 proteins (Nebert,
1979; Nebert and Negishi, 1982). More conservative estimates
place the number two orders of magnitude lower (Lu and West,
1980). Nucleotide sequencing of P-450 cDNA will undoubtedly

provide the best opportunity to understand polymorphic variation of P-450 proteins in laboratory animals.

   The almost total sequencing of two phenobarbital-inducible
rat P-450 cDNA clones (Fujii-Kuriyama et al., 1982) must herald
a new and exciting era in P-450 research. Nevertheless, we are
not optimistic that these techniques can be readily applied to
the problem of genetically variable human cytochromes P-450, at
least not for some time. We are still faced with the challenge
of being able to identify human P-450 phenotypes because of
their proven importance in understanding adverse drug reactions
(Ritchie et al., 1980; Smith and Idle, 1981; Shah et al., 1982)
and their potential importance in cancer etiology (Ritchie and
Idle, 1982). Section II will review the use of drug probes in
humans, with emphasis given to those proven polymorphic oxidative pathways. Section III will deal with the application of
these approaches to specific cancer problems and review our experiences to date.

II. DRUG PROBES FOR GENETICALLY VARIABLE METABOLIC OXIDATION

A. Background

   Considerable variation in carcinogen metabolism and activation has been demonstrated in vitro using biopsies of human
liver, placenta, macrophages, and cultured skin and lymphocytes
(for a review see Conney, 1981). Additionally, correlations
between drug and carcinogen metabolism in human liver biopsies
have been made, the most striking of which was that between
benzo[a]pyrene metabolism to fluorescent phenols and antipyrine
4-hydroxylation ($n = 48$, $r = .91$; Conney, 1981). One possible
limitation is envisaged in deriving correlations of this nature
using small amounts of biological material, and that is, by
necessity only one substrate concentration can be used. There-

fore, if the metabolizing cytochrome in one patient has a radically different K_m to that from another, then very different
degrees of saturation will obtain; that is, one patient's reaction may be proceeding at near its V_{max} and another's at only
a small fraction of it.   Thus, human variability in tissue mono-
oxygenation may be greater than is often observed.

Antipyrine emerged for a multitude of reasons as the candidate probe to assess interindividual differences in human
metabolic oxidation.   It has many features that commend it, but
unfortunately it is a very low-affinity substrate for human
P-450 monooxygenases, with a K_m for each of the known metabolic
pathways of about 10^{-2} M (Boobis et al., 1981).   This can be
interpreted as meaning that differences in antipyrine clearance
reflect purely differences in total hepatic V_{max}, which themselves reflect differences in total functional enzyme content,
at best a fourfold variation (see Section II,B).   If the source
of variation is a genetic polymorphism, producing a different
affinity (K_m) cytochrome in each phenotype, then antipyrine
could not be expected to detect such differences.   It is therefore hardly surprising that in spite of the voluminous literature concerning the drug, no genetic polymorphism of antipyrine
metabolism or disposition has ever been recorded.   Indeed,
there is now considerable doubt that the plasma clearance of
the drug is under detectable polygenic control with a measurable
heritability (Blain et al., 1982), an opinion that is at some
variance with the accepted tenet.

In order to investigate polymorphic cytochromes P-450, a
new generation of probes is required.   We believe the first of
these for potential use in humans has already been described
and arises from the number of human genetic polymorphisms in
metabolic oxidation that have emerged during the last 6 years,
each of which is reviewed in the following sections.

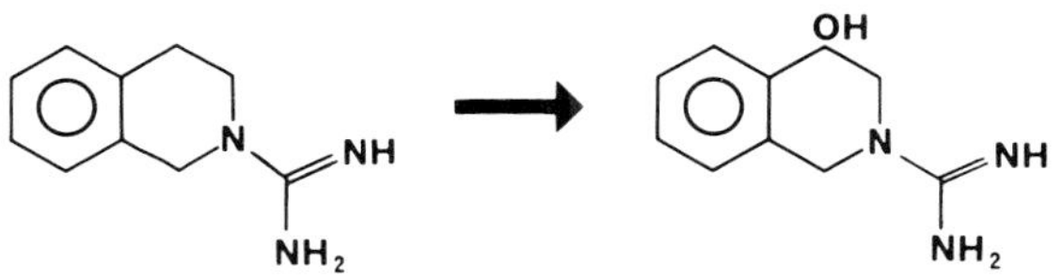

Fig. 1.   Debrisoquine 4-hydroxylation.

B.   Debrisoquine

Genetic polymorphism of debrisoquine 4-hydroxylation was first described in 1977 by Mahgoub *et al.* This study and an extended one (Evans *et al.*, 1980) demonstrated the existence of two human phenotypes for this reaction, on the basis of the urinary ratio of drug to metabolite measured by a simple gas chromatographic procedure (Idle *et al.*, 1979).   In the United Kingdom, approximately 1 in 10 white subjects is a recessive for impaired debrisoquine 4-hydroxylation (Fig. 1) and metabolizes less than 5% of an administered dose of 10 mg.   Consequently, recessives are identified as those persons with metabolic ratios (debrisoquine:4-hydroxydebrisoquine) greater than the antimodal value of 12.6.   In our laboratories, we have investigated 2224 healthy unrelated subjects for debrisoquine metabolism.   The frequency distribution histogram of metabolic ratio in this population is shown in Fig. 2.   Ethnic variation in the frequency of recessives is observed (Idle and Smith, 1980), and several pharmacokinetic, therapeutic, and toxicological implications of this polymorphism have been described elsewhere (Ritchie *et al.*, 1980; Smith and Idle, 1981; Shah *et al.*, 1982).

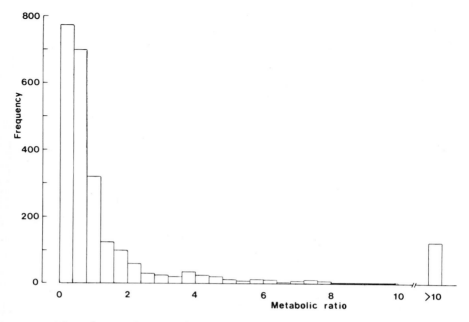

Fig. 2. Polymorphic 4-hydroxylation of debrisoquine in humans (n = 2224), represented as a frequency distribution of the metabolic ratio (see text). Recessives are shown as a single bar with values >10.

C. Sparteine

    Sparteine is a quinolizidine alkaloid, found in various lupin species, which was used as both an oxytocic and antiarrhythmic drug. In humans, it is thought to be metabolized to its N^1-oxide, which then undergoes dehydration to 2- and 5-dehydrosparteine, the principal urinary metabolites (Eichelbaum et al., 1978). Our own investigations of sparteine metabolism have been unable to substantiate these findings, particularly with respect to the number and nature of the human metabolites (Fig. 3). Nevertheless, by determining the ratio sparteine:2- + 5-dehydrosparteine in urine, Eichelbaum et al. (1978) have demonstrated a genetic polymor-

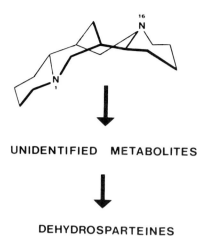

UNIDENTIFIED METABOLITES

DEHYDROSPARTEINES

Fig. 3.   Sparteine dehydrogenation.

phism in sparteine disposition. As for debrisoquine, deficient
metabolism was recessive. Figure 4 shows the distribution of
this ratio for 196 unrelated British whites, about 7% of whom
are recessives. All these subjects were also investigated
with debrisoquine, and it would appear that their sparteine and
debrisoquine phenotypes coincide (Harmer *et al.*, 1983).

D.   Phenformin

Phenformin is a biguanide hypoglycemic drug that may be
used safely in most people who suffer from maturity-onset dia-
betes. In some susceptible patients it may induce adverse
reactions including the often fatal condition lactic acidosis
(Cohen and Woods, 1976). Phenformin is metabolized almost exclusively in humans to 4-hydroxyphenformin (Fig. 5), drug and
metabolite being eliminated unconjugated in urine (Beckman,
1968). Human polymorphism of phenformin 4-hydroxylation was
first observed by Idle and Islam (1981) in a population of
Saudi females. Subsequently, in a study of 195 unrelated

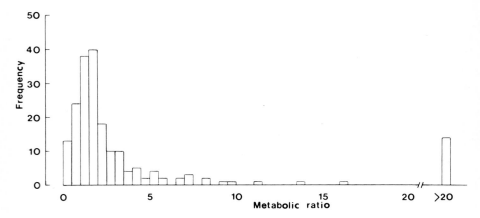

Fig. 4.   Polymorphic sparteine dehydrogenation in humans
(n = 196), represented as a frequency distribution of the metabolic ratio (sparteine:2- + 5-dehydrosparteine).   Recessives
are shown as a single bar with values >20.

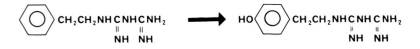

Fig. 5.   Phenformin 4-hydroxylation.

British whites and 27 families, it was confirmed that two phenotypes exist for phenformin metabolism, about 9% being recessive deficient metabolizers (Fig. 6; Oates et al., 1982).
In this latter study, 101 of the subjects were also investigated with debrisoquine.   Again both phenformin and debrisoquine phenotypes were apparently coincidental.

E.   S-Carboxymethyl-L-cysteine

     S-Carboxymethyl-L-cysteine is an amino acid derivative
used clinically as a mucolytic drug.   Although its metabolism

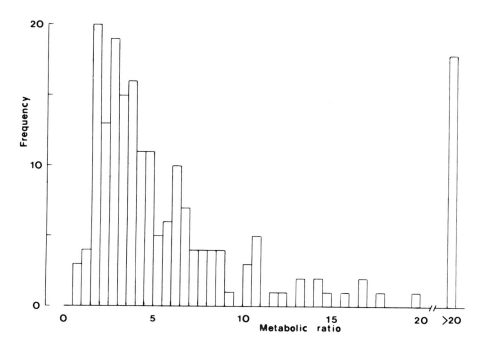

Fig. 6. Polymorphic phenformin 4-hydroxylation in humans (*n* = 195), represented as a frequency distribution of the metabolic ratio (phenformin:4-hydroxyphenformin). Recessives are shown as a single bar with values >20.

in humans is somewhat complex for such a small molecule, four distinct *S*-oxides can be discerned: of the parent compound, the decarboxylated metabolite, the *N*-acetylated metabolite, and the decarboxylated/*N*-acetylated metabolite (Fig. 7). The urinary ratio (drug + metabolites - *S*-oxides):*S*-oxides is polymorphic in humans (Waring *et al.*, 1982). As yet unpublished studies would suggest that impaired sulfoxidation (about 12% of British whites; see Fig. 8) of *S*-carboxymethyl-*L*-cysteine is recessive and that the sulfoxidation phenotypes do not coincide with those for debrisoquine oxidation. Additionally, we are aware of evidence that these two polymorphisms are linked. This is a potentially important development, be-

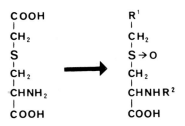

Fig. 7. *S*-Carboxymethyl-*L*-cysteine sulfoxidation. Four *S*-oxides are eliminated in human urine: the *S*-oxides of the parent drug (R^1 = COOH, R^2 = H), of the decarboxylated metabolite (R^1 = R^2 = H), of the *N*-acetylated metabolite (R^1 = COOH, R^2 = $COCH_3$), and of the decarboxylated/*N*-acetylated metabolite (R^1 = H, R^2 = $COCH_3$).

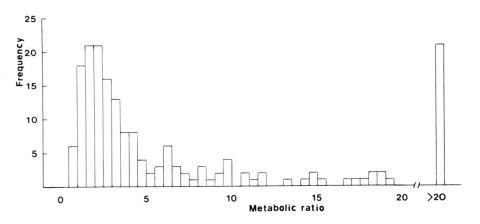

Fig. 8. Polymorphic *S*-carboxymethyl-*L*-cysteine sulfoxidation in humans (n = 181), represented as a frequency distribution of the metabolic ratio (drug + metabolites - sulfoxides):sulfoxides. Recessives are shown as a single bar with values >20.

cause it may allow us for the first time to consider haplotypes rather than phenotypes for human drug oxidation. If so, such data may shed light on the organization of *P*-450 genes in humans.

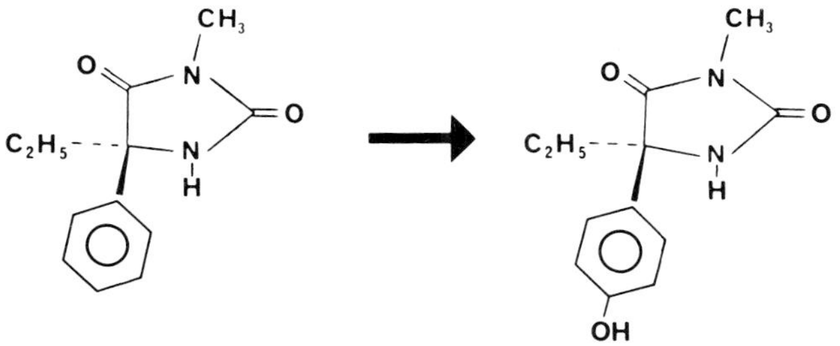

Fig. 9. S-Mephenytoin 4-hydroxylation.

F. Mephenytoin

Mephenytoin is a racemic 5,5-disubstituted hydantoin used as an antiepileptic drug in humans. When administered as such, the R and S isomers are handled quite differently by the body's metabolizing enzymes. R-Mephenytoin is N-demethylated, whereas the S isomer undergoes aromatic hydroxylation (Kupfer et al., 1982a; Fig. 9). A genetically determined deficiency of S-mephenytoin hydroxylation has been described by Kupfer et al. (1979), which in their family pedigree was inherited as a recessive character. Subsequent studies by Kupfer and colleagues in Bern, Switzerland indicate that this metabolic defect is a genetic variant of high incidence (~3%) in the German Swiss population (Kupfer et al., 1981). Of even greater interest was their observation that their study population contained 17 recessives for debrisoquine 4-hydroxylation, of whom 15 had a normal and extensive hydroxylation of S-mephenytoin, and only two had this latter reaction impaired. These findings show clearly that the polymorphisms of mephenytoin and debrisoquine are not coincidental and make it extremely unlikely that there is any appreciable genetic linkage between the two.

To date five genetic polymorphisms of drug oxidation have been characterized for humans. Those involving debrisoquine, sparteine, and phenformin metabolism would appear to arise from

allelomorphism at the same gene locus. However, independent,
closely linked loci cannot be ruled out, because the frequency
of recombinants may be so low as to defy detection by the kind
of investigation described in this section, involving hundreds
(and not thousands) of phenotype determinations•in volunteers.
It seems to us highly remote that very large populations can
be studied with many polymorphically metabolized substrates,
and thus we must seek alternative approaches to the problem of
understanding the microorganization of human P-450 genes. This
dilemma will be returned to in Section IV,B.

III. EXPERIMENTAL APPROACHES USING DRUG PROBES

A. Retrospective Study of the Cancer Patient

The metabolism *in vivo* of many drugs has now been shown
to be impaired or relatively so in recessive deficient metabolizers of debrisoquine (see Ritchie and Idle, 1982). It
seemed quite a reasonable hypothesis that the oxidative metabolism of certain chemical carcinogens might also proceed more
slowly in such persons. Activation and detoxication of these
substances would therefore be expected to be different also.
Providing that the disease itself did not introduce artifacts
into the phenotype determination, we believed that the simplest
line of investigation was to phenotype patients presenting
with carcinoma and compare our findings with those derived from
healthy isoethnic populations, where possible matched controls.
Because much more is known about the metabolism and pharmacogenetics of debrisoquine than any other polymorphically oxi-
dized substrate, we chose this as our phenotyping tool. As a
pharmacogenetic approach to cancer etiology in our laboratories, we have concentrated on the following disease states:
(1) bronchial carcinoma in smokers, (2) hepatocellular carcino-

ma in Africans, and (3) endemic nephropathy and renal tumors in Bulgarians. The last of these falls outside the scope of this chapter. An outline of the findings in the first two groups will be given here.

1. Bronchial Carcinoma in Smokers

Smoking is beyond doubt the primary cause of bronchial carcinoma. Many substances have been identified in cigarette smoke that are mutagenic and/or carcinogenic in test systems. Among these occur the polycyclic aromatic hydrocarbons and nitrosamines, both groups of which can be considered to be procarcinogens, requiring metabolic oxidation within the tissues to activate them to the ultimate electrophilic mutagens (Miller and Miller, 1977). If such reactions are prosecuted by polymorphic cytochromes P-450, genetic variants of which might have little or no catalytic activity with respect to the activation of certain procarcinogens, then by utilizing selective drug probes for such cytochromes we might be able to discern phenotypic differences between cancer and control patients. It would be naive to expect to observe large differences between such groups on the basis of phenotyping for a single polymorphic cytochrome. A myriad of other host factors, metabolic and nonmetabolic, must contribute to individual susceptibility to bronchial carcinoma.

In collaboration with Riad Ayesh and Martin Hetzel of the Chest Unit, Whittington Hospital, London, we have been investigating primary bronchial carcinoma patients and age-matched smoking controls. Data presented here is from untreated patients, that is, those in whom interference from the presence of other drugs during the phenotyping test is minimized. Fuller details of this study are reported elsewhere (Hetzel *et al.*, 1982). From this population of 120 bronchial carcinoma patients and 140 age-matched smoking controls, we have selected

the highest cigarette-consuming quintile in the control group
(102 ± 29 pack years; n = 28) and the lowest cigarette-
consuming quintile in the cancer group (28.4 ± 5.9 pack years;
n = 24) for comparison. Figure 10 shows the distribution of
the debrisoquine metabolic ratio (see Section II,B) in these
two groups who have radically different susceptibilities to
cigarette smoke. The median values (indicated by the arrows)
are around 1.0 and 0.3 for control and cancer, respectively.
This means that in the phenotyping test, whereas the median
control patient metabolized 50% of the probe drug, the median
cancer patient metabolized 77%. This difference is significant
as judged by the Wilcoxon rank sum test (p = .034). These
quintiles were selected to overcome the problem of enzyme induction by cigarettes. We now have unpublished evidence that
populations of cigarette smokers have a marginally higher debrisoquine metabolism (lower metabolic ratios) than their non-
smoking counterparts. Were it not for this phenomenon of enzyme induction, we contend that the metabolic differences between the two quintiles shown in Fig. 10 would be even greater,
because the controls have consumed on average 3.6 times as much
cigarette smoke as the cancer patients.

Although debrisoquine hydroxylation seems to be effected
by a single polymorphic cytochrome, carcinogen metabolism must
be considerably more complex. Without considering the additional etiological factors, such as promotion and DNA repair, which
must contribute toward individual susceptibility, we must take
stock of the contribution to both activation and detoxication
of alternative polymorphic cytochromes P-450. In this case,
S-carboxymethyl-L-cysteine and mephenytoin (Sections II,E and
II,F) may provide information, additional to debrisoquine,
about the role of polymorphic cytochromes in cancer induction.
Nevertheless, debrisoquine itself is showing some promise in
this respect.

2. Hepatocellular Carcinoma in Africans

Our reasons for investigating hepatocellular carcinoma in Africans have been given in detail elsewhere (Idle *et al.*, 1981; Ritchie and Idle, 1982). We believe that this is one of the carcinomas in which the number of causative factors is low and can probably be reduced to aflatoxin exposure and HBAg infection. Aflatoxin B_1 (AFB_1) is metabolized to AFB_1 8,9-oxide by both cytochromes *P*-450 and *P*-448 (Yoshizawa *et al.*, 1982), this metabolite being the ultimate mutagen that modifies DNA (Swenson *et al.*, 1977). Our studies, using debrisoquine, of cancer patients and controls in Ibadan, Nigeria have shown major differences between these groups in their ability to metabolize the drug, cancer patients being considerably faster debrisoquine hydroxylators than controls. As we have argued before (Idle *et al.*, 1981), we do not consider the presence of a solid hepatoma or HBAg to be the cause of artifactually enhanced debrisoquine metabolism. On the contrary, one would expect both tumor and virus to impair hepatic oxidation processes if anything. Nevertheless, these factors require further investigation.

B. Prospective Studies

The approach to uncovering genetically variable metabolic host factors just outlined does not lend itself readily to the prospective study of tumorigenesis. Phenotypes for drug oxidation are not routinely determined on hospital admission, for example, as are various hematological phenotypes, although we would argue that, from the point of view of preventing many of the serious adverse drug reactions in hospitalized patients, it would be useful to know which of a physician's 1 in 10 patients had a defective metabolism of a battery of drugs. Even a medical student would not consider administering A, B, or

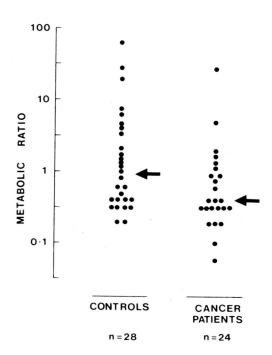

Fig. 10. Distribution of the debrisoquine metabolic ratio (see text, Section II,B) for the highest cigarette-consuming quintile of control subjects (102 ± 29 pack years; n = 28) and the lowest cigarette-consuming quintile of bronchial carcinoma patients (28.4 ± 5.9 pack years; n = 24). Arrows indicate medians (∿1.0 for controls, 0.3 for cancer patients.

Rh-antigenic blood to a patient who was phenotypically O Rh-ve! Such routine screening of patients with respect to hepatic drug-metabolizing function awaits the development of considerably less cumbersome phenotyping procedures than exist at present.

From the cancer research viewpoint, animal modeling probably provides the best way forward at present. Prospective study of the cause-and-effect relationships between polymorphic cytochromes P-450 and cancer should be attainable in valid animal models.

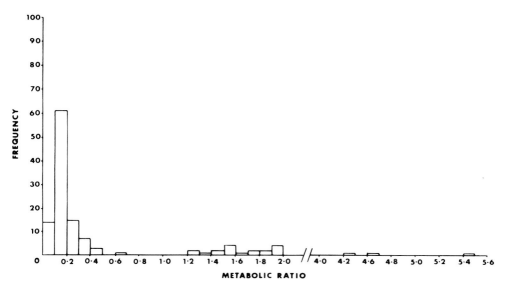

Fig. 11.   Polymorphic debrisoquine 4-hydroxylation in the rat (*n* = 121), represented as a frequency distribution of the metabolic ratio (see text, Section II,B).   Deficient hydroxylation phenotype (values 1.2 - 5.5) comprises only females of the DA strain, none of which appear in the extensive hydroxylation phenotype (values 0.07-0.7).

C.   Animal Modeling

In the course of a systematic search for debrisoquine hydroxylation phenotypes in the rat, Sabah Al-Dabbagh, a graduate student working in our laboratories, uncovered a genetic polymorphism analogous to that in humans (Al-Dabbagh *et al.*, 1981). A bimodal distribution of the debrisoquine metabolic ratio (see Section II,B) is observed (Fig. 11).   All animals comprising the defective metabolism mode were females of the DA strain.   No female DA was found in the major extensive metabolism mode. Breeding studies using female DA and male Lewis (an extensive metabolizing animal) rats show clearly the existence of two rat phenotypes for debrisoquine metabolism, the deficient metabolism phenotype being recessive (Fig. 12), as it is in humans.

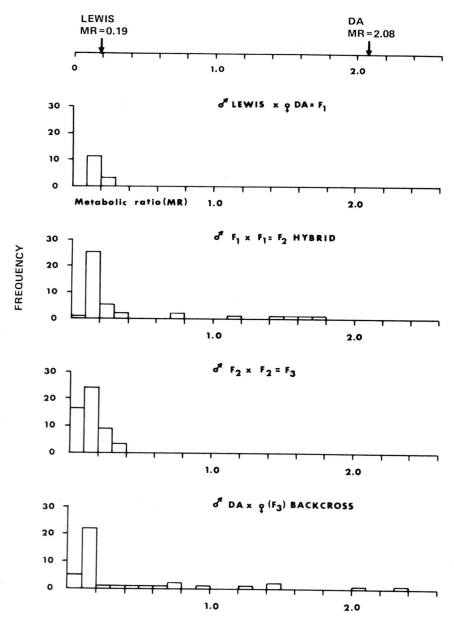

Fig. 12.   Breeding studies between female DA (deficient hydroxylation phenotype) and male Lewis (extensive hydroxylation phenotype) rats, showing that the DA characteristic is recessive. Mean metabolic ratios (see text, Section II,B) for parental strains are shown (top).

The female DA rat represents a novel opportunity to investigate the modulation of chemical carcinogenesis by an identifiable genetic factor. We will illustrate this statement with as yet unpublished data from our collaborative studies with Drs. G. E. Neal and T. A. Connors, M.R.C. Toxicology Unit, Carshalton, England. In these investigations, female DA and Fischer rats (deficient and extensive oxidation phenotypes, respectively) were fed AFB_1 (4 ppm) in their diet for 4 months. After a further 12 months the animals were culled and their livers examined histologically for signs of toxicity. While all Fischer rats had multiple solid hepatomas, none of the DA rats did, merely having degenerative foci and hyperplastic nodules. Investigation of DA × Lewis F_1 and F_2 progeny is under way to establish whether or not AFB_1 sensitivity in rats can be attributed directly to the polymorphism or is genetically linked to it. We are sanguine that the rat polymorphism will find increasing use in biomedical research, as a tool for investigating the implications of polymorphic metabolic oxidation.

IV. PERSPECTIVES

A. Substrate Screening

If progress is made in the future at the same rate as in the past, using only the historical methods and approaches, it will take us several decades to comprehend the number of drugs and other exogenous chemicals that are substrates for human polymorphic cytochromes P-450. More rapid screening procedures are required that can identify or eliminate new candidates from among, for example, the catalog of known mutagens and carcinogens. We are fairly certain that such a method, to identify substrates for the polymorphic cytochrome that metabolizes debrisoquine, sparteine, and phenformin already exists. This method again utilizes the analogous rat polymorphism, but this time *in vitro*.

If hepatic microsomal fractions from hydroxylation-deficient and normal rats are subjected to difference spectral investigations using the polymorphically metabolized substrates debrisoquine, sparteine, and phenformin, an interesting inter-phenotype variation is seen. Normal hydroxylating rat micro-somes (Lewis, Fischer, or Sprague-Dawley strains) give a type I (blue shift) difference spectrum, arising from drug binding to a single site on *P*-450, with dissociation constants of 0.5 to 10 μM. Microsomes from hydroxylation-deficient rats (female DA) elicit no spectral binding at all, and only at very high drug concentrations can a weak Type I interaction be seen (Kupfer *et al.*, 1982b). It may be possible that such spectral studies could provide a means of identifying new polymorphic substrates, obviating direct and laborious human investigation with drugs. In the case of carcinogens, this may represent a real advance, because *in vivo* carcinogen testing is costly and time consuming in animals and impossible in humans.

B. Subject Screening

How do we realistically identify persons most at risk from the effects of chemical carcinogens because of phenotypic dif-ferences in their activating enzymes? The principal points have been touched on already, and some future urgent needs can be listed as follows:

1. The systematic search for new examples of genetic polymorphisms in metabolic oxidation

2. Determination of the degree of linkage between known and new allelomorphic loci, leading to a better under-standing of the organization of human *P*-450 genes

3. Development of simpler tests for human P-450 phenotypes and haplotypes that would lend themselves to
   · wider usage

4. An increased understanding of the modification of
   phenotypes by the environment, including the effects
   of enzyme induction

5. Determination of P-450 phenotypes in epidemiological
   studies

6. Isolation and characterization of the polymorphic cytochromes P-450 from human and rat, leading toward a
   more rational classification of these enzymes based
   on their substrate selectivity

ACKNOWLEDGMENTS

We are grateful to the Cancer Research Campaign (London)
for their generous financial support. Our thanks are also extended to Lawrence Wakile and Sabah Al-Dabbagh for allowing us
to use their unpublished Figs. 11 and 12.

REFERENCES

Al-Dabbagh, S. G., Idle, J. R., and Smith, R. L. (1981). *J.
    Pharm. Pharmacol. 33,* 161-164.
Beckman, R. (1968). *Ann. N.Y. Acad. Sci. 148,* 820-832.
Blain, P. G., Mucklow, J. C., Wood, P., Roberts, D. F., and
    Rawlins, M. D. (1982). *Br. Med. J. 284,* 150-152.
Boobis, A. R., Brodie, M. J., Kahn, G. C., Toverud, E.-L.,
    Blair, I. A., Murray, S., and Davies, D. S. (1981). *Br.
    J. Clin. Pharmacol. 12,* 771-777.
Cohen, R. D., and Woods, H. F. (1976). "Clinical and Biochemi-
    cal Aspects of Lactic Acidosis." Blackwell, Oxford.
Conney, A. H. (1981). *In* "Accomplishments in Cancer Research
    1980" (H. H. Hiatt, J. D. Watson, and J. A. Winsten,
    eds.), pp. 605-627. Cold Spring Harbor Lab., Cold Spring
    Harbor, New York.

Eichelbaum, M., Spannbrucker, N., and Dengler, H. J. (1978).
    In "Biological Oxidation of Nitrogen" (J. W. Gorrod, ed.),
    pp. 113-118. Elsevier-North Holland, Amsterdam.
Evans, D. A. P., Mahgoub, A., Sloan, T. P., Idle, J. R., and
    Smith, R. L. (1980). *J. Med. Genet. 17,* 102-105.
Evered, D., and Lawrenson, G. (eds.) (1980). *Ciba Found. Symp.
    76.*
Fujii-Kuriyama, Y., Mizukami, Y., Kawajiri, K., Sogawa, K., and
    Murumatsu, M. (1982). *Proc. Natl. Acad. Sci. USA 79,*
    2793-2797.
Harmer, D., Evans, D. A. P., Ritchie, J. C., Idle, J. R., and
    Smith, R. L. (1983). *J. Med. Genet.,* in press.
Hetzel, M. R., Law, M., Keal, E. E., Sloan, T. P., Idle, J. R.,
    and Smith, R. L. (1982). *In* "Cellular Biology of the
    Lung" (G. Cumming and G. Bonsignore, eds.), pp. 448-457.
    Plenum, New York.
Idle, J. R., and Islam, S. I. (1981). *Br. J. Pharmacol. 73,*
    177P-178P.
Idle, J. R., and Smith, R. L. (1980). *In* "Toxicology in the
    Tropics" (R. L. Smith and E. A. Bababunmi, eds.), pp.
    239-253. Taylor & Francis, London.
Idle, J. R., Mahgoub, A., Angelo, M. M., Dring, L. G.,
    Lancaster, R., and Smith, R. L. (1979). *Br. J. Clin.
    Pharmacol. 7,* 257-266.
Idle, J. R., Mahgoub, A., Sloan, T. P., Smith, R. L.,
    Mbanefo, C. O., and Bababunmi, E. A. (1981). *Cancer
    Lett. (Shannon, Irel.) 11,* 331-338.
Kupfer, A., Desmond, P., Schenker, S., and Branch, R. A.
    (1979). *Pharmacologist 21,* 173.
Kupfer, A., Dick, B., and Preisig, R. (1981). *Hepatology
    (Baltimore) 1,* 524.
Kupfer, A., Desmond, P. V., Schenker, S., and Branch, R.
    (1982a). *J. Pharmacol. Exp. Ther. 221,* 590-597.
Kupfer, A., Al-Dabbagh, S. G., Ritchie, J. C., Idle, J. R., and
    Smith, R. L. (1982b). *Biochem. Pharmacol. 31,* 3193-3199.
Lu, A. Y. H., and West, S. B. (1980). *Pharmacol. Rev. 31,*
    277-295.
Mahgoub, A., Idle, J. R., Dring, L. G., Lancaster, R., and
    Smith, R. L. (1977). *Lancet ii,* 584-586.
Miller, J. A., and Miller, E. C. (1977). *In* "Origins of Human
    Cancer" (H. H. Hiatt, J. D. Watson, and J. A. Winsten,
    eds.), pp. 605-627. Cold Spring Harbor Lab., Cold Spring
    Harbor, New York.
Nebert, D. W. (1979). *Mol. Cell. Biochem. 27,* 27-46.
Nebert, D. W., and Jensen, N. M. (1979). *CRC Crit. Rev.
    Biochem. 6,* 401-438.
Nebert, D. W., and Negishi, M. (1982). *Biochem. Pharmacol. 31,*
    2311-2317.

Oates, N. S., Shah, R. R., Idle, J. R., and Smith, R. L. (1982). *Clin. Pharmacol. Ther. 32,* 81-89.

Ritchie, J. C., and Idle, J. R. (1982). *In* "Host Factors in Carcinogenesis" (H. Bartsch and B. Armstrong, eds.), pp. 381-394. International Agency for Research on Cancer, Lyon, France.

Ritchie, J. C., Sloan, T. P., Idle, J. R., and Smith, R. L. (1980). *Ciba Found. Symp. 76,* 219-244.

Robinson, J. R., Gonsidine, N., and Nebert, D. W. (1974). *J. Biol. Chem. 249,* 5851-5859.

Shah, R. R., Oates, N. S., Idle, J. R., Smith, R. L., and Lockhart, J. D. F. (1982). *Br. Med. J. 284,* 295-299.

Smith, R. L., and Idle, J. R. (1981). *In* "Drug Reactions and the Liver" (M. Davis, J. M. Tredger, and R. Williams, eds.), pp. 95-104. Pitman, London.

Swenson, D. H., Lin, J. K., Miller, E. C., and Miller, J. A. (1977). *Cancer Res. 37,* 172-181.

Vainio, H., and Hietanen, E. (1980). *In* "Concepts in Drug Metabolism" (P. Jenner and B. Testa, eds.), Part A, pp. 251-284. Dekker, New York.

Waring, R. H., Mitchell, S. C., Idle, J. R., and Smith, R. L. (1982). *Biochem. Pharmacol. 31,* 3151-3154.

Yoshizawa, H., Uchimaru, R., Kamataki, T., Kato, R., and Ueno, Y. (1982). *Cancer Res. 42,* 1120-1124.

36

POSSIBLE ROLES OF FUNGAL INFECTION AND MYCOTOXIN IN HUMAN ESOPHAGEAL CARCINOGENESIS

Chu-Chieh Hsia

Department of Pathology
Cancer Institute
Chinese Acacemy of Medical Sciences
Beijing, People's Republic of China

I.   INTRODUCTION

Esophageal carcinoma is the second most common cancer in
China. An area with high incidence of esophageal carcinoma,
Linxian (a county in northern Honan province) is located
along the Tai-Haun mountains. In a certain township the incidence has reached 273 in 100,000 people/year, which is the
highest incidence reported in the world.

Our previous studies on esophageal biopsies and cytological smears in Linxian showed that fungal infections were often
associated with hyperplasia or dysplasia of the esophageal epithelium in patients with severe dysplasia or early esophageal
cancer. The majority of these invading fungi were *Candida*
spp. The staple foodstuffs of local inhabitants in Linxian
were often contaminated by fungi of *Fusarium* genus. Our
present studies are focused on these questions: What are the
roles of these fungal infections and mycotoxin in esophageal
carcinogenesis? Is there any interaction between fungi and
the nitrosamines that have been suspected to be causative factors in esophageal cancer?

Fungal infections and mycotoxin exposure may play an important role in esophageal carcinogenesis. Consistent with
this hypothesis, our experimental and epidemiological studies
suggest esophageal carcinogenesis is most likely a multifactorial and multistage process.

II.   MATERIALS AND METHODS

A.   Esophageal Biopsies

Biopsies were taken under fiberoptic esophagoscopy in
Linxian. Routine paraffin sections were stained with hematoxylin and eosin, periodic acid Schiff's and Gomori's methenamine
silver reactions.

B.   Serum Anti-*Candida* Antibody Assays

Anti-*Candida* antibody titers were determined by indirect immunofluorescence (Hsia *et al.*, 1979), indirect immunoperoxidase (Wang *et al.*, 1982), and cell agglutination technique. Anti-*Candida* antiserum of rabbit was used as a positive control.

C.   Organ Cultures of Esophageal Mucosa

Human fetal esophagus was obtained from fetuses mostly aborted by water balloon technique at fetal age 3-9 months. Human adult esophageal mucosa was obtained from surgical specimens with esophageal cancer. Specimens were placed in 4°C L-15 medium and were cut into explants of 0.3 to 0.5 cm^2.

The culture medium 199 or 1640 was supplemented with glutamine, insulin, hydrocortisone, Hepes, and 5% newborn calf serum. Culture dishes were put into a chamber with a mixture of 45% O_2, 50% N_2, and 5% CO_2 on a rocker platform at 36.5 to 37°C.

D.   Electron Microscopy

1.   Transmission Electron Microscopy (TEM)

Fresh tissues were fixed in a mixture of 4% glutaraldehyde and 1% formaldehyde in 0.1 M phosphate buffer, pH 7.4, then postfixed in 1% osmium tetroxide in 0.1 M phosphate buffer, pH 7.2, for 2 h. After dehydration in a graded series of acetone, the samples were embedded in Epon 812, sectioned by a LKB 8800 ultramicrotome, and observed under Hitachi 600 transmission electron microscope.

2.   Scanning Electron Microscopy (SEM)

Fresh tissues were first fixed in 2% glutaraldehyde and postfixed in 1% osmium tetroxide. After fixation, the specimens were dehydrated in a graded series of ethanol and critical point-dried from CO_2. The specimens were sputter-coated with

gold prior to examination in a Camscan 3-30 ACV scanning electron microscope.

III.   RESULTS

A.   Fungal Infection of Esophagus and Its Relationship to
     Esophageal Dysplasia and Carcinoma

1. *Clinicopathological Studies*
     The relative incidence of esophagitis in Linxian is rather
high; 13.5% of a series of 1635 adults examined by cytological
smears were positive for esophagitis (Shen *et al.*, 1964). We hav
diagnosed 60 cases of esophagitis in a consecutive series of 300
esophageal biopsies in patients in Linxian (Hsia *et al.*, 1978,
and unpublished data). The relative incidence of esophagitis in
local inhabitants over 26 years of age in Linxian was found to
be 20% (Hsia *et al.*, unpublished data). A high incidence of
esophagitis has also been found in a high-incidence area of
esophageal carcinoma in northern Iran (Crespi *et al.*, 1979).
     Our further studies of the nature of the esophagitis in
Linxian revealed that many cases of esophagitis were caused by
the combined infections of bacteria and fungi. In the biopsies
of 60 cases of esophagitis, 15 had fungal invasions in the mucosa as identified by periodic acid Schiff's (PAS) or Gomori's
methenamine silver (GMS) stains in pathological sections. In
biopsy studies we have found that fungal infections were
present in about 40 to 50% of dysplastic epithelium in patients
with severe dysplasia or early cancer of the esophagus. The
presence of fungal infections in the normal epithelium was almost negligible (Hsia and Tsao, 1978).
     Patients with fungal esophagitis had clinical symptoms
very similar to patients with early esophageal carcinoma. The
patients may have mild dysphagia, substernal pains, and a

feeling of dryness in the throat, among other signs. Radiological examinations of the esophagus show stiffness at certain segments, disruption of mucosal lines, and sometimes even small filling defects. Using fiberoptic esophagoscopy, we located 80% of lesions in the middle third segment of the esophagus, which is also the major segment of predilection for esophageal carcinoma (in which 73.6% of cases are located in the middle third). The lesions may be present as erosions, roughness of mucosa, plaques, and, more rarely, as leukoplakia. These lesions are very similar to those of early esophageal carcinoma. The average age of patients with fungal esophagitis is about 46 years old, 7 years younger than the average age of patients with early esophageal carcinoma.

The fungal esophagitis we found in Linxian in normal working inhabitants is very different from those acute or invasive cases of candidiasis usually seen in terminally ill patients. The former lesions are discrete and multifocal, usually limited to the mucosa of the esophagus. The superficial layers of esophageal epithelium are usually thickened to various degrees and are invaded by mycelia and spores of fungi in epithelium with few lymphocytes and leukocytes present. Prominent inflammatory reactions are found in the lamina propria underneath the foci of fungal infections. Sometimes the superficial layers of epithelium are highly thickened, many times thicker than normal, with numerous mycelia and spores invading the epithelium (Fig. 1). More than half the invading fungi are *Candida,* according to morphology. In a few patients we have found more than one species of fungi in the same patient. The epithelia adjacent to or underneath the foci of fungal infections may show different features, from mild, moderate, or severe dysplasia to carcinoma *in situ.* In some specimens of early esophageal cancers, we found multiple foci of cancerous lesions intermingled with lesions of fungal esophagitis. Thus chronic fungal esophagitis was often the background lesion of esophageal cancer.

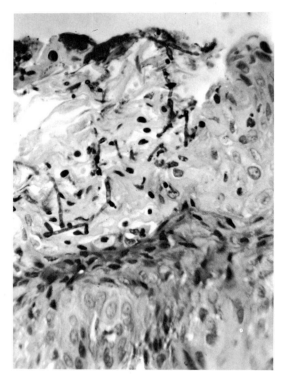

Fig. 1. *Candida* esophagitis in the noncancerous portion of early esophageal carcinoma. Numerous *Candida* cells have invaded the thickened epithelium. Nuclei of epithelial cells adjacent and beneath the *Candida* infection are enlarged and dysplastic (PAS, ×400).

2. *Electron-Microscopic Studies*

Electron-microscopic examinations of the lesions of candidal esophagitis showed that most of the candidal organisms are seen to invade in the intercellular spaces of esophageal epithelium together with numerous bacteria, and occasionally *Candida* cells were observed in the cytoplasm of esophageal epithelial cells (Fig. 2). Some species of fungal mycelia may invade through several layers of epithelial cells. Most of the *Candida* cells are round or oval with few pseudomycelia. They have very thick walls with short microvilli on the sur-

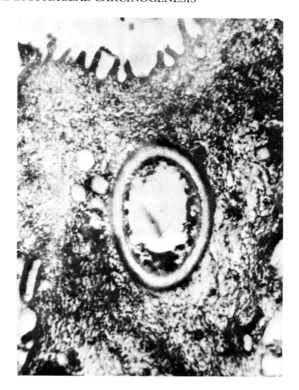

Fig. 2.   Electron micrograph of esophageal epithelium of
Candida esophagitis.   *Candida* cell (center) is seen in the
cytoplasm of epithelial cells (x15,000).

face, and some mitochondria and dense bodies inside the cells
(Hsia and Tsao, 1978).

3.   Isolation and Identification of Fungi

Tissues from surgical specimens of esophageal cancer and
saline washings from cytological balloons of patients with
fungal esophagitis were cultured on Sabouraud's medium.   Fungal
growth was isolated in 15 of 51 cases with cancer; 13 (26%)
belonged to the *Candida* genus and 12 were *C. albicans*.   No
fungal growth was observed in cancer cases (3) treated by pre-
surgical radiotherapy.   In 46 cases of fungal esophagitis, 16
(34.8%) of 18 isolates were *Candida*, and among them 15 were

C. albicans. Other species are *Aspergillus versicolor* (one
from cancer and one from esophagitis), penicillin, and other
aspergilli.

B.   Seroepidemiological Studies of Fungal Infection

     Comparative studies on pathological sections of biopsies
and sera anti-*Candida* antibody titers detected by indirect immunofluorescence technique showed that most patients with
fungal invasions in esophageal epithelium had high serum titers of anti-*Candida* antibody, whereas those individuals without fungal invasions in esophageal biopsies usually had very
low titers, as seen in the majority of normal people. In our
first series of 130 individuals using immunofluorescence technique, 80% of patients with severe dysplasia or early esophageal carcinoma in Linxian had high anti-*Candida* antibody titers
(Hsia *et al.*, 1979). Identical results were found in another
series of individuals using immunoperoxidase technique (Wang
et al., 1982). Results of an extended series of studies using
cell agglutination technique are shown in Fig. 3. These three
series included a total number of 969 individuals. These results suggested that in patients with severe dysplasia or early
esophageal carcinoma, *Candida* infections were more frequent than
in normal individuals. The relative incidence of *Candida* infection was also higher in Linxian than that in a lower incidence
area such as Beijing. The average percentage of normal persons
with high titers in the age group 31-50 years is 24% in Linxian
inhabitants and 3.8% in Beijing, that is, 6.4-fold higher in
Linxian. In this age group, the percentage of high titer in
Linxian males is 18.9, whereas that in Beijing males is 0
(Table I). The difference of percentage of high titer in the
high- and low-incidence area is most significant among the male
31- to 50-year age group. The percentage of persons with a
negative reaction is 20% in Linxian and 59% in Beijing.

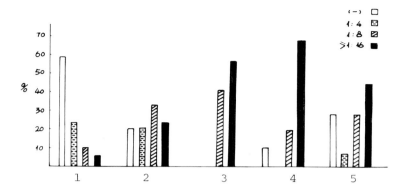

Fig. 3. Comparison of percentage of persons with high
Candida agglutinin titer in different groups of individuals in
high- and low-incidence areas of esophageal carcinoma.
(1) Beijing normal population; (2) Linxian inhabitants;
(3) Linxian patients with severe epithelial dysplasia of esophagus; (4) Linxian esophageal cancer patients at early and median stage; (5) esophageal cancer patients at advanced stage.

TABLE I. Comparison of Individuals with Higher Titer of Serum
          Candida Agglutinin in Different Age Groups and Sexes
          in Linxian County and Beijing

	Male (%)			Female (%)		
Location	21-30	31-50	>51	21-30	31-50	>51
Linxian	12.5	18.9	14.4	60.0	35.2	22.2
Beijing	4.3	0	n.d.[a]	15.4	8.3	n.d.

[a]n.d., *Not detected.*

It also appears that more than half the infections in
early adult life persist beyond 51 years of age. These data
support our previous suggestion that *Candida* infections of the
esophagus in Linxian may be a long-term persistent chronic infection. The high incidence of esophageal carcinoma in Linxian
might be related in part to the higher incidence of *Candida*

infections in that area. We suspect that *Candida* infection
may have an etiological relationship to severe dysplasia and
cancer of the esophagus. Some authors had reported a case of
esophageal candidiasis with cutaneous candidiasis in a 14-year-
old. The patient died of esophageal cancer at the age of 38.
These authors suspected that the cancer might have developed
from chronic esophageal candidiasis (Kugelman *et al.*, 1963).
It had been reported that not fewer than 6 of 10 patients with
chronic oral candidiasis finally developed oral cancers (Cawson
1959). Studies of possible roles of these pathogenic fungi
that invade esophageal epithelium in esophageal carcinogenesis
is an important and interesting new approach.

C.   Preliminary Prospective Studies of Relation of Fungal In-
     fection and Esophageal Dysplasia and Carcinoma

     In order to investigate further the relation between fungal
infection and esophageal cancer, a preliminary prospective study
in two production brigades with a high incidence of esophageal
cancer in Linxian has been carried out. Sera *Candida* agglutinin
in 435 unselected normal inhabitants over the age of 26 were
determined by cell agglutination technique.

     In 435 normal adults, 24% had high titers of *Candida* ag-
glutinin. Forty-eight unselected inhabitants with high *Candida*
agglutinin titers accepted further cytological examinations of
the esophagus, and some were further examined by X ray 8 months
after serological tests. All 48 individuals proved to have esophagitis, most of them are of moderate to severe degree. The
results of clinical examinations of these 48 persons are shown
in Table II. Four patients were proven to have esophageal carcinoma by both cytological and X-ray examinations: Two patients
were in early stages, one in median, and one in late stage, but
none showed superficial lymph node metastases. The clinical

TABLE II. Clinical Examinations of 48 Cases with High *Candida* Agglutinin Titers

Diagnosis	Age group					Total number	Average age	Relative Incidence (%)
	30-40	41-50	51-60	61-70	>71			
Cancer	0	1	1	1	1	4	59.3	8.3
Suspected cancer	1	1	1	0	0	3	48.0	6.3
Severe dysplasia	12	6	8	5	1	32	48.7	66.7
Mild dysplasia	3	4	0	0	0	7	39.6	14.6
No dysplasia	1	1	0	0	0	2	42.5	4.2
Inflammation	17	13	10	6	2	48	47.9	100.0
Total	17	13	10	6	2	48	47.9	100.0

TABLE III. Clinical Information of Four Cases of Esophageal Carcinoma Detected in 48 Persons with High *Candida* Agglutinin Titers

Patient number	Sex	Age	Cytology	X Ray result	Clinical stage
1	M	63	Sq. Ca[a]	Irregularities of mucosal lines	Subclinical
2	F	44	Sq. Ca	Filling defect less than 3 cm long	Early clinical
3	M	71	Sq. Ca	Filling defect about 4 cm long	Median clinical
4	M	59	Sq. Ca	Filling defect 7-8 cm long	Late, without metastases of superficial lymph nodes

[a]squamous cell carcinoma.

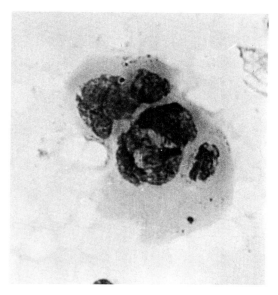

Fig. 4.   Cancer cells found in cytological smears of a female patient of 44 years of age with high serum *Candida* agglutinin and esophagitis.

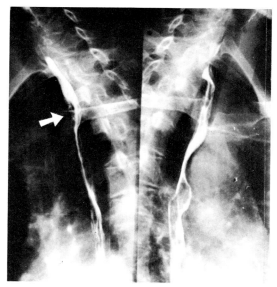

Fig. 5.   X-Ray film of esophagus of the same patient as in Fig. 4, showing filling defect less than 3 cm long in the upper segment of esophagus at clinically early stage.

data of these four cancer patients are shown in Table III. The
patients have no noticeable symptoms and are working normally
in the commune. The cytology and X ray of a female cancer patient in early stages are shown in Figs. 4 and 5. It is important to note that three fourths of the cancers found in this
prospective study are of early and median stage, and among them
half are of early stage. In comparison, more than 99% of the
patients who come to the clinics are at late stage. The prognosis for patients at early stage is much better than that for
advanced-stage patients. Five-year survival rate of esophageal
cancer of early stage after surgery is about 90%, whereas that
of advanced stage is only about 25%. The average age of patients with mild dysplasia is 10 years younger than that of patients with severe dysplasia and 20 years younger than patients
with esophageal cancer. These data suggest that severe dysplasia of the esophageal epithelium may be a precancerous lesion
of esophageal cancer.

Of 11,011 individuals with normal esophageal epithelium,
examined by cytology that had been followed up for several
years, 13 cases (0.118%) developed esophageal cancer (Coordinating Groups for the Research of Esophageal Carcinoma, 1975).
The relative incidence of esophageal cancer in patients with
Candida esophagitis was 8.3% in a follow-up of 8 months, a
figure much higher than that in persons with normal esophagi.

In addition, 3 cases of suspected esophageal cancer (6.3%)
and 32 cases of severe dysplasia of esophageal epithelium
(66.7%) were found in this group. The cancer and precancerous
lesions constitute a total of 81.3% in 48 patients.

Isolation of fungi from cytological balloon were carried
out on Sabouraud's agar medium. A single kind of fungal
growth was evident on 34% of the specimens: *C. albicans*.

The preceding data give strong support to our previous
hypothesis that fungal esophagitis may play an important role

in the dysplastic and malignant change of esophageal epithelium.
We speculate that *Candida* esophagitis may be one of the etiological factors of esophageal carcinoma in Linxian. Besides the
etiological significance, serological detection of anti-*Candida*
antibody may probably also be used as a simple effective and
acceptable screening technique for cancer and precancerous lesions in the high-incidence area of esophageal cancer, Linxian.
Prospective studies on a larger scale are in progress.

D. Effects of T_2 Toxin, a Trichothecene Metabolite of
   Fusarium, on Human Fetal and Adult Esophageal Epithelium
   in Organ Culture

   In Linxian, as a result of the bad weather and natural conditions, cereals, especially corn, are seriously infected with
mold; *Fusarium* genus was the most common fungal contaminant,
and residents usually consume a lot of this moldy food in combination with pickled vegetables. Ingestion of corn inoculated
with *Fusarium sporotrichiella* has induced papilloma in the
forestomachs of rats (Chang and Hue, 1965). T_2 Toxin, a trichothecene produced by many species of *Fusarium,* caused inflammation and necrosis of oral mucosa in chickens (Chi and Mirocha,
1978). Intragastric administration of T_2 toxin induced tumors
of various organs and hyperplasia of basal epithelial cells of
the esophagus in rats (Schoental *et al.,* 1979). Studies have
shown that T_2 toxin caused single-strand DNA breaks in lymphocytes (Lafarge-Frayssinet *et al.,* 1981). T_2 Toxin is one of
the many mycotoxins that possibly exist in *Fusarium*-contaminated
cereals. During ingestion of the contaminated food, mycotoxins
come in direct contact with the esophageal mucosa. We have
speculated that the esophagitis, esophageal hyperplasia and
dysplasia, and oral leukoplakia often seen in Linxian inhabitants may be related in part to the action of some mycotoxin.

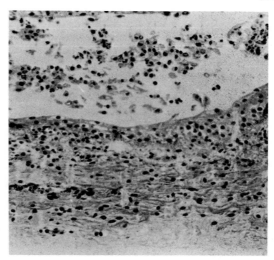

Fig. 6.   Light micrograph of esophageal explant of human
fetus after action by T2 toxin (0.4 ng/ml) for 6 days.   Area
of focal necrosis, most of epithelium sloughed off (H + E,
×200).

Whether T_2 toxin has toxic or proliferative effects on human
esophageal epithelium has not been reported.   So we tested the
effects of various concentrations of T_2 toxin on human fetal
and adult esophageal mucosa in organ culture.

Techniques for long-term organ culture of normal adult
esophageal mucosa have been developed by Hillman *et al.* (1980).
We have successfully cultured explants of human fetal (3 to 9
months fetal age) and adult esophagis using techniques according to Hillman *et al.* in culture medium 199 or 1640 for as long
as about 3 months (C. C. Hsia and C. C. Harris, 1983).

1.   Effects of T_2 Toxin on Human Fetal Esophagus

a.   Light-microscopic Observations. T_2 toxin has both cytotoxic and proliferative effects on human fetal esophagus.
The effects depend on dosage and duration of exposure.   Dosage
of 0.01 to 0.1 ng/ml medium for 4 to 6 days has mild effects
on esophageal epithelium, that is, thinning or mild hyperplasia

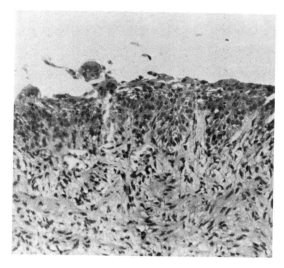

Fig. 7. Light micrograph of esophageal explant of human fetus after action by T$_2$ toxin (0.4 ng/ml) for 6 days. Some superficial epithelial cells are sloughing off. The basal cells show multifocal papillary proliferation growing downward into the lamina propria (H + E, ×200).

of the epithelium and mild superficial focal necrosis of epithelial cells. Dosage of 0.2 to 1.2 ng/ml for 4 to 8 days had both toxic and proliferative effects. Sometimes cytotoxic and proliferative effects may be seen in the same or different areas of epithelium of one explant. The cytotoxic effects are expressed as focal necrosis and sloughing off of whole or some layers of epithelium (Fig. 6). The proliferative effects are expressed as basal hyperplasia, dysplasia, increase of mitotic figures, and presence of atypical mitotic figures; the latter was never seen in control explants. The basal cell hyperplasia or dysplasia is multifocal, the basal cells proliferating to form papillae or small masses extending into the lamina propria (Fig. 7). Because T$_2$ toxin induces atypical mitosis in esophageal epithelium, we suggest that T$_2$ may have effects on DNA or chromosome structure of esophageal epithelium, and may have mutagenic and/or promoting effects in esophageal carcinogenesis.

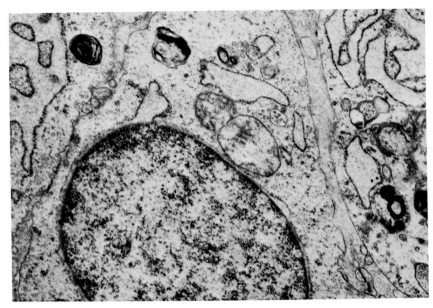

Fig. 8. Electron micrograph of epithelial cells (intermediate layer) of human fetal esophageal explant after action
by T_2 toxin (0.4 ng/ml) for 6 days. The number of organelles
has decreased; there are mitochondrial degeneration, myelin
figures formation, and rough endoplasmic reticulum dilatation
(16-day culture, ×12,000).

When larger doses of 2 to 4 ng/ml T_2 toxin were present
in the medium for 4 to 6 days, the whole layer of epithelium
became necrotic and sloughed off, or only a thin layer of epithelium was left.

    b. *Transmission electron-microscopic observations*. The
superficial cells of epithelium showed various degrees of necrotic changes (0.1-0.2 ng/ml T_2 toxin). In some cells the mitochondria and rough endoplasmic reticulum were destroyed, and intracellular and intercellular vacuolation were very prominent.
The epithelial cells of deeper layers usually had mild changes
with irregular and enlarged nuclei and sometimes degenerative
changes in the mitochondria.

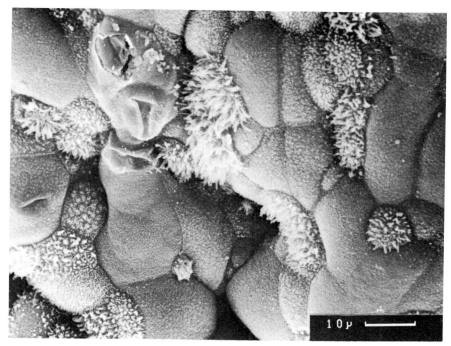

Fig. 9. Scanning electron micrograph of explants of human fetal esophagus after action by T_2 toxin (0.1 ng/ml) for 6 days. Some cells are ciliated. Some of the epithelial cells are swollen and ruptured (16-day culture).

When 0.4 ng/ml T_2 toxin was present in medium, the superficial layers of epithelium usually showed various degrees of necrotic changes, and the intermediate and deep layers showed hyperplastic or dysplastic changes. The contours of nuclei might become irregular; the ratio of nuclei to cytoplasm increased. Sometimes the cell nuclei had deep indentations and prominent nucleoli. The organelles of cytoplasm showed various degrees of degeneration or destruction (Fig. 8). Mitochondria and rough endoplasmic reticulum increased in some cells.

   c. *Scanning electron-microscopic observations.* In control explants of 16-day culture, the surface epithelial cells are polygonal with prominent intercellular margins. The cell sur-

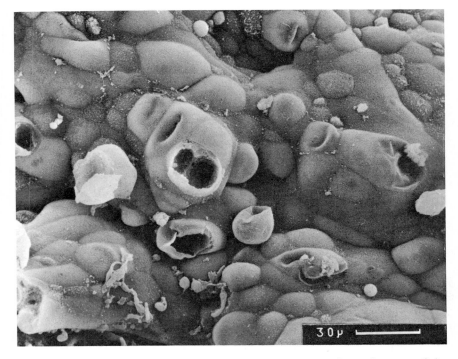

Fig. 10. Scanning electron micrograph of explants of human
fetal esophagus after action by T_2 toxin (0.4 ng/ml) for 6 days.
The surface of epithelium has become very irregular. Cells are
crowded together because of proliferation. Some superficial
cells are broken because of the cytotoxic effect (16-day culture).

faces are more or less flat with a little convexity. When
0.1 ng/ml of T_2 toxin was present in medium for 4 to 6 days, the
superficial cells of epithelium became irregular. Some cells
are polygonal and sometimes become more or less round. Some
cells are swollen with smooth or ruptured surfaces (Fig. 9).

Focal proliferations of cells are dominant with few ruptured cells on the surface after the explants were exposed to T
toxin (0.4 ng/ml) for 4 to 6 days. The proliferated cells gath-
ered in small groups. The whole surface is very irregular. The
surface of cells are more or less smooth with convex contours
(Fig. 10).

The whole surface of epithelium sloughs off in most of the explants, and only debris of cells remains sticking to the fibrous meshwork of the lamina propria after exposure to 2 to 4 ng/ml of T_2 toxin for 4 to 6 days.

2. *Effects of T_2 Toxin on Human Adult Esophagus*

Human adult esophageal epithelium was obtained from the "normal portion" of surgical specimens of esophageal carcinoma (20 cases). After culture for 3 days, T_2 toxin was added to the medium at 0.4, 1, 2, or 4 µg/ml for 24 h. The whole surface epithelium of all explants become necrotic. The epithelial cells of esophageal glands were also necrotic and accumulated in the lumens of glands. When the explants were exposed to T_2 toxin (4-40 ng/ml) for 2 days, the whole layers of epithelium become necrotic and sloughed in three fourths of the cases. In one fourth of the cases most of the epithelial layers became necrotic, and in some explants the epithelial layer became very thin and flat. Basal cell proliferation, dysplasia, or focal hyperplasia of epithelium were also seen at the same time in half of the explants. In one fourth of the cases, increase of mitotic figures and atypical mitosis were seen.

Necrosis of esophageal glands was also very prominent, and many necrotic cells accumulated in the lumen. When the explants were exposed to T_2 toxin (0.2-1.2 ng/ml) for 4 to 6 days, proliferative effects could be observed in about 60% of cases, with proliferation of basal cells being the most common type. The basal cells grow downward and form papillae or cords extending into the lamina propria. Atypical mitotic figures may be present in these papillae. Superficial focal necrosis and basal cell proliferation can occasionally be seen in the same area of epithelium.

As a conclusion, the effects of T_2 toxin on human fetal and adult esophagus are quite similar, although the percentage of

explants with proliferative effects in human adult esophagus
seems higher than that in fetal tissues. In contrast, the percentage of cases with atypical mitosis in T_2-treated explants
seems to be higher in fetal esophagus than that in human adults.
Short exposure to larger doses caused necrosis and sloughing
off of the most part or whole layer of epithelium. Small doses
of median exposure time caused proliferative changes with a mild
degree of necrosis or degeneration of the superficial layers of
epithelium. Interindividual variations are very prominent.

IV. CHEMICAL AND MICROBIAL INTERACTION IN ESOPHAGEAL CARCINOGEN

     Many species of bacteria and some species of fungi can re-
duce nitrate to nitrite, thereby enhancing the formation of nitrosamines (Ayanaba and Alexander, 1973; Uibu et al., 1978).
Can these microorganisms colonized in epithelia of patients
with fungal esophagitis play a role in formation of certain
chemical carcinogens? Because C. albicans is the most common
fungi isolated from fungal esophagitis and esophageal cancer,
we tested the ability of C. albicans to form N-nitrosobenzyl-
methylamine (NBMA), a strong carcinogen that selectively induces esophageal cancer in rats and mice (Druckrey et al.,
1967), from its precursors in vitro. Benzylmethylamine (BMA),
the precursor of NBMA, has been identified as a variety of
foods, especially vegetables, at levels as high as 16 ppm
(Neurath et al., 1977). Nitrite and its precursor nitrate
were commonly found in the drinking water and food in Linxian,
and the level of salivary nitrite was often increased in patients with esophageal epithelial dysplasia or carcinoma. Our
studies have established the ability of C. albicans to augment
the nitrosative formation of NBMA from its precursors (Hsia et
al., 1981). When stationary or exponentially growing cultures

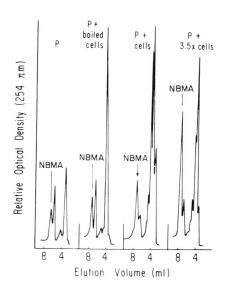

Fig. 11.   HPLC curves of NBMA formation under different
conditions with pH controlled at 6.8.   NBMA, benzylmethylnitro-
samine; P, precursors only; P + boiled cells, precursors plus
Candida cells boiled for 15 min; P + cells, precursors plus
7.4×10^7 *Candida* cells.   P + 3.5 x cells, precursors plus
26×10^7 *Candida* cells.

of *C. albicans* were cultured with BMA and $NaNO_2$, a significant

increase in the amount of NBMA was found in these cultures com-

pared to precursors-only controls.   The identity of the NBMA

was confirmed by high-performance liquid chromatographic (HPLC)

coelution with authentic NBMA in three solvent systems and by

mass spectroscopy.   The amount of NBMA synthesized depended on

the number of *Candida* cells.   Boiled *Candida* cells and condi-

tioned medium were not effective in enhancing nitrosation

(Fig. 11).

    C. albicans produces various acidic metabolites that cause

decrease of pH of the media.   The nitrosation of NBMA signifi-

cantly depends on pH.   At pH values above 7.4, the amounts of

NBMA detected were very low and near the limit of sensitivity

of the methods employed.   Significant amounts were found with

TABLE IV. Effects of pH of Media and Formation of NBMA from Its Precursors by *C. albicans*

Experiment number	pH	Components	Number of cells (× 10^7)	Incubation time (h)	Buffer Concentration (M)	NBMA formed (μg/5 ml)
1	6.8	BMA + NaNO$_2$	--	48	0.08	30.7 ± 5.1
		BMA + NaNO$_2$ + live Candida cells	7.4	48	0.08	62.1 ± 3.3
			26	48	0.08	110.2 ± 22.6
		BMA + NaNO$_2$ + conditioned medium	--	48	0.08	34.1 ± 18.9
		BMA + NaNO$_2$ + boiled Candida cells	7.4	48	0.08	32.0 ± 4.0
2	7.4	BMA + NaNO$_2$	--	24	0.12	1.9 ± 0.1
	7.4 decreased to 7.2[a]	BMA + NaNO$_2$	--	48	0.038	8.4 ± 2.7
	7.4 decreased to 6.1[a]	BMA + NaNO$_2$ + live Candida cells	12.0	48	0.038	121.3 ± 19.6
3	8.0 at end of incubation	BMA + NaNO$_2$	--	48	None	1.3
	6.8 at end of incubation	BMA + NaNO$_2$ + live Candida cells	4.5	48	None	75.0

[a]

greater acidity over the pH range of 7.4 to 3.5 (2.6 $\mu M/24$ h at pH 7.4, 19.9 $\mu M/24$ h at pH 6.8, 253.7 $\mu M/24$ h at pH 5.6, 928 $\mu M/24$ h at pH 3.5). When *Candida* was cultured with BMA and $NaNO_2$ with 0.038 M buffer, pH of the media decreased from 7.4 to 6.1, and NBMA formation increased to about 30-fold of that in precursors-only controls at pH 7.4 (Table IV). Our results indicate that the combined effect of cell-mediated nitrosation and reduction in pH could cause a 30- to 50-fold enhancement of rate of formation of NBMA from its precursors. Generation of nitrosamine in close proximity to the target tissue, especially under conditions of poor fluid circulation, could result in a concentration sufficient to initiate tumorigenesis. Initiation by carcinogen *in situ* will be much more efficient and the threshold will be much lower than by those carcinogens possibly ingested with food or water. We speculate that the foci of fungal and bacterial infection in esophageal epithelium might be one of the sites of endogenous synthesis for nitrosamines or other carcinogens. The new approach to *in situ* formation of carcinogen and its local action on target cells deserves further studies.

V. POSSIBLE ROLE OF FUNGAL INFECTION AND MYCOTOXIN IN MULTI-FACTORIAL AND MULTISTAGE ESOPHAGEAL CARCINOGENESIS

Carcinogenesis is now generally recognized as a multistage process (Berenblum, 1974; Slaga et al., 1978). On the basis of our previous studies in Linxian, we speculate that esophageal carcinogenesis is multifactorial and multistaged. For esophageal cancer, the existence of background diseases such as esophagitis, simple hyperplasia, or mild dysplasia of esophageal epithelium probably acts as a predisposing host factor. Nutritional factors, especially deficiency in vitamins

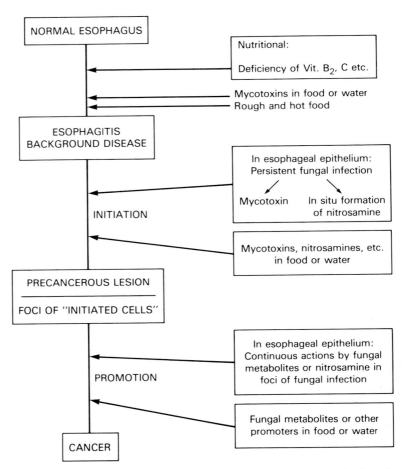

Fig. 12. Diagram of possible role of fungal infection and mycotoxin in multifactorial and multistage esophageal carcinogenesis in Linxian county.

B_2 and C, mycotoxins in moldy food, and roughness of food, may be responsible for the development of background diseases. We have proposed the following hypothesis for the possible role of fungal infection and mycotoxin and other factors in esophageal carcinogenesis (Fig. 12). In the presence of background diseases, the basal cells of epithelium usually become hyperplastic, during which the DNA synthesis is increased. When the chances of dissociation of double chains of DNA increase, there are more chances of inducing initiation by carcinogens. The background diseases may be further complicated by fungal infections. Fungal esophagitis may play a role in esophageal carcinogenesis in three ways: (1) it might induce a chronic persistent inflammation that stimulates basal cell hyperplasia and dysplasia; (2) the fungi and bacteria colonized in esophageal epithelium may enhance the endogenous synthesis of nitrosamines or other carcinogens *in situ,* which may act as initiators; and (3) the metabolites of fungi invading the epithelium may have initiating or promoting effects directly on esophageal epithelium. Our investigations in Linxian have added support to our speculations.

The initiating agents might come from two sources: foci of fungal infections and carcinogens and/or their precursors in food or drinking water. The initiators from these sources might act at the weak points of the esophagus with long-term background diseases (esophagitis) and induced multiple foci of initiated cells. These initiated cells are difficult to identify and can be considered as latent cancerous lesions. They will not progress to cancer unless exposed to further prolonged action of promoters. The promoters may also come from the two sources previously mentioned as initiators.

Our studies, just discussed, have shown that mycotoxins such as T_2 toxin have both cytotoxic and proliferative effects on esophageal epithelium; thus they may play roles at different stages of esophageal carcinogenesis. Because T_2 toxin causes necrosis of epithelium *in vitro*, it is possible that it could induce esophagitis *in vivo*. T_2 Toxin can induce proliferation of epithelium *in vitro*; it is possible that it has promoting effects in esophageal carcinogenesis. T_2 Toxin could induce atypical mitosis of esophageal epithelium *in vitro*; therefore it is possible that it has a certain degree of mutagenic potential *in vivo*.

Nutritional factors may also play roles in the stage of initiation. For example, vitamin C could block the endogenous synthesis of nitrosamines. Vitamin A might protect DNA to some extent from action by chemical carcinogens. Esophageal carcinoma is the end product of complicated combined effects of multiple factors acting at different stages.

Because esophageal carcinogenesis is complicated, it remains to be explored by further investigation.

REFERENCES

Ayanaba, A., and Alexander, M. (1973). *Appl. Microbiol. 25,* 862-868.
Berenblum, I. (1974). "Carcinogenesis as a Biological Problem." North-Holland, Amsterdam.
Cawson, R. A. (1959). *Proc. R. Soc. Med. 62,* 610-614.
Chang, B. G., and Heu, M. C. (1965). *Chung-hua Ping Li Hsueh Tsa Chih (Chin. J. Pathol.) 9,* 51-53.
Chi, M. S., and Mirocha, C. J. (1978). *Poult. Sci. 57,* 807-808.
Coordinating Groups for the Research of Esophageal Carcinoma (1975). *Chin. Med. J. (Peking Engl. Ed.) 1,* 110-116.
Crespi, M., Munoz, N., Grassi, A., Aramesh, B., Amiri, G., Mojtabai, A., and Casale, V. (1979). *Lancet 2,* 217-220.
Druckrey, H., Preussmann, R., Ivankovic, S., and Schmahl, D. (1967). *Z. Krebsforsch. 69,* 103-201.
Hillman, E. A., Vocci, M. J., Schurch, W., Harris, C. C., and Trump, B. F. (1980). *Methods Cell Biol. 21,* 332-348.
Hsia, C. C., and Tsao, I. Y. (1978). *Chung-hua I Hsueh Tsa Chih (Peking) (Natl. Med. J. China) 58,* 392-396.
Hsia, C. C., Wang, K. C., Zue, W. T., and Lu, S. C. (1978). "Scientific Reports from 1958-1978," pp. 860-867. Cancer Inst. Chinese Acad. Med. Sci., Beijing.
Hsia, C. C., Sun, T. T., and Lu, S. C. (1979). *Chung-hua Zhong Liu Tsa Chih (Chin. J. Oncol.) 1,* 190-194.
Hsia, C. C., Sun, T. T., Wang, Y. Y., Anderson, L. M., Armstrong, D., and Good, R. A. (1981). *Proc. Natl. Acad. Sci. USA 78,* 1878-1881.
Hsia, C. C., Tsao, S. K., Tsing, T. H., and Lu, S. C. (1983). *Chung-hua Zhong Liu Tsa Chih (Chin. J. Oncol.),* in press.
Hsia, C. C., and Harris, C. C. (1983). *Carcinogenesis,* in press

Kugelman, T. P., Cripps, D. J., and Harrell, E. R. (1963).
    Arch. Dermatol. *88*, 150-157.
Lafarge-Frayssinet, C., Decloitre, F., Mousset, S., Martin, M.,
    and Frayssinet, C. (1981). *Mutat. Res.* *88*, 115-123.
Neurath, G. B., Dunger, M., Pein, F. G., Ambrosius, D., and
    Schreiber, O. (1977). *Food Cosmet. Toxicol.* *15*, 275-282.
Schoental, R., Joffe, A. Z., and Yagen, B. (1979). *Cancer Res.*
    39, 2179-2184.
Sheng, C., Chiu, S. L., Liu, F. Y., and Lian, T. S. (1964).
    Chung-hua Ping Li Hsueh Tsa Chih (Chin. J. Pathol.)
    (Suppl.), 407-409.
Slaga, T. J., Sivak, A., and Boutwell, R. K. (1978). "Mechanism
    of Tumor Promotion and Cocarcinogenesis." Raven, New York.
Uibu, J., Bogovski, P., and Tauts, O. (1978). *In* "Environmental
    Aspects of N-Nitroso Compounds" (E. A. Walker and M.
    Castegnaro, eds.), pp. 247-256, IARC Publ. No. 19. IARC
    Sci. Publ., Lyon, France.
Wang, Y. Y., Hsia, C. C., Lu, S. C., and Sun, T. T. (1982).
    Chung-hua Zhong Liu Tsa Chih (Chin. J. Oncol.) *4*, 86-88.

37

INTERDISCIPLINARY STUDIES IN THE EVALUATION OF PERSONS AT HIGH RISK OF CANCER

William A. Blattner, Mark H. Greene, and James J. Goedert

Family Studies Section
Environmental Epidemiology Branch
National Cancer Institute
Bethesda, Maryland

Dean L. Mann

Office of the Director
Division of Biology and Diagnosis
National Cancer Institute
Bethesda, Maryland

I.   INTRODUCTION

Genetic factors are well established in the etiology of
cancer (Mulvihill, 1977), and study of familial cancer syndromes provides opportunities for evaluating a role for host-
genetic susceptibility (Blattner, 1977). Claims that up to
90% of cancers are due to environmental risk factors are based
on studies of international variation in cancer incidence
(Haenszel and Kurihara, 1968) and do not take into account the
role of risk modifiers such as individual host-genetic susceptibility (Harris *et al.*, 1980; Fraumeni, 1982). The interdisciplinary approach involves collaboration between etiologically
oriented clinician/epidemiologists and similarly minded laboratory investigators (Blattner, 1977). Studies of persons at high
risk of cancer, identified by virtue of environmental exposures,
genetic traits, or family history of cancer, offer unique opportunities for understanding cancer risk mechanisms. Etio-
logic leads developed at the bedside provide the catalyst
for developing clinico-laboratory protocols that test hypotheses concerning host susceptibility and host-environmental
interaction.

Because this process begins at the bedside, a checklist
of questions that help identify high-risk patients has been
developed (Mulvihill, 1975). The questions to consider are

1.   What are the demographic features of the patient?
     Is the tumor occurring at an unusual site or at a
     younger or older age than expected?
2.   Are there potentially relevant environmental exposures?
3.   Are there identifiable host factors such as a positive
     family history, antecedent disease, or laboratory ab-
     normality?

Examples in which this approach has promoted our understanding
of host susceptibility mechanisms are presented here.

II.   HEREDITARY MELANOMA: A MODEL FOR INTERDISCIPLINARY
      STUDIES OF CANCER-PRONE FAMILIES

Melanoma-prone families are an ideal study group for
clarifying host susceptibility factors and mechanisms of melanoma pathogenesis. Preliminary studies of such families led
to the recognition of a new preneoplastic syndrome. Originally
this was designated the "B-K mole syndrome," named after families "B" and "K," the first two kindreds evaluated (Clark et
al., 1978; Greene et al., 1978; Reimer et al., 1978; Greene
and Fraumeni, 1979). Subsequently, we introduced the more precise and descriptive term, dysplastic nevus syndrome (DNS),
when it became clear that cytological atypia, or dysplasia of
melanocytes, was the hallmark of these lesions (Greene et al.,
1980b; Elder et al., 1981). The following is a summary of the
current status of this syndrome, based on detailed clinical
and laboratory studies conducted on 401 members of 14 melanoma-
prone families.

By way of background, the typical Caucasian has 25-40 common acquired nevi on his/her skin. These lesions begin as pin-
point macules that expand circumferentially, evolve into a pigmented papule, and eventually lose their pigmentation. Such
lesions may disappear completely in the later years of life.
In general nevi are small, round, uniformly pigmented (tan,
brown), have a smooth border, and predominate on sun-exposed
skin above the waist (Elder et al., 1981).

In contrast, dysplastic nevi (DN) are generally more numerous than normal and are larger than 5 mm in diameter; they have
irregular borders, a persistent macular component, and varie-
gated pigmentation (pink hues are frequent). Not infrequently,
they occur on the scalp, breast, and buttock, sites generally
spared by ordinary nevi (Reimer et al., 1978; Greene et al.,
1978, 1980a; Elder et al., 1981). Our original report on this

subject emphasized the large number of morphologically atypical
nevi found in affected patients (Reimer *et al.*, 1978). As our
experience has grown, it has become clear that the number of
abnormal nevi varies over a broad range, from isolated lesions
to many hundred. It is now apparent that *abnormal morphology
of individual nevi* is the salient clinical feature of the DNS
(Greene *et al.*, 1980a; Elder *et al.*, 1981). In examining an
affected patient, nevus to nevus variability is common; and individual nevi cannot be placed along the normal developmental
spectrum of common acquired nevi (CAN) outlined previously.
Clinically, DN display a morphology that occupies a middle
ground between CAN on the one hand and fully developed, invasive
cutaneous malignant melanoma (CMM) on the other. In fact,
biopsy may be required to distinguish a severely dysplastic
nevus from early CMM.

Our largely cross-sectional observations indicate that dysplastic nevi are absent at birth. An increased number of morphologically normal nevi in childhood may be the first detectable abnormality, but the characteristic clinical features of
dysplastic nevi usually are not recognizable until the onset of
adolescence. Unlike common acquired nevi, new dysplastic nevi
continue to appear throughout adult life. Occasionally, in
high-risk families, we have observed lesions such as this on the
scalp of preadolescent children with normal skin (Tucker *et al.*,
1983). Severely dysplastic scalp nevi of this type clearly have
malignant potential, and because the hair makes these lesions
difficult to monitor, we advocate their routine removal. This
is in contrast to dysplastic nevi elsewhere on the skin, which
are readily followed and need be removed only when changing in
a suspicious fashion. The back is the most common site for dysplastic nevi in both sexes. All 14 families studied were affected by the DNS, albeit in varying degrees (Greene *et al.*,
1980a). It is only a matter of time, however, before melanoma-

prone kindreds lacking this phenotype are found. Approximately 40% of the adult first-degree blood relatives of the melanoma patients in these families also had dysplastic nevi. That the DNS comprises the substrate upon which hereditary CMM arises has now been confirmed by other investigators in the United States (Lynch et al., 1978), Australia (Ramsay et al., 1982), England (Dowd and Everale, 1979), Germany (Braun-Falco et al., 1979; Bork et al., 1981), Japan (Sakamoto et al., 1977), and Czechoslovakia (Stava, 1980).

Histologically, the sine qua non of DN is cytological atypia, that is, dysplasia of melanocytes. This is invariably accompanied by a lymphocytic infiltrate and a pattern of fibrous bands that span from rete ridge to rete ridge (the latter designated lamellar fibroplasia) (Clark et al., 1978; Elder et al., 1981). Two morphological patterns of dysplasia are currently recognized: (1) epithelioid, in which the dysplastic melanocytes are in clusters or nests, and (2) lentiginous, in which dysplastic melanocytes form a sheet along the dermal-epidermal junction. Dysplastic melanocytes are significantly larger than normal melanocytes when studied by conventional light microscopy (Rhodes et al., 1982), and they show striking ultrastructural similarities to the malignant melanocytes of radial growth phase superficial spreading melanoma (W. H. Clark, D. E. Elder, and M. H. Greene, unpublished).

Our clinical studies have documented that, like other familial cancers, hereditary CMM is characterized by a younger than usual age at disease onset and a predisposition to multiple, independent primary tumors. Thus, of the 67 hereditary CMM patients in our 14 high-risk families, 43% were under age 30 at first melanoma diagnosis, compared with a mean age of 50 in unselected CMM patients. The youngest patient in our series was 12 years old. Among these hereditary cases, 44% had more than one primary CMM, with 11 separate primaries the most observed

in a single patient (Greene *et al.*, 1980a). Most melanomas
were of the superficial spreading type, the majority of which
were very thin (i.e., ≤ 0.76 mm) and thus amenable to surgical
cure. Over 90% of the hereditary CMM patients examined to
date have also had the DNS. Detailed histological evaluation
of these hereditary neoplasms revealed a dysplastic precursor
at the tumor margin in 69% of cases, compared to one third of
unselected melanomas (Elder *et al.*, 1981). The percentage of
melanomas with an identifiable dysplastic precursor lesion ex-
ceeds 95%, if one limits consideration to prospectively diagnosed cases (see later), lesions sufficiently new in their
natural history so as not to have overgrown a preexisting
nevus.

One of the most gratifying aspects of this study from a
clinical point of view has been the diagnosis of 31 new primary melanomas in 17 study patients. All but one of these malignancies measured ≤ 0.76 mm in thickness, and these have a high
probability of surgical cure. All newly diagnosed hereditary
CMM developed in family members with the DNS; none occurred in
family members with normal skin. Thus it is clear that careful dermatological evaluation of high-risk family members (i.e.,
those with the DNS) can facilitate early diagnosis of CMM at a
point in its natural history when mortality can be avoided.

One advantage to a study of this size is that it permits
application of various quantitative analytical techniques. For
example, one might reasonably inquire as to the extent of risk
of melanoma in these families. Using general population rates
to compute expected values (Boice *et al.*, 1980), computing
person years of observation (Monson, 1974), and excluding the
2 melanoma cases from each family that were required for study
participation, 39 persons developed melanoma. Because fewer
than 0.5 cases of CMM would be expected, it is clear that members of CMM-prone families are at least 100 times more likely

to develop this specific cancer than are their age-, race-, and sex-matched counterparts in the general population. The magnitude of this risk is not surprising, because segregation analysis of the melanoma trait in these families documented a Mendelian autosomal dominant mode of inheritance (Greene et al., 1983). Linkage analysis has revealed a correlation between CMM/DNS and the Rh locus (lod score = 2.00), suggesting that a melanoma susceptibility gene may be located on the short arm of chromosome 1.

These families provide an invaluable opportunity to conduct laboratory studies designed to elucidate mechanisms of CMM pathogenesis. For example, we have described borderline low T-cell levels and decreased mixed leukocyte culture response to an allogeneic stimulator pool in members of these families (Dean et al., 1979). Peripheral blood mononuclear cells isolated from family members "recognize" melanoma tumor antigens in vitro (Vandenbark et al., 1979), and their sera frequently contain circulating immune complexes and antimelanoma antibodies (T. Philips and M. H. Greene, unpublished). Australian investigators have reported depressed natural killer cell function in this setting (Hersey et al., 1979). Because a variety of immunosuppressed patient groups are at increased risk of melanoma (Greene et al., 1981), these observations are quite provocative. Precisely how they contribute to the risk of hereditary CMM is currently unclear, but a search for ultraviolet-induced immune dysfunction might prove fruitful in view of reported animal models for such effects (Picus et al., 1981; Fisher and Kripke, 1982).

The contribution of sensitivity to ultraviolet (UV) radiation and other environmental carcinogens have also been assessed in this study cohort. Using cultured skin fibroblasts from patients with multiple primary hereditary melanomas and the DNS, cellular response to injury induced by various carcinogens was evaluated using a colony-forming assay of cell survival. Six

fibroblast strains representing five separate families have been
studied *in vitro*. Their survival following exposure to graded
doses of toxic ionizing radiation was normal. In contrast,
all six strains displayed a 1.2- to 2.3-fold decrease in survival following exposure to 254-nm UV radiation (Smith *et al.*,
1982) (Fig. 1). Three of the six strains were also sensitive
to the effects of 4-nitroquinoline oxide, a UV-mimetic chemical
carcinogen (Smith *et al.*, 1983). Both induction of DNA repair
synthesis and inhibition of de novo DNA synthesis were normal
in these cells, indicating that these strains are proficient
in the repair of thymine dimers. Australian investigators have
reported similar UV sensitivity using lymphoblastoid cell lines
from melanoma-prone family members, and have suggested that
this sensitivity segregates in high-risk families in a pattern
consistent with autosomal dominant inheritance (Ramsay *et al.*,
1982). The mechanism of this UV sensitivity is as yet unde-
termined, but it is clearly different from that observed in patients with xeroderma pigmentosum. Given the known association
between UV radiation and melanoma risk, this observation is
particularly exciting and is under active additional study.

    Lest one conclude that these observations are only of
passing interest, based as they are on a small subgroup of patients drawn from a pool of persons with a relatively rare
malignancy, the broader relevance of these studies deserves
emphasis. Having identified the DNS in the setting of hereditary melanoma, we subsequently evaluated a series of unrelated
CMM patients, all of whom had a negative family history for
CMM, and found that a fraction of them had on their skin nevi
that were clinically and histologically indistinguishable from
those observed in high-risk family members (Elder *et al.*,
1980). This observation has been confirmed by other investigators, both in this country (Rhodes *et al.*, 1980; Rahbari and

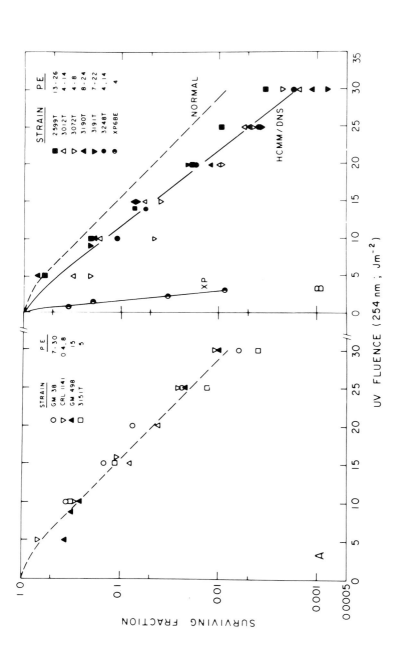

Fig. 1. Survival of colony-forming ability of normal fibroblast strains (a) and
six HCMM/DNS fibroblast strains (b) as a function of UV irradiation (254 nm).
(a) represents the mean response of the indicated normal strains and is reproduced in
(a) represents the mean response of the indicated normal strains and is reproduced in (b). Each
point represents the mean surviving fraction for the varying members of determinations (from 1 to
4) made on each cell line. Some points are offset for clarity. SE <10%; PE, plating efficiency
(%). From Smith *et al.* (1982) with permission.

Mehregan, 1981) and abroad (Scheibner *et al.*, 1981). We desig-
nate this the sporadic (nonfamilial) variant of the DNS (Greene
et al., 1980b; Elder *et al.*, 1980).

Thus the study of high-risk families has led to the recognition of what now appears to be the most common precursor to
melanoma, be it familial or sporadic. Furthermore, nevus surveys in various cohorts of noncancer patients have suggested
that from 2 to 4% of such persons have dysplastic nevi (Rhodes
et al., 1980; Scheibner *et al.*, 1981). Neither of these reports
has appeared in full manuscript form, so a detailed consideration of their methods has not yet been possible, but it seems
certain that DN will turn out to be much more prevalent in the
general population than previously estimated. Further support
for this notion is found in the observation that the CMM that
arise in immunosuppressed renal transplant recipients, a group
known to be at high melanoma risk, evolve from dysplastic nevi
(Greene *et al.*, 1981).

In summary, it is now reasonable to accept familial melanoma as a hereditary disorder. Careful monitoring of melanoma
families with the DNS has resulted in the diagnosis of a substantial number of potentially curable melanomas. DN thus constitutes a clinical marker that permits identification of and
improved prognosis for persons at high risk. Management guidelines for use by health professionals and for family members
and their physicians have been developed, as have series of edu-
cational videotapes dealing with various aspects of the DNS
(Fraser, 1982).

The identification of the DNS has moved our ability to
recognize melanoma a quantum step earlier in its natural history, a significant advance toward the eventual control of this
potentially lethal disease. Laboratory studies in this context
have provided a number of important clues to the etiology and
pathogenesis of human malignant melanoma. The sequence of

hyperplasia, dysplasia, neoplasia that has been described in
many other human and experimental tumor systems can be seen to
pertain to the melanocyte as well. Given its location on the
skin's surface, where its evolution can be directly observed,
the melanocyte has become an invaluable model for the study of
human carcinogenesis.

III. ECOGENETICS AND HOST SUSCEPTIBILITY

Environmental factors, particularly cigarette smoking and
certain industrial chemicals such as aromatic amines, are well-
documented risk factors in the etiology of bladder cancer (Blot
and Fraumeni, 1978). Other nonoccupanional chemicals, such as
nitrosamines, are shown to be bladder carcinogens in animal experiments but have not been conclusively associated with human
bladder cancer (Price, 1971). Experimental studies, however,
suggest that susceptibility may be modified by intrinsic host
variation in metabolic processing of putative carcinogens.
Examples of this are risks of bladder cancer associated with
the *N*-acetyltransferase phenotype (Lower *et al.*, 1979) and the
elevation of urinary glucuronidase, a lysosomal enzyme (Boyland
et al., 1955).

The members of a bladder cancer-prone family (Fig. 2),
first reported by the National Cancer Institute in 1967
(Fraumeni and Thomas, 1967), were followed up to evaluate the
predictability of the previously mentioned and other risk factors (Blattner *et al.*, 1983). The occurrence of familial urinary bladder cancer appears to be rare, in that only 13 familial
clusters have been reported. Not surprisingly, little is known
about the etiology of familial bladder cancer. Environmental
factors have been linked as causative agents to a large proportion of human bladder cancer (Wynder and Gori, 1977). Although

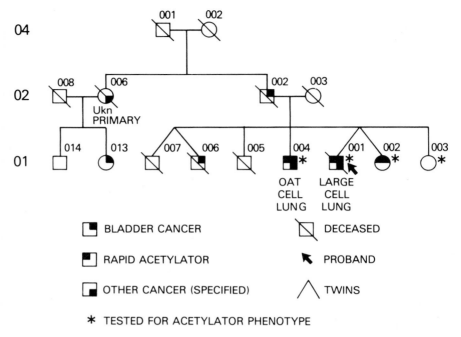

Fig. 2. Pedigree of bladder cancer-prone family.
☐, male; ○, female.

environmental carcinogens play a significant etiological role,
genetic influences seem to play an important role as well. In
many of the previously reported familial cases, heavy occupational exposures and/or cigarette smoking histories were noted,
suggesting the interaction of host and environmental factors.
In our family, all cases with bladder cancer gave strong positive smoking histories, although in one case there was a long
latent period between the discontinuance of smoking and diagnosis. Additional evidence for a smoking-related etiology was
the occurrence of second primary lung carcinoma in the proband
and his brother. In the case of familial lung cancer, host
susceptibility to environmental agents has also been implicated
(Goffman *et al*., 1982). However, this is the first familial aggregation reported with dual primary lung and bladder tumors,
where putative ecogenetic factors are implicated in both tumors.

The concept of ecogenetics focuses on developing epidemiological approaches for quantifying host susceptibility
mechanisms. Such studies in lung and bladder are likely to be
fruitful given the role for environmental factors in the etiology of these tumors.

Metabolic approaches are particularly applicable for understanding ecogenetic interaction, especially in cases where an
environmentally linked cancer occurs excessively in a family
(Mulvihill, 1976). One example of an ecogenetic interaction
having a possible causative role is the metabolism of aromatic
amines. Arylamines have long been implicated as having a strong
etiological role in the development of human bladder cancer
(Clayson and Cooper, 1970). It has been documented that latent
carcinogenic arylamines require metabolic activation by enzyme
systems that can be viewed as components of detoxification pathways with respect to arylamine-induced bladder carcinogenesis.
However, the relationships are complex because of the interaction of various pathways in the generation of intermediate metabolites, some of which act as carcinogens for either bladder or
liver (Lower et al., 1979). It has been postulated that the
rapid N-acetyltransferase phenotype is associated with rapid
detoxification of arylamines, resulting in protection from
bladder cancer (Lower et al., 1979). In this family all bladder
cases were rapid acetylators, whereas the unaffected sib was a
slow acetylator (Blattner et al., 1983). This result is not
what would be expected on the basis of the conventional thinking
about the role of N-acetyltransferase enzymes in the etiology of
bladder cancer. One explanation for this paradox is that the
acetylator phenotype per se is not the major risk determinant;
rather, some other genetic pathway, linked to this enzyme system on the same chromosome, might influence host susceptibility
to bladder carcinogens.

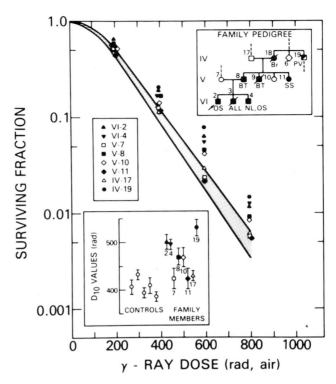

Fig. 3. Abbreviated pedigree and survival curves for fibroblasts exposed to graded doses of toxic ionizing radiation. The stippled area indicates the range in the mean survival response of five normal strains. The number designations in the family pedigree (insert top right) and the scattergram of D_{10} values (insert bottom left) calculated from the survival data are those used previously. D_{10} values of the five controls are shown in the scattergram in the order GM38, 1461-T, 2270-T, 2650-T, 3151-T, from left to right. Each point represents the mean of two to five experiments, and their standard errors were routinely less than 10%. Points for strains V-7 and V-8 are the means of duplicate tests with the two independent biopsies. OS, osteogenic sarcoma; ALL, acute lymphoblastic leukemia; NL, bilateral malignant neurilemmoma; SS, soft tissue sarcoma; BT, brain tumor; BR, breast cancer; PV, polycythemia vera. Symbols in the pedigree: solid, cancer; half solid, polycythemia vera; open, normal. From Bech-Hansen *et al.* (1981) with permission.

None of the molecular epidemiological assays employed in this family provide a clear or conclusive answer to why members of this family are at risk for bladder cancer. Clearly these patients and their offspring bear close follow-up. In addition, as new methods of *in vitro* study of metabolic pathways are developed, families such as this, where bedside observations provide etiological clues, should furnish new insights into the role of host susceptibility factors in tumorigenesis.

In the mid-1960s F. P. Li and J. F. Fraumeni were intrigued by the occurrence of rhabdomyosarcoma in a child and acute leukemia in his father. Epidemiological detective work led to the discovery of a distant branch in which other similar cancers occurred (Li, 1977). In addition, three families with a similar pattern suggested a syndrome characterized by the occurrence of bony and soft tissue sarcoma, breast cancer, brain cancer, and leukemia (Li and Fraumeni, 1969). The family shown in Fig. 3 came to our attention because of the occurrence of childhood neoplasms (osteosarcoma, bilateral malignant neurolemmoma, and acute lymphocytic leukemia) in three brothers (Blattner *et al.*, 1979). Over the next few years the father of these boys developed a low-grade astrocytoma, and their paternal aunt developed leiomyosarcoma.

In our initial study, a genealogical search identified a total of 16 cases of cancer among the descendants of the proband's great-great-great-grandmother. This included a previously unsuspected cluster of similar neoplasms in a distant branch of the family. The constellation of tumors in the family included bony and soft tissue sarcomas, brain and neural tumors, leukemia, and breast carcinoma, and occurred in a pattern suggesting the action of an incompletely penetrant autosomal dominant gene with pleiotrophic effects (Blattner *et al.*, 1979).

However, possible ecogenetic interaction in several cases
where environmental exposures seemed to have contributed to individual tumor development, led us to collaborate with
M. C. Patterson to study the effects of γ radiation on *in vitro*
DNA repair. The first two patients to be studied were (1) a
paternal great uncle of the proband who had polycythemia vera
and an occupational history of chemical and radiation exposure
and (2) the brother of the proband who developed osteosarcoma
of the lumbar vertebra in the site of prior radiotherapy.
When exposed to graded doses of radiation, skin fibroblasts
from these patients demonstrated an unusual survival pattern--
their cells were resistant to the killing effects of γ radiation (Fig. 3; Bech-Hansen *et al.*, 1981). Other relatives in
the cancer-prone lineage, but not their spouses, over three
generations demonstrated a similar pattern. This novel radiation phenotype could be a manifestation of a basic cellular defect, predisposing to a variety of tumors in members of this
family. Thus, *in vitro* radioresistance, like radiosensitivity,
may be a phenotype of a mechanism that increases cancer risk in
humans.

IV.   HOST-SUSCEPTIBILITY MECHANISMS

In 1973, two adolescent brothers developed acute lymphocytic leukemia within 3 weeks of each other (Blattner *et al.*,
1978). Clinically the brothers had almost identical courses
of disease. Both responded to chemotherapy and had relatively
late disease relapses. One brother recently died from infectious complications of his recurrent disease. At the time

that these brothers were diagnosed it was surmised, on clinical grounds, that a shared susceptibility to a common environmental exposure might be important. Although studies have attempted to identify an etiological agent, none has been found.

However, immunogenetic studies have provided important insights into the role of host susceptibility. HLA typing was performed on family members, and the two leukemic sibs were found to be HLA identical. In addition, sera from mothers of leukemic children contained antibodies to B-cell alloantigen markers that were linked to the major histocompatibility complex. By pedigree analysis of these reactions and the fortuitous occurrence of recombinants in one material haplotype, it was possible to trace these leukemia-associated reactions through the family tree and demonstrate that the sibs were homozygous for these specificities (Blattner et al., 1978). Follow-up has confirmed that these HLA reactions are linked to a specific HLA Dr4 and a variant of Dw4 called DB31. In this case, the HLA pattern in these siblings resembles the occurrence of immunologically associated leukemia in certain strains of mice. In the murine model, homozygosity for defective H-2-associated immune response genes, results in increased risk for acute leukemia, whereas heterozygosity allows the mouse to mount an adequate immune response (Lilly and Pincus, 1973). This response gene function is linked to leukemia susceptibility and resembles the mechanism that appears to underlie the defect in the X-linked immunodeficiency syndrome described by Purtillo et al. (1981).

Evidence that HLA-associated defective immune-regulatory genes may play a role in the pathogenesis of lymphoproliferative malignancy is also seen in the report of a family prone to

Waldenstrom's macroglobulinemia (WM) and autoimmune disease
(Blattner *et al.*, 1980). This family first came to our attention because of the occurrence of WM in two brothers. Laboratory testing in 22 members of the family confirmed the diagnosis
of WM in a third sibling and their father, as well as clinical
and subclinical autoimmunity. We found that one HLA haplotype
(A2, B8, DrW3) was present in all family members with WM and
clinical thyroid disease, and in all but one with subclinical
autoantibodies. In this family, the B-cell alloantigens Ia 172
and 350, previously associated with sicca syndrome, were identified in all family members with the HLA haplotype. This is
interesting in view of the exceptionally high risk of histiocytic lymphoma and WM in sicca syndrome patients. We postulate
that the susceptibility to WM and autoimmune disease in this
family results from a defect in the immune-regulatory system.
In particular, a new class of immune-suppressor genes linked to
similar disorders in mice may provide a model for understanding
how a common abnormality predisposes to autoimmunity and lymphoproliferative malignancy (Naor, 1979).

V.   ACQUIRED IMMUNODEFICIENCY AND CANCER RISK

   Recognition of the acquired immunodeficiency syndrome among
male homosexuals and some other groups has shown the value of
interdisciplinary studies in identifying precursor abnormalities
in high-risk populations.

   An outbreak of a rare malignancy, Kaposi sarcoma, a para-
sitic pneumonia caused by *Pneumocystis carinii,* and other unusual opportunistic infections appeared during 1981 among previ-

ously healthy homosexual men and intravenous drug addicts (Gottlieb *et al.*, 1981a; Hymes *et al.*, 1981; Friedman-Kien *et al.*, 1981). The cases were highly clustered in time and space, with New York City, San Francisco, and Los Angeles being the predominant areas affected. Immunological evaluation of the affected individuals typically demonstrated evidence of cytomegalovirus (CMV) infection, anergy to a battery of delayed-hypersensitivity recall antigens, poor *in vitro* lymphocyte function tests, profound depletion of helper T cells with reversal of the helper:suppressor (H:S) T-lymphocyte ratio, and normal or high levels of circulating immunoglobulins with preservation of B-cell function (Gottlieb *et al.*, 1981b; Masur *et al.*, 1981). These laboratory findings, accompanied by the precedent of Kaposi sarcoma and opportunistic infections in iatrogenically immunosuppressed patients, pointed to a new syndrome of acquired immunodeficiency (AID) that predisposed to cancer and other life-threatening diseases (Walzer *et al.*, 1974; Safai and Good, 1981).

The syndrome is lethal with median life expectancy of less than 1 year. There were several postulated causes, including use of recreational drugs like amyl nitrite (AN), hyperinfection with cytomegalovirus, or a new biological agent (Sigell *et al.*, 1978; Durack, 1981).

Attempting to make optimal use of the etiological clues and available laboratory markers, a multidisciplinary team of epidemiologists, immunologists, and virologists conducted a pilot study in the autumn of 1981 on 15 asymptomatic homosexual men in New York City (Goedert *et al.*, 1982). Their ages ranged from 29 to 53 years (median, 39 years). Eleven were white, four were black, and all were in apparent good health. On two occasions the subjects completed epidemiological questionnaires, had a physical examination by a medical oncologist, and donated blood, urine, saliva, and throat swabs. The latter specimens were plated for viral isolation, and seperated serum and peripheral blood lymphocytes were cryopreserved for subsequent analysis.

Seven of the healthy homosexual men said they had never or had infrequently used AN (fewer than 10 doses ever). The other eight used AN one or two times per month; only four of eight had used AN before 1975. AN users reported more sexual partners (median, 16 per year) than nonusers (median, 7 per year); the two groups were similar with respect to age, race, socioeconomic status, length of homosexual activity, frequency of use of other drugs, history of hepatitis and syphilis, and palpable lymphadenopathy. None of the subjects had a clinical history of CMV or infectious mononucleosis.

All 15 healthy men had normal complete blood counts, differentials, and estimated total T-cell counts (range OKT3-positive cells, 68-86%). Seven of the eight AN users had low H:S ratios (range, 0.71-1.07); all seven had an excess of OKT8-positive (suppressor) cells (range, 36-53%), and four also had a deficit of OKT4-positive (helper) cells (range, 31-38%). H:S ratios were similar (range, 0.65-0.99) at the second examination 2 months later in six AN users who had used the drug more than once during the study period; all six still had an excess of suppressor cells, and five also had a deficit of helper cells. In two AN users with very low H:S ratios, CMV was cultured from the urine. In contrast, six of the seven non-users had normal H:S ratios (1.22-2.32 at first examination, 1.34-3.17 after 2 months), and CMV was not isolated from any of the AN nonusers. H:S ratios were not significantly correlated with number of sexual partners or with physical findings in this cohort. However, other investigators in New York have re-

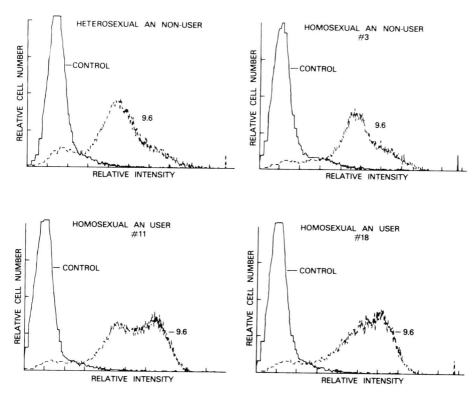

Fig. 4. Fluorescent-antibody profile (log plot) with the monoclonal antibody reagent 9.6 against the peripheral blood mononuclear cells of four healthy men. In the two lower plots, the cells from regular AN users (subjects 11 and 18) demonstrate a rightward shift high-intensity fluorescence with reagent 9.6.

ported low H:S ratios in homosexual men with lymphadenopathy or other prodromal symptoms, and in study subjects with more than 100 sex partners/year (Kornfeld et al., 1982).

The fluorescence profiles of all eight regular AN users to a pan-T monoclonal antibody 9.6 (which detects the sheep E-rosette receptor) showed an abnormal biomodal peak due to an increase in a densely staining subpopulation (Fig. 4; Goedert et al., 1982). There was a similar shift in the profiles of

two of the nonusers, but the other five nonusers had normal
fluorescence profiles. A similar shift toward a more densely
staining pattern was observed among the AN users when OKT8,
which detects suppressor lymphocytes, was used. Mean fluorescence with OKT8 was significantly higher for the eight AN
users than the seven nonusers.

Subsequent follow-up of the cohort confirms a persistence
of abnormal helper:suppressor ratios in the amyl nitrite users
over a 6-month period despite the fact that AN usage was somewhat reduced. These data provide preliminary evidence that
AN-induced immunosuppression, together with repeated CMV exposure, predisposes homosexual men to *P. carinii pneumonia* and
to Kaposi Sarcoma. Although we found no link between AN-
induced immunosuppression and any HLA or DR loci, the very high
prevalence of immunological abnormalities among homosexual men
suggests that as yet unidentified host and environmental characteristics may contribute to the comparatively rare occurrences
of *P. carinii* pneumonia and cancer. Further study is needed to
disentangle the roles of AN, viruses, and other factors in the
development of immunodeficiency, opportunistic infections, and
Kaposi sarcoma, with a particular eye toward new immunosuppres-
sive environmental agents, including viruses.

VI. SUMMARY AND CONCLUSION

The interdisciplinary approach involves collaboration between etiologically oriented clinician/epidemiologists and
similarly minded laboratory investigators. Studies of persons
at high risk of cancer, identified by virtue of environmental
exposure, or genetic trait or family history of cancer, offer
unique opportunities for understanding cancer risk mechanisms.
Etiological leads developed at the bedside provide the catalyst

for developing clinico-laboratory protocols that test hypotheses concerning host susceptibility and host-environmental interaction.

The studies summarized here represent examples of interdisciplinary studies of families and other high risk-populations that have provided important opportunities for understanding mechanisms of cancer risk. The future of such studies is favorable because of the advent of newer molecular biological, somatic cell, and gene cloning techniques. The approach could be considered a pilot for studying the role of host factors in human cancer with broad application to cancer etiology and environmental carcinogenesis.

REFERENCES

Bech-Hansen, N. T., Blattner, W. A., Sell, B. M., McKeen, E. A., Lampkin, B. C., Fraumeni, J. F., Jr., and Patterson, M. C. *(1981). *Lancet 1,* 1335-1337.

Blattner, W. A. (1977). *In* "Genetics of Human Cancer" (J. J. Mulvihill, R. W. Miller, and E. Frei, eds.), pp. 269-280. Raven Press, New York.

Blattner, W. A., Naiman, J. L., Mann, D. L., Wimer, R. S., Dean, J. H., and Fraumeni, J. F., Jr. (1978). *Ann. Intern. Med. 89,* 173-176.

Blattner, W. A., McGuire, D. B., Mulvihill, J. J., Lampkin, B. C., Hanaian, J., and Fraumeni, J. F., Jr. (1979). *JAMA J. Am. Med. Assoc. 24,* 259-261.

Blattner, W. A., Garber, J. E., Mann, D. L., McKeen, E. A., Henson, R., McGuire, D. B., Fisher, W. B., Bauman, A. W., Goldin, L. R., and Fraumeni, J. F., Jr. (1980). *Ann. Intern. Med. 93,* 830-832.

Blattner, W. A., Saunders, R. J., McGuire, D. B., Lower, G., Paigen, K., and Fraumeni, J. F. (1983). Submitted for publication.

Blot, W. J., and Fraumeni, J. F. (1978). *J. Natl. Cancer Inst. (U.S.) 61,* 1017-1023.

Boice, J. D., Greene, M. H., Keehn, R., Higgins, G., and Fraumeni, J. F. (1980). *J. Natl. Cancer Inst. (U.S.) 64,* 501-511.

Bork, K., Brauninger, W., and Nake, A. (1981). *Dermatologica 162,* 191-196.

Boyland, E., Wallace, D. M., and Williams, D. C. (1955). *Br. J. Cancer 9*, 62-79.

Braun-Falco, V. O., Landthaler, M., and Ryckmanns, F. (1979). *Fortschr. Med. 97*, 1489-1494.

Clark, W., Reimer, R., Greene, M. H., Ainsworth, A., and Mastrangelo, M. (1978). *Arch. Dermatol. 114*, 732-738.

Clayson, D. B., and Cooper, E. H. (1970). *Adv. Cancer Res. 13*, 271-381.

Dean, J., Greene, M. H., Reimer, R., LeSane, F., McKeen, E. A., Mulvihill, J. J., Blattner, W. A., Herberman, R., and Fraumeni, J. F. (1979). *J. Natl. Cancer Inst. (U.S.) 63*, 1139-1145.

Dowd, P., and Everale, J. (1979). *Br. J. Dermatol. 17*, 32-33.

Durack, D. T. (1981). *N. Engl. J. Med. 305*, 1465-1467.

Elder, D. E., Goldman, L., Goldman, E., Greene, M. H., and Clark, W. H. (1980). *Cancer (Philadelphia) 46*, 1787-1794.

Elder, D. E., Greene, M. H., Bondi, E., and Clark, W. H. (1981). *In* "Pathology of Malignant Melanoma" (A. B. Ackerman, ed.), pp. 185-215. Masson, New York.

Fisher, M. S., and Kripke, M. L. (1982). *Science (Washington, D.C.) 216*, 113-114.

Fraser, M. C. (1982). *Cancer Nurs. 5*, 351-360.

Fraumeni, J. F., Jr. (1982). *In* "Cancer Medicine" (J. F. Holland and E. Frei, eds.), pp. 5-12. Lea & Febiger, Philadelphia, Pennsylvania.

Fraumeni, J. F., and Thomas, L. B. (1967). *JAMA J. Am. Med. Assoc. 201*, 507-509.

Friedman, S. M., Felman, Y. M., Rothenberg, R., Dritz, S., Braff, E., Fannin, S., Heindl, I., Sikes, R. K., Gunn, R. A., and Roberts, M. A. (1981). *Morbid Mortal Weekly Rep. 30*, 409-410.

Friedman-Kien, A., Laubenstein, L., Marmor, M., Hymes, K., Green, J., Ragaz, A., Gottleib, J., Muggia, F., Demopoulas, R., Weintraub, M., Williams, D., Oliveri, R., Marmer, J., Wallace, J., Halperin, I., Gillooley, J. F., Prose, N., Klein, E., Vogel, J., Safai, B., Myskowski, P., Urmacher, C., Koziner, B., Nisce, L., Kris, M., Armstrong, D., Gold, J., Mildran, D., Tapper, M., Weissman, J. B., Rothenberg, R., Friedman, S. M., Siegal, F. P., Groundwater, J., Gilmore, J., Coleman, D., Follansbee, S., Gullett, J., Stegman, S. J., Wofsy, C., Bush, D., Drew, L., Braff, E., Dritz, S., Klein, M., Preiksaitis, J. K., Gottleib, M. S., and Jung, R. (1981). *Morbid Mortal Weekly Rep. 30*, 305-308.

Goedert, J. J., Wallen, W. C., Mann, D. L., Strong, D. M., Blattner, W. A., Neuland, C. Y., Greene, M. H., Murray, C., and Fraumeni, J. F., Jr. (1982). *Lancet i*, 412-416.

Goffman, T. E., Hassinger, D. D., and Mulvihill, J. J. (1982). *JAMA J. Am. Med. Assoc. 247*, 1020-1023.

Gottlieb, M. S., Schanker, H. M., Fan, P. T., Saxon, A.,
    Weisman, J. D., and Pozalski, I. (1981a). *Morbid Mortal
    Weekly Rep.* 30, 250-252.
Gottlieb, M. S., Schroff, R., Schanker, H. M., Weisman, J. D.,
    Fan, P. T., Wolf, R. F., and Saxon, A. (1981b). *N. Engl.
    J. Med.* 305, 1425-1431.
Greene, M. H., and Fraumeni, J. F. (1979). *In* "Human Malignant
    Melanoma" (W. H. Clark, L. Goldman, and M. Mastrangelo,
    eds.), pp. 139-166. Stratton, New York.
Greene, M. H., Reimer, R., Clark, W., and Mastrangelo, M.
    (1978). *Semin. Oncol.* 5, 85-87.
Greene, M. H., Clark, W. H., Kraemer, K. H., Fraser, M.,
    Elder, D. E., McGuire, D., and Dresdale, A. (1980a).
    Proc. Annu. Meet. Am. Soc. Clin. Oncol. 11th, Abstr. C-21,
    p. 323.
Greene, M. H., Clark, W. H., Jr., Tucker, M. A., Elder, D. E.,
    Kraemer, K. H., Fraser, M. C., Bondi, E. E., Guerry, D.,
    Tuthill, R., Hamilton, R., and LaRossa, D. (1980b).
    Lancet 2, 1024.
Greene, M. H., Young, T. I., and Clark, W. H., Jr. (1981).
    Lancet 1, 1196-1198.
Greene, M. H., Goldin, L. R., Clark, W. H., Jr., Lovrien, E.,
    Kraemer, K. H., Tucker, M. A., Elder, D. E., Fraser, M. C.,
    and Rowe, S. (1983). *Proc. Natl. Acad. Sci.*, in press.
Haenszel, W., and Kurihara, M. (1968). *J. Natl. Cancer Inst.
    (U.S.)* 40, 43-68.
Harris, C. C., Mulvihill, J. J., Thorgeirsson, S. S., and
    Minna, J. D. (1980). *Ann. Intern. Med.* 92, 809-825.
Hersey, P., Edwards, A., Honeyman, M., and McCarthy, W. H.
    (1979). *Br. J. Cancer 40*, 113-122.
Hymes, K. B., Cheung, T., Greene, J. B., Prose, N. S., Marcus,
    A., Ballard, H., William, D. C., and Laubstein, L. J.
    (1981). *Lancet ii*, 598-600.
Kornfeld, H., Vande Stouwe, R. A., Lange, M., Reddy, M. M.,
    and Grieco, M. H. (1982). *N. Engl. J. Med.* 307, 729-731.
Li, F. P. (1977). *In* "Genetics of Human Cancer" (J. J.
    Mulvihill, R. W. Miller, and J. F. Fraumeni, Jr., eds.),
    pp. 263-268. Raven, New York.
Li, F. P., and Fraumeni, J. F. (1969). *Ann. Intern. Med.* 71,
    747-751.
Lilly, F., and Pincus, T. (1973). *Adv. Cancer Res.* 17, 231-
    277.
Lower, G. M., Nilson, T., Nelson, C. E., Wolf, H., Gamsky,
    T. E., and Bryan, G. T. (1979). *EHP Environ. Health
    Perspect.* 29, 71-79.
Lynch, H. T., Frichot, B. C., and Lynch, J. F. (1978). *J.
    Med. Genet.* 15, 352-356.

Masur, H., Michelis, M. A., Greene, J. B., Onorato, I., Vande
    Stouwe, R. A., Holzman, R. S., Wormser, G., Brettman, L.,
    Lange, M., Murray, H. W., and Cunningham-Rudle, S. (1981).
    N. Engl. J. Med. 305, 1431-1438.

Monson, R. R. (1974). *Comp. Biomed. Res. 7,* 325-332.

Mulvihill, J. J. (1975). *In* "Persons at High Risk of Cancer:
    An Approach to Cancer Etiology and Control" (J. F.
    Fraumeni, Jr., ed.), pp. 3-37. Academic Press, New York.

Mulvihill, J. J. (1976). *J. Natl. Cancer Inst. (U.S.) 57,*
    3-7.

Mulvihill, J. J. (1977). *In* "Genetics of Human Cancer" (J. J.
    Mulvihill, R. W. Miller, and J. F. Fraumeni, Jr., eds.),
    pp. 137-143. Raven, New York.

Naor, D. (1979). *Adv. Cancer Res. 29,* 45-125.

Picus, J., Germain, R. N., Fox, J. J., Greene, M. I., Benacer-
    rof, B., and Letvin, N. L. (1981). *Cell. Immunol. 63,*
    300-307.

Price, J. M. (1971). *In* "Benign and Malignant Tumors of the
    Bladder" (E. Maltry, ed.), pp. 189-261. Med. Exam. Publ.,
    Flushing, New York.

Purtillo, D. T., Sakamoto, K., Saemundsen, A. K., Sullivan, J.
    L., Synnerholm, A., Anvret, M., Pritchard, J., Sloper, C.,
    Sieff, C., Pincott, J., Pachman, L., Rich, K., Cruzi, F.,
    Cornet, J. A., Collins, R., Barnes, N., Knight, J.,
    Sandstedt, B., and Klein, G. (1981). *Cancer Res. 41,*
    4226-4236.

Rahbari, H., and Mehregan, A. H. (1981). *Arch. Dermatol. 117,*
    329-331.

Ramsay, R. G., Chen, P., Imray, F. P., Kidson, C., Lavin, M. F.,
    and Hockey, A. (1982). *Cancer Res. 42,* 2909-2912.

Reimer, R., Clark, W., Greene, M. H., Ainsworth, A., and
    Fraumeni, J. F. (1978). *JAMA J. Am. Med. Assoc. 239,*
    744-746.

Rhodes, A. R., Sober, A. J., Mihm, M. C., and Fitzpatrick, T. B.
    (1980). *Clin. Res. 28,* 252A.

Rhodes, A. R., Melski, J. W., Sober, A. J., Harrist, T. J.,
    Fitzpatrick, T. B., and Mihm, M. C. (1982). *Clin. Res.
    30,* 265A.

Safai, B., and Good, R. A. (1981). *CA. 31,* 1-12.

Sakamoto, G., Sugano, H., Kasuga, T., Horigoe, N., Kumata, H.,
    and Funabaski, T. (1977). *Gan no Rinsho 23,* 857-861.

Scheibner, A., Milton, G. W., McCarthy, W. H., and Shaw, H.
    (1981). *Aust. N.Z. J. Surg. 51,* 386.

Siegal, F. P., Lopez, C., Hammer, G. S., *et al.* (1981). *N.
    Engl. J. Med. 305,* 1439-1444.

Smith, P. J., Greene, M. H., Devlin, D. A., McKeen, E. A., and
    Paterson, M. C. (1982). *Int. J. Cancer 30,* 39-45.

Smith, P. J., Greene, M. H., Adams, D., and Paterson, M. C.
    (1983). *Carcinogenesis,* in press.

Stava, Z. (1980). *Cs Dermatol.* *55,* 344-345.

Tucker, M. A., Greene, M. H., Clark, W. H., Kraemer, K. H., Fraser, M. C., and Elder, D. E. (1983). *J. Pediatrics,* in press.

Vandenbark, A., Greene, M. H., Burger, D., Vetto, M., and Reimer, R. (1979). *J. Natl. Cancer Inst. (U.S.) 63,* 1147-1151.

Walzer, P. D., Perl, D. P., Krogstad, D. J., Rawson, P. G., and Schultz, M. G. (1974). *Ann. Intern. Med. 80,* 83-93.

Wynder, E. L., and Gori, G. B. (1977). *J. Natl. Cancer Inst. (U.S.) 58,* 825-832.

38

CONCLUDING REMARKS: ROLE OF CARCINOGENS, COCARCINOGENS, AND HOST FACTORS IN CANCER RISK

Curtis C. Harris

Laboratory of Human Carcinogenesis
Division of Cancer Cause and Prevention
National Cancer Institute
Bethesda, Maryland

I.   INTRODUCTION

Cancer, like most diseases, is the result of a complex interaction between host and environment. The three major categories of determinants of cancer risk are carcinogens, cocarcinogens, and host factors (Table I). I prefer simple and broad
definitions of these three categories. A carcinogen is a chemical, physical, or biological agent that causes cancer. A cocar-

TABLE I. Determinants of Human Cancer Risk

Class	Example	Primary target site for cancer
Carcinogens		
Chemical		
Direct acting	Mustard gas	Lung
Indirect acting	2-Naphthylamine	Bladder
Complex mixture	Tobacco smoke	Lung
Physical		
Fiber	Asbestos	Pleura
Metal	Nickel compounds	Nasal cavity
Radiation	Ultraviolet light	Skin
Viral		
RNA	T-Cell leukemia virus (?)	Hemopoietic system
DNA	Epstein-Barr virus (?)	Hemopoietic system
	Hepatitis B virus (?)	Liver
Cocarcinogens		
Chemical	Ethanol[a]	Esophagus
Physical	Asbestos[a]	Bronchus
Viral	Hepatitis B virus[b]	Liver
Predisposing host factors		
Genetic		
Single gene	Xeroderma pigmentosum	Skin
Polygenic	Familial breast cancer	Breast
Chromosomal	Trisomy 21	Hemopoietic system
Acquired		
Infectious	Schistosomiasis	Bladder
Noninfectious inflammatory conditions	Ulcerative colitis	Colon
Nutritional	Plummer-Vinson syndrome (?)	Esophagus
Trauma	Lye	Esophagus

[a]Interactive effects with carcinogen, tobacco smoke.
[b]Interactive effects with carcinogen (e.g., aflatoxin B_1).

cinogen augments the oncogenic potential of a carcinogen. Tumor promoters are a specific category of cocarcinogens that induce tumor development only after both initiation by a genotoxic agent and repeated applications of the tumor promoter

(Pitot et al., 1982; Hennings, 1983).[1] Host factors, genetic
and acquired, determine the oncogenic susceptibility of an animal exposed to carcinogens and/or cocarcinogens. As illustrated
in the Venn diagram (Fig. 1), one could envision high risk of
cancer occurring in either an individual with a predisposing
host factor who is exposed to small amounts of a carcinogen such
as a person with the autosomal recessive disease xeroderma pigmentosum, who develops skin cancer when exposed to small doses
of sunlight (Cleaver et al., 1982), or an individual who has no
predisposition and is chronically exposed to large amounts of
carcinogen(s) and cocarcinogen(s), such as a dye worker who develops bladder cancer after being exposed to high doses of aromatic amines (Case et al., 1954).

Although these examples are at the two extremes, calculations based on epidemiological data also suggest the hypothesis
that a 100-fold difference in host susceptibility to carcinogens
exists in the general population (Doll, 1978; Peto, 1980). As
will be discussed later, experimental data from the laboratory
and the clinic are also consistent but do not as yet prove
this hypothesis.

After developing experimental systems during the early
decades of this century in which cancers were produced by either
complex mixtures of carcinogens (e.g., coal tar) or biological
preparations (e.g., tumor filtrates), cancer researchers have
taken a reductionistic approach and focused their attention on
identifying and studying the effects of individual agents. In
the field of chemical carcinogenesis, this attention has over
the last few decades shifted to cocarcinogens and tumor promoters. Interest in and studies of host factors has always been
present but seemingly to a lesser degree.

[1]*In an effort to be concise, many of the references listed
are reviews that are sources of more extensive discussions and
citations.*

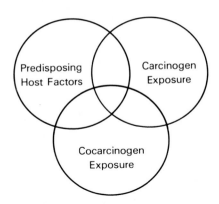

Fig. 1.   Major determinants of cancer risk are shown in
this Venn diagram.   The size and contribution of each category
of determinant will vary with each individual.

In this chapter the role of host factors in carcinogenesis
will be emphasized.

II.   *IN VITRO* MODELS OF HUMAN CARCINOGENESIS

Host factors have been traditionally studied by two approaches: clinical investigations and animal models.   As a
bridge between these approaches, we have developed a strategy
illustrated in Fig. 2.   An important facet of this strategy is
the capability to compare responses as well as mechanisms between experimental animals and humans at the molecular, cellular, and tissue levels of biological organization.

Substantial progress has been made in the last few years
in the methodology to culture human epithelial tissues and
cells (Table II).   Tissues from the major sites of human cancer
can be maintained *in vitro* for periods of weeks to over 1 year
(Harris *et al.*, 1980).   Because of the advantages listed in
Table III, chemically defined media have been developed to culture human tissues (bronchus, esophagus, colon, and pancreatic

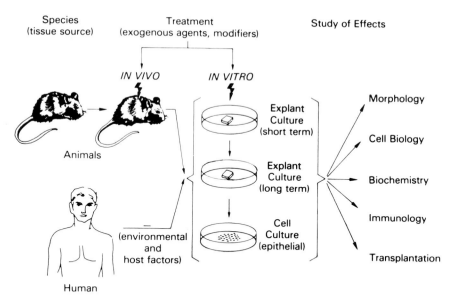

Fig. 2.   Experimental approach for comparative studies of carcinogenesis in tissues and cells from humans and experimental animals.

duct).   In addition, clonal growth of epithelial cells from either the bronchus (Lechner *et al.*, 1982) or epidermis (Tsao *et al.*, 1982) in chemically defined, serum-free media has been achieved.   These major advancements will aid scientists in all of the biomedical sciences including cancer research.   Impressive results in the culture of specific types of human carcinoma cells have also been obtained (Gazdar *et al.*, 1982; Bongemann and Jones, Chapter 5).

In vitro carcinogenesis studies will provide opportunities to test hypotheses directly in human tissues and cells. As noted in this volume, *in vitro* transformation of human cells by chemical, physical, and viral agents has been accomplished in the last decade.   Although these carcinogen-exposed cells frequently display a transformed phenotype *in vitro* (e.g., increased saturation density, prolonged life span in culture,

TABLE II.   Culture and Xenotransplantation of Normal Human Epithelial Tissues and Cells[a]

Cancer Sites	Explant	Epithelial cell culture		Xenotrans- plantation
		Primary	Clonal	
Breast	3[b]	+	+	+
Bronchus	12	+	+	+
Colon	0.8	+		+
Prostate	3	+	+	+
Esophagus	3	+	+	+
Bladder	4	+	+	+
Skin	3	+	+	+
Uterus, corpus	2	+	+	+
Stomach	2	+		
Pancreatic duct	3	+	+	+
Uterus, cervix	4	+	+	+
Liver	0.8	+	+	+

[a]Compiled from Harris et al. (1980); Sun and Wang (Chapter 31); E. Kaighn, (personal communication); C.-C. Hsia (personal communication).

[b]Months in culture; tissues from adults except for fetal liver.

TABLE III.   Advantages of Chemically Defined Media to Culture
Human Epithelial Cells

Less variability when compared to media containing serum
Identification of specific growth factors
Selective growth of differentiated normal and malignant cells
Identification of specific inducers of differentiation
Ease of isolation and analysis of secreted cellular products

and/or anchorage independence), they most generally have a finite life span *in vitro* and rarely form progressively grow-ing, invasive cancers when xenotransplanted in athymic *nude* mice.   One could formulate a hypothesis that these cells are partially transformed, that is, premalignant.   Because this is a new field of study, rapid advances are to be expected.

III.   INTERINDIVIDUAL DIFFERENCES IN HUMAN CARCINOGENESIS

Observational study of biology has taught us that people differ. Charles Darwin (1859) noted, "No one supposes that all the individuals of the same species are cast in the very same mould. The individuals differences are very important to us." Ernst Mayr (1982, p. 55) has stated, "In biology, one rarely deals with classes of identical entities, but nearly always studies populations consisting of unique individuals. This is true for every level of the hierarchy, from cells to ecosystems."

In the field of experimental carcinogenesis, differences in oncogenic susceptibility have been shown among both individuals in an outbred population (Boutwell, 1964) and, more clearly, different strains of inbred animals (Slaga et al., 1982); each strain can be considered to be a surrogate for a single individual in an outbred population. These differences can have a genetic basis. For example, susceptibility either to polycyclic aromatic hydrocarbons (Nebert et al., 1982) or to 1,2-dimethylhydrazine (Diwan and Blackman, 1980) varies in different strains of inbred mice. Similar differences have been observed in the oncogenic susceptibility of inbred rats to the hepatocarcinogenicity of aflatoxin B_1 in which female DA rats are much less susceptible when compared to most other strains, for example, Fischer 344 and Wistar (Idle and Ritchie, Chapter 35). Interstrain differences in susceptibility to either oncogenic viruses or physical carcinogens are also well known (Essex et al., 1980; Vogel and Turner, 1982).

Examples of genetic or acquired host factors associated with increased cancer risk in humans are shown in Tables I, IV, and V. Instead of choosing a rare condition such as xeroderma pigmentosum, Bloom syndrome, or familial polyposis, in which a genetically determined increased risk of cancer has been well

TABLE IV.   Examples of Acquired Diseases and Conditions Associated with Increased Cancer Risk[a]

Acquired disease	Cancer
Hepatitis B	Liver
Osteomyelitis	Skin
Schistosomiasis	Bladder
Ulcerative colitis	Intestine
Crohn disease	Intestine
Sarcoidosis	Lung, lymphoid
Diabetes mellitus	Pancreas
Stein-Leventhal syndrome	Uterus
Plummer-Vinson syndrome (iron deficiency)	Esophagus
Burns (thermal, caustic)	Skin, esophagus
Scar (tuberculosis)	Lung
Pernicious anemia	Stomach
Benign nevi (on palms of hands and soles of feet)	Melanoma

[a]*Adapted from Templeton (1975).*

documented (Table V), let us examine the role of host factors
in a group of common cancers, that is, those of the lung.

A.   Lung Cancer Epidemiology

Epidemiology has provided us with a number of important
facts.   Cigarette smoke is the most common cause of lung cancer.   The first interindividual difference is simply stated as
"to smoke or not to smoke."   This individual decision has been
extensively investigated by psychologists in which a number of
important factors have been identified including personality
type of the individual, smoking habits of other family members,
especially parents and siblings, peer pressure, exposure to
prosmoking versus antismoking advertising, and education (U.S.
Public Health Service, 1982).   Once an individual starts smoking, both psychological and physiological factors determine in
part whether or not the person continues to smoke and the number

TABLE V.   Interindividual Differences in Host Carcinogenesis Factors[a]

Examples of host factors	Increased risk (-fold)	Cancer site
Xeroderma pigmentosum	>1000	Skin
Dyskeratosis congenita	667	Buccal mucosa and pharynx
	125	Digestive system
Bloom syndrome	294	Digestive system
	286	Buccal mucosa and pharynx
	154	Hemopoietic and lymphoreticular systems
Klinefelter syndrome	66	Breast
Cryptorchid testes	33	Testes
Down syndrome	11	Lymphoreticular system
Ulcerative colitis	10	Colon
HLA-A2	5	Nasopharynx
Atrophic gastritis	4	Stomach
Familial history of cancer	3	Breast, lung, colon, stomach
Sarcoidosis	3	Lung

[a]From Feinberg and Coffey (1982); Henderson et al. (1976); Mulvihill (1975).

of cigarettes consumed. Nicotine dependence is considered to be one of the major physiological factors. Small doses of nicotine stimulate the central nervous system, but large doses depress it. Therefore, heavy smokers may become dependent on smoking because of its tranquilizing effect. Assuming that interindividual differences to nicotine dependence exist, and this seems to be the case (Russell, 1976; Russell et al., 1980), do these interindividual variations have a genetic basis? A definite answer to this important question is not known.

Age is an important host factor in lung cancer caused by cigarette smoking. If one starts smoking as a teenager, risk

TABLE VI.   Relative Risk of Death from Lung Cancer Among Male
            Cigarette Smokers According to the Age at Which
            They Began Smoking

Age when smoking started	Relative risk[a]
<15	16.8
15-19	14.7
20-24	10.1
>25	4.1

[a]*Relative risk to a risk of 1.0 for nonsmokers.*

of lung cancer is substantially greater than in someone who
starts at 25 years of age, even when the total amount of smoking is the same (Table VI) (U.S. Public Health Service, 1982).
This age-related risk factor(s) has not been identified.   However, hormonal changes are likely candidates.

A family history of lung cancer (Tokuhata and Lilienfeld,
1963) and/or chronic obstructive lung disease (Cohen et al.,
1977) in first-degree relatives is associated with an increased
risk of lung cancer in both smokers and nonsmokers.   The precise
contribution of genetic factors compared to environmental factors is uncertain, especially in light of the evidence that
children exposed to their parent's tobacco smoke have increased
frequency of respiratory infections (Harlap and Davies, 1974),
and passive smokers may sustain pulmonary dysfunction (White and
Froels, 1980) and be at increased risk for lung cancer (U.S.
Public Health Service, 1982).

B.   Lung Cancer Pathophysiology

A consideration of the pathobiological effects of tobacco
smoke on the respiratory tract encompasses principles in physics,
anatomy, genetics, physiology, and pathology.   Examples of the
various biological and pathological effects of tobacco smoke are

TABLE VII.   Biological and Pathological Effects of Tobacco
             Smoke

Level of biological organization	Examples of effects
Macromolecule	Inactivate α_1-antitrypsin
	Induced aryl-hydrocarbon hydroxylase
	Inhibit adenylate kinase, succinate dehydrogenase, cytochrome oxidase, and NADH diaphorase
Organelle	Swollen endoplastic reticulum
	Nuclear and nucleolar pleomorphism
	Abnormal cilia morphology and function
Cell	Ciliary loss
	Brown pigment granules and lysosome accumulation
	Necrosis
	Mutation
	Neoplastic transformation
Tissue	Intercellular permeability at luminal tight junctions
	Mucous cell hyperplasia
	Loss of cell polarity
	Squamous metaplasia
	Neoplasia
Organ	Pulmonary macrophage accumulation
	Emphysema
	Cancer
Organism	Carbon monoxide intoxication
	Allergy with histamine release
	Diminished behavioral response to external stimuli
	Increased Levels of carcinoembryonic antigen
	Cancer with metastasis

listed in Table VII. Tobacco smoke is a complex mixture of
gases and particulates that contains approximately 2000 constituents including chemicals, metals, and radionuclides, some
of which are carcinogenic and/or cocarcinogenic in experimental
animals. The respiratory tract has a surface area of approximately 200 m^2, and each of us inhales approximately 15,000

liters of air daily. A gradient exists in the size of particulates and their deposition in the lung. Particulates of
<2 μm in diameter reach the alveolus, whereas larger particu-
lates are deposited in the upper respiratory tract. The respiratory tree is a multibranched structure, and turbulence of
the inspired air and deposition of particulates occur at points
of bifurcation. It may not be incidental that carcinoma *in
situ* is also frequently observed at bifurcations (Auerbach *et
al.*, 1961).

Once inhaled, the particulates are frequently engulfed by
pulmonary macrophages, and both free and ingested particulates
in macrophages are swept up the mucociliary transport system.
The two major components of this essential host defense are
mucous blanket and ciliary action moving the blanket in a
proximal direction. The properties and constituents of mucus
are being defined (Chantler *et al.*, 1982). Increased viscosity
can lead to mucus stasis and luminal plugs. α_1-Antitrypsin
(AAT) and other antiproteases have been shown to be important
constituents of mucus. The amount of this glycoprotein is under both genetic and environmental control. Individuals who
are homozygous for the mutants Z or S have a reduced amount of
AAT and are at increased risk to develop emphysema (Lieberman,
1974). Tobacco smoke also reduces the effective amount of AAT
by oxidation of its reactive methionine. However, there is no
evidence that individuals with the abnormal phenotype of AAT
are at increased risk of lung cancer; in fact, patients with
lung cancer have abnormally high plasma levels of AAT (Harris
et al., 1976).

Ciliary action is also under genetic and environmental
control. The immotile-cilia syndrome is inherited as an autosomal recessive at a frequency of 1 per 16,000 (Afzelius, 1976).
Patients with this syndrome do not necessarily have immotile
cilia, but their cilia function ineffectively and they commonly

have chronic respiratory infections. It is not known if these individuals and/or heterozygous carriers are at increased cancer risk. In the general population, 50-fold interindividual differences in clearance rates of particulates have been observed (Cammer *et al.*, 1972; Wilkey *et al.*, 1980; Hubert *et al.*, 1982). Studies of monozygotic and dizygotic twins indicate that genetic factors have a major influence on this important host defense (Cammer *et al.*, 1972).

Environmental factors may be ciliatoxic and/or cause loss of ciliated cells. Cigarette smoke contains several known ciliatoxic agents, including formaldehyde and acrolein, and mucociliary transport is inhibited in smokers (U.S. Public Health Service, 1982). Cigarette smoke also causes defects in tight junctions at the intercellular luminal surface of the epithelium, loss of ciliated cells, and squamous metaplasia. Cilia with an aberrant morphology have been observed in the respiratory epithelium of patients with lung cancer (McDowell *et al.*, 1976) and in animal models of respiratory carcinogenesis (Harris *et al.*, 1974). Squamous metaplasia is also a common response to infectious agents, vitamin A deficiency, and occupational toxic gases. These conditions have been shown to increase the incidence of lung cancer caused by chemical carcinogens in animal models (Nettesheim and Griesemer, 1978; Harris, 1978). Epidemiological data suggest that the risk of lung cancer is enhanced in individuals who are deficient in vitamin A (Bjelke, 1975; Shekelle *et al.*, 1981). Because viral infections with influenza, respiratory syncytial virus, and adenovirus are very common, their potential as cocarcinogens cannot be easily ascertained by epidemiological studies. *In vitro* models using cultured human bronchial tissue and epithelial cells offer the opportunity to test this hypothesis.

Cigarette smoke enhances the number of pulmonary alveolar macrophages by 3- to 10-fold. Although these phagocytic cells

are important scavengers of foreign material, including particulates, macrophages and leukocytes may also damage the lung
by releasing superoxides and proteases (Gadek *et al.*, 1979).
Moreover, cultured human pulmonary macrophages can engulf
benzo[a]pyrene-coated ferric oxide, deabsorb the benzo[a]pyrene
from the ferric oxide, and release benzo[a]pyrene, its proximate carcinogenic metabolite (7,8-diol), and mutagenic metabolites into the extracellular space (Hsu *et al.*, 1979). In
addition, a wide interindividual difference in macrophage-
mediated mutagenicity is observed. These results are consistent with the hypothesis that pulmonary macrophages could act
in concert with the bronchial epithelium in the metabolic activation of chemical carcinogens.

C. Carcinogen Metabolism, DNA Damage, and DNA Repair in
    Bronchial Epithelium

Once the carcinogen reaches the bronchial epithelium via
(1) the inspired air, (2) release from pulmonary macrophages,
and/or (3) a systemic route from the blood, one can speculate
that the carcinogen may exert its oncogenic effects at the cell
surface and/or at intracellular sites. To reach intracellular
sites (e.g., DNA), the chemical must be passively and/or actively transported into the target cell. Transport of carcinogens and cocarcinogens into cells mediated by a cytosol receptor can be an important determinant of tissue response (Knutson
and Poland, 1982; Nebert *et al.*, 1982). Once in the cell, most
chemical carcinogens must be enzymatically activated into
electrophiles that covalently bind to cellular macromolecules
(Miller, 1979). Competing deactivation pathways are also
present, so that one can formulate the hypothesis that tumor
initiation and therefore cancer risk are determined in part by
the metabolic balance between activation and deactivation of

TABLE VIII. Binding of Chemical Carcinogens to DNA in Cultured Human Bronchus[a]

Chemical carcinogen	Binding value[b]
Polycyclic aromatic hydrocarbons (1.5 µM)	
Benzo[a]pyrene 7,8-diol	471 (3)
7,12-Dimethylbenz[a]anthracene	118 (28)
3-Methylcholanthrene	34 (2)
Benzo[a]pyrene	32 (15)
Dibenz[a,h]anthracene	28 (4)
Mycotoxin (1.5 µM)	
Aflatoxin B_1	14 (17)
N-Nitrosamines (100 µM)	
N-Nitrosodimethylamine	906 (15)
N-Nitrosodiethylamine	264 (4)
N-Nitrosopyrrolidine	183 (4)
Others	
1,2-Dimethylhydrazine (100 µM)	675 (4)
2-Acetylaminofluorene (1.5 µM)	73 (13)

[a]The explants were cultured for 7 days in a chemically defined medium prior to addition of the radioactively labeled carcinogens. After incubation for 24 h, the mucosa were removed and the DNA isolated and purified either by CsCl gradient centrifugation or by hydroxylapatite chromatography.

[b]pmol carcinogens bound/10 mg DNA. Numbers in parentheses are numbers of cases studied.

chemical procarcinogens. Although studies in experimental animals are consistent with this simplistic hypothesis, epidemiological data are insufficient to reach a similar conclusion in humans. Investigations in biochemical epidemiology are providing important information that will aid in testing this hypothesis.

Several chemical classes of carcinogens are enzymatically activated to metabolites that bind to DNA in cultured human bronchial explants (Table VIII). These chemicals were chosen for study because they are (a) constituents of tobacco smoke (e.g., benzo[a]pyrene and N-nitrosodimethylamine), (b) environmental pollutants, (e.g., benzo[a]pyrene and aflatoxin B_1), and/or (c) carcinogens, (e.g., 7,12-dimethylbenz[a]anthracene and 2-acetylaminofluorene) that have been extensively studied in the laboratory. In addition to metabolic pathways, the major carcinogen-DNA adducts isolated from cultured human tissues have been identified for several of these procarcinogens (Fig. 3). In each case so far studied (Harris et al., 1983), the adducts are identical to those found in experimental animals in which the chemical has been shown to be carcinogenic. Although this observation supports the extrapolation of carcinogenesis data from experimental animals to the human situation, studies with additional carcinogens are needed before one can be assured that this generalization is correct.

The quantity of carcinogen-DNA adducts formed has been shown to vary 50- to 150-fold among cultured tissues from different people (Table IX). These interindividual differences are of the same order of magnitude as those found in pharmacogenetic studies of drug metabolism. Evidence is accumulating that certain carcinogens and drugs may be metabolically activated by the same mixed-function oxidase (Idle and Ritchie, Chapter 35). Such drugs may prove to be useful in probing the genetic polymorphism of carcinogen metabolism.

We have also measured interindividual variation in activation of carcinogens by using a human tissue-mediated mutagenesis assay (Hsu et al., 1978). A wide variation in human bronchi-mediated frequencies of ouabain-resistant mutation and sister chromatid exchanges in cocultivated Chinese hamster V-79 cells was found. A highly statistically significant correlation between mutation frequency in the V-79 cells and amount of carcinogen-DNA adducts in the bronchial mucosa was observed.

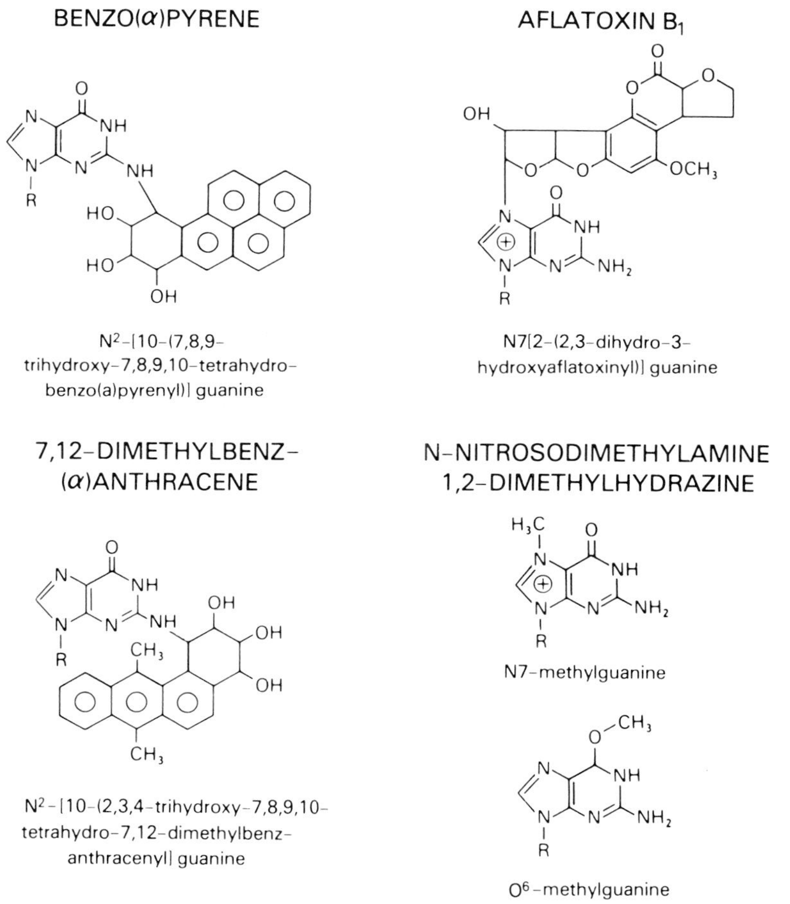

BENZO(α)PYRENE

N²-[10-(7,8,9-
trihydroxy-7,8,9,10-tetrahydro-
benzo(a)pyrenyl)] guanine

AFLATOXIN B₁

N7[2-(2,3-dihydro-3-
hydroxyaflatoxinyl)] guanine

**7,12-DIMETHYLBENZ-
(α)ANTHRACENE**

N²-[10-(2,3,4-trihydroxy-7,8,9,10-
tetrahydro-7,12-dimethylbenz-
anthracenyl] guanine

**N-NITROSODIMETHYLAMINE
1,2-DIMETHYLHYDRAZINE**

N7-methylguanine

O⁶-methylguanine

Fig. 3. Examples of major carcinogen-DNA adducts formed in cultured human tissues and cells.

These findings further support the contention that carcinogen metabolism and DNA damage have important biological implications.

Once carcinogen-DNA adducts are formed, DNA repair processes may remove the adduct. Although the rates of removal and the interindividual variation are being investigated, the

TABLE IX.   Interindividual Differences in DNA-Binding Values
            of Chemical Carcinogens in Cultured Human Epithelial
            Tissue[a]

Tissue	Benzo[a]pyrene (1.5 µM)	Aflatoxin B_1 (1.5 µM)	N-Nitrosodimethylamine (100 µM)
Bronchus	75	120	60
Esophagus	99	70	90
Colon	130	150	145
Bladder	68	90	n.t.
Endometrium	70	n.t.[b]	n.t.

[a]*From Harris et al. (1982); Kaufman et al. (Chapter 19);
Daniel et al. (1983).*
[b]*n.t., Not tested.*

fidelity of the various DNA repair pathways are not as yet
known.   This variation in removal rates of adducts and in activities of DNA repair enzymes may be substantial and biologically
significant (Setlow, Chapter 10).   Extreme deficiencies in DNA
repair are known, and xeroderma pigmentosum is of course the
classical example of a condition deficient in excision repair.
Although the various complementation groups of xeroderma pigmentosum vary in their deficiencies in DNA repair (Cleaver et
al., 1982), the variation in the general population is just now
being systematically investigated.   Setlow and co-workers
(Chapter 10) have observed an approximately eightfold variation
in O^6-methyltransferase activity in lymphocytes from 44 donors.
We have observed two- to threefold differences in lung or colon
tissues from a smaller number of people (R. Grafstrom, A. Pegg,
and C. C. Harris, unpublished).   When compared to rodents,
human tissues and cells have more than fivefold levels of both
O^6-methyltransferase activity and excision repair capability
(Montesano et al., 1982; R. Grafstrom, unpublished).   One can

predict that studies measuring O^6-methyltransferase and other DNA repair enzymes in larger human populations will uncover even wider variations. The biological significance of variations in rates and fidelity of DNA repair will obviously require further study.

IV. COCARCINOGENESIS AND TUMOR PROMOTION

The foregoing discussion emphasizes our current understanding of the determinants of the initial events in lung carcinogenesis. We know comparatively less about the mechanism(s) of cocarcinogenesis including tumor promotion.

Extensive reviews of the experimental data pertaining to the concepts of tumor initiation, tumor promotion, and tumor progression are available (Foulds, 1975; Farber, 1981; Weinstein, 1982; Pitot et al., 1982; Yuspa and Harris, 1982). Mouse skin carcinogenesis has provided us the most information concerning tumor initiation and promotion. As investigators become enamored with biochemical and molecular effects of tumor promoters [e.g., 12-O-tetradecanoylphorbol-13-acetate (TPA)], it is easy to lose sight of the biology of mouse skin carcinogenesis. For example, papillomas, the primary tumor type produced by initiation-promotion protocols, are benign tumors that frequently regress, and this frequency varies among strains and regimens of exposure to carcinogens and promoters (Boutwell, 1964). The progression of papillomas to carcinomas is an infrequent event that can be substantially increased by once again exposing the papillomas to initiating agents as well as complete carcinogens (Hennings, 1983). Therefore, conversion of promoter-dependent cells to autonomous malignant cells may require a second mutagenic step and/or chromosomal change (Fig. 4).

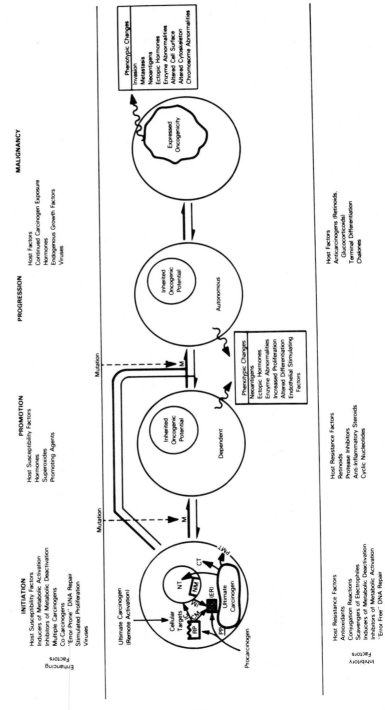

Fig. 4. Schematic representation of chemical carcinogenesis. The circles represent cells at various stages in the process of malignant transformation by chemicals. On the left a normal cell is exposed to procarcinogens. As the carcinogen enters the cell it may go directly to cytoplasmic (endoplasmic reticulum, ER) or nuclear (nuclear membrane, NM) sites of constitutive metabolic activity. Alternatively, procarcinogens may complex with a receptor protein (RP), form an inducer complex (IC), and derepress genes controlling enzymatic activity, leading to induction of metabolism (IM). Metabolically activated (electrophilic) ultimate carcinogens may complex with other proteins (PP) which prevent immediate degradation or covalent interactions at nearby sites. Ultimate carcinogenic species will interact with a variety of target molecules in the nucleis (NT), in the cytoplasm (CT), or at the plasma membrane (PMT). Carcinogens may also be metabolized in one cell and delivered to other cells in activated form. In both cases interaction with critical cellular targets, possibly DNA, in a precise way is required for initiation. A number of endogenous and exogenous factors will also influence the probability that the carcinogen-cellular interaction will lead to a permanent state of "initiation" of carcinogenesis. Similarly endogenous and exogenous factors determine the level of preneoplastic progression (→), depicted here for schematic purposes as two cells but representing a series of progressive changes. Each preneoplastic change may be stable for long periods and may even revert (→) to a more dependent stage under the proper conditions. As progression toward malignancy continues, the preneoplastic cell becomes more autonomous (perhaps secondary to another mutagenic and/or clastogenic event). A number of phenotypic alterations (⟷) become apparent during this prolonged process, and the clone zize of preneoplastic cells increases. Ultimately progression results in a malignant clone with clinical expression of cancer. Adapted from Yuspa and Harris (1982).

961

Mice may be very susceptible to promoter-induced progression from benign to malignant growth due to inherent chromosomal instability of murine cells compared to those of primates. Papillomas and the subsequent carcinomas are clonal growths, that is, derived from single cells. Therefore, promoting agents and conditions must allow selective growth of initiated cells. Most researchers have assumed that promoting agents act directly on initiated cells. The enhanced transformation frequency of mouse 10T1/2 fibroblasts exposed to carcinogens and the mimicry of the *in vitro* transformed cell phenotype, both caused by TPA, support this assumption (Heidelberger, 1982). However, *in vitro* studies with normal epithelial cells from rodents (Yuspa *et al.*, 1982) and humans (Grunberger *et al.*, Chapter 8; J. Willey and C. C. Harris, unpublished) provide evidence that TPA can be a potent inducer of terminal differentiation. Therefore, one can propose that TPA enhances the terminal differentiation of the noninitiated, normal cells and the initiated cells are less responsive, so that they gain a selective advantage leading to progressive clonal growth. In fact, it seems most likely that promoting agents have important effects on both initiated and noninitiated cells that results in either the formation of a papilloma or its functional equivalent in the ordered community of cells in the epithelium. Finally, tumor promoters have been shown to have pronounced organ and species specificity. Therefore, interspecies extrapolations are uncertain and the identification of agents and conditions that cause tumor promotion in human tissues and cells is an area of high priority.

Sentinal concepts in experimental carcinogenesis are being applied to human carcinogenesis. Epidemiological data are consistent with the hypothesis that lung cancer caused by tobacco smoke fits the tumor initiation-promotion model (Doll and Peto, 1978). As shown in the mouse model of skin carcinogenesis, tobacco smoke contains both initiators and promoters (Wynder and Hoffmann, 1979).

Interindividual differences in oncogenic susceptibility to tumor promoters and cocarcinogens in humans have not as yet been identified. Studies in experimental animals (Boutwell, 1964; Pitot et al., 1982) indicate the likelihood that individual and tissue differences will be found in the human population. These experimental investigations have shown that stocks and strains of mice vary widely in their sensitivity to skin carcinogenesis by promoting agents (Boutwell, 1964; Slaga et al., 1982). Although sensitivity to the tumor-initiating potential of polycyclic aromatic hydrocarbons is positively correlated with their binding to specific sites in cellular DNA, the critical targets of tumor promoters have not been identified in spite of the myriad and pleiotrophic effects produced by promoting agents (Weinstein, 1982).

Epithelial carcinogenesis can be conceptually considered to be a progressive sequence of morphological stages each with an increasing probability for expression of malignancy. Serial cytological examination in animal models (Schreiber et al., 1975) and in patients (Auerbach et al., 1961; Saccomanno et al., 1971) indicates that the morphological stages are hyperplasia, atypical metaplasia, in situ carcinoma, and microinvasive carcinoma. The pathobiological cellular phenotypes in these histological lesions is being investigated in vitro using cultured rat trachea (Nettesheim et al., 1982) and human bronchi (Lechner et al., 1983). Nettesheim and co-workers (1982) have found that rat tracheal cells in hyperplastic and metaplastic lesions caused by carcinogens have a low probability for progression to tumorigenicity, and with subtumorigenic doses of carcinogens these lesions often revert to normal-appearing epithelium. In contrast, when cells in these histological lesions are dispersed and cultured as single cells, a small percentage of the clonogenic cells continue to grow in vitro and are resistant to inducers of terminal differentiation. After several subculturings,

the cells develop anchorage-independent growth and eventually
become tumorigenic. Similar observations have been made by
Yuspa and co-workers (1982) in their studies of *in vitro* carcinogenesis using mouse epidermal cells. We have also observed
that carcinogen-altered epithelia of human tissues frequently
revert to a normal-appearing epithelium when the tissues are
xenotransplanted into athymic *nude* mice. Clinical investigations have also demonstrated that these preneoplastic histological lesions regress when individuals stop smoking cigarettes
(U.S. Public Health Service, 1982). However, the experimental
studies just discussed indicate that preneoplastic cells may
persist even though the histological lesions have regressed.

V.   TUMOR PROGRESSION

    Evaluation of epidemiological data suggests that interin-
dividual differences in tumor progression may exist. For
example, "incidental" cancers are frequently found at autopsy
of people dying in their seventh and eight decades. These
small carcinomas occur at several tissue sites including prostate, pancreas, breast, thyroid, and lung (Sugano, 1980; Pour
et al., 1981). One can speculate that host defenses prevent
these cancers from progressively growing and forming metastases (Wheelock *et al.,* 1981). Alternatively, the cancers may
have an intrinsic slow growth and/or the host has not been exposed to sufficient dose of the appropriate endogenous or exogenous tumor promoter, such as prolactin in breast carcinogenesis or asbestos in bronchogenic carcinogenesis.
    Investigation of tumor progression is being conducted in
animal models and to a limited extent in the clinic. The
pathogenesis of carcinomas at many organ sites has been extensively investigated in animal models (Farber, 1982; Yuspa and

Harris, 1982). In experimental animals, respiratory carcinogenesis is clearly a multistage process (Kuschner and Laskin,
1970; Nettesheim and Griesemer, 1978; Harris, 1978; Becci et
al., 1979). As noted previously, clinical studies have shown
a similar sequence of morphological changes. Most cancers are
subpopulations of cells with wide biological and morphological
diversity. Metastasis is an obvious example of biological diversity of cancer cells (Fidler and Hart, 1982). Although the
various stages have been morphologically, and in some cases
biologically, identified, the mechanism(s) responsible for the
progression from one stage to the next is essentially unknown.

VI. PERSPECTIVES

Examples of host-environment interactions in human carcinogenesis have been recognized for several centuries. In addition
to interactions considered to be important in lung carcinogenesis reviewed here, others are described in this volume. It
seems likely that liver cancer in Africa and the People's
Republic of China is caused by the interactive effects of chemical carcinogens such as aflatoxin B_1, and cocarcinogens such as
hepatitis B virus, in an individual who is predisposed to the
development of chronic active hepatitis (Sun and Wang, Chapter
31; Robinson et al., Chapter 30). Lymphomas induced by Epstein-
Barr virus seem to occur primarily in individuals who have
either a genetic or acquired immune deficiency (Portilo et al.,
Chapter 29). A classic example is the increased risk of cancer
found in patients with xeroderma pigmentosum (Cleaver et al.,
1982). The host factors important in the oncogenic susceptibility to the retrovirus associated with T-cell leukemia have
not as yet been identified.

Bronowski (1973) has stated that "the hardest part is not to answer but to conceive the question" and "That is the essence of science: ask an impertinent question, and you are on the way to the pertinent answer."

It is fair to note that each generation of scientists rediscovers the critical questions formulated by previous generations. Fortunately for us, additional information obtained from within our field of investigation--and importantly from peripheral fields--and advances in experimental methodology, allow us to refine these questions into ones that can be investigated. Technical advancements in molecular and cell biology, methods to culture human epithelial tissues and cells, development of animal models, and so on, provide exciting new opportunities for investigators.

Some questions of current interest to me in the area of carcinogenesis are listed below.

1. Why do rodent cells frequently "spontaneously" transform *in vitro*, whereas primate cells, including human, rarely, if ever, "spontaneously" transform to malignant cells?

2. Which phenotypic traits of cultured cells predict tumorigenicity *in vivo*?

3. What are the critical functions of proto-oncogene and *c*-oncogene products?

4. Do carcinogens and cocarcinogens cause gene rearrangements in human cells that are important in carcinogenesis?

5. Can one make valid qualitative and quantitative extrapolations of the effects and mechanisms of carcinogens, cocarcinogens, and tumor promoters among cell types, tissues, and animal species?

6. How wide is the interindividual variation among humans in responsiveness to tumor promoters?

7. Where are the primary cellular and molecular sites of
    action of physical carcinogens?

Scientists, including contributors to this volume, are address-
ing many of these questions as well as others of fundamental
importance to the understanding of human carcinogenesis.

REFERENCES

Afzelius, B. A. (1976). *Science (Washington, D.C.) 193,* 317-
    319.
Auerbach, O., Stout, A., and Hammond, E. (1961). *New Engl. J.
    Med. 265,* 253-259.
Becci, P., McDowell, E., and Trump, B. F. (1979). *J. Natl.
    Cancer Inst. (U.S.) 61,* 607-618.
Bjelke, E. (1975). *Int. J. Cancer 15,* 561-565.
Boutwell, R. K. (1964). *Prog. Exp. Tumor Res. 4,* 207-250.
Bronowski, J. (1973). "The Ascent of Man." Little, Brown,
    Boston, Massachusetts.
Cammer, P., Philipson, K., and Friberg, L. (1972). *Arch.
    Environ. Health 24,* 82-87.
Case, R. A., Hosker, M. E., McDonald, D. B., and Pearson, J. T.
    (1954). *Br. J. Ind. Med. 11,* 193-205.
Chantler, E. N., Elder, J. B., and Elstein, M. (1982). *Adv.
    Exp. Med. Biol. 144,* 441-472.
Cleaver, J. E., Bodell, W. J., Gruenert, D. C., Kapp, L. N.,
    Kaufmann, W. K., Park, S. D., and Zelle, B. (1982). *In*
    "Mechanisms of Chemical Carcinogenesis" (C. C. Harris and
    P. A. Cerutti, eds.), pp. 409-418. Liss, New York.
Cohen, B. H., Graves, C. G., Levy, D. A., Permutt, S., Diamond,
    E. L., Kreiss, P., Menkes, H. A., Quaskey, S., and
    Tockman, M. S. (1977). *Lancet 2,* 523-527.
Daniel, F. B., Stoner, G. D., and Schut, H. A. J. (1983). *In*
    "Individual Susceptibility to Genotoxic Agents in Human
    Population" (F. J. deSerre and R. Pero, eds.). Plenum,
    New York, in press.
Darwin, C. (1859). "The Origin of the Species." Murray, London.
Diwan, B. A., and Blackman, K. E. (1980). *Cancer Lett.
    (Shannon, Irel.) 9,* 111-115.
Doll, R. (1978). *Cancer Res. 38,* 3573-3583.
Doll, R., and Peto, R. (1978). *J. Epidemiol. Community Health
    32,* 301-313.
Essex, M., Todaro, G., and zur Hausen, H. (eds.) (1980).
    "Viruses in Naturally Occurring Cancers." Cold Spring
    Harbor Lab., Cold Spring Harbor, New York.

Farber, E. (1981). *New Engl. J. Med. 305*, 1379-1389.

Feinberg, A. P., and Coffey, D. S. (1982). *Cancer Res. 42*, 3252-3254.

Fidler, I. J., and Hart, I. R. (1982). *Science (Washington, D.C.) 217*, 998-1002.

Foulds, J. (1975). "Neoplastic Development." Academic Press, New York.

Gadek, J. E., Fells, G. A., and Crystal, R. G. (1979). *Science (Washington, D.C.) 206*, 1315-1317.

Gazdar, A. F., Carney, D. N., and Minna, J. D. (1982). *In* "Lung Cancer 1982" (S. Ishikawa, Y. Hayata, and K. Suemasu, eds.), pp. 14-30. Excerpta Medica, Amsterdam.

Harlap, S., and Davies, A. M. (1974). *Lancet 1*, ʋ29-532.

Harris, C. C. (1978). *In* "Lung Cancer: Clinical Diagnosis and Treatment" (M. Straus, ed.), pp. 1-17. Grune & Stratton, New York.

Harris, C. C., Kaufman, D., Jackson, F., Smith, J., Dedick, P., and Saffiotti, U. (1974). *J. Pathol. 114*, 17-19.

Harris, C. C., Cohen, M., Connor, R., Primack, A., Saccomanno, G., and Talamo, R. (1976). *Cancer (Philadelphia) 38*, 1655-1657.

Harris, C. C., Trump, B. F., and Stoner, G. D. (eds.) (1980). *Methods Cell Biol.*

Harris, C. C., Trump, B. F., Grafstrom, R. C., and Autrup, H. (1982). *In* "Mechanisms of Chemical Carcinogenesis" (C. C. Harris and P. Cerutti, eds.), pp. 289-298. Liss, New York.

Harris, C. C., Grafstrom, R. C., Shamsuddin, A., Sinopoli, N. T., Trump, B. F., and Autrup, H. (1983). *In* "Biochemical Basis of Chemical Carcinogenesis" (H. Greim, R. Jung, M. Kramer, H. Marguardt, and F. Oesch, eds.), Raven, New York, in press.

Heidelberger, C. (1982). *In* "Mechanisms of Chemical Carcinogenesis" (C. C. Harris and P. A. Cerutti, eds.), pp. 563-573. Liss, New York.

Henderson, B. E., Louie, E., Jing, J. S., Buell, M. S., and Murray, B. G. (1976). *New Engl. J. Med. 295*, 1101-1106.

Hennings, H. (1983). *In* "Pathophysiology of Dermatologic Disease" (H. P. Baden and N. A. Soter, eds.), McGraw-Hill, New York, in press.

Hsu, I. C., Autrup, H., Stoner, G. D., Trump, B. F., Selkirk, J. K., and Harris, C. C. (1978). *Proc. Natl. Acad. Sci. USA 75*, 2003-2007.

Hsu, I. C., Harris, C. C., Trump, B. F., Shafer, P. W., and Yamaguchi, M. (1979). *J. Clin. Invest. 64*, 1245-1252.

Hubert, H. B., Fabsitz, R. R., Feinleid, M., and Gwinn, C. (1982). *Am. Rev. Respir. Dis. 125*, 409-415.

Knutson, J. C., and Poland, A. (1982). *Cell 30*, 225-234.

Kuschner, M., and Laskin, S. (1970). *In* "Morphology of Experimental Respiratory Carcinogenesis" (P. Nettesheim, M. G. Hanna, and J. W. Deatherage, eds.), pp. 203-227. Nat. Tech. Information Service, Springfield, Virginia.

Lechner, J. F., Haugen, A., McClendon, I. A., and Pettis, E. W. (1982). *In Vitro 18*, 633-642.

Lieberman, J. (1974). *Med. Clin. North Am. 57*, 691-714.

Mayr, E. (1982). "The Growth of Biological Thought." Harvard Univ. Press, Cambridge, Massachusetts.

McDowell, E., Barrett, L., Harris, C. C., and Trump, B. F. (1976). *Arch. Pathol. 100*, 429-436.

Miller, E. C. (1979). *Cancer Res. 38*, 1479-1498.

Montesano, R., Bresil, M., Blanche-Martel, G., Pegg, A. E., and Margison, E. (1982). *Proc. Symp. Organ Species Specificity Chem. Carcinog.*, pp. 531-543.

Mulvihill, J. J. (1975). *In* "Persons at High Risk of Cancer" (J. F. Fraumeni, Jr., ed.), pp. 3-37. Academic Press, New York.

Nebert, D. J., Negishi, M., Lang, M. A., Hjelmeland, L. M., and Eisen, H. J. (1982). *Adv. Genet. 21*, 2-52.

Nettesheim, P., and Griesemer, R. A. (1978). *In* "Pathogenesis and Therapy of Lung Cancer" (C. C. Harris, ed.), pp. 75-188. Dekker, New York.

Nettesheim, P., Terzaghi, M., Klein-Szanto, A. J. P. (1982). *In* "Mechanisms in Chemical Carcinogenesis" (C. C. Harris and P. Cerutti, eds.), pp. 473-489. Liss, New York.

Peto, J. (1980). *Banbury Rep*. No. 4, 203-213.

Pitot, H. C., Goldsworthy, T., and Moran, S. (1982). *In* "Mechanisms of Chemical Carcinogenesis" (C. C. Harris and P. A. Cerutti, eds.), pp. 141-154. Liss, New York.

Pour, P. M., Sayed, S., and Sayed, G. (1981). *Am. J. Clin. Pathol. 77*, 137-152.

Russell, M. A. H. (1976). *Res. Adv. Alcohol Drug Probl. 3*, 1-47.

Russell, M. A. H., Jarvis, M., Iyer, R., and Feyerabend, C. (1980). *Br. Med. J.* Apr. 5, 972-976.

Saccomanno, G., Archer, V. E., and Auerbach, O. (1971). *Cancer (Philadelphia) 27*, 515-523.

Schreiber, H., Schreiber, K., and Martin, D. H. (1975). *J. Natl. Cancer Inst. (U.S.) 54*, 187-197.

Shekelle, R. B., Liu, S., Raynor, W. J., Jr., Lepper, M., Maliza, C., and Rossof, A. H. (1981). *Lancet* Nov. 28, 1186-1190.

Slaga, T. J., Fischer, S. M., Weeks, C. E., Klein-Szanto, A. J. P., and Reiners, J. (1982). *In* "Mechanisms of Chemical Carcinogenesis" (C. C. Harris and P. A. Cerutti, eds.), pp. 207-227. Liss, New York.

Sugano, H. (1980). *Trans. Soc. Pathol. Jpn. 69*, 27-57.

Templeton, A. C. (1975). *In* "Persons at High Risk of Cancer" (J. F. Fraumeni, Jr., ed.), pp. 69-848. Academic Press, New York.

Tokuhata, G., and Lilienfeld, A. (1963). *J. Natl. Cancer Inst. (U.S.) 30,* 289-298.

Tsao, M. C., Walthall, B. J., and Ham, R. G. (1982). *J. Cell. Physiol. 110,* 219-229.

US Public Health Service (1982). "The Health Consequences of Smoking, A Report from the Surgeon General," Publ. No. HSM 71-7513. Dept. of Health, Education & Welfare, Washington, D.C.

Vogel, H. J., Jr., and Turner, J. E. (1982). *Radiat. Res. 89,* 264.

Weinstein, I. B. (1982). *In* "Mechanisms of Chemical Carcinogenesis" (C. C. Harris and P. A. Cerutti, eds.), pp. 107-128. Liss, New York.

Wheelock, E. F., Weinhold, K. J., and Levich, J. (1981). *Adv. Cancer Res. 34,* 107-139.

White, J. R., and Froels, H. F. (1980). *N. Engl. J. Med. 302,* 720-732.

Wilkey, D. D., Lee, P. S., Hass, F. J., Gerrity, T. R., Yeates, D. B., and Lourenzo, R. V. (1980). *Arch. Environ. Health 35,* 294-303.

Wynder, E. L., and Hoffmann, D. (1979). *N. Engl. J. Med. 300,* 894-902.

Yuspa, S. H., and Harris, C. C. (1982). *In* "Cancer Epidemiology and Prevention" (D. Schottenfeld and J. F. Fraumeni, Jr., eds.), pp. 23-43. Saunders, Philadelphia, Pennsylvania.

Yuspa, S. H., Hennings, H., and Lichti, U. (1982). *In* "Mechanisms of Chemical Carcinogenesis" (C. C. Harris and P. Cerutti, eds.), pp. 169-181. Liss, New York.

Index

U